The Handbook of Chicana/o Psychology
and Mental Health

The Handbook of Chicana/o Psychology and Mental Health

Edited by

Roberto J. Velásquez
San Diego State University

Leticia M. Arellano
University of La Verne

Brian W. McNeill
Washington State University

LEA LAWRENCE ERLBAUM ASSOCIATES, PUBLISHERS
2004 Mahwah, New Jersey   London

Lawrence Erlbaum Associates, Inc., Publishers
10 Industrial Avenue
Mahwah, New Jersey 07430

Cover art by Malaquias Montoya. Adapted with permission by
the Julian Samora Research Institute, Michigan State University.

Cover design by Kathryn Houghtaling Lacey.

Library of Congress Cataloging-in-Publication Data

The handbook of Chicana/o psychology and mental health / Roberto J. Velásquez,
Leticia M. Arellano, Brian McNeill, editors.
    p.   cm.
    Includes bibliographical references and index.
    ISBN 0–8058–4158-X (alk. paper) — ISBN 0–8058–4159–8 (pbk. : alk. paper)
    1. Mexican Americans—Psychology—Handbooks, manuals, etc. 2. Mexican
Americans—Mental health services—Handbooks, manuals, etc. I. Velásquez, Roberto.
II. Arellano, Leticia M. III. McNeill, Brian.
    RC451.5.M48H36 2004
    362.2'089'68073—dc21
                                              2003045646

To the memory of the late Martha E. Bernal,
an appreciation of whose life follows the preface.

To my children Diego and Diana, my mother Maria Luz,
and the memory of my father, Ventura. I would also like to thank
the quintessential Chicano band, Los Lobos, for their inspiration.
Este libro esta dedicado a mis hijos, Diego y Diana, mi madre, Maria Luz,
y la memoria de mi padre, Ventura. Quiero darle las gracias
al grupo musico, Los Lobos, por su inspiracion.

Roberto Velásquez

To my family, thank you for your constant love and support.
To our creator, who always gives me strength.
Para mi familia, gracias por tu constante amor y apoyo.
A nuestro creador, quien siempre me sostiene.

Leticia M. Arellano

For my Mexican family, especially my Chicana mother.
Para mi familia Mexicana, especialmente mi madre Chicana.

Brian W. McNeill

Contributors

Leticia M. Arellano, University of La Verne
Patricia Arredondo, Arizona State University
Christina Ayala-Alcantar, California State University, Northridge
Louise Baca, Argosy University, Phoenix
Manuel Barrera, Jr., Arizona State University
Martha E. Bernal, Arizona State University
Erika Bracamontes, Michigan State University
Maria Patricia Burton, San Diego State University
J. Manuel Casas, University of California, Santa Barbara
Jeanett Castellanos, University of California, Irvine
Felipe González Castro, Arizona State University
Joseph M. Cervantes, California State University, Fullerton
Richard C. Cervantes, Behavioral Assessment, Inc.
Carla Victoria Corral, University of California, Santa Barbara
Israel Cuéllar, Julian Samora Research Institute, Michigan State University
Maria Félix-Ortiz, Florida International University, Miami
A. Cristina Fernandez, Arizona State University
Yolanda Flores Niemann, Washington State University, Tri-Cities
Yvette G. Flores-Ortiz, University of California, Davis
Maria Garrido, University of Rhode Island
Alberta M. Gloria, University of Wisconsin, Madison
Nancy A. Gonzales, Arizona State University
Martin Harris, Vanguard University
Nilda Teresa Hernandez, Yavapai College
Patricia Hernandez, Argosy University, Phoenix
Steven R. López, University of California, Los Angeles
Vera Lopez, Arizona State University
Brian W. McNeill, Washington State University
Kurt C. Organista, University of California, Berkeley
Fernando Ortiz, Washington State University
Loreto R. Prieto, University of Akron
Stephen M. Quintana, University of Wisconsin, Madison
Jason Duque Raley, University of California, Santa Barbara

Manual Ramirez III, University of Texas, Austin
Teresa Renteria, Vanguard University
Richard A. Rodriguez, University of Colorado, Boulder
Theresa A. Segura-Herrera, University of Wisconsin, Madison
Roxana I. Siles, Michigan State University
Lisa I. Sweatt, California Polytechnic State University, San Luis Obispo
Melba J. T. Vasquez, Vasquez & Associates Mental Health Services
Roberto J. Velásquez, San Diego State University
Elizabeth M. Vera, Loyola University, Chicago
Amy Weisman, University of Miami
Jerre White, Vanguard University
Cynthia A. Yamokoski, University of Akron

Contents

Preface

Latina/os are now the largest and fastest growing minority group in the United States, representing approximately 33 million in the year 2000, and two thirds of them are Chicana/os. However, there are major differences among Latino subgroups in terms of their cultural characteristics, immigration experiences, history, socioeconomic levels, and other important factors. It is no longer appropriate to negate these differences or to assume that all Latinos share similar psychological issues (McNeill et al., 2001).

However, despite their increasingly strong presence, as a distinct population, they face various challenges such as low educational attainment rates. Approximately 51% are high school graduates and less than 7% have obtained a bachelor's or higher degree. Chicana/os are also confronted with harsh economic conditions, such as poverty, unemployment, and underemployment: For instance, 24% of Chicana/os lived below the poverty level in 1999 (Therrien & Ramirez, 2000).

Chicana/os, through recent legislation in many states, have been denied affirmative action and access to key institutions. Chicana/os' use of their native language has also recently been legislated in English-only movements. Many *Mejicana/os* now living in the United States remain undocumented, marginalized, and oppressed. Even apart from economic and educational factors, problems stemming from immigration and migration, high rates of substance use, gang involvement, high incarceration rates, racism, sexism and homophobia, single-parent households, domestic violence, and separation from family all contribute to Chicana/os' risk for psychological and medical disorders.

The relevance of this book, at this time in our history, is critical for many reasons. The last book on the psychology of Chicana/os (Martinez & Mendoza, *Chicano Psychology,* second edition, 1984) was published nearly 20 years ago as a second edition of a book originally published in 1977 (Martinez, 1977). Both editions followed conferences in a small series organized by Chicana/o psychologists as pioneering efforts to stimulate the development of theory and research. The first conference, "Increasing Educational Opportunities for Chicana/os Psychology," was held at the University of California, Riverside in 1973. At this meeting, papers highlighted concerns and necessary changes in psychology to ensure that Chicana/os were largely represented at the undergraduate and graduate levels. This conference was held at the height of the Chicana/o civil rights movement and reflected changes taking place on many university campuses such as Chicana/o Studies programs, Chicana/o student organizations, and high school walkouts in California and Texas (Navarro, 1995).

The second conference, First Symposium on Chicano Psychology, was held in 1976 at the University of California, Irvine. This conference focused on areas of research including bilingual education, the IQ controversy, and culturally sensitive mental health services. Given the increase in the number of Chicana/os enrolled in Ph. D. programs, graduate students were also represented. The proceedings of the conference were published in *Chicano Psychology* (Martinez, 1977). Another outcome of the conference was the legendary National Conference of Hispanic Psychologists, also known as the Lake Arrowhead Meeting.

The third conference, Second Symposium on Chicano Psychology, was held in 1982 at the University of California, Riverside. Like those of the second conference, conference proceedings were published in the second edition of *Chicano Psychology* (Martinez & Mendoza, 1984). Unfortunately, the conference was held in the context of the decline of the Chicana/o civil rights movement and severe cutbacks in social programs during the Reagan and Bush administrations. The rollbacks in social programs were also felt on university campuses across the country, as ethnic studies programs were scaled back. Unfortunately, efforts to recruit minority students into graduate programs of psychology were reduced.

After a gap of 16 years, a fourth conference, "Innovations in Chicana/o Psychology: Looking Towards the 21st Century," was held at Michigan State University. The primary aims of the conference were to present a forum for the presentation of state-of-the-art psychological research on Chicana/os and to increase the coverage of previously neglected issues, such as Chicanas and students. Chicanas, underrepresented in previous conference programs, also participated in workshops, presentations, and panel discussions, and a special poster session was included to highlight the work of students. Many generations were represented by the approximately 400 conference participants. A special feature of the conference was a tribute to pioneering Chicana/o psychologists who mentored those who followed.

We designed this Handbook with four goals in mind: First, we wanted to present current empirically based data on the mental health and health status of Chicana/os. Mainstream psychologists have often argued that a subfield of Chicana/o psychology is not needed or that the absence of empirical data makes a psychology of Chicana/os irrelevant or unecessary. The data that are presented in this volume clearly rebut these arguments.

Second, we wanted to showcase the talent that has laid the foundation of a psychology of the Chicana/o experience. Today, as in the past, many mainstream psychology journals refuse to publish research that relates to ethnicity or race or that argues for the need for culture-driven psychologies. We have invited many young scholars to present their work in this book to disseminate their innovative ideas, ideas that we hope will now resonate in a wider world.

Third, we wanted to pay tribute to many of the psychologists who were present at the beginning, who fought the many battles to establish Chicana/o psychology as a legitimate field of study. We invited many of these pioneers to contribute to this book by presenting summaries of their life's work. We also acknowledge the work of others in the section entitled "About Other Pioneers in Chicana/o Psychology" at the end of this volume.

Fourth, we wanted to include a balance of male and female contributors in order to offer the important perspective of gender, and made every effort to do so. Although the numbers of Chicana psychologists continues to increase, only one Chicana, Maria Nieto Senour (1977), contributed to the first edition of *Chicano Psychology* (Martinez, 1977). Her chapter on La Chicana remains a classic treatise on the experience of being a Chicana. In this volume, we present diverse perspectives on the Chicana experience.

Any working theory of Chicana/o psychology must reflect the diversity of the Chicana/o community, which varies with respect to ethnic identity, age, religion, citizenship, sexual orientation, theoretical orientation, and education. The contributors also bring a diversity of experiences to their task. Some are academics, while others are practitioners, or both. Many of the pioneers have directed major research institutes or programs devoted to the study of Chicana/os, others have founded journals. Still others have been leaders and activists in professional organizations such as the American Psychological Association. At least three authors have held public office in their communities.

The Handbook is divided into six main sections on general issues, assessment, intervention with individual men and women, intervention with families, risks and prevention, and new directions, respectively. An epilogue contributed by the late Martha E. Bernal reflects on the challenges Chicana/o psychologists have faced and continue to face as they seek both to reinforce the research and theoretical base of Chicana/o psychology and to serve their people.

In the text, we use the terms *Mexican American* and *Chicana/o* interchangeably. As noted by McNeill et al. (2001), there are a variety of labels of self-identification utilized by Americans of Mexican descent that may vary by generation or region. However, it is in the spirit of past conferences and publications that we proudly use the identifying labels *Chicano* and the feminine equivalent *Chicana,* as these terms are associated with the sociopolitical and civil rights *movimiento* (movement) born in the late 1960s and reflect a political awareness of resistance, defiance, and ethnic pride.

We hope that students and psychologists use this Handbook to enhance their understanding of the psychology of Chicana/os and are encouraged by it to add, themselves, to the growing body of relevant literature. We dedicate our efforts in creating this volume to the memory of the late Martha E. Bernal, a mentor to so many of us. An appreciation of her life and works by Melba J. T. Vasquez follows.

Roberto J. Velásquez, San Diego State University
Leticia M. Arellano, University of La Verne
Brian W. McNeill, Washington State University

SPECIAL ACKNOWLEDGMENT

The editors would like to acknowledge the tireless efforts of Virgina Cardon for her assistance in the typing and preparation of this book. ¡Mil gracias Virgina!

REFERENCES

Martinez, J. L. (Ed.). (1977). *Chicano psychology.* New York: Academic Press.

Martinez, J. L., & Mendoza, R. H. (Eds.). (1984). *Chicano psychology* (2nd ed.). New York: Academic Press.

McNeill, B. W., Prieto, L., Niemann, Y. F., Pizarro, M., Vera, E. M., & Gómez, S. (2001). Current directions in Chicana/o psychology. *The Counseling Psychologist, 29,* 5–17.

Navarro, A. (1995). *Mexican American Youth Organization.* Austin: University of Texas Press.

Nieto Senour, M. (1977). Psychology of the Chicana. In J. L. Martinez, Jr. (Ed.), *Chicano psychology* (pp. 329–342). New York: Academic Press.

Therrien, M., & Ramirez, R. R. (2000). *The Hispanic population in the United States: March 2000* (Current Population Report No. P20-535). Washington, DC: U.S. Bureau of the Census.

An Appreciation of Dr. Martha E. Bernal (1931–2001)

Melba J. T. Vasquez
Vasquez & Associates, Mental Health Services
Austin, TX

The authors have chosen to dedicate this book to Dr. Martha E. Bernal. It is fitting that many of us honor her in various ways. She was the first known Chicana in the United States to earn a doctorate in psychology, in 1962 from Indiana University in Bloomington. The focus of her research during the first part of her career was parent-training approaches for behaviorally deviant children. Later, it shifted to the ethnic identity of Mexican American children. Dr. Bernal presented numerous papers at professional conferences and published approximately 60 articles, book chapters, and several books. She served as a member of the editorial board of several journals and also worked as a guest editor of various special issues. In the early 1970s, she dedicated herself to the goal of ensuring that more Chicana/os had the opportunity to receive graduate training and she worked to increase ethnic minority recruitment and retention and to improve training across the spectrum of minority groups. Her seminal articles in *The American Psychologist* and *The Counseling Psychologist* documented the dearth of minority graduate students and faculty members in psychology departments throughout the United States.

Dr. Bernal implemented a variety of strategies to achieve her goals. She received an NIMH Minority Clinical Training Grant and served as the director of that program at the University of Denver. At Arizona State University, she helped sponsor an annual Ethnic Identity Symposium for several years, which was attended by some of the leading researchers and students in the field. She and her colleague, George Knight, along with graduate and undergraduate students, worked to develop a methodology for measuring ethnic identity, collected normative data, and studied its developmental course as well as its correlates in Mexican American children. Her work has been widely cited, and has had a tremendous impact in the field.

Dr. Bernal was a pioneer in using her research knowledge to advocate for change. She promoted awareness of the importance of ethnic minority psychology to the leadership of psychology organizations. She was one of a handful of Chicana/o psychologists who met at American Psychological Association conventions to lobby

APA on ethnic minority concerns and issues. She continued to promote a minority agenda at other major conferences, such as the Vail Conference, where she was the only Latina participant, and the Lake Arrowhead Conference, where she presented one of the principal papers formally detailing recommendations for increasing the numbers of Chicana/os in psychology. Her recommendations at the Dulles Conference contributed to the development of the APA Board of Ethnic Minority Affairs (BEMA). She was involved in drafting its by-laws and in the rest of the complex process involved in establishing it. Once BEMA was established, she served on its Education and Training Committee. One of the founders of the Hispanic Psychological Association, she served as its second president, as well as treasurer, and was an active member of its executive committee from its beginning.

Despite health problems, which forced her to drop out of leadership activities for a period of time, she served on the Commission on Ethnic Minority, Recruitment, Retention, and Training (CEMRRAT) appointed by former APA President Ron Fox and chaired by former APA President Dick Suinn. She subsequently served on the Board for the Advancement of Psychology in the Public Interest CEMRRAT 2 Task Force, which oversaw the implementation of CEMRRAT's recommendations. At the time of her death, she was serving on the APA Committee of Gay, Lesbian, and Bisexual Concerns.

Dr. Bernal received numerous awards, including the Distinguished Life Achievement Award from APA Division 45, the Society for the Psychological Study of Ethnic Minority Issues, and the Hispanic Research Center Lifetime Award from Arizona State University. She was honored as one of four "Pioneer Senior Women of Color" at the first National Multicultural Conference and Summit held in Newport Beach, California, in 1999. She received the Carolyn Attneave award for life-long contributions to ethnic minority psychology and received the highly esteemed Distinguished Contribution to Psychology in the Public Interest Award at the American Psychological Association in 2001, which honored the full range of her research and professional activities.

Dr. Bernal influenced many colleagues, young professionals, and students. She was willing to be a situational mentor for many students and professionals across the country at times. She directly and indirectly provided guidance and inspiration to a wide range and number of psychologists of color, both men and women. She will be missed, but her influence will endure in the lives of all of those she touched.

Being and Becoming a Chicana/o:
General Issues

Mestiza/o and Chicana/o Psychology: Theory, Research, and Application

Manuel Ramirez III
University of Texas, Austin

The purpose of this chapter is to discuss the history of and recent developments in Chicana/o psychology and to point out new directions for theory and research. The concept of mestizaje (multicultural-multiracial world view) and the seven basic tenets of Chicana/o psychology are introduced.

WHAT IS CHICANA/O PSYCHOLOGY?

Chicana/o psychology is a psychology grounded in the tradition of the famous African American educator and civil rights leader, W. E. B. DuBois, and the first Chicano psychologist, George I. Sanchez. It is also a psychology based on the work of many subsequent Chicana and Chicano psychologists whose research has been devoted to they study of Chicanas and Chicanos as well as other multiracial-multicultural peoples in the Americas. The principal objective of Chicana/o psychology is to develop new concepts and strategies for understanding the struggles, trials, and tribulations of persons of Mexican descent as well as those of all of the cultural and genetic Mestizo peoples living in the United States.

Chicana/o psychology is a multicultural-multiracial field of study illuminated by the mestiza/o world view that has challenged the restrictive and exclusionary perspectives of North American and western European psychology. The first to articulate this world view was the Mexican philosopher-politician-educator Jose Vasconcellos. In his major works entitled *La Raza Cosmica* (1925) and *Indologia* (1927), Vasconcellos extolled the advantages offered by the synthesis of racial and cultural diversity through the amalgamation process of "mestizoisation." He argued that the genetic and cultural amalgamation of different races and cultures in Latin America offered the promise of a more enlightened way of life for all the peoples of the world. Vasconcellos believed that the Mestiza/o, the product of the synthesis of the Native American Indian and European groups in the Americas, was the end result of the intial stages in the development of the ideal citizen of the world: "Our major hope for salvation is found in the fact that we are not a pure race, but an aggregation of races in formation, an aggregation that can produce a race more powerful than those which are the products of only one race" (1927, p. 1202).

Taking Vasconcellos's perspective, the pioneers of Chicana/o psychology have questioned and changed the concepts, theories, and strategies of the larger field of psychology—and reached out to other fields, including sociology, anthropology, history, education, theology, political science, and Chicana/o studies—in an effort to create a more inclusive and socially responsible psychological science that is reflective of our new global society. This new psychology seeks to liberate those who are disenfranchised in society by eradicating stereotypes and denigrating images and other negative influences on people who are considered to be different, freeing them from feelings of inferiority, insecurity, uncertainty, and dependence. Chicana/o psychology seeks to produce research that is methodologically sound, but also congruent with and useful to those who need it most, *la gente* "the people."

Chicana/o psychology also aims to address societal problems—racism, sexism, and ageism—that affect those who feel different and who are alienated from mainstream American society. Other objectives include empowering individuals, families, and communities to combat poverty, crime, lack of education, and internalized racism and improving ethnic pride and self-esteem.

WHAT CHICANA/O PSYCHOLOGY IS NOT

It is not merely a subfield of psychology, nor is it based solely on Anglo or western European models of behavior and development. While recognizing that some mainstream psychological concepts and constructs may be useful in understanding multicultural-multiracial people, Chicana/o psychology emphasizes that all conceptual frameworks need to be carefully scrutinized before they are applied. The new multicultural-multiracial psychology is not a psychology of racial and cultural superiority; it offers new perspectives on reality that can enhance and enrich mainstream psychological theory and research.

TENETS OF CHICANA/O PSYCHOLOGY

The fundamental tenets of Chicana/o psychology were derived from the knowledge and experience of the mestizo peoples in the Americas. They reflect the developmental forces that influenced the cultures of Native American Indian, African American, Asian American, and European peoples. There are seven principles of underlying the Mestiza/o world view:

1. The person is an open system. In the Mestiza/o world view, the person is inseparable from the physical and social environments in which he or she lives. Traits, characteristics, skills, perceptions of the world, and philosophies of life evolve by meeting the environmental challenges the person encounters. Information and knowledge derived from others and the environment is regarded as modifying, incorporating, and influencing the dynamics of the person. The individual modifies and affects others and the environment as he or she interacts with these elements. In this ecological context, person-environment fit is the primary criterion for determining the quality of human adaptation.

2. The spiritual world holds the key to destiny, personal identity, and life mission. In addition, spiritualism serves to link the individual with supernatural forces in the cosmos from the Mestiza/o perspective and can influence individual and group or collective destiny. The developmental emphasis is on achieving control over the supernatural by attaining self-control and self-knowledge as well as on enlisting the help of a person or spirit who can mediate between the supernatural and the individual. A strong identification with the group to whom the individual belongs is also important because the group can provide access to knowledge concerning the maintenance of a proper balance between the individual and the supernatural.

Persons believed to have special knowledge, access to supernatural powers, or possession of these powers play an important role in personality development and functioning. For example, wisdom is highly valued in Chicana/o culture and is often sought from "special persons" within the community, including curandera/os, espiritistas, shamans, and clergy. These individuals all assist people in their search for self-knowledge and identity, provide treatment, and advise individuals experiencing personal conflicts, existential crises, or adjustment problems. In many communities, contemporary Chicana/o psychologists take on the role of such special persons and are frequently sought out for consultation regarding such issues. It is also important to note that the community is likely to view the Chicana/o psychologist as a person who has many powers, often magical, spiritual, or psychological.

In addition, some aspects of the Mestiza/o world view have been influenced by the belief that, through achieving communication with the spiritual world, a person can experience a vision or a dream that may provide an adult identity, a life mission, and a spirit-helper to facilitate the attainment of life goals. For example, it is very common among Chicana/os to talk about their deceased relatives in the present tense and to find solace and comfort in honoring the presence of these relatives in everyday life. Spirituality is also perceived to play an important role in achieving harmony with and protection from negative supernatural forces. Not only does religion provide models with which to identify and codes of conduct that facilitate the achievement of meaning in life and death, it also provides confession as a means of achieving reconciliation with the self and the supernatural.

3. Community identity and responsibility to the group are of central importance in development. In the Mestiza/o world view, the individual is socialized to develop a strong sense of responsibility to the group, whether it is the family community or ethnic group. Individuals come to feel that they are always representative of the group. In contemporary times, this is especially the case with Chicanos and Chicanas who have obtained high levels of education and who are highly valued and esteemed by their respective communities. The statement "I am the people" is often used by members of Native American Indian groups because identity cannot be separated into individual and group levels. LaFramboise (1983) observed that a central value of Native American cultures is the importance of close ties to the homeland and extended family. She reported that this value is inculcated in children because the entire community participates in the socialization and parenting processes. Community socialization is familiar to Chicana/os, who are socialized not only by the immediate family, but also by the extended family and the community. Identification with family and community is encouraged through extended family involvement in modeling and instruction in cultural traditions and rituals. This mode of socialization among Native American Indians is most evident in the powwows (Parfit & Harvey, 1994) that are held regularly by the Indian nations of North America. Powwows serve to maintain a sense of community by teaching and reinforcing traditions and values to the young and by keeping the culture alive.

From the Mestiza/o world view, the individual is seen as embedded in the context of the family group. Recognition of the important role of family identity, or familism, within the social sciences and helping professions has been one of the major contributions of the Native American Indian cultures of the Americas and the world. For example, as much as a Chicana/o may attempt to separate from family, this can never be fully accomplished because of built-in psychological mechanisms that keep that person joined to the family.

4. The foundations of a good adjustment to life (mental health) are liberation, justice, freedom, and empowerment. The history of the cultures of mixed ethnic peoples is one of struggles against political, social, and economic oppression; the stories surrounding these struggles are important to the education and socialization of children. The heroes of these struggles are held up as models for young children and adolescents and also serve to pull the individual back home, especially when the person is alienated. Poverty, human misery, racism, linguistic barriers, repression of individual rights, state-sanctioned brutality, and equality of opportunity are all visible realities for people of mixed heritage. For example, if one is to study the effects of colonization on a Chicana/o community, one important factor that must be understood is that of police-community relations. These factors also affect the socialization of individuals; they are the principal reason for the pragmatic orientation of a Mestiza/o, multicultural-multiracial psychology. The Native American Indian nations of North America have influenced the development of Mestiza/o psychology because, unlike many European societies, Native American communities are free of rulers, slavery, and social classes based on land or materialistic ownership. Indeed, many early European ethnographers and philosophers frequently described American Indian societies as just, equitable, and democratic when compared to various European societies (Weatherford, 1988).

5. Total development of abilities and skills is achieved through self-challenge. A prominent Native American Indian belief is that self-challenge and endurance of pain, hardship, hunger, and frustration encourage the development of an individual's full potential. Children are encouraged to seek out competitive situations and the goal of education is the full development of capacity. Lee (1976) observed that Native Americans were historically taught "to engage themselves in the elements—to meet them with an answering strength. If a torrential rain fell, they learned to strip and run out in it, however cool the weather. Little boys were trained to walk with men for miles through heavy snow drifts in the face of biting winds, and to take pride in the hardship endured" (p. 53). One of the principal goals of such self-challenge is to learn restraint and self-control. LaFramboise (1983) reported that, in Native American Indian cultures, respect is accorded those individuals who are self-disciplined.

In the Mestiza/o view, personality is the sum total of the experiences of coping with life's challenges and problems—environmental, social, and personal. The life history of every person is a series of lessons resulting from successes and failures in meeting these diverse challenges. Specifically, the nature and quality of experiences with life challenges and change determine the degree to which the person is open to and accepting of pluralism and diversity in his or her environment. For instance, individuals who are open to, or accepting of, diversity view it as the key to surviving rapid and radical change. Conversely, individuals who are not accepting of diversity become protective, self-centered, and easily threatened by diversity and change.

6. The search for self-knowledge, individual identity, and life meaning is a primary goal. Both the Mayas and the Nahuatl-speaking peoples of the Valley of Mexico historically believed that an individual comes to earth without a face and without an identity. Identities were achieved through socialization and education. In order to develop an identity, it was believed a person had to have self-control and personal strength, which was believed to lead to the development of free will. What the Nahuas called "self-admonishment," knowing for oneself what one should be, was the major goal of education. Leon-Portilla (1963) observed that the Nahuas, even more than the Greeks, recognized the relationship between identity and change of self-image through their conception of the self as being in constant motion and change.

7. Duality of origin and life in the universe and education within the family play a central role in personality development. The psychological concept of the duality of origin and life emerged from the cultures of Indian nations of Central and South America and the Caribbean. Polar opposites—male and female, religion and war, poetry and math—were often fused in the cultures of the Nahuas and Mayans. In the religion of the Nahuas, the god Ometeotl represents the dual nature of the culture. Ometeotl is androgynous—both father and mother of the other gods. (There many other male-female deities contained in the religion of the Nahuas.) Duality is further present in other aspects of the Nahua and Mayan cultures, such as the association of science with mysticism as reflected in the time theory of the Mayans and the calendaric diagnoses of the Nahuas. In addition, these cultures regarded education as the key to the proper development of the personality and of free will. Education was believed to be the responsibility of both the parents and the philosophers (the *tlamatinime*). Parents educated their children up to about age 15, when they entered a school to be taught by the tlamatinime. Education was formalized and mandatory.

The basic tenets of Chicana/o psychology given above were first represented in the work of pioneer social scientists who rebelled against the limited perspectives on personality typical of North American/western European psychology.

HISTORY OF CHICANA/O PSYCHOLOGY: PIONEERS

As early as 1903, African American educator and civil rights leader, W. E. B. DuBois, articulated the goals of multicultural-multiracial development as it applied to African Americans. Indeed, these same goals hold for all peoples of the world:

amalgamation as individuals merge their "double self" (such as African American and American) into a better and truer self. DuBois (1989) outlined his hope:

> In this merging he wishes neither of the older selves to be lost. He would not Africanize America, for America has much to teach the world and Africa. He would not bleach his Negro soul in a flood of White Americanism, for he knows that Negro blood has a message for the world. He simply wishes to make it possible for a man to be both a Negro and an American. (p. 17)

The first Latino scholar to address the injustices perpetrated by psychological research that employed biased tests of intelligence with Chicana/o children was George I. Sanchez (1932, 1934). Sanchez argued that it was necessary to consider language and culture in assessing intellectual or cognitive functioning in children of ethnic minority groups. He concluded that the entire intelligence-testing movement was based on erroneous information from genetics and heredity in order to champion the superiority of one race over another. In his works, Sanchez also referred to Native Americans and Latinos, both of whom possessed indigenous roots, as "forgotten Americans" (1948, 1967) whose needs were being ignored by the larger society.

In 1953, a type of psychotherapy for neuroses emerging from Japanese culture came to light: Morita therapy (Kondo, 1953). This is the first reported instance of a type of mental health treatment that did not originate from Anglo or western European culture. The therapy borrowed extensively from Zen and encouraged patients to cultivate an attitude toward life that was appropriate for them.

In 1967, Franz Fanon highlighted the insidious impact of colonization and oppression on people throughout the world, arguing that colonization not only served as a tool for oppressing people, but also was perhaps the best instrument for cutting away or eliminating culture, rituals, and belief systems from those who were colonized. Other negative consequences pointed out by Fanon included the destruction of religious or spiritual beliefs, the destabilization of families and communities, and the ultimate destruction of the human spirit. Fanon argued that identification with the aggressor would often serve as one means of maintaining colonization, or a colonization-like mentality, for many subsequent generations. He warned that western European psychologies, including the theories of Freud and Jung, were based on oppression, subjugation, and destruction (Bulhan, 1985).

Attneave (1969) recognized the need to encourage and reinforce the reciprocal support of Native American Indian extended families living in urban environments as a treatment model for Native Americans and others of mixed heritage. Speck and Attneave (1969) collaborated to establish a model, entitled "social network therapy." This model employed approaches used by medicine men, specifically, the involvement of family and community, in treatment to restore wholeness and harmony in the client. For example, the concept of *retribalization* was introduced to restore a vital element of the relationship and pattern that had been lost to the family and community. This social network consisted of the nuclear family and all kin of each member, as well as friends, neighbors, work associates, and significant helpers from churches, schools, social agencies, and institutions who were willing to help. This group, or network, served to revive or create a healthy social matrix, which then dealt with the distress and predicaments of the members far more quickly and effectively than any outside professional could ever hope to do.

In the academic year 1968 to 1969, I taught the first organized course in Chicana/o psychology at Pitzer College of the Claremont Colleges in Claremont, California. This new course was entitled "The Psychology of the Chicano Child." The course was based on the family values of the Mexican American and Mexican cultures and reviewed the psychological, anthropological, and sociological research that had been done with Latinos of Mexican origin up to that point in time. In March of 1973 the National Institute of Mental Health (NIMH) awarded a grant to Alfredo Castaneda (who had been my mentor at the University of Texas, Austin) and to myself to examine the underrepresentation of Latinos in psychology. The project had two objectives: (a) to conduct a national survey of all psychology departments in the United States to assess Chicana/o representation and recruitment and (b) to convene a national conference to address the issues that emerged from the findings of the survey. The data collected revealed that only 15 of 1,335 faculty positions in psychology departments were held by Chicanas and Chicanos. The number of Mexican American graduate students enrolled in MA programs was 51 and those in doctoral programs numbered only 37. Of the 254 institutions of higher education that responded to the survey, only 24 offered some form of financial assistance to students of Mexican descent. The national conference that followed the survey was held at the University of California, Riverside in May of 1973 and was entitled "Increasing Educational Opportunities in Psychology for Mexican Americans." Many of the pioneers of Chicana/o psychologists were present at that conference—Martha Bernal, Art Ruiz, Maria Nieto Senour, Joe Martinez, and Amado Padilla. Also attending were several undergraduate students who went on to achieve their doctorates and became major contributors to the field, such as Ray Buriel and Alex Gonzalez. The findings and recommendations made at this first conference were incorporated into an informational manual for undergraduates entitled *Chicanos and Psychology* (Ramirez & Gonzalez, 1974), which was distributed nationwide.

In 1973, Amado Padilla and Art Ruiz published their book entitled *Latino Mental Health: A Review of the Literature* (1973b). The research reviewed in this book, most of which had been presented at the Riverside conference, served to shape the research and training agenda of the Spanish Speaking Mental Health Research Center funded by NIMH at UCLA. This center also gave birth to the *Hispanic Journal of the Behavioral Sciences*, edited by Amado Padilla.

The passage of the Bilingual Education Act and the initiation of the Office of Bilingual Education and of Project Follow Through in the U.S. Office of Education made research funds available to Chicana/o psychologists who were interested in studying children and adolescents of Mexican descent. In 1974, Alfredo Castañeda and I summarized the findings of most of the research that had been done with Chicana/o children and families in our book entitled *Cultural Democracy, Bicognitive Development, and Education*, which provided the first psychological conceptual framework based on the Mestiza/o world view. The bicultural-bicognitive model we presented had a significant impact on teacher training programs as well as on graduate programs in psychology and education throughout the country.

Another major landmark in the development of Chicana/o psychology was the publication of the book edited by Joe Martinez entitled *Chicano Psychology*, published in 1977, a compilation of the papers that had been presented at the second national Chicana/o conference held at Irvine, California in 1975. A second edition of this book was edited by Martinez and Mendoza and published in 1984 following the third conference on Chicana/o psychology held at UC, Riverside in 1982. The present volume presents the contributions made at the two most recent conferences—at Michigan State University in 1998 and at San Antonio, Texas in 2000.

The most recent conference at Michigan State University in 1998, organized by Roberto Velasquez and Leticia Arellano, celebrating the 25th year of Chicana/o and Mestiza/o psychology, revived national interest in the new field that had remained dormant since 1984. This recent conference provided the impetus to examine the professional advancements of our field and to examine other areas that warrant consideration. Several books and publications on Chicana/o and Mestiza/o psychology and numerous volumes of the *Hispanic Journal of the Behavioral Sciences* have been published, yet growth of Chicana/o faculty and graduate students in departments of psychology has stagnated, as reported in this volume by Martha Bernal (Epilogue). The effects of anti-affirmative action efforts that culminated in the Hopwood Case and the passage of Proposition 187 in California have had a negative effect on diversity in higher education. It is also disturbing that Chicana/o research was found to be significantly underrepresented in APA journals in a study by Castro and Ramirez (1996). Nevertheless, some progress has been made in theory, research, and application.

In order to properly assess the degree of progress made in the development of a Chicana/o-Mestiza/o-Multicultural psychology, I reviewed publications in the area of cultural diversity in psychology and evaluated them with respect to the guidelines for Mestiza/o-multicultural scholarship in my book entitled *Multicultural/Multiracial Psychology* (1998). This is by no means an exhaustive literature review, but merely an attempt to select a few representative works in the theory, research, and practice of Chicana/o-Mestiza/o psychology that have appeared within the last 25 years.

RECENT DEVELOPMENTS IN CHICANA/O THEORY

Work in theory has expanded on the pioneering work of Dubois (1989), an African American sociologist who first introduced the notion of bicultural identities for people of color in the United States. A second contribution by Dubois that has also had a significant impact on Chicana/o theory is his idea of Pan-Africanism, which has contributed to a Pan-Latin Americanist perspective for Chicana/os and Mestiza/os. A natural outgrowth of the Pan-Latin Americanist perspective was the liberation theology of Paolo Freire (1970), which influenced the work of Martin-Baro (1985) in El Salvador, a prosocial action approach to the study of the Latin American peasant, which in turn influenced the participative approach to scholarship of Fals Borda (1987) in Colombia.

Also important was the work of the Jewish American scholars Kallen (1924) and Draschler (1920). Together with the work of Dubois, it influenced the introduction of the cultural democracy theory in conceptualizing the psychology of people of color in the United States (Ramirez & Castañeda, 1974). Casteñeda and I focused on the important relationship that cultural values, as reflected in family socialization practices, have on the bicultural and bicognitive development of Mestiza/o children. The mixed-race psychology paradigm introduced by Maria Root (1992) also provided a perspective on the unique experiences and paths to identity development observed in children of mixed race.

The ideas of Trimble (1981) regarding the Native American Indian concept of harmony, with the environment and the person as an open system have been critical in understanding the development and psychological adjustment of Mestiza/os. Thus, ecology is central in personality development and functioning. LaFramboise (1983) observed that a crucial value of Native American cultures is close ties to the homeland and the extended family. La Framboise and her colleagues also provided a very important summary of the different models used to conceptualize biculturalism among people of color (LaFramboise et al., 1993).

RECENT DEVELOPMENTS IN RESEARCH

In accordance with the guidelines for Chicana/o-Mestiza/o-multicultural scholarship laid out in my book entitled *Multicultural/Multiracial Psychology* (1998, Appendix Table 1), the following investigations in the last 25 years have made significant contributions to the development of a new psychology of *la raza*. Diaz-Guerrero has been one of the major pioneers. His research on the psychology of the Mexican has focused on values, or what he refers to as "historico-sociocultural premises" (1972). Research on bilingualism has also been very important. The early works by Lopez et al. (1974), Garcia (1997), and Padilla & Padilla (1977) helped to dispel the notion that Mestiza/os suffered intellectually because of language interference.

Another critical issue, generation level, was first targeted by Ray Buriel (1975, 1993a, 1993b). Buriel pointed out that most of the research conducted on Mestiza/os was confounded because the generation level of participants was not being taken into account. Buriel and his colleagues were also able to demonstrate that generation level was related to critical variables such as school achievement and ethnic identity (Buriel, Calzada, & Vasquez, 1982). Research on ethnic identity was also greatly enhanced by the work of Bernal and her colleagues (Ocampo, Knight, & Bernal, 1997).

Another important focus was biculturalism-multiculturalism. Alfredo Castañeda and I published work in this area in 1974 and Szapocznick and Kurtines (1993) did similar work with Cuban Americans. The recent work by Maria Root and her colleagues (Root, 1992) added the dimension of mixed race to the investigation of multicultural identity.

The Mestiza/o guidelines for research have also been presented in two very important publications on cross-cultural research by Vega (1992) and Betancourt and Lopez (1993). Both address important issues. Finally, in addition to the contributions of scholars from several generations to this volume, progress in research in Chicana/o psychology is evidenced by recent articles published in mainstream journals. These include those in a special issue of the *Journal of Multicultural Counseling and Development* entitled "Counseling Mexican Americans/Chicanos" (Velásquez, 1997), as well as a major contribution of *The Counseling Psychologist* on current directions in Chicana/o psychology by McNeill et al. (2001). Other important contributions related to the training of researchers and practitioners in issues of Chicana/os and Mestiza/os are noted by McNeill, Prieto, Ortiz, and Yamokoski (Chap. 20).

RECENT DEVELOPMENTS IN PRACTICE

Mestiza/os have suffered extensively from the application of Anglo and western European psychology. Children have been unjustly labeled as mentally retarded, culturally inappropriate mental health services have been provided, and opportunities in higher education institutions have been limited, because Chicana/o learning styles have been ignored. Examination of Appendix B provides general guidelines for working with Mestiza/os. The areas in which progress has been made in the last 25 years include primary prevention, assessment, therapy, and acculturation.

In the area of primary prevention, Sylvia Ramirez et al. (1994) has conducted important research on multicultural consultation in the schools. Lopez (1996) developed a model for school consultation based on the philosophy of cultural democracy and the concept of bicognitive development introduced by Ramirez and Castañeda (1974). Manuel Casas et al. (1998) is implementing a model for intervention with Chicana/o families and children who are at risk for educational and psychosocial problems. The pioneering work of Felipe Castro developing culturally oriented tobacco abuse prevention interventions in Chicana/o youth (see Castro, Maddahian, Newcomb, & Bentler, 1987, and chap. 18, this volume) has also given Mestiza/o psychology a central role. Castro has also done important work on heart disease and cancer (Castro, Cota, & Vega, 1999).

Assessment has always been of critical importance to Mestiza/o people. The misclassification of Mestiza/o children and adolescents and the misdiagnosis of clients of all ages have been central issues in Chicana/o-Mestiza/o mental health (Padilla & Ruiz, 1973a; Ramirez & Gonzalez, 1973). The work of Steve Lopez and his colleagues has been particularly seminal. Lopez and Nuñez (1987) concluded that the sets of diagnostic criteria in current use and interview schedules for schizophrenia and affective and personality disorders pay little attention to cultural factors. They make some general recommendations for addressing cultural considerations when making diagnoses. Steve Franco (1996) found that Chicana/o cultural values as assessed through the Family Attitudes Scale (Ramirez & Carrasco, 1996) were related to how adolescent Mexican Americans performed on different neuropsychological tests. Velásquez, Mendoza, Nezami, Castillo-Canez, Pace, Choney, Gomez, and Miles (2000) argued for the use of acculturation, gender, socioeconomic status, ethnic identity, and language variables when interpreting the MMPI-2 with Mestiza/os. Assessment issues also become central in the study of acculturation and acculturative stress.

Underutilization of mental health services (Cuellar & Schnee, 1987) has long been recognized as a major problem in Mestiza/o communities. Recent research by Castro (1996) and Trees (1997) identified the important role of culture in the type of mental health services that Mestiza/o people view as appropriate for their mental health needs, and also offered insights into why Latina/os and Filipina/os underutilize mental health services based on Anglo and western European values.

Attneave (1969) was the first to recognize the need for encouraging and reinforcing the reciprocal support of Native American Indian extended families living in urban environments as a viable treatment model for Native American and others of mixed heritage. She entitled this treatment "network therapy."

Lopez (2002) introduced a model of culturally competent psychotherapy that integrates a cultural perspective. The model encompasses four domains of clinical practice: engagement, assessment, theory, and methods that require the clinician to work within both mainstream and Chicano cultures. Szapocznick and his colleagues (Szapocznick, Scopetta, & King, 1978, 1993) adapted a European treatment family therapy approach, that of Salvador Minuchin (1974), for use with people of mixed heritage. Their approach employed a focus on family values and bicultural processes. Rogler and Cooney (1984) developed a community program to serve troubled Puerto Rican adolescents in the South Bronx. The major goal of the program was to counter-act the stressful effects of single-parent households and family disorganization by providing symbolic families for the clients. Carrasco, Garza-Louis, and King (1996) developed an approach to psychotherapy with Latino male sex offenders that focuses on values relating to gender role definition, in particular the definition of machismo. Working with Latina/o families in San Antonio, Cervantes and Ramirez (1995) focused on the importance of spirituality in family therapy. They also emphasized the philosophy of curanderismo as an important mindset for the therapist working with these families. Baron (1981) evolved a model for counseling Chicana/o college students that emphasizes the importance of acculturation, ethnic or racial identity development, and gender role socialization. The model employs the concept of "interactive culture strain" as a unifying framework that captures the dynamic interplay of the aforementioned variables. Ramirez (1994; 1999) introduced a multicultural model of psychotherapy and counseling for Mestiza/os that can be applied to individuals, couples, and families. The theoretical basis of the model has its origins in cross-cultural mental health and in the psychology of liberation that evolved from developments in the psychologies of ethnic minorities, other colonized populations, and women.

How can we assure the continued success and evolution of Chicana/o-Mestiza/o psychology? One necessary requirement is that we continue to be skeptical of Anglo and western European psychology, or, as Franz Fanon referred to it, the psychology of oppression (cf. Bulham, 1985). In a paper presented at a conference sponsored by the International Union of Psychologists and the Mexican Society of Social Psychology in Merida, Mexico (1994), I observed that, like the warning on cigarette packages, North American and western European psychology should be introduced to Mestiza/os with the following words of caution: "Warning—this psychology could be harmful to your self-esteem and to the well-being of your people" (p. 3).

Second, we need to make changes in psychology departments in colleges and universities, as they have been the most resistant to diversity and to the needs of people of color. Far too many minority psychologists have left faculty positions in psychology departments for more hospitable environments, such as schools of education. The loss of Chicana/o faculty is alarming, particularly at a time when the number of minority graduate students and faculty is dropping dramatically (see chap. 20, this volume). We need to continue to recruit undergraduate and graduate minority students into psychology programs and we need to make curriculum changes in psychology training programs that truly reflect the new world order, one in which people of color and multicultural and multiracial people are in the majority.

Third, we need to support the drive to establish guidelines that will ensure cultural competence in the provision of mental health services. If these guidelines are not adopted by state and national professional associations, managed care companies, and licensing boards, Chicana/os and Mestiza/os in this country will continue to be underserved and malserved with respect to their mental health needs.

Finally, as psychologists, social scientists, and educational and mental health professionals, we need to model ourselves after DuBois, Sanchez, and Attneave. Like these pioneers, we need to be the uncompromising opposition in society. We cannot afford to be accommodationists because freedom and self-respect cannot be negotiated or compromised.

REFERENCES

Attneave, C. L. (1969). Therapy in tribal settings and urban network intervention. *Family Process, 8,* 192–210.

Baron, A., Jr. (1981). *Explorations in Chicano psychology.* New York: Praeger.

Bernal, M. E., & Knight, G. P. (1993). *Ethnic identity: Formation and transmission among Hispanics and other minorities.* Albany, NY: State University of New York Press.

Betancourt, H., & Lopez, S. R. (1993). The study of culture, ethnicity, and race in American psychology. *American Psychologist, 28,* 629–637.

Bulhan, H. A. (1985). *Franz Fanon and the psychology of oppression.* New York: Plenum.

Buriel, R. (1975). Cognitive styles among three generations of Mexican American children. *Journal of Cross-Cultural Psychology, 10,* 417–429.

Buriel, R. (1993a). Acculturation, respect for actual differences, and biculturalism among three generations of Mexican American and Euro American school children. *Journal of Genetic Psychology, 145,* 531–543.

Buriel, R. (1993b). Childrearing orientations in Mexican American families: The influence of generation and sociocultural factors. *Journal of Marriage and Family, 55,* 987–1000.

Buriel, R., Calzada, S., & Vasquez, R. (1982). The relationship of traditional American culture to adjustment and delinquency among three generations of Mexican American male adolescents. *Hispanic Journal of the Behavioral Sciences, 14,* 41–55.

Carrasco, N., Garza-Louis, D., & King, R. (1996). The Hispanic sex offender: Machismo and cultural values. In A. B. Jones (Ed.), *Yearbook for the sex offender: Correctional, treatment and legal practice* (pp. 4–5). Plymouth, MA: Spring.

Casas, J. M., Bimbela, A., Corral, C. R., Yanez, I., Swaim, R. C., Wayman, J. C., & Bates, S. (1998). Cigarette and smokeless tobacco use among Mexican and nonimmigrant Mexican American youth. *Hispanic Journal of Behavioral Sciences, 20,* 102–121.

Castro, A. (1996). *Mexican-American values and their impact on mental health care.* Unpublished doctoral dissertation, University of Texas, Austin.

Castro, A., & Ramirez, M. (1996). *The Latino representation in the psychological literature: A 25-year review of six APA journals.* Unpublished manuscript.

Castro, E. G., Maddahian, E., Newcomb, M. D., & Bentler, P. M. (1987). A multivariate model of the determinants of cigarette smoking among adolescents. *Journal of Health and Social Behavior, 28,* 273–289.

Castro, F. G., Cota, M. K., & Vega, S. (1999). Health promotion in Latino populations: Program planning, development and evaluation. In R. M. Huff & M. V. Kline (Eds.), *Promoting health in multicultural populations: A handbook for practitioners* (pp. 137–168). Thousand Oaks, CA: Sage.

Cervantes, J. M., & Ramirez, O. (1995). Spirituality and family dynamics in psychotherapy with Latino children. In K. P. Monteiro (Ed.), *Ethnicity and psychology* (pp. 103–128). Dubuque, IA: Kendall-Hunt.

Cuellar, I. B., & Schnee, S. B. (1987). An examination of the utilization characteristics of clients of Mexican origin served by the Texas Department of Mental Health and Mental Retardation. In R. Rodriguez & M. Coleman Tolbert (Eds.), *Mental health issues of the Mexican-origin population in Texas.* Austin, TX: Hogg Foundation for Mental Health.

Diaz-Guerrero, R. (1972). *Hacia una teoria historico-biopsico-sociocultural del comportamiento humano.* Mexico, D.F.: Trillas.

Drachsler, J. (1920). *Democracy and assimilation: The blending of immigrant heritages in America.* New York: McMillan.

DuBois, W. E. B. (1989). *The souls of Black folk.* New York: Bantam. (Original work published 1903)

Fals Borda, O. (1987). *Investigacion-accion participativa en Colombia* [Participative Action Research in Columbia]. Bogota, Columbia: Punta de Lanza.

Fanon, F. (1967). *Black skin, white masks.* New York: Grove.

Franco, S. L. (1996). *Neuropsychological test performance of Mexican American and Anglo American high school students from communities of the U. S.-Mexican border region of south Texas.* Unpublished doctoral dissertation, University of Texas, Austin.

Freire, P. (1970). *Pedogagy of the oppressed.* New York: Seabury Press.

Garcia, E. E. (1977). The study of early childhood bilingualism: Strategies for linguistic transfer research. In J. L. Martinez (Ed.), *Chicano psycology* (pp. 141–151). New York: Academic Press.

Kallen, H. M. (1924). *Culture and democracy in the United States.* New York: Boni and Liveright.

Keefe, S. E., & Padilla, A. M. (1987). *Chicano ethnicity.* Albuquerque, NM: University of New Mexico Press.

Kondo, A. (1953). Morita therapy: A Japanese therapy for neurosis. *American Journal of Psychoanalysis, 13,* 31–37.

LaFramboise, T. (1983). *Assertion training with American Indians.* Las Cruces, NM: ERIC Clearinghouse on Rural Education and Small Schools.

LaFramboise, T., Coleman, H. L. K., & Gerton, J. (1993). Psychological impact of biculturalism: evidence and theory. *Psychological Bulletin, 114,* 395–412.

Lee, D. (1976). *Valuing the self: What we can learn from other cultures.* Englewood Cliffs, NJ: Prentice-Hall.

Leon-Portilla, M. (1963). *Aztec thought and culture: A study of the ancient Nahuatl mind.* Norman, OK: University of Oklahoma Press.

Lopez, M., Hicks, R. E., & Young, R. K. (1974). The linguistic interdependence of bilinguals. *Journal of Experimental Psychology, 102,* 981–983.

Lopez, S., & Nuñez, J. A. (1987). Cultural factors considered in selected diagnostic criteria and interview schedules. *Journal of Abnormal Psychology, 96,* 270–272.

Lopez, S. L. (2002, October). *Conceptions of culture: Implications for clinical research and practice with Latinos.* Contribution presented at the meeting of the Latino Psychology 2002 conference, Providence, RI.

Lopez, V. (1996, May). *A multicultural approach to consultation.* Poster session presented at the student conference at University of Texas, Austin School of Education, Austin, TX.

Martin-Baro, I. (1985). *Accion e ideologia* [Action and ideology]. San Salvador: Universidad Centro Americana.

Martinez, J. (Ed.). (1977). *Chicano psychology.* New York: Academic Press.

Martinez, J. L., & Mendoza, R. H. (1984). *Chicano psychology* (2nd ed.). New York: Academic Press.

McNeill, B. W., Prieto, L. P., Niemann, Y. F., Pizzarro, M., Vera, E. M., & Gomez, S. P. (2001). Current directions in Chicana/o psychology. *The Counseling Psychologist, 29,* 5–17.

Minuchin, S. (1974). *Families and family therapy.* Cambridge, MA: Harvard University Press.

Ocampo, K. A., Knight, G. P., & Bernal, M. E. (1997). The development of cognitive abilities and social identities in children: The case of ethnic identity. *International Journal of Behavioral Development, 21,* 479–500.

Padilla, A. M., & Ruiz, R. (1973a). *Latino mental health.* (Department of Health, Education, and Welfare Publication No. MSM 73-9143). Washington, DC: U. S. Government Printing Office.

Padilla, A. M., & Ruiz, R. A. (1973b). *Latino mental health: A review of the literature.* Washington, DC: U.S. Government Printing Office.

Padilla, E. R., & Padilla, A. M. (1977). *Transcultural psychiatry: An Hispanic perspective.* Los Angeles, CA: Spanish Speaking Mental Health Research Center.

Parfit, M., & Harvey, A. D. (1994, June). Powwow. *National Geographic, 85*(6), 88–113.

Ramirez, M. (1994). *Psychotherapy and counseling with minorities: A cognitive approach to individual and cultural differences.* Needham Heights, MA: Allyn and Bacon.

Ramirez, M. (1998). *Multicultural/multiracial psychology: Mestizo perspectives in personality and mental health.* Northvale, NJ: Aronson.

Ramirez, M., & Carrasco, N. (1996). Revision of the Family Attitude Scale. Unpublished manuscript. Austin, TX.

Ramirez, M., & Castañeda, A. (1974). *Cultural democracy, bicognitive development, and education.* New York: Academic Press.

Ramirez, M., & Gonzalez, A. (1973). Mexican Americans and intelligence testing. In N. M. Mangold (Ed.), *La Causa Chicana: The Movement for Justice* [The Chicano cause: The movement for justice] (pp. 137–147). New York: Family Service Association of America.

Ramirez, M., & Gonzalez, A. (1974). *Chicanos and psychology.* New York: Family Service Association of America.

Ramirez, S., Wassef, A., Paniagua, F., & Kinskey, A. (1994). Perceptions of mental health providers concerning cultural factors in the evaluation of Hispanic children and adolescents. *Hispanic Journal of Behavioral Sciences, 16,* 28–42.

Rogler, L. H., & Cooney, S. R. (1984). *Puerto Rican families in New York City: Intergenerational processes* (Hispanic Research Center Monograph No. 11). Maplewood, NJ: Waterfront.

Root, M. P. P. (Ed.). (1992). *Racially mixed people in America.* Newbury Park, CA: Sage.

Sanchez, G. I. (1932). Group differences and Spanish-speaking children—A critical review. *Journal of Applied Psychology, 16,* 549–558.

Sanchez, G. I. (1934). Bilingualism and mental measures: A word of caution. *Journal of Applied Psychology, 18,* 756–772.

Sanchez, G. I. (1948). *The people: A study of the Navajos.* Washington, DC: United States Indian Service.

Sanchez, G. I. (1967). *Forgotten people: A study of New Mexicans.* Albuquerque, NM: Calvin Horn.

Speck, R., & Attneave, C. L. (1974). *Family networks.* New York: Vintage.

Szapocznik, J., & Kurtines, W. M. (1993). Family psychology and cultural diversity: Opportunity for theory, research, and application. *American Psychologist, 48,* 400–407.

Szapocznik, J., Scopetta, M. A., & King, O. E. (1978). Theory and practice in matching treatment to the special characteristics and problems of Cuban immigrants. *Journal of Community Psychology, 6,* 112–122.

Trees, J. (1997). *Filipino American values and mental health attitudes.* Unpublished manuscript, University of Texas, Austin.

Trimble, J. E. (1981). Value differentials and their importance in counseling American Indians. In P. P. Pederson, J. G. Draguns, W. J. Lonner, & J. E. Trimble (Eds.), *Counseling across cultures* (2nd ed., pp. 203–226). Honolulu: University of Hawai'i Press.

Vasconcellos, J. (1925). *La raza cosmica: Mision de la raza iberoamericana* [The cosmic race: Mission of the Iberoamerican race]. Mexico, D.F.: Espasa-Calpe Mexicaña SA.

Vasconcellos, J. (1927). *Indologia: Una interpretacion de la cultura iberoamericano* [The study of Indian cultures: An interpretation of Iberoamerican culture]. Barcelona, Spain: Agencia Mundial de Liberia.

Vega, W. A. (1992). Theoretical and pragmatic implications of cultural diversity for community research. *American Journal of Community Psychology, 20,* 375–391.

Velásquez, R. J. (Ed.). (1997). Counseling Mexican Americans/Chicanos [Special issue]. *Journal of Multicultural Counseling and Development, 25*(2).

Velásquez, R. J., Mendoza, S., Nezami, E., Castillo-Canez, I., Pace, T., Choney, S. K., Gomez, F. C., & Miles, L. E. (2000). Culturally competent use of the Minnesota Multiphasic Personality Inventory–2 with minorities. In I. Cuellar & F. A. Paniagua (Eds.), *Handbook of multicultual mental health* (pp. 389–417). San Diego, CA: Academic Press.

Weatherford, J. (1988). Indian givers: How the Indians of the Americas transformed the world. New York: Fawcett Columbine.

Appendix A

HOW WELL DOES THE STUDY OR PROGRAM MEET MULTICULTURAL/MULTIRACIAL STANDARDS?

Each of the following standards is evaluated on a scale of 1 (not at all characteristic) to 5 (very characteristic).

Theory or Conceptual Framework

1. Degree to which the theory or conceptual framework is consistent with Mestizo multicultural-multiracial world view.

Participants

2. Degree to which participants reflect intracultural diversity of target group or groups.
3. Degree to which SES, linguistic, generational status, and acculturation-multiculturation information were taken into consideration in selection of participants.
4. If two or more groups were compared, degree to which groups are comparable.

Instruments

5. Degree to which content of the instruments was reflective of the Mestizo view.
6. Degree to which structure of the instruments was reflective of the Mestizo view.
7. Degree to which demands that the instruments made on the participants were consistent with the Mestizo view.

Data Collection and Interpretation

8. Degree to which data were collected in a historical, social, economic, political, cultural, and religious or spiritual context.
9. Degree to which data were interpreted in a historical, social, economic, political, cultural, and religious or spiritual context.

Note. From *Multicultural/Multiracial Psychology: Mestizo Perspectives in Personality and Mental Health* (p. 109), by Manuel Ramirez III, 1998, Northvale, NJ: Jason Aronson. Adapted with permission.

Appendix B

HOW WELL DOES THE STUDY OR PROGRAM FOCUS ON THE MESTIZO POPULATIONS?

Theory or Conceptual Framework

1. The theory or conceptual framework does not reflect notions of superiority with regard to culture, race, gender, genetics, physical disabilities, or sexual orientation.
2. The theory or conceptual framework emerged from the native culture or value system of the people who are being studied or on which the program is being implemented.

Participants

3. The participants reflect the intracultural diversity of the groups that are the object of the research or intervention.
4. SES, linguistic, generational status, and multiracial-multicultural variables were considered in the selection of participants.
5. Groups being compared are comparable (SES, generational, and educational levels are common confounds).

Instruments and Intervention Procedures

6. The content of the instrument is reflective of the Mestizo multicultural-multiracial world view.
7. The structure of the instrument is reflective of the Mestizo view.
8. The demands of the instruments or procedures of the intervention made on the participants are consistent with the Mestizo world view.

9. The instruments and the procedures reflect approaches that are part of the native culture(s), for example, story telling, life histories, respect for nature, spirituality, and a sense of community and humanity.

Methodology

10. Employs multiple methods and multiple measures.
11. Uses qualitative as well as quantitative methodology.

Data Collection

12. Data are collected without deceiving, demeaning, or embarrassing participants.
13. Data collection uses participant observation or approaches that are potentially beneficial (empowering) to the participants (Almeida Acosta & Sanchez, 1985).
14. Data are interpreted in the context of historical, political, religious, economic, and social perspectives.

Data Analysis

15. Statistical procedures used allow findings to be placed in the context of historical, political, religious, economic, and social perspectives.

Researchers/Intervenors

16. The researchers or intervenors conduct self-analysis to determine the degree of similarity or difference between their values and world views and those of the participants on which the intervention plan is being implemented.

Note: From *Multicultural/Multiracial Psychology: Mestizo Perspectives in Personality and Mental Health* (p. 128), by Manuel Ramirez III, 1998, Northvale, NJ: Jason Aronson. Adapted with permission.

Acculturation:
A Psychological Construct of Continuing
Relevance for Chicana/o Psychology

Israel Cuéllar
Roxana I. Siles
Erika Bracamontes
Julian Samora Research Institute
Michigan State University

INTRODUCTION

This chapter reviews the construct of acculturation, its measurement, and its relevance not just to the psychology of Chicana/os, but also to that of all persons who live and develop in multicultural or pluralistic environments. It is well understood that there are many complex and interesting changes resulting from different cultures coming into continuous contact with each other. Historically, great centers of trade, growth, and prosperity resulted from this convergence as well as longlasting and, unfortunately, apparent irresolvable conflicts. Chicana/os are caught between two cultures (the cultures of Mexico and of the United States). They experience different degrees of exposure to these two large complex cultural systems over time and integrate different aspects of these cultures throughout their lifespan. There are no fixed outcomes from acculturation processes: They are interdependent, transactional, and ecological and depend on numerous types of variables, including but not limited to environmental and contextual, individual personality, status, sociocultural, and political. Acculturation outcomes at the individual level are very much like personality characteristics: They are difficult to define, occur along continuous dimensions or degrees, are generally multidimensional in nature, and are influenced by both genetic and cultural factors. Chicana/o social scientists, including psychologists, have played an important role in understanding acculturation processes, their influences, measurement, and importance with respect to psychological well-being and development.

DEFINITION AND HISTORY

Acculturation began as an anthropological construct, evolving out of a body of literature on culture change and culture contact that was popular at the turn of the century. One publication was an article on Yaqui and Apache Indians as they moved through four theoretical linear stages of acculturation: Savagery, Barbarism, Civilization, and finally Enlightenment (McGee, 1898), another the changing roles of females in the Antler Indian culture through contact with Whites (Mead, 1932). This literature was largely qualitative and ethnographic. Anthropologists struggled with a definition of acculturation as its conceptual definition became increasingly all encompassing. The Social Science Research Council appointed a team of experts to clarify the definition of what was included in the construct of acculturation. According to their published report in the *American Anthropologist*, "acculturation comprehends those phenomena which result when groups of individuals having different cultures come into continuous first-hand contact, with subsequent changes in the original cultural patterns of either or both groups" (Redfield, Linton, & Herskovitz, 1936, p. 149). This definition, as noted, included macro- to micro-level changes and phenomena, it was not exclusionary and it also included all that might change as a result of people from different cultures coming into contact. This distinction was important because anthropologists and psychologists soon followed by making it clear that psychological processes were a part of acculturation phenomena. Robert C. Pierce (a research psychologist) along with M. Margaret Clark and Christie W. Kiefer (both anthropologists) laid the groundwork for the first empirical measure of acculturation at the individual psychological level (Pierce, Clark, & Kiefer, 1972). Prior to their research, others had made serious efforts to measure cognitive ideologies relevant to acculturation. For example, Levinson and Huffman (1955) developed the Traditional Family Ideologies Scale and Kluckholm and Strodtbeck (1961) created the Values Orientation Scale. These cognitive references of acculturation were not identified as "acculturation measures" per se but were, nonetheless, examples of measures that assessed cultural changes at the psychological level.

Several works by Chicana/o psychologists in the late 1970s were instrumental in focusing research on Chicana/os in the developing field of psychological acculturation. The first was the introduction of the Measure of Acculturation for Chicano Adolescents (Olmedo, Martinez, & Martinez, 1978; Olmedo & Padilla, 1978), the second was the *American Psychologist* article entitled "Acculturation: A psychometric perspective" by Olmedo (1979), and the third was the book entitled *Acculturation: Theory, Models, and Some New Findings* (Padilla, 1980). This book contained several important chapters, including contributions from Padilla (1980), which had very seminal theoretical and applied influences such as the idea of acculturative typologies. These three publications led to a proliferation of measures and research on acculturation, not only on Chicana/os, but through paradigmatic measures on acculturation in any two ethnic-cultural groups. (For a selected listing of trends and a chronology of acculturation and various ethnicity measures between 1955 and 1995, see Cuéllar, 2000c, and Roysircar-Sodowsky & Maestas, 2000.)

Ethnic identity as a concept and construct was growing in parallel to the concept of acculturation. How ethnic identity and acculturation relate to each other was, and continues to be, of much theoretical interest. Clark, Kaufman, and Pierce (1976), Cohen (1978), and Padilla (1980) argued that ethnic identity was a part of acculturation phenomena or, as Cohen noted, ethnicity arises from a situation of contact between different cultural groups. Ethnic identity is often discussed in terms of what determines what. Ethnic identity models and their measurement became the focus of acculturation research in the 1980s and 1990s. Some of the representative ethnic identity models developed were Phinney's Ethnic Identity Development Model (Phinney, 1989), Cross' (1991) Psychological Nigrescence Model, Helms' (1990) Racial Identity Model, and Knight-Bernal's Social Cognitive Model of Ethnic Identity Development (Knight, Bernal, Garza, & Cota, 1993). (Examples of ethnic identity measures were the Multigroup Ethnic Identity Measure or MEIM, Phinney, 1992, and the Ethnic Identity Questionnaire, Bernal, Knight, Ocampo, Garza, & Cota, 1993.)

A very significant methodological and theoretical contribution in the assessment of acculturation was made with what has been labeled variously as the "Two-culture Matrix Model" (McFee, 1968; Ruiz, Casas, & Padilla, 1977; see also Keefe & Padilla, 1987), the "Orthogonal Model" (Oetting & Beauvais, 1991), or the "Two-Dimensional Model" (Buriel, 1993). In these models, each culture is conceived as a separate axis and their interaction as forming a matrix. Each person undergoing acculturation may vary independently in his or her exposure, acceptance, rejection, or adaptation with respect to each of the two cultures. This methodological advancement led to the psychometric assessment of bicultural adaptations including forms of integration and marginalization for the first time.

Among the contributions of acculturation research, both on and by Chicana/os and others in the field of acculturation, was the notion that the cultural context in which individuals grow up determines who they are, how they identify themselves, their psychological characteristics, and their sense of well-being. Berry (1994), a world-renowned giant in the field of acculturation, noted that acculturation processes, defined as those processes that allow one "to move toward a culture," change people in various ways and are commonly associated with some form of stress. In order to comprehend the influences of acculturation on the self, an ecological construction of culture and the individual is required (Cuéllar, 2000a).

BRIEF REVIEW OF LITERATURE ON CHICANA/OS AND LATINA/OS AND ACCULTURATION

A review conducted by the authors of this chapter of published articles on MEDLINE and PsycINFO searches using "Acculturation and Hispanics" as keywords over the period of 1966 to 2001 found 996 ($n = 743$ unduplicated) articles. The largest category (40% or 401 hits) was that of health, followed by alcohol use (10.6% or 106 hits). Mental health represented 9.4% or 94 hits. A total of 56% (564) of the hits were found on MEDLINE and 44% (432) on the PsycINFO database. When other ethnic groups were included, the number of hits was truly incredible ($n = 4,122$) given the very limited interest in the subject of acculturation by psychologists prior to 1970.

Culture, Acculturation, and Mental Health

The concept of illness is far broader than that of disease and includes psychosocial and sociocultural influences, not traditionally thought of as being part of a disease (Kleinman, 1988). The lack of understanding of this difference hampered the understanding of the role of culture on health for many years. Culture has a profound impact on illness as well as disease, although not as directly on the latter. With the introduction of the biopsychosocial model (Engel, 1977), a formal understanding of the role of psychosocial-cultural variables became more generally accepted. The influences of culture on mental health and its treatment have now been well documented (National Institute of Mental Health [NIMH], 1995; Cuéllar & Paniagua, 2000). Cultural influences have been found to be associated with numerous symptoms of well-being and adjustment and have etiological influence on many mental disorders as noted in the *Diagnostic and Statistical Manual of Mental Disorders-IV* (American Psychological Association, 1994). Clearly the role of culture and pathology extends far beyond specific culture-bound syndromes.

The relationship of acculturation to mental health has been increasingly researched and reviewed (Berry & Kim, 1988; Negy & Woods, 1992b; NIMH, 1995; Rogler, Cortes, & Malgady, 1991). The experience of living simultaneously within more than one cultural context has led to much speculation about coping with present, as well as potential, cultural conflicts, particularly for members of racial, cultural, and ethnic minority groups. Speculation about the relation of acculturation to mental health can be traced to Stonequist's hypothesis (1935, 1937), which stipulated that being caught between two cultural groups, particularly with regard to "the system of mores," leads to mental tension and possible changes in self-concept or ethnic identity. Stonequist believed that psychologically marginalized individuals were at greater risk for, and experienced more, mental health related problems. Accommodations reached during acculturation processes can also have positive effects, including forms of biculturalism that lessen experiences of conflict (NIMH, p. 103). Very little is known about accommodations to acculturation with respect to their relative distribution, how they come about, or how they increase or decrease risk and vulnerability to health and mental health problems.

Mental Health and Acculturation of Latina/o Hispanics

There are increasing amounts of data pertaining to the effects of acculturation on Latina/o mental health. In fact, this area of research comprises the second largest number of hits when the words "acculturation," "Hispanic," and "mental health" are entered using the MEDLINE and PsycINFO databases. In the field of mental health, the three most common areas of research are depression, alienation and stress, and overall mental status. Not only have studies on these topics increased in number, variety, and complexity, but they have also become more intense as they elucidate either unequivocal or conflicting trends in this area of research.

Stemming from this extensive field of research are important trends that provide a better understanding of the overall mental status of Latina/os. For example, Mexican-born immigrants have consistently better mental health profiles then U.S.-born Mexican Americans when socioeconomic variables are controlled for (Escobar et al., 1988; Escobar, Hoyos-Nervi, & Gara, 2000). Among Mexican-born persons living in the U.S., less acculturated Mexican Americans have healthier psychological profiles than more acculturated Mexican Americans. A second consistent trend in this field is that "biculturalism," or an intermediate level of acculturation among Latina/os, is "the least detrimental to Latina/os' mental health" (Miranda & Umhoefer, 1998, p. 159). Another publication by Miranda supports previous work on the subject suggesting that "bicultural" Latina/os have better mental health profiles than both less and more acculturated Latina/os (Miranda, 1995). These studies emerge from the idea that depression increases and social interest decreases with increasing levels of acculturation (Miranda; Miranda & Umhoefer, 1998).

Depression is probably the most commonly studied and conflicting aspect of Latina/o mental health. For example, Zamarian et al. (1992) pointed to a strong inverse relationship between acculturation and depression: They explain that apparent retention of Mexican culture without concomitant attempts to incorporate aspects of the dominant culture results in the most vulnerable position to depression. Recent work in this area by Gonzalez, Haan, and Hinton (2001) supports the idea that less acculturated Mexican Americans have a higher risk of depression than their highly acculturated counterparts. Along the same line, however, the evidence suggests that depression does not directly correlate with acculturation (Griffith, 1983). In fact, Griffith stated that socioeconomic status can best explain mental conditions such as anxiety among Latina/os. In accordance with this finding, subsequent research by Canabal and Quiles (1995) demonstrates that socioeconomic variables, including education, age, and employment, have a significantly stronger correlation than acculturation with depression among Latina/os. Interestingly, a dissertational study by Duran (1995) suggests that more acculturated Latinas exhibit a higher degree of somatization of depressive symptoms than less acculturated Latinas. The same study then explains that somatization is a cultural modality to elicit support and, consequently, is not associated with depression among less acculturated individuals.

Data on "alienation" and its effects on stress among Latina/os offer a complex and confounding view of the effects of alienation among Latina/os. For example, one study by Kaplan and Marks (1990) suggested that distress symptoms increase significantly with higher levels of acculturation among young adults, but not among older adults. The same study then asserted that higher levels of acculturation are directly correlated with more feelings of alienation and discrimination among young Latina/os. On the contrary, Negy and Woods (1992b) showed that feelings of alienation have an inverse relationship with increasing levels of acculturation.

Immigration and Mental Health

The Immigrant Paradigm of Acculturation has as its subject an adult immigrant living in the U.S. who acquires characteristics of the host culture in order to adapt, function, and prosper in the new culture (cf. Cuéllar, 2000b). For many second-, third-, and fourth-generation minority group members, acculturation experiences are bicultural and the Immigrant Paradigm does not apply, but the Minority Paradigm of Acculturation does. In the Minority Paradigm of Acculturation, the minority individual is "acculturating" and "enculturating" with regards to at least two cultures throughout his or her lifespan. The Minority Paradigm emphasizes biculturalism and bicognitive adaptation and subjects are required to acculturate simultaneously, but in varying degrees, to both their ethnic traditional culture and mainstream American culture.

A subject of growing interest in acculturation research is the effect of American culture on the immigrant who is undergoing acculturation based on the Immigrant Paradigm of Acculturation. Suarez-Orozco (1997) noted that an increasing number of studies show that the new immigrant from Mexico displays better mental health and a healthier attitude toward wanting to do well in school and graduate from college than third-generation U.S.-born Chicana/os.

Suarez-Orozco (1997) was not the only investigator to note that new immigrants sometimes have better mental health than more acculturated Chicana/os. Vega et al. (1998) compared adjusted lifetime prevalence rates for various mental disorders using the Composite International Diagnostic Inventory (CIDI) of Mexican immigrants with native-born Mexican Americans. The results show that the native-born lifetime prevalence rate for any disorder (48.1%) is twice that of the immigrants (24.9%). Vega et al. also concluded that short-term-stay immigrants (< 13 years) have almost half the lifetime prevalence rates for any disorder than long-term immigrants, those having lived in the U.S. for more than 13 years. In comparing the lifetime prevalence rates for Mexicans in Mexico City with short-term immigrants, long-term immigrants, and native-born Mexican-origin populations, they found that prevalence rates increase with increased acculturation to the U.S. culture. Additionally, they discovered that individuals of Mexican origin who were born and raised in the U.S. or who had lived the longest there had higher prevalence rates of depression, affective disorders, and psychiatric disorders than those who were born in Mexico or who had lived the longest in Mexico.

Obesity and Related Diseases and Acculturation in Latina/o Hispanics

An important health concern affecting the increasing mortality rates of the Hispanic population is the upsurge of hypertension and diabetes. Despite the significance of diabetes and cardiovascular-related diseases for Latina/os, these problems are not heavily represented in current research.

The current literature findings on nutrition and acculturation appears to demonstrate a positive correlation between acculturation towards the U.S. culture and better nutrition. For example, Woodruff, Zaslow, Candelaria, and Elder (1997) showed that Hispanics who identified themselves as being highly acculturated were more likely to avoid fat, cholesterol, and high-calorie foods in their diet. Those Latina/os who fell under the less acculturated group were more likely to eat fruits, rice, beans, meat, and fried foods and to drink whole milk than more acculturated Latina/os (Otero-Sabogal, Sabogal, Perez-Stable, & Hiatt, 1995).

In addition to healthier food consumption, the highly acculturated Latina/os exhibited more knowledge about nutrition. Vega, Sallis, Patterson, Atkins, and Nader (1987) showed that Hispanic children with high parental acculturation levels have an increased awareness of health behavior knowledge and are likely to be more knowledgeable about the importance of exercise.

Given their lack of awareness about a healthy lifestyle, it should follow that less acculturated Latina/os are more obese than those in the highly acculturated group, but some of the literature on obesity appears to contradict this hypothesis (Hazuda, Haffner, Stern, & Eifler, 1988). In Hispanic males and females obesity and acculturation are inversely related. In a related study, Khan, Sobal, and Martorell (1997) found that Latinas with a greater preference for speaking English (highly acculturated group) have a reduced Body Mass Index in comparison to the less acculturated group.

Interestingly enough, Sundquist and Winkleby's (2001) findings were conflicting. They used an individual's waist circumference to monitor obesity and found that acculturation status was positively associated with waist circumference and abdominal obesity: subjects in mostly highly acculturated group had the largest waist circumference. In addition to being more obese, this study found that the highly acculturated group was more likely to suffer from non-insulin-dependent diabetes, hypertension, or high fat and cholesterol levels.

In terms of diseases, most studies found that acculturation led to higher rates of hypertension and that it was a greater predictor of hypertension than socioeconomic status (Espino & Maldonado, 1990). Markides, Lee, and Ray (1993) suggested that middle-aged Latino men in the moderate acculturated group had higher rates of hypertension than men in the less acculturated group.

The influence of acculturation and diabetes proves to be inconclusive. Stern et al. (1991) pointed out that the prevalence of type II diabetes declines with acculturation toward the values, attitudes and behaviors of American society. Other evidence suggests that greater acculturation, higher educational attainment, and higher diabetes prevalence are associated (Weller et al., 1999).

From these contradictory findings, one can see that more research is needed in this area. Because cardiovascular disease is the leading cause of mortality for Latina/os, researchers must strive to find valid conclusions regarding the effects of acculturation on heart-related diseases such as hypertension and diabetes.

In addition to more research, there is also a need for the development of better scales for acculturation. Once again, the general trend of acculturation measurements seems to be the preferred language spoken. This type of scale proves to be inefficient for measuring the full realm of acculturation. In order to obtain a full scope of the Hispanic community, more work must focus on the health and development of this growing population within the American culture.

Substance Abuse and Acculturation in Chicana/o Hispanics

There are three major areas of interest in the study of Latino acculturation and substance abuse: alcohol use, tobacco use, and use of other drugs such as marijuana and crack cocaine. Current research shows an overwhelmingly large disparity between acculturation and the practices of substance use as well as an increase of substance abuse within the Latina population.

Research links an increase in the use and abuse of alcohol with a higher degree of acculturation. A common finding suggests that acculturation is positively correlated with the frequency of alcohol consumption as well as the probability of being a drinker (Black & Markides, 1993). In a study by Cherpitel (1992), Latinos with a higher level of acculturation were more likely to have an alcohol-related injury resulting in the need for hospital emergency care.

Studies have found that highly acculturated Latinos share drinking behaviors with the non-Hispanic White subjects, who tend to have a more liberal view of alcohol and its consumption (Marin, 1996). In research done by Neff, Hoppe, and Perea

(1987), less acculturated Mexican Americans consumed alcohol less frequently but in higher quantities than Whites. This suggests that less acculturated Mexican Americans consume higher amounts of alcohol, but less habitually than the more acculturated Mexican Americans.

Motivation behind drinking also varies for the acculturated groups. In the least acculturated group, expectations of emotional and behavioral impairment as well as an increase in social extroversion were found to motivate alcohol consumption (Marin, Posner, & Kinyon, 1993). Like non-Hispanic Whites, the more highly acculturated groups were not as likely to be motivated by social extroversion or ideas of escape, which led Neff et al. (1987) to conclude that less acculturated Latina/os are at higher risk for heavy, problem drinking.

Acculturation plays a further role in the differences of alcohol-related behaviors. Results of a study done by Hines and Caetano (1998) linked excessive alcohol consumption with risky sexual behavior: Less acculturated men engage in heavy drinking and are more likely to employ risky sexual behaviors than the highly acculturated group. This study also showed that less acculturated women engaged in riskier sexual behavior even though the highly acculturated group of Hispanic women consumed more alcohol.

The influence of American cultural values affects alcohol use more for acculturated females than for males. Evidence shows that acculturated females have more drinks in their lifetime, and more acculturated males and females are more likely to binge drink in the last 30 days than the less acculturated group (Lovato, Litrownik, Elder, & Nunez-Liriano, 1994). Findings suggest that there is more open-mindedness and validation for alcohol consumption with the more acculturated group of Latinas, leading to an increase in alcohol use.

Acculturation is also influential in tobacco use. Sabogal et al. (1989) found that more acculturated Hispanics have higher levels of nicotine addiction and smoke more cigarettes and that, among the highly acculturated Hispanics, the self-efficacy to avoid smoking and lower levels of addiction show that Hispanics as a whole are more likely to quit smoking and avoid relapse compared to non-Hispanic Whites.

Gender is another determining factor for smoking. Epstein, Botvin, and Diaz (1998) showed that adolescent Hispanic females smoke more frequently than adolescent males and that acculturation is an associated factor of smoking. In addition, smoking during pregnancy, low birth weight, and preterm delivery are associated with Latinas with a moderate level of acculturation more than less acculturated women (Wolff & Portis, 1996).

It has been found that the higher the level of acculturation, the lower the level of drug use (Garcia, 1999). Wagner-Echeagaray, Schuetz, Chilcoat, and Anthony (1994) pointed out that, among Mexican Americans, the higher the degree of acculturation, the less likely the subjects were to have used crack cocaine. In the case of marijuana use, however, the results differ: Adolescents who were more acculturated smoked marijuana more frequently than those who were less acculturated (Epstein, Botvin, & Diaz, 2001).

Many of the researchers dealing with acculturation and substance abuse failed to include the tools used to measure acculturation within their reports. The scales that were included were generally described as some form of linguistic acculturation, meaning that they rated acculturation based on whether the subject was interviewed in Spanish or English or if the subject spoke Spanish to his or her parents (Epstein et al., 2001). Other researchers, such as Lessenger (1997), used the Acculturation Rating Scale for Mexican Americans-II (ARSMA-II) to study the relation between acculturation and substance abuse.

Measuring acculturation based on language falls short of truly capturing a Latina/o's adoption of American culture, especially considering the current trend of code switching, where Latina/os combine English and Spanish in their speech. Thus, new research should focus on the development of new and legitimate methods to measure acculturation so that the various levels of acculturation can be taken into consideration.

As an overall trend, research demonstrates that acculturation may have negative effects on the Latino population. The increased use of substances, both legal and illegal, in association with the increased acculturation of Latinos presents a problem. Although we know that there is an increase in substance abuse, we do not know the reason why. Is it a result of stress? Is it an attempt to belong to the predominant culture? Now that research points out a disparity between the acculturated groups of Latina/os, it needs to search for the reasons why such changes occur in the adoption of American cultural values. With these answers in hand, more effective means of promoting drug awareness and successful treatment programs can be developed to prevent Latina/os from falling victim to substance abuse.

HIV and AIDS and Acculturation in Latina/o Hispanics

The relatively high number of HIV and AIDS cases among racial minorities indicates a need for the modification and improvement of campaign prevention efforts within these groups. In response to the epidemiological trends pertaining to HIV and AIDS and Latina/os, research has focused on the effects of acculturation and HIV and AIDS, especially during the 1990s. The published work concentrates on acculturation and its effects on high-risk behaviors and knowledge about the disease. For example, Marin and Marin (1990) indicated that less acculturated Latina/os had more erroneous beliefs about "casual" transmission and were less aware that someone can be infected without being ill. In accordance with this finding, Dawson (1995) concluded that acculturation serves as a predictor of AIDS-related beliefs of moralism, blame, and perceived control over contracting AIDS. Based on these data, one would then expect to see an inverse relationship between acculturation and high-risk behavior, but the literature suggests that this is not the case. According to some researchers, higher levels of acculturation augment risk behaviors for AIDS (Peragallo, 1996; Rapkin & Erickson, 1990) as well as the likelihood of being engaged in unsafe sexual practices (Marks, Cantero, & Simoni, 1998; Rapkin & Erickson).

An important characteristic of the studies found on the MEDLINE and PsycINFO databases is that they vary widely in methodology (e.g., sample size, age and gender of the subjects, type of surveys). Although this contributes to the diversity of research on the subject, it unfortunately confounds the results. The research on HIV and AIDS focuses largely on the need to target interventions in a culturally appropriate manner, but it also strives to improve the effectiveness of campaigns aimed at lowering the incidence of HIV transmission among Latina/os. One drawback is that, outside the realm of Latina/o knowledge and popular beliefs about HIV and AIDS, present research on trends pertaining to specific behavioral practices (e.g., condom use, sharing needles) is lacking.

A significant number of these studies, however, do not follow a standard form of measurement for the acculturation variable. Most published materials see acculturation in terms of language use and language preference, thereby minimizing the effects of other cultural components (e.g., customs and beliefs) on HIV and AIDS knowledge and risk behavior. They also hinder the cross-analysis of published materials among investigators. Accordingly, researchers are encouraged to continue their efforts to better understand the effects of acculturation on HIV and AIDS and to incorporate the use of standard measures or scales of acculturation.

Acculturation and Women's Health

The most commonly researched aspect of women's health is reproductive health, particularly breast and cervical cancer. In fact, most of the research materials found using the MEDLINE and PsycINFO search engines and the words "acculturation," "Hispanic," and "cancer" retrieved information relevant to pap smear and mammogram screening practices. Investigations in this area suggest that less acculturated women, especially Spanish-speaking women, have less knowledge about pap smear examinations and fewer cervical cancer screenings (Harmon, Castro, & Coe, 1996; O'Malley, Kerner, Johnson, & Mandelblatt, 1999; Peragallo, Fox, & Alba, 2000; Suarez, 1994; Suarez & Pulley, 1995). Ruiz, Marks, & Richardson (1992) studied the effects of acculturation on exposure to health information found in reading materials, television, and radio. They suggested that understanding and preference for the English language is positively correlated with exposure to "media-based health information," which, in turn, increases the knowledge and use of cancer screening practices among Latinas.

A second important trend in Latina women's health is that women with stronger traditional Mexican attitudes toward their family have increased rates of mammogram screenings (Suarez, 1994; Suarez & Pulley, 1995). Other studies state that access to health care (i.e., health insurance) and prior screening practices are more strongly associated with reproductive health screening among Latinas than acculturative factors (Zambrana, Breen, Fox, & Gutierrez-Mohamed, 1999). These findings have important implications for planning and designing effective programs to increase the utilization of breast and cervical cancer screening among Latinas in the U.S.

Like acculturation research on HIV and AIDS, the available literature on women's health uses various types of sample groups with respect to recruitment for participation, socioeconomic and demographic variables, and sample sizes. Although most of the materials relative to women's health emphasize the utilization of cancer screening programs, there are data that focus on other aspects of women's health and, more recently, on children's health. These include acculturation research on desired family size (Marin, Marin, & Padilla, 1981), attitudes about sex-role behavior (Kranau, Green, & Valencia-Weber, 1982), beliefs about breastfeeding (Thiel de Bocanegra, 1998), beliefs about immunization (Prislin, Suarez, Simspon, & Dyer, 1998), and low-birthweight (Scribner & Dwyer, 1989). It is noteworthy that a significant number of these published studies rely on information obtained from the Hispanic Health and Nutrition Examination Survey (HHANES) for data analysis.

Unlike acculturation studies that focus on HIV and AIDS, studies on cancer screening practices among Latinas use a variety of measures for acculturation. For example, Suarez and Pulley (1995) compared two different acculturation scales, namely, an abbreviated version of Cuéllar's Acculturation Rating Scale for Mexican Americans (ARSMA) and the Hazuda scale, in order to study cancer screening practices among older Mexican American women. Another study, Suarez (1994), used five different subscales, including: English use, English proficiency, value placed on culture, traditional family attitudes, and social interaction, as measures of acculturation. Despite the increasing use of acculturation scales, however, the most common determinant for acculturation in women's health research is use of the English language. Moreover, no studies with a focus on women's health found on the MEDLINE or PsycINFO search engines used the Orthogonal Model (Oetting & Beauvais, 1991) or the "Two-dimensional Model" (Buriel, 1993) as standard measures for acculturation.

Another significant limitation of previous research is the lack of information about the screening practices for other types of cancers, such as prostate cancer in men. Although there are data available on acculturation and its effects on diet and tobacco use, there are hardly any studies that focus directly on acculturation and colon cancer or lung cancer among Latina/os. The results of these studies would provide information for health practitioners, researchers, and campaign coordinators about health belief models and cancer screening practices for the Latino population.

ISSUES IN ACCULTURATION MEASUREMENT AND RESEARCH

The number one issue in acculturation measurement is still: How does one measure culture when culture is a construct whose very definition is unclear? The answer to this question is complicated by numerous factors, including the fact that there is no such thing as a pure culture. Rather, culture is an amorphous entity, neither static nor unidimensional. Although the components of culture (food, language, music, customs, beliefs, values, behaviors, gender roles, ideologies, beliefs, practices, etc.) are not definable as concrete entities with set parameters and descriptions, there are definable differences between and among cultures and their respective components.

Culture is a complex concept, much like personality and intelligence, difficult to define yet clearly important and useful as a psychological construct. A serious problem with the acculturation construct is that it can be misused or misdefined, leading to simplistic and erroneous assumptions about it and its influences. The myths surrounding culture abound and can be very problematic (Cuéllar & Glazer, 1996; Mumford, 1981). The development of acculturation scales exemplifies the misconstruction of culture. The very first scales had items like "Who was Pedro Infante?" measuring Mexican culture, which is comparable to "Who was Louis Armstrong"? on an American intelligence test. These items relating to education and history can become outdated very easily. The item "Who was Pedro Infante?" relates to cultural heritage, but not necessarily cultural identity. Likewise, language items may assess only one component of acculturation. Like the construct of intelligence, the construct of acculturation is composed of multiple factors, in which people demonstrate varying degrees of strengths, weaknesses, capacities, and abilities. There is no single test that assesses all the components of acculturation. Cognitions, emotions, and behaviors play a role in the processes of acculturation. Acculturation, like the construct of stress, is both an exogenous and an endogenous construct, that is, its influences can be external factors or variables that include macrochanges in the world around us. Acculturation can also be an endogenous concept in that it represents learned behavior, feelings, or thought processes (internalized referents of what has transpired in our outside world, of which we are a part). The internal referents of acculturation are the same as the psychological correlates that result from acquiring aspects of the culture(s) to which one is exposed. Verbal abilities appear to be particularly important in assessing both learning and acculturation, but nonverbal behaviors can be just as important.

One of the simplest and earliest definitions of culture was one proposed by Linton (1936): "learned behavior passed on from one generation to the next." Intelligence also once had a simple definition, provided by Binet and Simon (1905): "Intelligence is our capacity to make adaptations" to our environment. Likewise, personality was described as a "variety of characteristics whose unique organization define an individual" (Domino, 2000, p. 69). Although enormously complex and difficult to define and measure, the construct of acculturation, like the constructs of intelligence and personality, continues to have considerable construct validity and can be measured both reliably and validly when operationally defined.

NEW DIRECTIONS IN ACCULTURATION

Acculturative Typologies and Psychological Functioning

There have been few studies demonstrating the validity of typologies generated from orthogonal measurement, but this should soon change. The lead author of the present chapter has been involved in an ongoing program of acculturation research that demonstrates significant psychological differences in individuals representing various acculturative typologies. Two of these studies are briefly described here.

Study 1. This study was carried out on a sample of 1,865 freshmen students in southern Texas. These young adults, 95% of whom were of Mexican origin, were administered the ARSMA-II (Scale 1) and various other tests including measures of ethnic identity, self-esteem, loneliness, stress, and depression. These subjects were categorized into four acculturative typologies using the cutting scores defined by Cuéllar, Arnold, and Maldonado (1995). Only 46.2% (n = 865) were classified based on the four-way classification schema. The numbers and percentages classified were: traditional 12.5% (n = 235), marginal 8.9% (n = 167), highly integrated bicultural 19.6% (n = 368), and assimilated 5.1% (n = 368). Stress was measured using an abbreviated and adapted version of the Hispanic Stress Inventory (Cervantes, Padilla, & Salgado de Synder, 1991). Self-esteem was measured using an eight-item version of Rosenberg's (1965, 1979) self-esteem scale. Loneliness was measured using the Roberts UCLA Loneliness Scale-8 (RULS-8, Roberts, Lewinsohn, & Seely, 1993). Depression was measured using the DSM Scale for Depression-26 (DSD-26, Cuéllar & Rob-

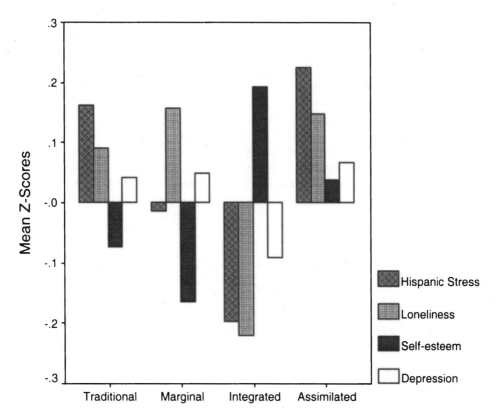

FIG. 2.1.   Study 1: Young Chicana/o Latina/o adults' acculturative types and psychological scores.

erts, 1997). The results in Fig. 2.1 show significant differences in patterns for each of the typologies based on psychological functioning. Specifically, significant differences were found for stress, $F(3, 757) = 6.09$, $p = < .0005$; loneliness, $F(3, 844) = 6.47$, $p = < .0005$; and self-esteem, $F(3, 860) = 5.298$, p = < .0005. Depression was not found to vary significantly among the groups.

The results from Study 1 show convincingly that each acculturative typology has a distinct psychological profile and mental health risk. The low acculturation or marginal acculturative typology shows the highest risk and the highly integrated bicultural typology shows the lowest risk or best psychological profile.

Study 2.   This study involved 2,686 Hispanic adolescents also from the Lower Rio Grande Valley of southern Texas along the U.S.-Mexico border. These adolescents were administered an abbreviated 12-item version of Scale 1 of the ARSMA-II, along with several measures of psychosocial functioning including ethnic identity, stress, depression, and family social support. These students were categorized into four acculturative typologies using the same cutting scores defined by Cuéllar, Arnold, and Maldonado (1995). A total of 1,651 subjects were classified, representing 61.5% of the total. Representation by typology was as follows: traditional 8.4% ($n = 226$), marginal 25.8% ($n = 694$), highly integrated bicultural 5.1% ($n = 138$), assimilated 22.1% (n = 593). Ethnic identity was measured using the Multigroup Ethnic Identity Measure (MEIM, Phinney, 1992). Self-esteem was measured by the eight-item Abbreviated Rosenberg Scale; stress was measured using a 26-item event scale assessing stressful events related to school, family, friends, and neighborhood. Depression was measured using the DSM Scale for Depression (DSD-26) and social support was measured by the Multidimensional Scale of Perceived Social Support (Zimet, Dahlem, Zimet, & Farley, 1988).

The results are shown in Fig. 2.2. Clear patterns are discernable for the various typologies by psychological functioning with the high bicultural typology showing the most favorable pattern and the marginal typology showing the highest risk pattern. The differences among the four typologies were significant for each of the four dependent measures. One-way ANOVA analyses were as follows: self-esteem, $F(3,1445)$ = 17.72, p < .0005; depression, $F(3,1245)$ = 4.37, p < .05; social support, $F(3,1009)$ = 14.264, p < .0005; ethnic identity, $F(3,1375)$ = 17.847, p < .0005; stress, $F(3,1016)$ = 3.468, p < .05.

The results from Study 2 showed that each acculturative typology appears to have a distinct profile with respect to risk for mental health and adjustment problems. However, the findings in Study 1 and Study 2 are not consistent across all dependent measures. The highly biculturals in the adolescent sample represented a much lower percentage of all typologies than at the young adult level. Yet, the highly bicultural

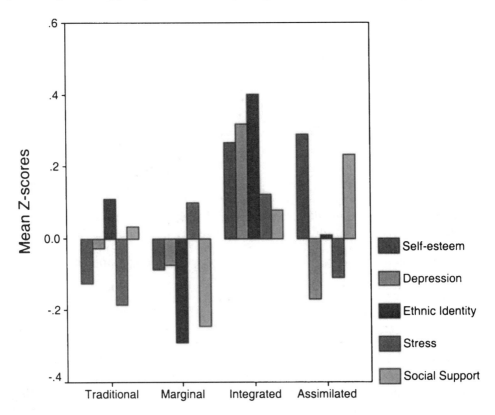

FIG. 2.2.   Chicana/o Latina/o adolescents.

typology in both studies stood out as clearly having a better overall profile than the other three typologies. Likewise, the marginal typology appeared to be at greater risk in both samples. Clearly the highly bicultural typology has the better sense of ethnic identity, but an interesting finding is that the highly bicultural group in the adolescent sample reported higher stress and depression despite having higher self-esteem and social support.

A point to consider with respect to both Study 1 and 2 is that linear correlations between acculturation and the various measures used did not reveal other than a few weak significant relations. The point is that the relations of acculturation and mental health are not always linear and the use of orthogonal measures of acculturation is needed in order to fully reveal and understand them.

Acculturation as a Moderator Variable in Clinical Practice

A growing area of interest is the use of acculturation measures to assist in developing or providing culturally appropriate and competent health and mental health care. Because not all Chicana/o Latinos are the same, they should not be stereotyped or treated in the same way. Therefore, it becomes necessary to assess the acculturation characteristics of the client in order to apply the most culturally tailored and appropriate services. Professional assessment practices in psychology mandate providing linguistically and culturally appropriate services to linguistically and culturally diverse populations. Acculturation assessment provides a means to assist in these practices, although the methodologies and approaches are still in the developmental stages. Acculturation scores can be used for assigning clinicians to match for understanding, language, culture, and sensitivity. This practice has been going on informally for years and is now becoming more widely practiced as it has some clear benefits in terms of effectiveness of and compliance with treatment.

In order to make assignments to treatment in response to culturally competent practices, acculturation assessment is justifiable and useful. The history of intellectual and personality assessment reveals a gradual increase in understanding of the influence of such variables as gender, socioeconomic status, and ethnicity on the norms, standardization, and psychometrics of psychological tests. One approach has been to eliminate items that reflect bias (differential item functioning) against a particular subgroup, another has been to develop representative standardization for normative reference groups. Other methods have developed separate normative groups using the same instrument, an emic measure of the construct being developed with a specific cultural group, or various combinations of each of these approaches. Although these approaches appear useful, they are very expensive, work intensive, and often very difficult to achieve. An alternate approach suggested by Dana (1993) is to use moderator variables to achieve these aims. Acculturation measurement is used as a gauge to assess the extent to which the person (i.e., Chicana/o) being assessed differs from the normative sample used in the development of a particular instrument (Cuéllar, 1998, 2000c). The scores on the standardized instrument are adjusted or corrected for culture according to the direction and strength of the correlation between acculturation and the psychological construct being assessed. Obviously, this "correction for culture" is an index that requires some empirical foundation in order to perform or calculate. However, this does not prevent clinicians from making a clinical judgment as to the direction and magnitude of such a correction. This clinical judgment can be justified on the basis that the null hypothesis (that there is no effect for culture) is no longer defensible.

The intent of the present chapter has been to provide a brief review of the continuing relevance of the construct of acculturation to both the field of psychology and the subspecialty of Chicana/o psychology. Chicana/o psychology has taken an important lead in the development and construction of acculturation instruments and in furthering the understanding of the role of culture and ethnicity on human development, psychological adjustment, mental health, health, and treatment. There has been an explosion in the development of measures of acculturation and ethnic identity in minorities, not just in the U.S., but throughout the world. As the U.S. and other countries experience increased globalization and cultural pluralism, the study of multicultural personality development has gained significance. Of increased concern is how multicultural environments affect human development and functioning. The field of Chicana/o psychology, through its enlightenment of acculturation processes, has played an important role in furthering understanding of cultural influences on such important areas as: appropriate utilization of services, health disparities, folk illness ideologies, appropriate assessment and treatment, stages of ethnic identity, mental health, substance abuse, manifestation of symptoms, culture-bound syndromes, gender roles, and cultural competence, among numerous others. Additionally, acculturation has important ramifications for the fields of cross-cultural, clinical, and community psychology. It is our conclusion that there is strong evidence for the continuing relevance of the construct of acculturation for both psychology and Chicana/o psychology.

REFERENCES

American Psychiatric Association. (1994). *Diagnostic and statistical manual of mental disorders* (4th ed). Washington, DC: Author.

Bernal, M. E., Knight, G. P., Ocampo, K. A., Garza, C. A., & Cota, M. K. (1993). Development of Mexican American identity. In M. E. Bernal & G. P. Knight (Eds.), *Ethnic identity: Formation and transmission among Hispanics and other minorities* (pp. 32-46). Albany: State University of New York Press.

Berry, J. (1994). Acculturative stress. In W. J. Lonner & R. Malpass (Eds.), *Psychology and culture* (pp. 211–215). Needham Heights, MA: Allyn and Bacon.

Berry, J., & Kim, U. (1988). Acculturation and mental health. In P. Dasen, J. W. Berry, & N. Sartorious (Eds.), *Health and cross-cultural psychology: Towards application* (pp. 207–236). London: Sage.

Binet, A., & Simon, T. (1905). Méthodes nouvelles pour le diagnostic du niveau intellectuel des anormaux. *L'Année Psychologique, 11*, 191–244.

Black, S. A., & Markides, K. S. (1993). Acculturation and alcohol consumption in Puerto Rican, Cuban-American, and Mexican American women in the United States. *American Journal of Public Health, 83*, 890–893.

Buriel, R. (1993). Acculturation, respect for cultural differences, and biculturalism among three generations of Mexican American and Euro American school children. *Journal of Genetic Psychology, 154*, 531–543.

Canabal, M. E., & Quiles, J. A. (1995). Acculturation and socioeconomic factors as determinants of depression among Puerto Ricans in the United States. *Social Behavior and Personality, 23*, 235–248.

Cervantes, R. C., Padilla, A. M., & Salgado de Snyder, V. M. (1991). The Hispanic Stress Inventory: A culturally relevant approach to psychosocial assessment. *Psychological Assessment, 3*, 438–447.

Cherpitel, C. J. (1992). Acculturation, alcohol consumption, and casualities among United States Hispanics in the emergency room. *International Journal of the Addictions, 27,* 1067–1077.

Clark, M., Kaufman, S., & Pierce, R. (1976). Explorations of acculturation: Toward a model of ethnic identity. *Human Organization, 35,* 231–238.

Cohen, R. (1978). Ethnicity: Problem and focus in anthropology. *Annual Review of Anthropology, 7,* 379–403.

Cross, W. (1991). *Shades of Black: Diversity in African American identity.* Philadelphia: Temple University Press.

Cuéllar, I. (1998). Cross-cultural clinical psychological assessment of Hispanic Americans. *Journal of Personality Assessment, 70,* 71–86.

Cuéllar, I. (2000a). Acculturation and mental health: Ecological transactional relations of adjustment. In I. Cuéllar & F. A. Paniagua (Eds.), *Handbook of multicultural mental health: Assessment and treatment of diverse populations* (pp. 45- 62). San Diego, CA: Academic Press.

Cuéllar, I. (2000b). Acculturation and mental health: Ecological transactional relations of adjustment. In I. Cuéllar & F. A. Paniagua (Eds.), *Multicultural mental health* (pp. 45–62). San Diego, CA: Academic Press.

Cuéllar, I. (2000c). Acculturation as a moderator of personality and psychological assessment. In R. Dana (Ed.), *Handbook of cross-cultural and multicultural personality assessment* (pp. 113–129). Mahwah, NJ: Lawrence Erlbaum Associates.

Cuéllar, I., Arnold, B., & Maldonado, R. (1995). The Acculturation Rating Scale for Mexican Americans-II: A revision of the original ARSMA scale. *Hispanic Journal of Behavioral Sciences, 17*(3), 275–304.

Cuéllar, I., & Glazer, M. (1996). The impact of culture on the family. In M. Harway (Ed.), *Treating the changing family: Handling normative and unusual events* (pp. 17–36). New York: Wiley and Sons.

Cuéllar, I., & Paniagua, F. A. (2000). *Handbook of multicultural mental health: Assessment and treatment of diverse populations.* San Diego, CA: Academic Press.

Cuéllar, I., & Roberts, R. E. (1997). Relations of depression, acculturation, and socioeconomic status in a Latino sample. *Hispanic Journal of Behavioral Sciences, 19*(2), 230–238.

Dana, R. (1993). *Multicultural assessment perspectives for professional psychology.* Boston: Allyn and Bacon.

Dawson, E. J. (1995). Acculturation as a predictor of parents' and children's attitudes and knowledge of HIV/AIDS in a multicultural population. *Sciences and Engineering, 56,* 0564.

Duran, D. G. (1995). The impact of depression, psychological factors, cultural determinants, and the patient/care-provider relationship on somatic complaints of the distressed Latina. *Dissertation Abstracts International, 56*(6A), 2428.

Engel, G. L. (1977). Need for a new medical model—Challenge for medicine. *Science, 196*(4286), 129–136.

Epstein, J. A., Botvin, G. J., & Diaz, T. (1998). Linguistic acculturation and gender effects on smoking among Hispanic youth. *Preventative Medicine: An International Journal Devoted to Practice and Theory, 27,* 683–689.

Epstein, J. A., Botvin, G. J., & Diaz, T. (2001). Linguistic acculturation associated with higher marijuana and polydrug use among Hispanic adolescents. *Substance Abuse and Misuse, 36,* 477–499.

Escobar, J. I., Hoyos-Nervi, C., & Gara, M. A. (2000). Immigration and mental health: Mexican Americans in the United States. *Harvard Review of Psychiatry, 8,* 64–72.

Escobar, J. I., Karno, M., Burnam, A., Hough, R. L., & Golding, J. (1988). Distribution of major mental disorders in an US metropolis. *ACTA Psychiatrica Scandinavica, 78*(Suppl. 344), 45–53.

Espino, D. V., & Maldonado, D. (1990). Hypertension and acculturation in elderly Mexican Americans: Results from 1982–84 Hispanic HANES. *Journal of Gerontology, 45,* 209–213.

Garcia, S. E. (1999). Substance abuse, acculturation, and alienation among Hispanic adolescents. *Dissertation Abstracts International, 60,* 3B.

Gonzalez, H. M., Haan, M. N., & Hinton, L. (2001). Acculturation and the prevalence of depression in older Mexican Americans: Baseline results of the Sacramento area Latino study on aging. *Journal of the American Geriatrics Society, 49,* 948–953.

Gowen, L. K., Hayward, C., Killien, J. D., Robinson, T. N., & Taylor, C. B. (1999). Acculturation and eating disorder symptoms in adolescent girls. *Journal of Research on Adolescence, 9,* 67–83.

Griffith, J. (1983). Relationship between acculturation and psychological impairment in adult Mexican Americans. *Hispanic Journal of Behavioral Sciences, 5,* 431–459.

Harmon, M. P., Castro, F. G., & Coe, K. (1996). Acculturation and cervical cancer knowledge, beliefs and behaviors of Hispanic women. *Women and Health, 24*(3), 37–58.

Hazuda, H. P., Haffner, S. M., Stern, M. P., & Eifler, C. W. (1998). Effects of acculturation and socioeconomic status on obesity and diabetes in Mexican Americans. *American Journal of Epidemiology, 128,* 1289–1301.

Helms, J. (1990). *Black and White racial identity: Theory, research, and practice.* New York: Oxford University Press.

Hines, A. M., & Caetano, R. (1998). Alcohol and AIDS-related behavior among Hispanics: Acculturation and gender differences. *AIDS Education and Prevention, 10,* 533–547.

Kaplan, M., & Marks, G. (1990). Adverse effects of acculturation: Psychological distress among Mexican American young adults. *Social Science and Medicine, 31,* 1313–1319.

Keefe, S. E., & Padilla, A. M. (1987). *Chicano ethnicity.* Albuquerque: University of New Mexico Press.

Khan, L. K., Sobal, J., & Martorell, R. (1997). Acculturation, socioeconomic status, and obesity in Mexican Americans, Cuban Americans, and Puerto Ricans. *International Journal of Obesity and Related Metabolic Disorders, 21*(2), 91–96.

Kleinman, A. (1988). *The illness narratives: Suffering, healing and the human condition.* New York: Basic Books.

Kluckholm, F. R., & Strodtbeck, F. L. (1961). *Variations in value orientations.* Homewood, IL: Dorsey.

Knight, G., Bernal, M., Garza, C., & Cota, M. K. (1993). A social cognitive model of ethnic identity and ethnically based behaviors. In M. E. Bernal & G. P. Knight (Eds.), *Ethnic identity: Formation and transmission among Hispanics and other minorities* (pp. 213-234). Albany: State University of New York Press.

Kranau, E. J., Green, V., & Valencia-Weber, G. (1982). Acculturation and the Hispanic woman: Attitudes toward women, sex-role attribution, sex-role behavior, and demographics. *Hispanic Journal of Behavioral Sciences, 4,* 21–40.

Lessenger, L. H. (1997). Use of Acculturation Rating Scale for Mexican Americans II with substance abuse patients. *Hispanic Journal of Behavioral Sciences, 19,* 387–398.

Levinson, D. J., & Huffman, P. E. (1955). Traditional Family Ideology Scale. *Journal of Personality, 23,* 251–273.

Linton, R. (1936). *The study of man.* New York: Appleton-Century.

Lovato, C. Y., Litrownik, A. J., Elder, J., & Nunez-Liriano, A. (1994). Cigarette and alcohol use among migrant Hispanic adolescents. *Family and Community Health, 16*(4), 18–31.

Marin, B. V., & Marin, G. (1990). Effects of acculturation on knowledge of AIDS and HIV among Hispanics. *Hispanic Journal of Behavioral Sciences, 12,* 110–121.

Marin, B. V., Marin, G., & Padilla, A. M. (1981). Attitudes and practices of low-income Hispanic contraceptors. *Spanish Speaking Mental Health Research Center Occasional Papers, 13,* 20.

Marin, G. (1996). Expectancies for drinking and excessive drinking among Mexican Americans and non-Hispanic Whites. *Addictive Behaviors, 21,* 491–507.

Marin, G., Posner, S. F., & Kinyon, J. B. (1993). Alcohol expectancies among Hispanics and non-Hispanic Whites: Role of drinking status and acculturation. *Hispanic Journal of Behavioral Sciences, 15,* 373–381.

Markides, K. S., Lee, D. J., & Ray, L. A. (1993). Acculturation and hypertension in Mexican Americans. *Ethnicity and Disease, 3,* 70–77.

Marks, G., Cantero, P. J., & Simoni, J. M. (1998). Is acculturation associated with sexual risk behaviors? An investigation of HIV-positive Latino men and women. *AIDS Care, 10,* 283–295.

McFee, M. (1968). The 150% man: A product of Blackfeet acculturation. *American Anthropologist, 70,* 1096–1103.

McGee, W. J. (1898). Piratical acculturation. *American Anthropologist, 11,* 243–249.

Mead, M. (1932). *The changing culture of an Indian tribe.* New York: Columbia University Press.

Miranda, A. O. (1995). Adlerian life styles and acculturation as predictors of the mental health in Hispanic adults. *Dissertation Abstracts International, 55,* 10A.

Miranda, A. O., & Umhoefer, D. L. (1998). Depression and social interest differences between Latinos in dissimilar acculturation stages. *Journal of Mental Health Counseling, 20,* 159–171.

Mumford, E. (1981). Culture: Life perspectives and the social meaning of illness. In R. C. Simon & H. Pardes (Eds.), *Understanding human behavior in health and illness* (pp. 271–280). Baltimore: Williams and Wilkins.

National Institute of Mental Health. (1995). *Basic behavioral science research for mental health: A report of the National Advisory Mental Health Council* (NIH Publication No. 95-3682). Washington, DC: U.S. Government Printing Office.

Neff, J. A., Hoppe, S. K., & Perea, P. (1987). Acculturation and alcohol use: Drinking patterns and problems among Anglo and Mexican American male drinkers. *Hispanic Journal of Behavioral Sciences, 9,* 151–181.

Negy, C., & Woods, D. J. (1992a). Mexican Americans' performance on the Psychological Screening Inventory as a function of acculturation level. *Journal of Clinical Psychology, 48,* 315–319.

Negy, C., & Woods, D. J. (1992b). The importance of acculturation in understanding research with Hispanic-Americans. *Hispanic Journal of Behavioral Sciences, 149*(2), 224–247.

Oetting, E. R., & Beauvais, F. (1991). Orthogonal cultural identification theory: The cultural identification of minority adolescents. *International Journal of the Addictions, 25,* 655–685.

Olmedo, E. L. (1979). Acculturation: A psychometric perspective. *American Psychologist, 34,* 1061–1070.

Olmedo, E. L., Martinez, J. L., & Martinez, S. R. (1978). Measure of acculturation for Chicano adolescents. *Psychological Reports, 42,* 159–170.

Olmedo, E. L., & Padilla, A. (1978). Empirical and construct validation of a measure of acculturation for Mexican Americans. *Journal of Social Psychology, 105,* 179–187.

O'Malley, A. S., Kerner, J., Johnson, A. E., & Mandelblatt, J. (1999). Acculturation and breast cancer screening among Hispanic women in New York City. *American Journal of Public Health, 89,* 219–227.

Otero-Sabogal, R., Sabogal, F., Perez-Stable, E. J., & Hiatt, R. A. (1995). Dietary practices, alcohol consumption, and smoking behavior: Ethnic, sex, and acculturation differences. *Journal of National Cancer Institute Monographs, 18,* 73–82.

Padilla, A. M. (1980). The role of cultural awareness and ethnic loyalty in acculturation. In A. M. Padilla (Ed.), *Acculturation: Theory, models and some new findings* (pp. 47–84). Boulder, CO: Westview.

Peragallo, N. (1996). Latino women and AIDS risk. *Public Health Nursing, 13,* 217–222.

Peragallo, N. P., Fox, P. G., & Alba, M. L. (2000). Acculturation and breast self-examination among immigrant Latina women in the USA. *International Nursing Review, 47,* 38–45.

Phinney, J. S. (1989). Stages of ethnic identity development in minority group adolescents. *Journal of Early Adolescence, 9,* 34–49.

Phinney, J. S. (1992). The Multigroup Ethnic Identity Measure: A new scale for use with diverse groups. *Journal of Adolescent Research, 7,* 156–176.

Pierce, R. C., Clark, M. M., & Kiefer, C. W. (1972). A "Bootstrap" Scaling Technique. *Human Organization, 31,* 403–410.

Prislin, R., Suarez, L., Simspon, D. M., & Dyer, J.A. (1998). When acculturation hurts: The case of immunization. *Social Science and Medicine, 47,* 1947–1956.

Rapkin, A. J., & Erickson, P. I. (1990). Differences in knowledge of and risk factors for AIDS between Hispanic and non-Hispanic women attending an urban family planning clinic. *AIDS, 4,* 889–899.

Redfield, R., Linton, R., & Herskovitz, M. J. (1936). Memorandum for the study of acculturation: Committee report to the Social Science Council. *American Anthropologist, 38,* 149–152.

Roberts, R. E., Lewinsohn, P. M., & Seely, J. R. (1993). A brief measure of loneliness suitable for use with adolescents. *Psychological Reports, 72,* 1379–1391.

Rogler, L. H., Cortes, D. E., & Malgady, R. G. (1991). Acculturation and mental health status among Hispanics. *American Psychologist, 46,* 585–597.

Rosenberg, M. (1965). *Society and the adolescent self-image.* Princeton: Princeton University Press.

Rosenberg, M. (1979). *Conceiving the self.* New York: Basic Books.

Roysircar-Sodowsky, G., & Maestas, M. V. (2000). Acculturation, ethnic identity, and acculturative stress: Evidence and measurement. In R. Dana (Ed.), *Handbook of cross-cultural and multicultural personality assessment* (pp. 131–172). Mahwah, NJ: Lawrence Erlbaum Associates.

Ruiz, M. S., Marks, G., & Richardson, J. L. (1992). Language acculturation and screening practices of elderly Hispanic women: The role of exposure to health-related information from the media. *Journal of Aging and Health, 4,* 268–281.

Ruiz, R. A., Casas, J. M., & Padilla, A. M. (1977). *Culturally relevant behavioristic counseling* (Occasional Paper No. 5). Los Angeles Spanish Speaking Mental Health Research Center, University of California, Los Angeles.

Sabogal, F., Otero-Sabogal, R., Perez-Stable, E. J., Marin, B. V., & Marin, G. (1989). Perceived self-efficacy to avoid cigarette smoking and addiction: Differences between Hispanics and non-Hispanic Whites. *Hispanic Journal of Behavioral Sciences, 11,* 136–147.

Scribner, R., & Dwyer, J. H. (1989). Acculturation and low birthweight among Latinos in the Hispanic HANES. *American Journal of Public Health, 79,* 1263–1267.

Stern, M. P., Knapp, J. A., Hazuda, H. P., Haffner, S. M., Patterson, J. K., & Mitchell, B. D. (1991). Genetic and environmental determinants of type II diabetes in Mexican Americans: Is there a descending limb to the modernization/diabetes relationship? *Diabetes Care, 14,* 649–654.

Stonequist, E. V. (1935). The problem of the marginal man. *American Journal of Sociology, 41,* 1–12.

Stonequist, E. V. (1937). *The marginal man: A study in personality and culture conflict.* New York: Russell and Russell.

Suarez, L. (1994). Pap smear and mammogram screening in Mexican American women: The effects of acculturation. *American Journal of Public Health, 84,* 742–746.

Suarez, L., & Pulley, L. (1995). Comparing acculturation scales and their relationship to cancer screening among older Mexican American women. *Journal of the National Cancer Institute Monographs, 18,* 41–47.

Suarez-Orozco, M. M. (1997). The cultural psychology of immigration. In A. Ugalde & G. Cardenas (Eds.), *Health and social services among international labor migrants* (pp. 131–149). Austin, TX: The Center for Mexican American Studies.

Sundquist, J., & Winkleby, M. (2001). Country of birth, acculturation status and abdominal obesity in a national sample of Mexican American women and men. *International Journal of Epidemiology, 29,* 470–477.

Thiel de Bocanegra, H. (1998). Breast-feeding in immigrant women: The role of social support and acculturation. *Hispanic Journal of Behavioral Sciences, 20,* 448–467.

Vega, W. A., Kolody, B., Aguilar-Gaxiola, S., Alderete, E., Catalano, R., & Caraveo-Anduaga, J. (1998). Lifetime prevalence of DSD-III-R psychiatric disorders among urban and rural Mexicans. *Archives of General Psychiatry, 55*(9), 771–778.

Vega, W. A., Sallis, J. F., Patterson, T., Atkins, C., & Nader, P. R. (1987). Assessing knowledge of cardiovascular health-related diet and exercise behaviors in Anglo- and Mexican Americans. *Preventive Medicine, 16*(5), 696–709.

Wagner-Echeagaray, F. A., Schuetz, C. G., Chilcoat, H. D., & Anthony, J. C. (1994). Degree of acculturation and the risk of crack cocaine smoking among Hispanic Americans. *American Journal of Public Health, 84*(11), 1825–1827.

Weller, S. C., Baer, R. D., Pachter, L. M., Trotter, R. T., Glazer, M., Garcia, J. E., & Klein, R. E. (1999). Latino beliefs about diabetes. *Diabetes Care, 22,* 722–728.

Wolff, C. B., & Portis, M. (1996). Smoking acculturation and pregnancy outcome among Mexican Americans. *Health Care for Women International, 17,* 563–574.

Woodruff, S. I., Zaslow, K. A., Candelaria, J., & Elder, J. P. (1997). Effects of gender and acculturation on nutrition-related factors among limited-English proficient Hispanic adults. *Ethnicity and Disease, 7,* 121–126.

Zamarian, K., Thackrey, M., Starrett, R. A., Brown, L. G., Lassman, D., & Blanchart, A. (1992). Acculturation and depression in Mexican American elderly. *Clinical Gerontologist, 11,* 109–121.

Zambrana, R. E., Breen, N., Fox, S. A., & Gutierrez-Mohamed, M. L. (1999). Use of cancer screening practices by Hispanic women: Analyses by subgroup. *Preventive Medicine, 29,* 466–477.

Zimet, G. D., Dahlem, N. W., Zimet, S. G., & Farley, G. K. (1988). The Multidimensional Scale of Perceived Social Support. *Journal of Personality Assessment, 52,* 30–41.

Ethnic Identity Development in Chicana/o Youth

Elizabeth M. Vera
Loyola University, Chicago

Stephen M. Quintana
University of Wisconsin, Madison

Children's racial and ethnic cognitions have been investigated for more than half a century. Such research has been linked to the study of ethnic prejudice and discrimination in children (Aboud, 1988; Allport, 1954; Clark & Clark, 1940; Katz, 1978; Quintana & Vera, 1999; Ramsey, 1987) and has influenced public policy on interracial relations (e.g., *Brown v. Board of Education*, 1954). Ethnic identity for Chicana/o children, as well as for other ethnic minority children, is believed to be particularly important not only in the development of identity in general, but also as a self-protective strategy for coping with prejudice, discrimination, and stigmatization (Crocker & Major, 1989; Cross, 1995; Parham & Helms, 1985). In the present chapter, components of ethnic identity development are defined and described and contextual influences related to ethnic identity developmental processes are presented. In addition, implications for practice and research are suggested.

It is important to understand ethnic identity in the broader context of identity development. Ethnic identity is part of the more complex construct of social identity. Tajfel (1974) defined social identity as a contextual understanding of the self based on the social realms in which one interacts. Contexts that influence social identity include cultural (i.e., race, ethnicity, and gender), familial, occupational, and peer contexts. Thus, social identity is a multifaceted perspective of the self that influences the way individuals explain and make sense of their lives. Social identity theory provides a framework for understanding how group membership influences interpersonal relations with members of one's own group and other groups (Bernal, Saenz, & Knight, 1991). Understanding the social identity and world view of clients is critical to the work of psychologists. Because childhood and adolescence in particular are life stages in which identity is very much a work in progress, working effectively with Chicana/o youth requires a grounding in the literature that has explored these issues.

DEFINITIONS OF ETHNIC IDENTITY

Ethnic identity is an important part of one's self-identity that differentiates members of one ethnic group from another (Bernal, Knight, Garza, Ocampo, & Cota, 1990). In addition to the formation of the self-concept, ethnic identity is also thought to be influential in the development of values, attitudes, and behaviors. Ethnic identity development begins in childhood and serves as the mechanism by which children attain an understanding of themselves as members of their ethnic group (e.g., Chicana/os). Hence, ethnic identity development is dynamic and involves a number of phases and requisite social-cognitive abilities.

COMPONENTS OF CHICANA/O ETHNIC IDENTITY

Leading scholars have identified a number of key components involved in ethnic identity development in children (Aboud, 1987; Bernal et al., 1990; Rotheram & Phinney, 1987). We discuss these components separately, although they are obviously interrelated.

Self-Identification

Perhaps the most simple form of ethnic identity involves self-identification or self-categorization into an ethnic group. Although rudimentary, the process of identifying oneself as a member of a social group has critical implications for the formation of social or ethnic groups (Tajfel, 1974). Identification with a social group tends to produce a psychological or social connection to other group members. From this identification process, members of a social group may show preferences toward others of the same social group. These processes are not specific to Chicana/os or even ethnic groups, but probably stem from universal human needs to affiliate with one or more human groups (Allport, 1954).

   The self-identification process for Chicana/o children is complex. Although most children begin to self-identify membership in a racial group relatively early in life (i.e., around 3 to 4 years of age), the identification into an ethnic group occurs later in childhood (i.e., around 5 to 7 years of age; Bernal, Knight, Ocampo, Garza, & Cota, 1993). Quintana (1994) found that some Mexican American children aged 7 and 8 were not able to identify their ethnic group membership. Self-identification of ethnicity is further complicated for young Chicana/o children because they may first self-identify racially as White and then later, in order to self-identify ethnically, they must differentiate their racial status (White) from their ethnicity (Chicana/o). Quintana found that many second graders identified both as White and Mexican American because, in the words of one child, they were not "Black." In preschool and early elementary school, many children may not have ethnic constancy, which is the understanding that ethnic status remains constant despite superficial changes (e.g., changes in appearance, clothing, or skin color). Indeed, one reason that children are believed to self-identify racially before self-identifying according to ethnicity is that most of the racial terms commonly used in the U.S. also have chromatic connotations (e.g., White or Black; Hirschfeld, 1994). There is some debate over when children use racial terms that also have chromatic connotations if they are using the terms to refer to race or to color. Quintana reasoned that, during middle elementary school, children understood nonchromatic racial and ethnic terms when the terms were reflective of literal or descriptive features of ethnicity, such as marking heritage (e.g., Mexican American or African American). Hence, existing research suggests that the developmental sequencing of children's understanding of racial and ethnic terms is based on ontologic complexity. Racial terms that are also chromatic are learned before ethnic terms that refer to less obvious features, but are still understandable to children (e.g., reference to family heritage). Following this logic, it would seem that children's understanding of the political connotations underlying the term *Chicana* or *Chicano* would occur developmentally later because understanding the political connotations is ontologically more complex.

Most of the research on Mexican American children has not focused on the development of a Chicana/o identification per se, but on self-identification of Hispanic or Mexican American labels (e.g., Bernal et al., 1993; Quintana, 1994). The ethnic term that young children first identify with may reveal the context in which they have learned it. For example, young children in the Quintana study who self-identified as Hispanic indicated that they had learned about the term at school, whereas those who self-identified as Mexican American reported learning about it from their families. Clearly, the nascent uses of an ethnic label result from how others have taught or socialized the children to label themselves. As children develop, they may be exposed to various alternatives for their self-identification and thereby have the opportunity to choose among various options for self-identification labels, such as *Chicana/o*, based on what suits them best (Matute-Bianchi, 1986). Because there are some regional differences, some children or youth may never self-identify as Chicana/os, particularly in Texas and parts of New Mexico where the term *Chicana/o* is used infrequently, even among adults.

Phenotypical Features.   Because of the mixed genetic ancestry of Chicana/o populations (Spanish, North African, Indigenous peoples of North America, etc.), there is wide variation in the expression of genetic ancestry among Chicana/os and other Latina/os. The phenotypical features that young Chicana/o children associate with their ethnic ancestry include skin, hair, and eye colorations, features that young children associate with their ethnic group status. Because some phenotypical characteristics of Chicana/os (e.g., skin complexion, eye and hair color) may be similar to those of other groups (e.g., Middle Eastern populations), young Chicana/o children may not be able to differentiate their ethnic group from others. Some adults from other ethnic groups may also confuse Chicana/o children with other groups of similar complexion and coloration. In the U.S., given that White and Black seem to define two opposite ends of a racial spectrum, all ethnic groups with Brown complexions and coloration may be lumped together somewhere in the middle.

As Chicana/o children mature, they develop a more differentiated understanding of the physical features associated with ethnicity and they may make fewer mistakes in classifying according to ethnicity. However, children's increased differentiation according to physical manifestations of race and ethnicity may contribute to their drawing distinctions within the Chicana/o ethnic group. Later in adolescence, for example, there may be some questioning of the ethnic authenticity of those who have light complexions. Moreover, the degree of discrimination that Chicana/os experience may depend in part on their phenotypical features, with those appearing more Caucasian probably experiencing discrimination less often from strangers and acquaintances than those appearing more indigenous. We discuss additional literature on this topic later in the chapter.

Cultural Heritage and Primary Cultural Characteristics.   A third component of ethnic identity for Chicana/os is their cultural heritage. The terms *Chicana* and *Chicano* first appeared among Mexican Americans who were not born in Mexico, but tended to be second- or third-generation Americans. Cultural ancestry comes with associated cultural behaviors, preferences, and values (Bernal et al., 1993). The root of many cultural features of Chicana/os can be traced to Mexico and Mexican traditions. Ogbu (1994) characterized primary cultural characteristics for minority groups to refer to those features that can be traced to the minority group's cultural or national origin. For Chicana/os and Mexican Americans, the primary cultural characteristics include food preferences, Mexican and religious (mostly Catholic-based) celebrations, and customs (Bernal et al.). Probably the most critical feature of cultural traditions are language patterns and preferences. Although most first- and many second-generation Mexican Americans may be Spanish language dominant or bilingual, English is likely to be dominant among those of third and later generations (Keefe & Padilla, 1987). Additionally, knowledge of Mexican history and the history of Mexican Americans and Chicana/os in the U.S. are significant cultural features.

There are also important social norms guiding role behavior within families and between family members and non-family members. Showing signs of respect to parents, sharing resources among immediate and extended family members, and acting in a way that maintains personal as well as family dignity are all role expectations for members of Chicano and Mexican American families (Bernal et al., 1993). There are also some traditional gender role socializations that includes different expectations for boys and men versus girls and women, although the tendency to adhere to gender role expectations varies for males and females, with males adhering at higher rates than females (Ocampo, Bernal, & Knight, 1993). The extent to which Chicana/os have maintained primary cultural features that originated in Mexico can be associated with their ethnic identity.

Secondary Cultural Characteristics.   Not all of the cultural characteristics of Chicanos can be traced to Mexico and Mexican traditions. According to Ogbu (1994), secondary cultural features are those characteristics of a minority group that have evolved in response to contact with a dominant or majority group. The use of the terms *Chicana* and *Chicano* in part reflects a response to the discrimination Mexican Americans experienced from Anglos. These terms involve the conversion of a stereotype into a mark of pride. Historically, Chicana/os formed gangs in the early 1900s as a way to protect themselves from U.S. servicemen who sometimes, for entertainment, cruised streets in Los Angeles to fight with Chicanos (Martinez, 1991). In this case, affiliation among urban Chicana/o youth was, in part, a response to the alienation experienced because of stigmatization. Values and attitudes (or behaviors) that develop as a result of oppressive experiences (e.g., opposition to English-only legislation) are considered to be secondary cultural characteristics.

Probably the most critical secondary cultural characteristic for Chicana/os is the recognition of prejudice and discrimination from mostly Anglos. Elementary school-aged Mexican American children recognize that they are the targets of discrimination from parents, teachers, police, and government officials (Quintana & Vera, 1999). Developing resilience against ethnic bias and discrimination can be a source of ethnic pride for Chicana/os. The achievement of success in the classroom, in business, in politics and in other arenas despite discrimination inspires other Chicana/os and remains an important feature of Chicana/os' ethnic identity and pride.

Intra-Ethnic Attitudes and Interactions.   An important feature of Chicana/o ethnic identity is their relations with and attitudes toward other Chicana/os. For young Chicana/os, this may be related to perceptions of similarity to other Chicana/os as well as preference to interact with Chicana/os (Bernal et al., 1993). In adolescence, intra-ethnic attitudes are associated with ethnic pride, a sense of acceptance and belonging (Phinney, 1992), and a sense of psychological, social, and ideological identification with Chicana/os as an ethnic group. Youth develop an ethnic group consciousness, which was described in a seminal manuscript by Arce (1981) and more recently by Quintana (1994). Arce (1981, p. 184) described three features of ethnic group consciousness:

> (a) questioning the legitimacy of the superordinate group [Anglos] to define the status of one's subordinated group [Chicana/os], (b) shifting the locus of responsibility for the group's oppressed position and status from blame of one's group to blame of the outgroup's prejudiced attitudes, and (c) changing the meaning of stereotypes attributed to one's group from negative to positive.

Quintana (1994) characterized an ethnic group consciousness as an awareness of the interconnectedness of members with the larger ethnic group such that the behavior of one member reflects on the entire group and that interethnic interactions (e.g., discrimination) involving one member are considered to have involved the entire ethnic group. Ethnic group consciousness is a critical feature of Chicana/os' ethnic identity.

Integrated Ethnic Identity.   Ethnic identity for Chicana/os involves an integration of all the previously described features: self-identification, phenotypical characteristics, primary and secondary cultural characteristics, interethnic and intra-ethnic relations and attitudes, and an ethnic group consciousness. Each of these factors contributes to Chicana/os' expression and psychological experience of ethnicity. The relative salience of any one of these features is likely to be determined by many contextual factors and the specific nature of each of is also determined by two broad factors that influence ethnic identity development for Chicana/os: social cognitive maturation and ethnic socialization.

Social Cognitive Maturation.   Research and theory with White and African American children has shown that cognitive maturation plays a critical role in the development of ethnic and racial identity (Aboud, 1987; Alejandro-Wright, 1985; Doyle, Beadet, & Aboud, 1988); Spencer, 1983. Research on Mexican American children has similarly shown that the development of ethnic cognition plays an important role in the development of ethnic identity (Bernal et al., 1993; Quintana, 1994; Quintana, Ybarra, Gonzalez-Doupe, & de Baessa, 2000). Bernal et al. developed a model of ethnic identity for Mexican American and Chicana/o children during early childhood, identifying five features of young children's ethnic identity that develop during the early elementary school level: ethnic self-identification, ethnic constancy, ethnic role behaviors, ethnic knowledge, and ethnic feelings and preferences. Ethnic self-identification and constancy refer to young Chicana/o children's ability to accurately identify membership in their ethnic group and their understanding that ethnic status remains constant across contexts or superficial transformations (e.g., altering one's hair color or skin tone), respectively. Ethnic role behaviors refer to children's engagement in ethnic-related behaviors (e.g., celebration of Mexican holidays and customs), including the understanding that these behaviors reflect their ethnic status. Ethnic knowledge refers to children's ability to differentiate ethnic practices, values, and activities according to ethnic group, for example, understanding which customs are more common for Mexicans than for Anglos. Finally, ethnic feelings and preferences refer to children's preferences and affective orientation toward their own ethnic group (e.g., preferring Chicana/o friends over non-Chicana/os).

Bernal et al. (1993) provided support for this model through the creative and innovative operationalization of each of these dimensions of ethnic identity. Building on this work, Knight, Bernal, Cota, Garza, and Ocampo (1993) found further support for strong relationships between parental socialization and ethnic teachings and each of these ethnic identity dimensions. In particular, families who retained their Mexican traditions and orientation were associated with children who had advanced levels of ethnic identity development. Bernal et al. also found strong correlations between chronological age and most components of ethnic identity, confirming the developmental nature of children's ethnic identity.

Extending Bernal et al.'s (1993) seminal work on ethnic identity, Quintana (1994) proposed a developmental model for Mexican American children's understanding of their ethnicity. Quintana's model extended Bernal et al.'s work through childhood and into adolescence. Specifically, he identified five levels of ethnic perspective-taking ability, which is essentially the reasoning or logic that children and adolescents use to construe their ethnic identification and interethnic and intra-ethnic relations (see Table 3.1). He found that, during preschool and into early elementary school, young Mexican American children defined their ethnicity based on superficial physical (e.g., skin, eye, and hair color) and prominent observable (e.g., language usage) features. Later in early childhood, children acquired an understanding of the literal features associated with ethnicity that include the five dimensions of ethnic identity identified by Bernal et al. During late elementary school, children assumed a social perspective on ethnicity, understanding some of the social dynamics of interethnic and intra-ethnic relations, including ethnic preferences as well as ethnic prejudice. In adolescence, youth develop an ethnic group consciousness from which they can explore and commit to particular features of a Chicana/o or Mexican American identity. Finally, in late adolescence and early adulthood, Chicana/os develop an

TABLE 3.1
Quintana's Model of Ethnic Perspective-Taking Ability

Level	Sublevel
0: Physicalistic and observable perspective	0a: Idiosyncratic terminology used for race, awareness of race, but not of nonobservable characteristics of ethnicity 0b: Increased accuracy in classifying races and ethnicities based on observable features
1: Literal perspective of ethnicity	1a: Beginning understanding of some of the relatively permanent, nonobservable aspects of ethnicity (e.g., language spoken, food preferences) 1b: Conception of the heritage or ancestry components of ethnicity; at both sublevels of 1, understanding of ethnicity remains fixed on nonsocial, somewhat abstract aspects of ethnicity directly connected to Mexico (e.g., Mexican food)
2: Nonliteral and social perspective of ethnicity	2a: Awareness of subtle aspects of ethnicity associated with ethnicity not directly tied to Mexico (e.g., social class issues) 2b: Integration of everyday social experiences related to ethnicity and awareness of ethnic prejudice
3: Group perspective of ethnicity	3a: Awareness of the impact of pervasive experiential influences associated with ethnicity 3b: Ethnic group consciousness
4: Multicultural perspective of ethnicity	4a: Diversity within ethnic groups and similarities across ethnic groups appreciated and integrated 4b: Awareness of diverse sociocultural influences on self and identity

Note. Copyright 1993 by Stephen M. Quintana. Reprinted with permission.

ethnic identity that integrates the variety of cultural experiences of their lives. The development of ethnic perspective-taking ability has been found to be predictive of specific ethnic cognition (i.e., Bernal et al.'s measure of ethnic knowledge) and scores on Phinney's (1992) measure of ethnic identity, as well as predicted by the children and youth's exposure to ethnic socialization (Quintana, Castañeda-English, & Ybarra, 1999; Quintana et al., 2000).

Ethnic Socialization

Children's families, peer groups, schools, and communities all influence the type and quantity of information and experiences relevant to the development of ethnic identity. Such socialization experiences have been the topic of research investigating enculturation, acculturation, and assimilation processes.

According to Knight, Bernal, Garza, Cota, and Ocampo (1993), enculturation is a process through which children learn they have specific, distinctive ethnic group membership, ethnic group behaviors (e.g., rituals, celebrations of holidays), and ethnic preferences (e.g., music, food, friends). In contrast, acculturation is the process by which Chicanas/os learn or adopt characteristics (e.g., behaviors, preferences) and practices from the mainstream culture. Examples of acculturation are when individuals become English dominant (or monolingual) or when mainstream rituals or behaviors are preferred over traditional Mexican and Chicana/o cultural practices (e.g., having a Sweet Sixteen party instead of the more traditional Quinceñera). Enculturation and acculturation dynamics influence the ethnic socialization of children and can result in the development of various ethnic identity statuses, such as assimilation, separation, integration (biculturalism), and marginalization.

Assimilation is often understood as the result of complete immersion in mainstream culture, whereby individuals lose all traces of their ethnic heritage and become indistinguishable from the dominant group (Keefe & Padilla, 1987). However, it does not follow that the outside world or society sees the individual as indistinguishable from the majority. Social assimilation, which can be defined as social, political, and economic equality or integration, has not occurred for Chicana/os and other racial and ethnic minorities (Pizarro & Vera, 2001), regardless of how much assimilation may have occurred at a personal level. However, individuals who were raised in communities (or families) where ethnic practices or behaviors were overtly or covertly shamed (e.g., being punished for speaking Spanish at school) would likely have been more strongly influenced by the pressure to assimilate toward the mainstream or pass for an Anglo. Separation is another ethnic identity status that is characterized by a rejection of the mainstream culture and complete immersion in one's ethnic culture. Integration, or biculturalism, occurs when an individual feels comfortable participating in mainstream culture while maintaining a positive commitment to his or her ethnic culture. Finally, marginalization occurs when one rejects both the mainstream and one's ethnic culture, resulting in a lack of identity commitment.

Although ethnic identity development is influenced by the aforementioned processes (i.e., enculturation, acculturation, and assimilation pressures), it is often within the family system that children experience their primary ethnic socialization. Therefore, factors such as parental level of acculturation and parental ethnic socialization efforts (Bernal et al., 1991; Phinney & Chavira, 1995; Quintana & Vera, 1999) are critical influences on children's ethnic identity formation. In the Quintana and Vera study, for example, parental level of acculturation was related to children's acquisition of ethnic behaviors. Thus, ethnic identity development, especially for children and adolescents, is heavily influenced by social and familial contexts that determine the level of enculturation and acculturation to which an individual is exposed.

It has been difficult to reach a consensus on the nature of the relationships between acculturation, enculturation, assimilation processes, and ethnic identity development in Chicana/os. Although some evidence exists that greater enculturation leads to higher ethnic knowledge or practice of ethnic behaviors (Bernal et al., 1991; Phinney & Chavira, 1995; Quintana & Vera, 1999), other research has shown that strong, positive ethnic identities are achieved in individuals who are highly acculturated (Cuéllar, Nyberg, Maldonado, & Roberts, 1997; Félix-Ortiz, Newcomb, & Myers, 1994; Keefe & Padilla, 1987). Thus, the relationships between acculturation, enculturation, and components of ethnic identity development do not seem to be linear and are in need of further empirical attention.

Racial Influences on Ethnic Identity Development

The complexity of Chicana/o ethnic identity is heightened by a consideration of racial identity issues. Racial identity refers to one's self-identification as a member of a racial group or groups (Helms, 1990). Though very little research has been done on the influence of race on Chicana/o social identity development, racial issues would seem to be inextricably related to ethnic identity, as is the case for other ethnic groups (Pizarro & Vera, 2001). Despite the fact that Chicanas/os are mixed-race individuals because of the history of the colonization of Mexico, they are classified as "White" within the legal system of the U.S. However, the early history of the U.S. demonstrates that Chicanas/os were not treated like Anglos in the southwest (DeLeon, 1983). This confusion regarding the racial status of Chicana/os, and the tendency for race and ethnicity to be confounded in psychological literature, has intimately connected the concepts of race and ethnicity for Chicanas/os.

Because Chicanas/os are a mix of indigenous and European peoples, their physical appearances vary. Those who are darker skinned and appear more phenotypically indigenous are likely to experience a different type of discrimination from Chicana/os who are lighter skinned, with more European features. It stands to reason that physical appearance is a part of one's self-concept and therefore affects one's ethnic and racial identity. It is important to mention that lighter skinned Chicana/os are not necessarily better off or protected from the within-group discrimination that occurs due to language usage and accents. More European-looking Chicana/os are sometimes accused of not "looking Mexican," whereas darker skinned Chicana/os are sometimes pejoratively called "indios" as a sign of disrespect. Issues of race within the Chicana/o community are undoubtedly complex and need further exploration by identity development researchers.

The limited research that has investigated racial differences among Chicanas/os has looked at the impact of racism on quality-of-life issues. For example, Relethford, Stern, Gaskill, and Hazuda (1983) found that skin color became progressively lighter along a continuum from lower to higher socioeconomic status in their Latina/o sample, which included Chicana/os. Arce, Murgia, and Frisbie (1987) also examined phenotypical differences among Chicana/os and found a correlation between darker skin tone, lower income level, and lower education level. The limited evidence that does exist would suggest that Chicana/os may indeed experience dual processes of ethnic and racial identity development and that racism has differential effects on individuals within the Chicano community. Studies that explore racial identity development among Chicana/os are sorely needed, especially given the multiracial nature of Chicana/os (Helms, 1990; Pizarro & Vera, 2001).

Models of Ethnic Identity Development in Chicana/o Children

During the 1990s, Martha Bernal, George Knight, and their colleagues made dramatic advances in the conceptualization and analysis of Chicana/o ethnic identity development. They attempted to explain the multiple processes that influence ethnic identity development in Chicana/o youth (Bernal et al., 1990), attending to multiple components of ethnic identity development and important contexts (family, community) that affect these processes in youth. Bernal et al. provided a model for operationalizing Chicana/o ethnic identity development that included the following dimensions: ethnic self-identification, ethnic constancy, use of ethnic role behaviors, ethnic knowledge, and ethnic preferences and feelings. Through interviews with young children that assessed each of these dimensions, Bernal et al. were able to uncover the earliest indications of Chicana/o ethnic identity development. They found that preschoolers have little understanding of their ethnic identity whereas older children begin to develop one. Specifically, ethnic awareness and identification occurred between the ages of 7 and 10 but ethnic constancy occurred between 8 and 10 for children in their sample. This research is significant as it provides a model for understanding and measuring early identity development, while also showing the emerging significance of ethnic identity in Chicana/o children's self-perceptions. According to Bernal et al.'s model, enculturation and acculturation work together to shape the ethnic identity and ethnic behaviors of children. The social ecology of the family (e.g., generation of migration, acculturation, parental ethnic identity, dominant language[s], familial cultural knowledge, and family structure) interacts with the ecology of the community in which they live, and these both work together to influence children's socialization. Familial agents, therefore, teach ethnic content, for example, while nonfamilial agents also communicate views about ethnicity and ethnic group membership. These factors, they suggested, shape the child's ethnic identity, which in turn shapes ethnic behaviors. Cognitive development is an overarching process that moderates the influence of various socialization agents and the extent to which such influences are manifested in ethnic behaviors. This model continues to influence the majority of research on ethnic identity development in Chicana/o children.

Models of Ethnic Identity Development in Chicana/o Adolescents

Jean Phinney is the most commonly associated researcher investigating ethnic identity development in adolescents in general. Phinney (1990, 1991, 1993) grounded most of her work in the writings of Erikson (1964, 1968), who focused on adolescence as the crucial time in life when youth go through a process of self-exploration that leads to a commitment to a personal identity. A critical aspect of this process, according to Erikson, is the development of a sense of continuity between the way others see the individual and the way the individual sees him- or herself. The result of this process yields an identity outcome status. These statuses were described by Marcia (1980) as: identity diffusion (individuals who have neither made a commitment to a particular identity nor experienced an identity conflict), identity foreclosure (those who have not explored identity and have made "premature" identity commitments), moratorium (those who are exploring identity options but have yet to make a commitment), and achieved identity (those who have explored identity in depth and have arrived at a well-grounded sense of self). Adolescents may move in and out of these statuses in a linear way (i.e., from diffusion to achievement).

Phinney (1993) conducted research with racial and ethnic minority adolescents, including Chicana/os, that asked them to discuss the degree to which they had addressed and resolved issues related to their ethnicity. Much of this research led to the development of the Multigroup Ethnic Identity Measure (MEIM), in which Phinney (1992) posited three components of ethnic identity: affirmation and belonging (i.e., the sense of group membership and attitudes toward the group such as attachment and pride), ethnic identity achievement (i.e., the extent to which a person has achieved a secure and confident sense of his or her ethnicity, including knowledge and understanding of the ethnic group), and ethnic behaviors (i.e., activities associated with group membership such as customs, traditions, and social interactions). Whereas feelings of affirmation and belonging and ethnic behaviors were seen as outcomes of ethnic identity development, ethnic identity achievement was conceptualized as representing a range of identity statuses similar to those articulated by Marcia (1980).

Phinney (1993) explained that the first stage of ethnic identity development is unexamined ethnic identity, where adolescents have given no thought to issues of ethnic identity (whether they are steeped in their own culture or trying to adopt mainstream culture) and she suggested that there are significant similarities between these youth and individuals that Marcia (1980) classified as having foreclosed or diffused identities. This unexamined stage continues until an identity crisis occurs whereby the next stage, ethnic identity search or moratorium, begins. No pivotal event is required to initiate this shift, but the search process is necessary to reaching an achieved identity. At this final stage, individuals are confident and comfortable with their ethnicity. An achieved identity status is proposed to be the most adaptive outcome, supported by research suggesting that adolescents with achieved identities have high self-esteem, strong ego identity, and healthy family and peer relationships (Phinney, 1989).

Although other models of racial and ethnic identity development exist in the literature, the majority of these models posit young adulthood as the starting point for identity development. The models of Bernal et al. (1990), Quintana (1994), and Phinney (1992), on the other hadn, are most applicable to Chicana/o children and adolescents.

Contextual Influences on Ethnic Identity Development

Ethnic identity development has been studied in relation to a host of contextual variables, including the family, peer group, and school setting. In some cases, the research has attempted to identify ways in which ethnic identity development is influenced by various contextual variables. In other cases, the relationship between ethnic identity development and overall indices of adjustment in various settings (e.g., academic achievement) has been the focus. Given the complexity of models of ethnic identity development in Chicana/os such as that of Bernal et al. (1990), it is likely that components of ethnic identity have complex, nonlinear relationships with many contextual variables that several studies have attempted to clarify.

Knight, Cota, and Bernal (1993) and Knight, Bernal, Cota, et al. (1993) investigated the relationship between Chicana/o children's ethnic socialization by their parents and their emerging ethnic identities. Results indicated that, generally: (a) parents' ethnic background, as reflected in their ethnic knowledge and ethnic preferences, influenced their teaching about Mexican culture; (b) parents' teaching about the Mexican culture influenced the multiple components of their children's ethnic identity; and (c) children's ethnic identity influenced their preferences (e.g., food, music, friends).

Knight, Bernal, Garza, Cota, and Ocampo (1993) also examined the relationships between parental socialization, ethnic identity, and cooperative, competitive, and individualistic behavior in Mexican American children. They found that mothers' ethnic background (i.e., mothers' ethnic knowledge and preferences) was directly related to teaching their children about Mexican culture (i.e., ethnic socialization). Mothers who had higher levels of knowledge about Mexican culture and who had preferences for more traditional Mexican activities (e.g., foods, music) taught their children more about Mexican culture and had more ethnically identified children. Ethnic socialization was then directly related to children's ethnic identity, which influenced their preferences for cooperative, competitive, and individualistic behavior with peers. Children who were more ethnically identified displayed greater concerns for others' resources and less concern for their own (i.e., cooperative preferences). They hypothesized that, when children are taught about their ethnic culture, they also internalize cultural values within their sense of who they are (Knight et al., 1993). These findings suggest that ethnic identity transcends the parameters of self-identification and personal preferences and includes the ways in which peer relationships are approached.

Family variables were also the primary focus of research investigating contextual influences on ethnic identity development in Chicanas/os by Phinney and Chavira (1995), who investigated the relationships between ethnic identity, parental ethnic socialization, and strategies for coping with racism. Chicana/o adolescents were included in the ethnically heterogeneous sample. Perhaps counterintuitively, the quantity of parental ethnic socialization efforts (i.e., the amount of time devoted to teaching about culture) was not found to be related to adolescents' ethnic identity attitudes. However, the authors did find that, when parents talked with their teenagers about the challenges of living in a diverse society, the adolescents reported higher ethnic identity scores. Perhaps the openness of communication between parents and their children on topics related to ethnicity is responsible for the more positive ethnic identity. Future research is needed in order to clarify how family processes influence the development of positive ethnic identity in youth.

Quintana and Vera (1999) found that parental background variables were associated with various aspects of ethnic identity in Mexican American children. Specifically, children's ethnic behavior was associated with both parental enculturation and parental acculturation levels. Direct ethnic socialization of children by their parents was significantly associated with children's acquisition of ethnic knowledge. These data suggest that parents can play a powerful role in shaping the ethnic climate into which their children are born and raised, and that this socialization influences the development of ethnic identity in children.

Bernal et al. (1991) reviewed research and theory on the relationships between ethnic identity and school adjustment in Mexican American youth. They concluded that, to the extent that "social contexts can be made friendlier, compatible, and more responsive to minority groups' social identities, academic achievement can be improved" (p. 147). Accordingly, for Mexican American youth, negative self-perceptions or ethnic identity would diminish morale and achievement in the classroom. If the relationship between feelings about ethnic group membership (i.e., feeling accepted in one's environment) and academic performance is indeed causal to some extent, there would be implications for interventions aimed at fostering cultural pride and heightening recognition of the positive contributions of members of the students' ethnic group (i.e., Chicanas/os, Tharp, 1994).

In an ethnographic study, Matute-Bianchi (1986) investigated the school performance of Chicanas/os in southern California, exploring relationships between self-labels and school perceptions, and offered conclusions similar to those of Bernal et al. (1991). Specifically, she found that youth preferring the term *Mexican* or *Mexicano* identified more with traditional Mexican culture than youth who preferred the term *Mexican American*. However, students who identified as either Mexican or Mexican American were perceived by teachers as more successful and achievement oriented than those who identified as Chicana/o or Chola/o. It was these teacher perceptions that Bianche-Matuti linked to subsequent student performance differences. In other words, students who were made to feel marginalized or whose teachers had lower expectations of them, via a self-fulfilling prophecy, had poorer academic performance. For example, seeing oneself as Mexican American may mean not seeing oneself as Chicana/o or Chola/o, especially if these groups are held in low esteem in particular contexts. This level of analysis may not generalize to communities where there is less politicization of ethnicity in the Mexican American population (e.g., areas of less concentration). However, Bianche-Matuti's research suggests that ethnic labeling may be more than just a function of personal and familial preferences.

Quintana, Vogel, and Ybarra (1991) conducted a meta-analysis of the literature examining psychological adjustment of Latinos (including Chicana/os) in post-secondary education. In many of these studies, ethnic identity variables were considered to be important predictors of academic success. One of the main findings was that cultural affiliation (e.g., participation in ethnic practices and behaviors) was negatively related to stress level in college students, whereas lower involvement in mainstream culture was related to higher levels of stress. This finding would suggest that greater ease in functioning in the dominant culture (i.e., bicultural competence) may make it easier for Chicana/o students to fit in and experience less stress. However, the studies considered in the meta-analysis often confounded the constructs of ethnic identity with indices of acculturation and acculturative stress. Both of the latter constructs are important in understanding the mental health of Chicana/os, but they are distinct concepts not always clearly related to ethnic identity development.

What is significant about the literature exploring the relationships among ethnic identity, acculturation, stress, and academic achievement is that it suggests that ethnic identity variables may have no direct relationship to academic success. Stress level may serve as a moderator. The stress that one experiences in one's immediate academic context may be influenced by the strength of one's ethnic identity (e.g., being on a predominantly White campus, experiencing discrimination because of one's participation in Mexican rituals or Chicana/o organizations). However, it is not the case that having a specific ethnic identity status or specific ethnic preferences is consistently related to quality-of-life issues for Chicanos.

In conclusion, the existing research on Chicana/o youth's ethnic identity development, though not prolific, suggests that familial influences are critical. The evidence suggests that familial variables may be most powerful during childhood, whereas other contextual factors become relevant in adolescence. We know much less about these other factors, however. It is possible that, as is typical of other aspects of adolescent development, the peer group becomes an equally influential context.

However, little research has investigated the influence of peer groups on ethnic identity development in Chicana/o youth. The research also reveals that the school context is important in the lives of Chicana/o youth. Matute-Bianchi (1986) looked at the power of teachers' perceptions of youth. However, it is not clear how ethnic identity development is tied to academic achievement. It has been argued that the receptivity of the school context is critical to the development of positive ethnic identity, but it is not clear that having a positive ethnic identity is always involved in academic success. In fact, some research has suggested that identifying with mainstream emphases on academic achievement may be at odds with having strong ethnic ties. Future research will be necessary to unravel the connections between family, peer, and school contexts across the childhood-adolescent lifespan.

What does existing research on ethnic identity development in Chicana/o youth suggest for delivering psychological services to this population? Some of the literature that has directly addressed this question has focused on older adolescents or young adults. For example, Ruiz (1990) presented a model that emphasizes strategies counselors can use to support Chicanas/os who are dealing with the struggles of identity achievement. Some clients may experience ethnic identity conflict, hold faulty beliefs about ethnicity, have a fragmented sense of ethnic identity, and need intervention and support to find greater acceptance of self, culture, and ethnicity. Counseling interventions might include the use of positive ethnic self-affirmations, along with participation in activities that promote ethnic appreciation and pride. The counselor may also address negative attitudes about race and ethnicity or find ways for a client to engage in meaningful community participation (e.g., joining a volunteer organization for tutoring Chicana/o children). The assumption in this literature is that helping a client move to a positive, explored, and resolved sense of ethnic identity is beneficial to one's mental health and adaptation.

The literature investigating academic achievement and ethnic identity suggests that the more children and adolescents feel a part of their learning environment, the less stress they experience. The lack of stress or feeling of belonging, then, would facilitate optimal academic performance (Bernal et al., 1993; Matute-Bianchi, 1986; Quintana & Vera, 1999).

The literature on interventions for children to enhance positive ethnic identity is meager (Quintana & Vera, 1999), however, based on the results of empirical investigations, it seems clear that the family context is a major focus for interventions with Chicana/o children. This is not to say that children could not benefit from individual or group interventions aimed at encouraging positive ethnic identification, but because the family sociology is so influential at this time, understanding parents' or caregivers' ethnic identities, their goals regarding ethnic socialization, and the family's rituals or traditions is critical to understanding children's ethnic identity development needs.

A general criticism of many identity development models is that they lack external validity because they decontextualize the development of ethnic identity from the development of other critical aspects of identity. In practice, these multiple aspects of identity co-exist and undergo simultaneous change across the lifespan. Chicana feminist writers (Anzaldúa, 1987; Castillo, 1994; Moraga, 1983) suggested the need to develop models that explain the interaction of gender and ethnicity in shaping the identities of Chicanas. Accordingly, they maintained that ethnic, racial, gender, sexual, and class identities must be integrated into the social identity scholarship. Identity construction and development for Chicana/os is a complicated process that is influenced by cultural variables of the client (e.g., age, gender, race), family variables (e.g., parental ethnic socialization), contextual variables (e.g., academic environment, community factors), and the dynamics of enculturation and acculturation forces. For this reason, placing individuals into categories of ethnic identity, though descriptive, may be overly simplistic. Additionally, there is a need to understand the pathways in which youth move from one stage or status to the next. For example, two individuals might have strong, positive ethnic identities that were constructed by different experiences. One might have an ethnic identity grounded primarily in very strong enculturation experiences, whereas another ethnic identity might be grounded in several recent experiences with racism that have led the individual to become immersed in Mexican culture as a means of resisting the messages conveyed by the racism encountered. Although the two individuals may be placed into the same category of ethnic identity, in many ways their identities are a result of divergent life experiences. Accurately conceptualizing the psychological strengths and needs of these individuals and developing more appropriate counseling strategies are ways to account for these differences.

Finally, lifespan issues as they pertain to ethnic identity development beyond childhood and adolescence must be integrated into model development. At this point, there is a solid body of research articulating the social cognitive processes that facilitate ethnic identity development in children and the powerful dynamics of the identity exploration that occurs in adolescence. As young adults become parents or immerse themselves in careers and the world of work, priorities shift and, as a result, so do self-perceptions. For example, as parents think about how to address issues of ethnicity and race in their young children, they undoubtedly must confront issues related to their own ethnic identities and ethnic socialization. In this sense, ethnic identity may be revisited and emerge with a greater or lesser importance. As issues of diversity become a more common part of the cannon of psychology, ethnic identity research and its application will become more and more critical to understanding the mental health and well-being of Chicanas/os and other ethnic minority populations.

REFERENCES

Aboud, F. E. (1987). The development of ethnic self-identification and attitudes. In J. S. Phinney & M. J. Rotheram (Eds.), *Children's ethnic socialization* (pp. 32–55). Newbury Park, CA: Sage.

Aboud, F. E. (1988). *Children and prejudice.* Cambridge, MA: Basil Blackwell.

Alejandro-Wright, M. N. (1985). The child's conception of racial classification: A socio-cognitive model. In M. B. Spencer, G. K. Brookins, & W. R. Allen (Eds.), *Beginnings: Social and affective development of Black children* (pp. 185–200). Hillsdale, NJ: Lawrence Erlbaum Associates.

Allport, G. W. (1954). *The nature of prejudice.* Cambridge, MA: Addison-Wesley.

Anzaldúa, G. (1987). *Borderlands/La Frontera: The new Mestiza.* San Francisco: Spinsters/Aunt Lute.

Arce, C. H. (1981). A reconsideration of Chicano culture and identity. *Daedalus, 110,* 177–192.

Arce, C. H., Murgia, E., & Frisbie, W. (1987). Phenotype and the life chances among Chicanos. *Hispanic Journal of Behavioral Sciences, 9,* 19–32.

Bernal, M. E., Knight, G. P., Garza, C. A., Ocampo, K. A., & Cota, M. K. (1990). The development of ethnic identity in Mexican American children. *Hispanic Journal of Behavioral Sciences, 12,* 3–24.

Bernal, M. E., Knight, G. P., Ocampo, K. A., Garza, C. A., & Cota, M. K. (1993). Development of Mexican American identity. In M. E. Bernal & G. P. Knight (Eds.), *Ethnic identity: Formation and transmission among Hispanics and other minorities* (pp. 31–46). Albany: State University of New York Press.

Bernal, M. E., Saenz, D. S., & Knight, G. P. (1991). Ethnic identity and adaptation of Mexican American youths in school settings. *Hispanic Journal of Behavioral Sciences, 13,* 131–154.

Brown vs. Board of Education, 347 US483 (1954).

Castillo, A. (1994). *Massacre of the dreamers: Essays on Xicanisma.* Albuquerque: University of New Mexico Press.

Clark, K. B., & Clark, M. P. (1940). Skin color as a factor in racial identification and preferences in Negro children. *Journal of Negro Education, 19,* 341–350.

Crocker, J., & Major, B. (1989). Social stigma and self-esteem: The self-protective properties of stigma. *Psychological Review, 96,* 608–630.

Cross, W. E., Jr., (1995). Oppositional identity and African American youth: Issues and prospects. In W. D. Hawley & A. W. Jackson (Eds), *Toward a common destiny: Improving peace and ethnic relations in America* (pp. 185–204). San Francisco: Jossey-Bass.

Cuéllar, I., Nyberg, B., Maldonado, R. E., & Roberts, R. E. (1997). Ethnic identity and acculturation in a young adult Mexican-origin population. *Journal of Community Psychology, 25,* 535–549.

DeLeon, A. (1983). *They called them greasers: Anglo attitudes toward Mexicans in Texas, 1821–1900.* Austin: University of Texas Press.

Doyle, A. B., Beadet, J., & Aboud, F. E. (1988). Developmental patterns in the flexibility of children's ethnic attitudes. *Journal of Cross-Cultural Psychology, 19,* 3–18.

Erikson, E. (1964). *Insight and responsibility.* New York: Norton.

Erikson, E. (1968). *Youth and crisis.* New York: Norton.

Félix-Ortiz, M., Newcomb, M., & Myers, H. (1994). A multidimensional measure of cultural identity for Latino and Latina adolescents. *Hispanic Journal of Behavioral Sciences, 16,* 99–115.

Helms, J. (1990). *Black and white racial identity: Theory, research, and practice.* New York: Greenwood.

Hirschfeld, L. A. (1994). The child's representation of human groups. *The Psychology of Learning and Motivation, 31,* 133–185.

Katz, P. A. (1978). The acquisition of racial attitudes in children. In P. A. Katz (Ed.), *Towards the elimination of racism* (pp. 447–461). New York: Pergamon Press.

Keefe, S. E., & Padilla, A. M. (1987). *Chicano ethnicity.* Albuquerque: University of New Mexico Press.

Knight, G. P., Bernal, M. E., Cota, M. K., Garza, C. A., & Ocampo, K. A. (1993). Family socialization and Mexican American identity and behavior. In M. E. Bernal and G. P. Knight (Eds.), *Ethnic identity* (pp. 105–129). Albany: State University of New York Press.

Knight, G. P., Bernal, M. E., Garza, C. A., Cota, M. K., & Ocampo, K. A. (1993). Family socialization and the ethnic identity of Mexican-American children. *Journal of Cross-Cultural Psychology, 24,* 99–114.

Knight, G. P., Cota, M. K., & Bernal, M. E., (1993). The socialization of cooperative, competitive, and individualistic preferences among Mexican American children: The mediating role of ethnic identity. *Hispanic Journal of Behavioral Sciences, 15,* 291–309.

Marcia, J. (1980). Identity in adolescence. In J. Adelson (Ed.), *Handbook of adolescent psychology* (pp. 159–187). New York: Wiley and Sons.

Martinez, E. (1991). *500 Years of Chicano history.* Albuquerque, NM: Southwest Organizing Press.

Matute-Bianchi, M. (1986). Ethnic identities and patterns of school success and failure among Mexican descent and Japanese descent students in a California high school: An ethnographic analysis. *American Journal of Education, 95,* 233–255.

Moraga, C. (1983). *Loving in the war years: Lo que nunca paso por sus labios.* Boston: South End Press.

Ocampo, K. A., Bernal, M. E., & Knight, G. P. (1993). Gender, race, and ethnicity: The sequencing of social constancies. In M. E. Bernal & G. P. Knight (Eds.), *Ethnic identity: Formation and transmission among Hispanics and other minorities* (pp 11–30). Albany: State University of New York Press.

Ogbu, J. U. (1994). From cultural difference to differences in cultural frame of reference. In P. M. Greenfield & R. R. Cocking (Eds.), *Cross-cultural roots of minority child development* (pp. 365–392). Hillsdale, NJ: Lawrence Erlbaum Associates.

Parham, T. A., & Helms, J. E. (1985). Relation of racial identity attitudes to self-actualization and affective states of Black students. *Journal of Counseling Psychology, 32,* 431–440.

Phinney, J. S. (1989). Stages of ethnic identity development in minority group adolescents. *Journal of Early Adolescence, 9*, 34–49.

Phinney, J. S. (1990). Ethnic identity in adolescents and adults: Review of research. *Psychological Bulletin, 108*, 499–514.

Phinney, J. S. (1991). Ethnic identity and self-esteem: A review and integration. *Hispanic Journal of Behavioral Sciences, 13*, 193–208.

Phinney, J. S. (1992). The multigroup ethnic identity measure: A new scale for use with adolescents and young adults from diverse groups. *Journal of Adolescent Research, 7*, 156–176.

Phinney, J. S. (1993). A three-stage model of ethnic identity development in adolescence. In M. E. Bernal & G. P. Knight (Eds.), *Ethnic identity: Formation and transmission among Hispanics and other minorities* (pp. 61–80). Albany: State University of New York Press.

Phinney, J. S., & Chavira, V. (1995). Parental ethnic socialization and adolescent coping with problems related to ethnicity. *Journal of Research on Adolescence, 5*, 31–53.

Pizarro, M., & Vera, E. M. (2001). Chicana/o ethnic identity research: Lessons for researchers and counselors. *The Counseling Psychologist, 29*, 91–117.

Quintana, S. M. (1994). A model of ethnic perspective-taking ability applied to Mexican American children and youth. *International Journal of Intercultural Relations, 18*, 419–448.

Quintana, S. M., Castañeda-English, P., & Ybarra, V. C. (1999). Role of perspective-taking ability and ethnic socialization in the development of adolescent ethnic identity. *Journal of Research on Adolescence, 9*, 161–184.

Quintana, S. M., & Vera, E. M. (1999). Latino children's understanding of ethnic prejudice: Educational implications. In S. Tomlinson (Ed.), *Building multicultural communities: Contributions from counseling psychology and higher education*. Newbury, CA: Sage.

Quintana, S. M., Vogel, M. C., & Ybarra, V. C. (1991). Meta-analysis of Latino students' adjustment in higher education. *Hispanic Journal of Behavioral Sciences, 13*, 155–168.

Quintana, S. M., Ybarra, V. C., Gonzalez-Doupe, P., & De Baessa, Y. (2000). Cross-cultural evaluation of ethnic perspective-taking ability: An exploratory investigation with U.S. Latino and Guatemalan Ladino children. *Cultural Diversity and Ethnic Minority Psychology, 6*, 334–351.

Ramsey, P. G. (1987). Young children's thinking about ethnic differences. In J. S. Phinney & M. J. Rotheram (Eds.), *Children's ethnic socialization* (pp. 56–72). Newbury Park, CA: Sage.

Relethford, J., Stern, M., Gaskill, S., & Hazuda, H. (1983). Social class, admixture, and skin color variation among Mexican Americans and Anglo Americans living in San Antonio, Texas. *American Journal of Physical Anthropology, 62*, 97–102.

Rotheram, M. J., & Phinney, J. (1987). Introduction: Definitions and perspectives in the study of children's ethnic socialization. In J. S. Phinney & M. J. Rotheram (Eds.), *Children's ethnic socialization* (pp. 10–28). Newbury Park, CA: Sage.

Ruiz, A. R. (1990). Ethnic identity: Crisis and resolution. *Journal of Multicultural Counseling and Development, 18*, 29–40.

Spencer, M. B. (1983). Children's cultural values and parental child rearing strategies. *Developmental Review, 3*, 351–370.

Tajfel, H. (1974). Social identity and intergroup behavior. *Social Science Information, 13*, 65–93.

Tharp, R. G. (1994). Intergroup differences among Native Americans in socialization and child cognition: An ethnogenetic analysis. In P. M. Greenfield & R. R. Cocking (Eds.), *Cross-cultural roots of minority child development* (pp. 87–106). Hillsdale, NJ: Lawrence Erlbaum Associates.

Stereotypes of Chicanas and Chicanos: Impact on Family Functioning, Individual Expectations, Goals, and Behavior

Yolanda Flores Niemann
Washington State University

Stereotypes are the definitive measure of Chicana/os. As societal, consensually held beliefs about the characteristics of Chicana/os, stereotypes prescribe behavior: They tell Chicana/os who they are supposed to be and how they are supposed to behave and allow them to pass judgment on themselves and others based on these prescriptions and expectations of behavior (Fiske & Taylor, 1991; Jones, 1997; Jussim, McCauley, & Lee, 1995). Stereotypes exist not only in the minds of individuals, but also in the "fabric of the society" itself (Stangor & Shaller, 2000, p. 68). As societal beliefs, they are very difficult to change. Stereotypes are insidiously powerful, as they not only affect outsiders' expectations, but also our expectations of ourselves (Cooley, 1902; Niemann & Dovidio, 1998; Pollak & Niemann, 1998, 1999; Steele, 1997). Consequently, we come to see ourselves in ways that we believe others see us such that stereotypes about who we are can become self-fulfilling prophecies (Cooley; Kanter, 1977; Pinel, in press; Steele, 1997).

The most prevalent stereotypes about Chicanas today are dichotomous images that have persisted for generations and have taken on mythical proportions. These images are grounded in the myths that originated in the conquest of the Aztecs and other indigenous groups in the early 1500s and the apparition of the Virgin de Guadalupe to a peasant Indian, Juan Diego, about 50 years after the conquest. These stereotypes have at their core beliefs about Marianismo, La Malinche, and Machismo concepts that define ethnic gender roles of Chicana/os.

This chapter examines the origins of prevalent overarching stereotypic categories about Chicana/os, and discusses how stereotypes within the Chicana/o community affect family relations, family functioning, and family members' goals and expectations. Certainly, out-group stereotypes and institutional racism also impact Chicana/os, but the power to affect gender role stereotypes lies most strongly within the

Chicana/o community, rather than in out-groups. Therefore, the present chapter focuses on the impact of within-group, cultural, and community stereotypes on Chicana/o family functioning and behaviors and expectations of individual family members.

LA MALINCHE AND MARIANISMO: BAD WOMEN AND GOOD WOMEN

The "good" Chicana is family and home oriented, nurturing, self-sacrificing, soft, passive, and submissive to her husband. The "bad" Chicana is self-centered, promiscuous, and, in general, the opposite of the "good" woman. According to prevalent myths, the original "bad" woman was Doña Marína, a 14-year-old indigenous girl who was given to Cortez as his slave, concubine, and translator. Doña Marína's translation skills are credited, in part, for Cortez' victory over the Aztecs. Reportedly, she also bore Cortez' child (Castillo, 1994). Doña Marína has come to be known as La Malinche, or the ultimate traitor and symbol of female transgression and treachery (Mirandé, 1985). Feminist scholars have recently countered that Doña Marína was only a 14-year-old child who had no say in what happened to her and who was raped by Cortez (Castillo). Nevertheless, the folklore persists in labeling her as a traitor who gave herself to the conqueror, thereby humiliating and emasculating the male (Mirandé). By connection and heritage, therefore, this myth also perpetuates the belief that all Latinas are potential whores and traitors and emasculators of men (Mirandé): "Even today, *malinchistas* are labels given to women who are perceived to betray their people" (Mirandé, p. 166). The writings of Octavio Paz (1985), Nobel Laureate of Mexico, support the general perception of the bad woman, *la mala mujer*, a woman who does not conform to the traditional female idea and assumes male attributes such as the independence of the macho. According to Paz, women are inherently inferior to men because they sexually submit to men. Paz echoes the prevalent attitude that Chicanas are to be judged on the basis of their perceived sexual behavior. The "bad woman" is, first and foremost, a sexual being. In stark contrast, the essence of a "good woman" is an asexual persona. Females dressed in a sexually revealing manner, female gang members, divorced women, and women's whose sexual identity is salient manifest today's bad woman image.

The myth of the "good" woman begins with the story of the Lady of Guadalupe (Rodriguez, 1994). According to legend, in 1531, in Tepeyac, called Guadalupe, an apparition identifying herself as the Virgin Mary, Mother of God, appeared to a peasant named Juan Diego. This apparition has come to be known as Our Lady of Guadalupe, or *La Virgen* (Rodriguez). This holy woman was and still is seen as the counterpart to *La Malinche*. She is all good, self-sacrificing, and nurturing. The story of the apparition provided a connection between indigenous and Spanish cultures and thus became the foundation of Mexican Christianity (Rodriguez). The Virgen de Guadalupe's actual apparition is debated, but her influential role in the culture is without question. That "good women" are still expected to aspire to be Virgin-like is a testament to her significance in the culture. This Virgen-based, "good woman" representation is known as *marianismo*. In today's application of the marianismo image, a girl remains pure, virginal, or nonsexual until she marries or becomes committed to her male lifelong partner. She is then expected to have children and center her life on her roles as wife and mother. Every other role is a distant priority to those relationships. Although she becomes a mother, her sexuality is never discussed.

The good versus bad dichotomies for descriptions of women exist in society at large, and within other ethnic and racial groups, not just for Chicanas. What is unique to the Chicana/o community is the reference to the Malinche and the Virgen and the exaggerated extremes created by those images. In spite of diversity among Chicanas (Zavella, 1997), the stereotype persists of the Chicana who is either good (motherly and nurturing) or bad (sexual, competing with other women to take men, or not conforming to traditional gender roles).

HOMBRES AND MACHOS: GOOD MEN AND BAD MEN

The counterpart to Marianismo is machismo, the stereotype that is associated with Chicano men. At first glance, machismo seems to describe one type of man. However, closer examination reveals that, much like the Malinche and Marianismo stereotypes of women, the meaning of machismo also presents a good-bad dichotomy of men.

The pathological model of machismo assumes that the male must live up to the dictates of being stronger, smarter, and better than women. He is expected to prove his masculinity in several ways. For instance, he must command respect from others for himself and his family and must have numerous girlfriends or mistresses. This model macho commands complete allegiance, respect, and submissiveness from his wife and children. He is authoritarian and creates dependence. Pathological views associate machismo with irresponsibility, inferiority, ineptitude, aggression, violence, and criminality, including rape (Mirandé, 1985). Today's cult of machismo, or the overbearing male, is seen as "compensation for powerlessness and weakness which become manifest as the impotent, powerless, colonized man turns his frustration and aggression inward toward his wife and family. Ultimately, machismo is but a futile attempt to prove one's masculinity" (Mirandé, p. 167). Paz (1985) concurs with this pathological view of the macho. He described the macho as having been born of the rape of Mexico by the conquerors, which accounts for his subsequent feelings of inferiority. Paz stated that Mexican men are self-described *hijos de la chingada* (sons of the raped one). The *Chingada* is the mythical mother of Mexico who was forcibly penetrated by the conquering Spaniard, thus producing a *nueva raza* (new race) of people now known as Mexicans. According to Paz, the original Chingada was Doña Marína. Some scholars (e.g., Anzaldúa, 1987) have argued that the negative macho image is a result of racist, distorted stereotyping of Chicanos and that, in reality, Chicano men are no different from men of other racial or ethnic groups within a patriarchal society.

The "good" macho man, the *hombre*, carries out his role within a patriarchal society compassionately. In this view, the macho's traits include pride, dignity, respect, and family responsibility (Anzaldúa, 1987). The positive macho man does not consume alcohol excessively or irresponsibly. He is not abusive to anyone weaker than himself. He treats his wife and children with respect and tenderness, but required firmness. He is a community leader who deserves respect from those he serves and protects. Although this relatively positive, social construction of the macho, hombre image is receiving increasing attention, some scholars (e.g., Castillo, 1994) have argued that there is no such thing as a positive macho image. In their view, all traits associated with machismo that maintain the idea of the man as the head and leader of the family are embedded in patriarchal ideals intended to subjugate women (e.g., Castillo).

HOW TO BE A CHICANA OR CHICANO: LEARNING STEREOTYPES

Stereotypes are grounded in racist, sexist, class-based, and homophobic ideologies that are continually reproduced, legitimized, and disseminated through the mass media, schools, workplaces, legislatures, and churches (Feagan, 2000, p. 32). The media may be a particularly powerful force in generating and maintaining stereotypes of Chicana/os (Duck, Hogg, & Terry, 2000). In the roles Chicana/o playwrights have created for *el teatro campesino,* the grassroots theatre of agricultural workers, the prevailing stereotype of the woman is virginal, soft, nurturing, and a long-suffering martyr and mother (Hurtado, 1995). In these plays, men are typically depicted in strong, macho images. In film, Chicanas are depicted as sensuous, hot, easy, or evil or as motherly women engaged in domestic chores. Chicanos are frequently portrayed as criminals (Cortés, 1997).

Social science researchers have also described Chicanas as one of two types: either home centered, submissive, docile, respectful, and usually modest in dress and behavior or rebellious, "independent, free moving women" (Humphrey, 1945, p. 75; cf. also Niemann, 2001). Recent portrayals of Chicana/os are self-belittling, strongly masochistic, self-sacrificing, submissive, docile, maternal, good cooks, passive, submissive, religious and promiscuous (Andrade, 1982; Niemann, Jennings, Rozelle, Baxter, & Sullivan, 1994) or hot, sexy, evil, and eager to take away other women's men (Cortés, 1997). Recent Chicano characters are virile, dominating, uneducated, unmannerly, lower class, poorly groomed, chauvinistic, and alcoholic (Andrade; Niemann et al.). These stereotypes reinforce the good-bad dichotomy for Chicanas and the macho image for men.

As consensually held societal beliefs, stereotypes are typically perpetuated by members of the stereotyped group as well as by the society at large (Fiske & Taylor, 1991; Niemann, Romero, Arredondo, & Rodriguez, 1999). In a study examining college students' open-ended descriptors of different groups (Niemann, 2001), traits that Chicana/os used to describe men and women of their group, but not White men and women, were, for men, lower class, hard working, family oriented, alcoholic, antagonistic, bad tempered, jealous, proud, masculine, criminal, and religious. Women were described as family oriented, determined, lower class, passive, antagonistic, loud, gifted at cooking, housewife, baby makers, having large families, marrying young, and lacking college education. Note that men's traits were consistent with the macho image, whereas those of women were primarily consistent with the Marianismo, good woman image. Research with non-college student community members reveals many of the same in-group traits provided by college students (Mindiola, Niemann, & Rodriguez, in press).

The stereotype of the Chicana who is submissive to her husband's wishes is also perpetrated by Chicanas themselves. Though evidence indicates that many Chicanas are empowered within the home, women continue to publicly proclaim and support patriarchal gendered norms, even when they no longer subscribe to or practice them (Del Castillo, 1996). Research shows a difference between what women say about men's and women's roles in the family and what men and women actually do in the family: the difference between *dicho y hecho* (what is said and what is done). For example, women may publicly state that men make the important decisions in the family and may stand by while men take the lead in a given situation. However, in private, women actually make many of the family decisions and hold much of the power within the family.

When Chicana working class housewives were asked to describe how they treat their husbands, they recited a list of *dos* and *do nots* of respectful behavior toward their mates. However, they admitted to violating such gender-appropriate behavior and made a distinction between being disrespectful in public or in front of their husbands and in private or behind their husbands' backs. Chicanas may claim to adhere to gendered norms to protect the male, macho image of their husbands (Del Castillo, 1996). Regardless of whether the women were employed, both husbands and wives stated that they believe that authority should reside within the husband or father of the family (Hurtado, 1995). This research with Chicano families concluded that wives still publicly adhered to the ideology of patriarchy, co-opting their own behavioral efforts to change traditional perceptions and definitions of men and women.

Stereotypic perceptions and attitudes are generated and maintained by a complex set of social ecological forces that seem to reveal a kernel of truth about groups (Jussim et al., 1995; Niemann, Pollak, Rogers, & O'Connor, 1998; Niemann & Secord, 1995; Oakes, Haslam, & Turner, 1994). From a social ecological perspective, the situating of women in domestic roles, excluding them from positions of authority, power, status, and influence, generates and sustains a stereotype of the traditional woman as unassertive, submissive to men, motherly, self-sacrificing, dependent, and domestic (Niemann et al., 1994; Niemann & Secord; Porter, 2000). The stereotype of men as economic providers, heads of their families, consistently strong, prideful, and disciplinarians of children and, at times, of their partners, leads to situating men in the more powerful positions within their families and communities (Castillo, 1994). Furthermore, the stereotype that men are the primary economic providers is sustained by a labor force pay structure that provides greater financial compensation for men than for women. It is also sustained by religious institutions and government structures in which more men than women are in elected and appointed positions. Because men and women are often restricted to such particular roles within confined contexts, those roles and associated behaviors then seem to reveal an essential truth about stereotypes such that women are good at mothering and housework, whereas men are the powerful leaders of the families. In this manner, stereotypes and social ecological contexts feed into and maintain each other.

MAINTENANCE OF STEREOTYPES
WITHIN THE FAMILY

Stereotype-consistent gender roles are acquired and maintained primarily within the family (Trager & Yarrow, 1952; Van Ausdale & Feagin, 2001; Worchel, 1999). By age 7, children's ideas and lay theories about groups remain constant (Cameron, Alvarez, Ruble, & Fuligni, 2001) and their essentialistic reasoning about groups is present (Hughes, 1997). The term *essentialism* refers to thinking about group members in terms of ostensibly inherent, static, and stereotypical traits, for example, men are powerful leaders and women are submissive to men. Parents shape their children's attitudes about other groups in many ways, including comments made directly to children or in their children's presence, for example, "Boys don't cry, "Good girls don't go out with boys," and "Who wears the pants in the family?"

In general, mothers are the primary conveyers of the culture (Castillo, 1994; Del Castillo, 1996; Rodriguez, 1997). Mothers' influence is such that the values of Hispanic mothers, but not fathers, are positively related to those of their children (Rodriguez, Ramirez, & Korman, 1999). Castillo argued that men are not born macho and that women play critical roles as the primary socializers of children, including teaching them gender roles. Although Chicanas experience a relatively low level of status and power in society relative to their male counterparts (Vasqúez, 1984, 1995), they do have social influence over children (Vasqúez, 1984, 1995), and the home, and they set parameters on children's behavior (Mirandé, 1985). Chicanas often pass on to their own children the philosophy that women are property that men can own (Castillo). They also pass on the information that all women are possible whores, jezebels, and betrayers and that the mother alone will not betray her son (Del Castillo). Within many families, parents teach the children that disobedience and nonconformance are equated with Malintzin, or Doña Marina (Alarcón, 1983).

In fact, gender roles are flexible, fluid, and responsive to environmental contexts. Girls are forming and joining gangs and women become heads of households more often. However, the stronger, more persistent voice is still given to traditional norms. The consequences of these community-held stereotypical gender roles can be destructive for family functioning and for individual family members.

FAMILISM (FAMILY)

Strong emphasis on *familism* is consistently seen in the literature as the most significant characteristic of the Chicano family (Hurtado, 1995; Mirandé, 1985): "A substantial body of research shows that Latinos not only ascribe to *familistic* norms, but practice them" (Hurtado, p. 50). Family values themselves, however, do not in themselves define gender roles. Where stereotypes come into play in *familism* is in the definitions of men's and women's roles within the families. Among Chicana/os, women's identities are defined on the basis of their roles as mothers and wives, that is, women are expected to exist solely within the family structure. As the foundation of the family unit, a Chicana must prioritize the needs of family members above her own (Rivera, 1994). Good Chicanas are expected to be completely devoted to their families, warm, and nurturing. They are expected to emulate the virtues of the revered cultural symbol, the Virgen de Guadalupe. The traits of family-centeredness and religiosity may reflect positively or negatively on group members, depending on the extent to which individuals' behavior is consistent with the traits:

> She is treasured as a self-sacrificing woman who will always look to the needs of others before her own. The influence of Catholicism throughout Latin America solidified this image within the community, where Latinas are expected to follow dogma and to be religious, conservative, and traditional in their beliefs. (Rivera, p. 5)

Chicanas who do not subscribe to traditional gender roles may be thought of as *vendidas* (traitors) within their ethnic community and alienated (Castillo, 1994; Garcia, 1989). This is especially true if they reject the Catholicism of their communities (Castillo). Chicanas have been attacked for developing a feminist discourse, considered a divisive ideology, and have been criticized for threatening solidarity with men and seen as a threat to the Chicano movement (Garcia; Pesquera & Segura, 1993).

Stereotypical gender roles have implications for Chicanas in other ways within the family. Adult Chicanas who are widowed or divorced are expected to remain single. When they date, they are judged critically as flaunting their sexuality. However, once they are seen as asexual elder women, Chicanas' power and authority within the family grows. Grandmothers are held in reverence within the Chicana/o community, but only as long as they remain in traditional roles, for example, grandmothers who agree to babysit their grandchildren (Facio, 1996):

> By encouraging definitions of Latinas as interconnected with and dependent upon status within a family unit structure, the Latino patriarchy denies Latinas individuality on the basis of gender. For Latinas, cultural norms and myths of national origin intersect with these patriarchal notions of a woman's role and identity. The result is an internal community-defined role, modified by external male centered paradigms. (Rivera, 1994, p. 5)

Similarly, Chicanos who do not fit traditional definitions of machismo or manhood risk not being perceived as "real men." Chicano boys are expected to grow up to be virile, commanding leaders of their families. Mothers are more likely to be pampering, indulgent, and permissive with their sons than with their daughters, especially during adolescence (Mirandé, 1985, p. 157). The general attitude is that girls must be restricted and protected, whereas the fledgling macho must be allowed to venture out of the home to test his wings and establish a masculine identity (Mirandé). Mothers also teach their sons that men must act "manly," and encourage extreme macho behavior that may result in adultery or wife abuse (Del Castillo, 1996). However, because men's traditional power is based on stereotypical definitions of empowered men with respect to economic or physical attributes, men gradually lose their power and authority as they age, unlike Chicanas. Elder Chicanos are often seen as lame and no longer "real men."

One of the most extreme examples of rigidly split gender roles occurs in the most collectively unempowered group: Mexican migrant workers (Valle, 1994). In this community, women take care of the food and home and men prepare automobiles for work. Women's work goes on most of the day and night, whereas men are able to obtain some rest during supper time or when women are cleaning up the home after supper. Poverty and uncertainty likely play a strong role in the maintenance of these rigid gender roles.

Meeting the Family

One salient example of how stereotypical gender roles are maintained in the family is one that my Chicano university students often discuss with me: what happens when they take their Chicana girlfriends home to meet their families. Most of the Chicana/o students who are coupled in college maintain what they consider to be egalitarian relationships. In their college apartments, both of them cook, clean, pay bills, and have joint responsibility for maintaining their households. When Chicanas go to their boyfriends' homes, they expect their Chicano boyfriends to have joint responsibility for any chores, most of which have to do with cleaning up after meals. Thus, when a Chicana begins to assist with cleaning the table and dishes after a meal, she expects her boyfriend to help.

However, when the boyfriends do assist, their family members often ridicule them and their mothers seem to become particularly upset that their sons are so ruled by their girlfriends. Students report that mothers often intercede and tell their sons to sit down and relax while expecting the girlfriends to assist with the dishes. If girlfriends insist on the boyfriends' participation in the chore, the Chicanos' family members may tell them that they are acting like women. Men are asked, "Who wears the pants in this relationship?" In general, young Chicanos report being soundly ridiculed by their families for participating in domestic chores along with their girlfriends. These men indicate that, usually, for that reason, they prefer not to tell their parents that they have an egalitarian relationship with their girlfriends. Some men report that, knowing their family's attitudes about gender roles, they do not even attempt to engage in chores with their girlfriends. They tell their girlfriends that they will lose respect if they participate in these chores. The girlfriends, on the other hand, want their Chicano boyfriends to take a stand with them in displaying an egalitarian relationship model. Invariably, these discrepancies in expectations and behaviors lead to tension in a young couple's relationship. Many of these couples have stated that, because of these traditional gender role expectations in their families, they dread the family visit and tension that results from it.

Young Chicana/os are expected to engage in behavior that will prepare them for their expected adult roles. They are judged according to whether or not they follow these expected behaviors. Those who do not are perceived as not fitting in, or as traitors to their families, and are often judged harshly for not adhering to stereotypical gender roles.

CHICANA ACTIVISM IN THE NAME OF THE FAMILY

One manner in which Chicanas rebel against the passive, submissive stereotype of their group is through their activism. What is consistent with the stereotype of the good Chicana, however, is that Chicanas' activism is almost always done in the interest of their families. For instance, the Mothers of East Los Angeles (MELA) fought against incinerators and prisons being placed in their neighborhoods and, thus, in proximity to their children (Pardo, 1990). The Chicanas who participated in the strike against Levi Strauss fought for wages that affected their families (Martinez, 1998). In New Mexico, Chicanas fought a major computer chip corporation that was disposing of dangerous waste in their neighborhoods and waters (Cordova, 1997). Throughout history, Chicanas have been involved in community activism in the names of their children. In spite of their successes, however, many of their husbands complain that their political organizing at work takes too much time and results in neglect of their families (Martinez).

SEXUAL BEHAVIORS AND ATTITUDES: MARRIAGE, PREGNANCY, AND ABORTION RATES AND STEREOTYPED GENDER ROLES

"Ladies, watch your chickens well for my rooster is on the loose." This Mexican folk saying, or *dicho,* expresses a mother's pride in her son's virility and manliness (Del Castillo, 1996). Within this *dicho* may lie one answer to a question that is frequently asked about the Chicana/o community: Given the conservative values of the community, especially relative to the sexual behavior of unmarried females, how do we account for the high pregnancy rate among unwed Chicanas? The *dicho* tells us that boys will be boys and are thus expected to engage in sexual activity. Whereas the *dicho* is consistent with the stereotype of the virile male, it conflicts with the stereotypical ideal of the "good woman," who is not expected to engage in sexual activity outside of marriage (Vega, 1995). A daughter's sexual purity is a major contributor of honor and dignity to the family and the female (Espin, 1994). In short, males are encouraged to "be men" and thus, sexually active, whereas girls are encouraged to remain virginal. These opposing messages cannot coexist within the same culture without negative, undesired consequences. In the case of Chicana/os, consequences of such conflicting messages likely underlie their sexual and reproductive behavior.

Over half (52%) of never-married Latinas aged 15 to 19 have had sex, compared with 61% of Latinos in the same group; 49% of Latinas 15 to 17 years old have had sex (Driscoll, Biggs, Brindis, & Yankah, 2001). Compared to White females, Chicanas have a higher pregnancy rate and marry at a younger age (Espin, 1994). In 1995, out of 1,000 pregnancies, 163 were among Latinas aged 15 to 19, compared to 72 out of 1,000 among Whites aged 15 to 19 (Driscoll et al.). In 1999, one in eleven 15- to 19-year-old Latinas gave birth (93 per 1,000) and Mexican-origin females had the highest birth rate of all Latina groups at 112 per 1,000 (Driscoll). Fifty-four percent of these females said birth was intended at conception. Chicanas are more likely than other groups to want to become parents while still in their teens. U.S.-born Mexican-origin girls hope to have their first child at an earlier age than do those born in Mexico (Driscoll).

The data on Chicana/o sexual activity cannot be explained by the presence of low socioeconomic status as its relationship with reproduction is weak (Driscoll et al., 2001). Additionally, there is little or no effect of parental education and welfare status on Chicanas' reproduction rate. Furthermore, controlling for socioeconomic status, Latinos are still only about half as likely to use contraception as White males (Driscoll et al.).

Stereotypes of Chicana/os and their expected roles within their communities help explain these data. First, although "good women" refrain from sexual behavior prior to marriage, the essentialized Chicana is first and foremost a mother. In the context of Chicanos pressuring them to engage in sexual activity, which is expected of males in the community, Chicanas are caught in a dilemma. If they choose to refrain from sexual activity, they stand to lose a part of their essential role—being partners to men and being mothers. On the other hand, if they engage in sexual activity, they lose their virginal, "good woman" status. However, if they lose the status of virgins, if they become mothers, they are still behaving in a manner consistent with their prescribed gender roles. That is, they ostensibly are not engaging in sexual activity for the purpose of personal pleasure or sexual satisfaction. As mothers, they are still qualifying as "good women," albeit outside of marriage. Research supports this argument: Although sexual activity among young women may not be sanctioned, once a pregnancy occurs, Latino families are more likely to encourage motherhood for their pregnant daughters (Driscoll et al., 2001). Relative to other subcultures in the U.S., Chicana/os more strongly value motherhood as an end in itself (Dore & Dumois, 1990). Chicanas internalize the expectation to be nurturers (Vasquez, 1998). At the same time, due largely to the stereotypical definitions of women, unwed mothers are seen as damaged goods, but their children are cared for. However, a woman can redeem herself by being a good mother to her children.

Chicanos are more likely to have engaged in sexual intercourse than Chicanas. They are also less likely to use condoms than members of other ethnic groups. One national study conducted in 1995 found that 58% of Latinos had used a condom the last time they had had sex, and 30% had used a condom regularly in the past year, compared to two thirds of Whites and three fourths of African American males (Driscoll et al., 2001). More recent research indicates that approximately 50% of Latino gay and bisexual men in the U.S., within a period of 1 year, had practiced unprotected anal intercourse (Díaz, 1998). Furthermore, this risky behavior continues to occur in the presence of substantial knowledge about HIV and AIDS and accurate perceptions of personal risk (Díaz). This relative lack of condom use is related to the definition of machismo, or manhood. A man's sexual prowess is a way to prove he is a man. However, among Latinos, use of condoms is associated with possible loss of penile erection. To prove one is a man, loss of penile erection must be avoided at all costs (Díaz). The relative lack of condom use puts Latinos and their partners at risk not only for pregnancy, but also for sexually transmitted diseases.

One study (Landrine, 1995) examined the contexts in which Chicana gang members engage in sexual activity and found that Chicanas dealing with the dilemma of attempting to comply with Chicanos' pressure to engage in sexual activity while still remaining virgins resolved their dilemma by engaging in risky behavior, specifically, by having unprotected anal sex.

> These young unmarried Latinas. . . . were engaging in anal intercourse in order to maintain their virginity. As unmarried, Roman Catholic, Mexican American women, they wanted to be (and men demanded that they be) virgins when they finally got married, but their boyfriends were demanding intercourse." (Landrine, p. 10).

In their minds, these women fulfilled their obligations as females and as good women. They technically remained virgins, but fulfilled what they perceived as their role as women who plan to become wives of Chicanos.

In summary, whereas Chicanas suffer the stigma associated with an unwed pregnancy, Chicanos who impregnate them are seen as merely being men. A Chicano who chooses not to marry the impregnated Chicana often does not suffer negative consequences for this decision. He has no obligation to marry a female who, by virtue of having sex with him, is no longer a "good woman" and potential marriage partner. On the other hand, for the male to practice safe sex through the use of a condom is to risk being seen as less than a man, an intolerable fate in a community that rigidly defines manliness. It is in this realm of sexual behavior and expectations that the stereotypes of Chicana/os have some of their most destructive effects within the Chicana/o community.

LABOR FORCE PARTICIPATION

Three issues are critical in understanding the construction of gender in the family: waged work, housework, and control over household income (Del Castillo, 1996). All three have at their core women's labor force participation (Del Castillo) as almost half of Chicanas are in the labor force. Their median earnings are lower than those of Chicano men, men from other ethnic or racial groups, and White, Asian, and African American women (Thomas, Herring, & Horton, 1995). Chicanas frequently hold jobs that are considered secondary, are often seasonal, and are characterized by low wages and few, if any, benefits (Segura, 1994). Equal pay contribution is difficult in a society that has institutionalized pay disparities between men and women. These pay discrepancies are exacerbated for Chicanas, who are often hired as expendable labor without benefits and opportunities for development (Hossfeld, 1994). Among Latina groups with children, those of Mexican descent are most likely to be in the labor force and are the least likely to be employed full time, year round and to have professional occupations. Mexican-descent women in the labor force are the most likely to be married and least likely to be divorced:

> The reality deviates sharply from the traditional ideology that relegates wives to full-time housewife status. Instead, wives justify their decision to work by stressing their roles as providers for their children and sometimes negotiate the decision to work within their families by taking part-time or season work." (Ortiz, 1995, p. 20)

Women's participation in the labor force is closely linked to their stereotypical family roles. However, Chicanas' employment creates domestic conflicts and role strains over their use of time and labor. Men who hold traditional views of gender roles still expect women to contribute to the family income, but husbands continue to want personal service, which they perceive to be dictated by women's primary roles as wives and mothers. Therefore, although labor force participation indicates a slight shift in gender roles, it seems to add to women's burden rather than enhancing their authority (Zavella, 1987).

Nevertheless, economic empowerment does relate to decision-making power in the family, as well as sharing of household duties. Economically empowered Chicanas use their power to displace ideal notions of gender-appropriate behavior and patriarchal dominance in the family (Del Castillo, 1996). The more money they make, the greater their decision-making power in the family and the greater the split of household duties between male and female partners (Del Castillo). Chicanos whose spouses contribute equally to the family income reluctantly comply in sharing household (Coltrane & Valdez, 1997). Indeed, Chicanas' authority to participate in family decisions increases as a result of working outside the home, but not as a result of Chicano men in these families voluntarily relinquishing power. Familism may therefore reinforce the gender subordination of women by placing a disproportionate burden on them (Hurtado, 1995, p. 50).

Stereotypes allow for this extra burden. Chicanas may be employed, but they are still seen primarily as wives and mothers. The stereotypes of Chicana/os reinforce patriarchy, which is supported by a division of labor by sex. This division of labor is also central to gendered stereotype maintenance. The stereotype that women are intended to be mothers and nurturers affects their experience in the labor force, including their pay and their positions. Similarly, the widespread hiring of Hispanic women as household servants contributes to the stereotype that Chicanas prefer types of work associated with low pay: a common racist ideology used by employers to justify hiring women in low-paying positions (Hossfeld, 1994; Segura, 1994).

For men, the reluctance (Coltrane & Valdez, 1997) to share in household responsibilities most likely results from their stereotypical definition of manhood, rather than the need to maintain power within the family unit. Within their communities, Chicanos have not been prepared for the role shifts in households with economically empowered women. The transition is often confusing, frustrating, and painful. Chicano men are painfully learning new gender roles that are being imposed upon them as women gain economic power. As they compromise their traditional, stereotypical gender roles, they must also face the ridicule of Chicana/os within their communities who still expect them to fit the rigid, stereotypical definitions of manhood.

At the same time, gender roles for men have not shifted consistently to the extent that they have for women. Men generally do not have the option to be unemployed, as the rigid definition of manliness demands that they provide economic support for their families. As a result, even though a man may be a better nurturer or parent than his wife, rigid role definitions do not give him the option to stay home. When men do become househusbands, it is usually the result of unexpected job loss, and most of these men are actively looking for work (Davis & Chavez, 1995). In their study of househusbands, Davis and Chavez found that the effect on men's self-concept of having to rely on their spouses for economic support depends largely on the acceptance of their status by family and friends: "When negativity is expressed, reeducation, joking and physical conflict are reported to result" (p. 270).

EDUCATIONAL VALUES, BEHAVIORS, AND STEREOTYPED GENDER ROLES

Community gender role stereotypes and accompanying expectations affect Chicana/os' educational pursuits. Recently reported data (Kristina Lane, Educating a Growing Community, *Black Issues in Higher Education, 18*[16]) indicate that 37% of all Hispanic 18- to 24-year-olds did not complete secondary schooling in 1999 and that these dropout rates have been consistent since 1985. Among Hispanic immigrants

25 years and older, 47% had a high school education. Only 18.7% of Hispanic 18- to 24-year-olds were enrolled in college in 1999, compared to 30.4% of Blacks and 39.4% of White non-Hispanics. In 2000, of students 25 years or older, 27.3% of Latina/os had less than a ninth-grade education, compared to 4.2% for Whites and 7.1% for Blacks. Among Latina/os, 46.4% had a high school diploma, compared to 60% for Whites, and 62% for Blacks. Statistics are also dim for college completion. Ten percent of Latina/os completed their bachelor's degree, compared to 28% of Whites and 16.5% of Blacks. Poverty is one factor that impacts Chicana/o higher educational pursuits, but socioeconomic status is not a significant predictor for grade point average. For Chicana/os, the motivational climate of the family is more important for educational achievement.

Vasquez (1997) stated that the "socialization process that often perpetuates or reinforces roles for girls and women results in a serious limitation of choices for them" (p. 456). Chicanas have less cultural and familial support for academic and career achievement (Gándara, 1995; Vasquez). Women experience role conflict as they attempt to balance the relative rewards and costs of marriage and children with an education (Vasquez). In the Chicana/o community, education is valued for men as a mechanism for self-improvement so that they can have a better job, make more money, and be economically responsible for their family (Mirandé & Enríquez, 1979; Niemann, Romero, & Arbona, 2000). Because men are traditionally responsible for the economic support of their families, women are not perceived to need a higher education. and may therefore experience a dilemma in choosing between their educational achievement and relationship goals, a dilemma referred to as the "double bind for the high achieving Chicana" (González, 1988, p. 367). Consistent with this work, Chicanas who are strongly ethnically identified and prefer to marry within their own group are more likely to experience psychological stress and perceive their educational achievements as threatening to men (Niemann et al.). Furthermore, because school achievement is stereotyped as a value of White culture, doing well in school takes on the connotation of "acting white" (Gándara, p. 5), which would be like being a traitor to one's community.

In her study of women who achieved higher education degrees, Valenzuela (1999) found that 50% cited the support of families as influential, with mothers most often cited as the most influential in shaping educational goals. For these women, families were exceptionally supportive of their educational goals. Even in these families, however, women were less likely to have mentors than male counterparts. Although parents encouraged both sons and daughters to achieve, they encouraged their sons more. Because men are expected to be providers, they are perceived to need education more than women. Indeed, Chicanas often sacrifice their own homework to help their boyfriends with theirs because they consider it more important that the boys do their work and do well than themselves.

As the stereotypical economic providers, however, Chicano males may feel more pressure than female counterparts to contribute to their families' economic well-being. The National Hispanic Institute (NHI) has documented a national trend over the last decade of females pursuing higher education in greater numbers than males (NHI President Ernesto Nieto, personal communication, November, 2001). Chicanas are also pursing more precollege programs and workshops than their male counterparts. The NHI has also found more gender role confusion among Chicanos than

Chicanas, which is leading to fewer men than women pursing higher education. The higher the education level of Chicana/os the less traditional their gender role attitudes (Hurtado, 1995). Therefore, it is important for both males and females to achieve higher education to effect consistent change in gender role expectations within the Chicana/o community.

SEXUAL IDENTITY AND STEREOTYPED GENDER ROLES

Chicana lesbians are the essentialized "bad women." By identifying as lesbian, they overtly identify themselves as sexual beings. Lesbians are a threat to the community "because their existence disrupts the established order of male dominance and raises the consciousness of many Chicana women regarding their own independence and control" (Trujillo, 1997, p. 281). They also disrupt the norms of the good woman: motherhood, religion, and suppression of sexuality. Chicana lesbians are, moreover, perceived as the ultimate sellouts to Anglo culture (Trujillo). For Chicana lesbians, coming out is very painful as fear of rejection of family and community is paramount (Trujillo); thus, they are among the most alienated of all community members, as other Chicanas do not want to associate with them for fear that they too will be perceived as lesbians or as traitors to the community. Their Catholic religion also does not sanction their homosexual lifestyle. All of these factors encourage the community to alienate and thus punish lesbians.

Latino gay and bisexual men often pay with their lives for adhering to their cultural, stereotypical perceptions of manhood. By June of 1996, 18% of all diagnosed AIDS cases in the U.S. were Latino (Díaz, 1998). Latino men who have sex with men constitute 51% of all these reported Latino male AIDS cases, with 59% of these cases being among men of Mexican descent (Díaz). It is likely that these data are conservative because approximately 20% of Latino AIDS cases have been incorrectly recorded as non-Latino Whites (Díaz). Men who have sex with men account for 44% of male Latino adolescent and adult AIDS cases (Driscoll et al., 2001). Furthermore, Latinos are less likely to discover they are HIV-positive until they have symptoms of AIDS (Driscoll et al.). As of 1990, 20% of U.S. women with AIDS and 23% of children with AIDS, were Latina/o (Nyamathi & Vasquez, 1995). Although a large percentage of these cases were related to drug use and needle sharing, unsafe sexual practices most likely add to these tragic statistics.

"Latino gay and bisexual men have had enormous difficulties adjusting to condom use and adopting less risky forms of sexual behavior" (Díaz, 1998, p. 29). Among Latino gay men, intentions to practice safe sex are often weakened or undermined by cultural factors related to definitions of manhood. Díaz stated, "A strong *machismo* discourse, widely diffused within the socialization practices of many Latino families, does associate masculinity with risk taking, low sexual control, and sexual prowess with multiple partners" (p. 4). He further noted that Latino boys learn that manhood is not a biological given, but must be proven from an early age with macho acts congruent with the culture's definition of masculinity and that "sexual penetration is a favored and well-defined act to prove masculinity" (Díaz, p. 4). Latino men are also given the message that homosexuals are failed men, or *Maricón,* the culturally equivalent word for *faggot,* a word that denounces those who are effeminate or who fail the masculinity test (Díaz). This stigma about homosexuality in the Chicana/o community often creates secrecy around homosexual behavior, which may be tied to a reluctance to come out and subsequent risky sexual behavior:

> When one considers the implications of *familism* for Latino homosexuals—namely, internalized homophobia, a sense of personal shame, the separation of sexuality and affective life, and the lack of a gay peer referent group—then it becomes clear how such cultural values might be strongly related to difficulties in the practice of safe sex. (Díaz, p. 110)

THE RELATIONSHIP BETWEEN INTIMATE PARTNER VIOLENCE AND STEREOTYPED GENDER ROLES

Chicanas, like women of other U.S. ethnic groups, suffer from domestic violence. A survey of 711 Latino families reported by Flores-Ortiz (1997) found that one out of eight Latino husbands physically assaulted his partner and that 7 out of every 100 Latinas were assaulted in a severe and potentially lethal way (kicked, punched, bitten, or choked). Hispanic women are murdered at rates of 2.89 per 100,000 compared to 2.09 for White women.

Domestic violence is a stereotypical, narrow, and unrealistic construct of Chicana womanhood (Rodriguez, 1997) that intersects with the stereotype of the man as the uncontested leader of the family. Culture-specific, stereotypical gender roles serve as norms of expected behavior that are then appropriated and used coercively to justify domestic violence against Chicanas (Flores-Ortiz, 1993; Rodriguez). Abusers use violence to punish Chicanas for not living up to their narrow expectations and to deter them from participating in roles outside their definition of "good" mother-wife. If a Chicana does attempt to get help, she is labeled a *vendida* or sellout (Rodriguez). Stereotypical expectations of Chicanos as uncontested leaders of their families, as demanding respect, and as the primary economic providers also justify men's violence against women. If a woman is seen as misbehaving (e.g., behaving in nontraditional ways), the man is obligated to punish her and keep her in line (Straus & Smith, 1989) on behalf of the community

Families that seem most at risk for domestic violence are those that adhere to frozen cultural patterns consisting of rigid, stereotyped values and behaviors (Flores-Ortiz, 1993). Chicanas themselves contribute to these destructive frozen patterns by engaging in the myth and stereotype of martyrdom: the idea that good women are either self-sacrificing, self-effacing, long-suffering martyrs or treacherous whores (Flores-Ortiz). As such, the socialization process in dysfunctional families tends to make women feel primarily responsible for the psychological, emotional, and physical well-being of their men. If they are beaten, they feel responsible for their own victimization:

> However, we must acknowledge that there is pressure to downplay these challenges in favor of lip-service to that "authenticated" cultural stereotype. . . . The symbolic power of that stereotype wields an ability to create and demand the perception of a more culturally authentic or potent expression of Chicana womanhood. (Rodriguez, 1997, p. 107)

Using broad claims to goodness and badness lends abusers symbolic claim and legit-imization for the restrictive violence.

Men are also victims of intimate partner violence, though to a lesser extent than women. In 1998, 85% of victims were women and 15% were men (Rennison, Welchans, & BJS Statisticians, 2000), although the data for men may be underre-ported. The constrictions around definitions of hombres and machos make it very difficult for men to either report the abuse or to receive help: If they report being vic-timized, they are no longer "real men." This is especially true if the perpetrator is a female. Stereotypical gender roles, then, affect men by justifying their violent behav-ior and by preventing them from attaining assistance when they are victims.

SEXUAL ABUSE AND STEREOTYPED GENDER ROLES

One in three Latina women reports incidents of sexual abuse, regardless of accultur-ation or citizen status, and across educational level, employment status, marital sta-tus, number of children, and neighborhood (Romero, Wyatt, Loeb, Carmona, & Solis, 1999). More than 80% of incidents occurred from the age of 7 years (Romero et al.) and 96% of the perpetrators were male. Almost half of the women were abused by persons within their family and two were abused by fathers or stepfathers. Fifty-one percent of the perpetrators were 20 years old or younger, 28% were between 21 and 39, and 21% were 40 or older. In another study, 15% of high school Latinas reported having been forced to have sex, as did 6% of Latino males (Driscoll et al., 2001. Eigh-teen percent of Latinas 15 to 44 reported that their first sexual experience was not voluntary (Driscoll et al., 2001). The rates of sexual abuse among Latinas are similar to those among African Americans and Whites (Romero et al.). What is different in the experience of Latinas is the tie to stereotypical gender roles within the family (Alarcón, 1983).

Stereotypes of appropriate female roles within families and of the role of men as the uncontested rulers of their homes underlie the experience of victims of sexual abuse in Chicano families. What happens in these families is normalized and hid-den under a mask of culture that defines the role of men and women: "*Familismo* becomes a rigidified code of behavioral expectations, distorted to insure compli-ance, secrecy, and submission under the guise of loyalty and respect to parental authority" (Flores-Ortiz, 1997, p. 58). Within this context, the dominated are isolated and rendered powerless, secrecy is labeled as good behavior, behavioral compliance motivated by terror is considered respect, and silent suffering of the abuse is reframed as loyalty (Flores-Ortiz). In the Chicano family, children are taught that "to be obedient/devoted is proof of love, especially for women and children" (Alar-cón, 1983, p. 186). There is more shaming of the victim in the Latina/o community, where she is seen as somehow at fault. In the family, young girls are sometimes not defined as victims of incest. The value of familism also contributes to Chicanas' ten-dency to deny their own needs to keep the family intact (Vasquez, 1995) lest they be viewed as traitors.

The rate of Chicano male sexual abuse has received little documentation. Driscoll et al. (2001) found that 6% of Chicanos were victims of sexual abuse. However, it seems likely that this number is inaccurate due to underreporting, as in the general population it is estimated that 20% of boys are sexually abused. Underreporting of abuse by Chicanos is consistent with maintaining their definition of manhood.

ALCOHOL ABUSE AND STEREOTYPES

Chicana/os' alcohol consumption is also related to community stereotypes and gender roles. Chicanos have some of the highest rates of alcohol consumption in the United States and are more liberal than other Latina/o groups regarding permission to drink enough to feel the effects of alcohol. They drink more and have a rate of problems associated with drinking two to eight times higher than other Latina/o groups (Caetano, 1988). Consistent with the good woman stereotype, Chicanas have the highest alcohol abstinence rates of all ethnic or racial groups (Caetano; Mora, 1997). Chicana/os' drinking behavior does not seem to be a trait retained from their country of origin. Caetano and Mora (1988) reported that both men and women in a Mexican sample drank "far less frequently than their counterparts in the U.S. sample" (p. 468). Abstention rates are higher for Mexican women in Mexico (66%) than for Chicanas (46%). Among women, 14% of Chicanas are either frequent high maximum or frequent heavy drinkers, compared to 1% of Mexicans. More Chicanos than Mexican men in Mexico reported frequent high maximum drinking or frequent heavy drinking (44% vs. 13%; Caetano & Mora). After 1 to 5 years of life in the U.S., Mexican-descent men who were born in Mexico already had changed drinking patterns from infrequent to more frequent drinker of large amounts, making their drinking similar to that of U.S.-born Chicanos (Caetano, 1988). For Mexican-descent women, alcohol consumption increases as women are in the U.S. for longer periods of time (Gilbert, 1987).

Limited progress has been made in understanding the antecedents of alcohol-related behavior. However, it is clear that, within the Chicana/o community, drinking by Chicano men is expected, whereas drinking among women is considered aberrant behavior (Gilbert, Mora, & Ferguson, 1994). The amount of alcohol consumed is related to expectations of consequences, with abstainers and light drinkers expecting negative emotional and behavioral consequences and more frequent drinkers expecting more positive outcomes (Marín, Posner, & Kinyon, 1993). Men and women who hold strong positive expectancies appear to drink more heavily and to experience more alcohol problems, though this relationship seems to be stronger among men than women (Cooper, Russell, Skinner, Frone, & Mudar, 1992). Gender role stereotypes also play a role, as all men are expected to consume alcohol, but only "bad women" are expected to drink (Niemann et al., 1994; Niemann & Lai, 1999).

Gender role stereotypes of Chicana/os have destructive effects on family functioning and on the behaviors and expectations of individual family members. Liberation from these rigid, limited norms and expectations requires breeching the good woman-bad woman dichotomy and macho/hombre definitions, providing Chicana/os with more options for personal identity and behavior. This requires changing definitions of male and female roles within the Chicana/o community. As Hurtado (1995) argued, for women to be described as fully human, the definitions of men also have to be expanded, especially within the culture. These restrictive gender roles keep men and women from pursuing their skills and gifts and, in general, from fulfilling their dreams when those dreams and goals do not reside within traditional gender role constraints and definitions.

It is not enough to challenge individual behavior, such as irresponsible sexual behavior, domestic violence, or alcohol consumption. Chicana/os must contest cultural platforms that, wittingly or unwittingly, exacerbate, justify, and condone these behaviors. To not contest these cultural stereotypes is to become complicit in the consequences. Chicana/os must de-essentialize Chicana/o men and women to give themselves the freedom to be individuals and to remove any justification of destructive behavior. In the language of Flores-Ortiz (1997), Chicana/os must unfreeze cultural norms and definitions about men and women.

In unfreezing rigid, stereotypical gender role descriptions, the community must also eliminate the dichotomous nature of Chicana/o gender role stereotypes. Stereotypes are dichotomous because, together, the bad and good stereotypes about men and women come much closer to defining a whole person than does either stereotype alone. The bad macho is the extreme of the good macho, that is, a respectful person becomes someone who demands respect at all costs, even to the extent of using violence. Such is the case with the extreme version of almost any trait: that it can begin as something positive and turn into something negative. Herein lies the solution to the diffusion of gender role stereotypes, especially those held within the community. Chicana/os must begin to see themselves as the complete human beings that they are. It must be acceptable and even expected for men and women to fulfill their dreams and pursue enhancement of their skills and competencies, whatever they may be. When Chicana/os reach a point where it is just as acceptable for men to be the primary nurturers in the family as it is for women, for either to be the primary bread winner, and for both to be sexual beings, they will no longer suffer the consequences of the negative effects of stereotypes on their daily lives, well-being, goals, and dreams. Furthermore, it is when Chicana/os respect themselves as complete human beings that members of other groups will also see them as heterogeneous, complete human beings.

REFERENCES

Adolph, C., Ramos, D. E., Linton, K. L. P., & Grimes, D. A. (1995). Pregnancy among Hispanic teenagers: Is good parental communication a deterrent? *Contraception, 51,* 303–306.

Alarcón, N. (1983). Chicana's feminist literature: A Re-vision through Malintzin/or Malintzin: Putting flesh back on the object. In C. Moraga & G. Anzaldúa (Eds.), *This bridge called my back: Writings by radical women of color* (pp. 182–190). New York: Kitchen Table, Women of Color Press.

Andrade, S. J. (1982). Social science stereotypes of the Mexican American woman: Policy implications for research. *Hispanic Journal of Behavioral Sciences, 4,* 223–244.

Anzaldúa, G. (1987). *Borderlands/la frontera.* San Francisco: Spinster/Aunt Lute.

Bargh, J. A., Chen, M., & Burrows, L. (1996). Automaticity of social behavior: Direct effects of trait construct and stereotype activation on action. *Journal of Personality and Social Psychology, 17,* 230–244.

Baumeister, L. M., Flores, E., & Marín, B. V. (1995). Sex information given to Latina adolescents by parents. *Health Education Research, 10,* 233–239.

Caetano, R. (1988). Alcohol use among Hispanic groups in the U.S. *American Journal of Drug and Alcohol Abuse, 14,* 293–308.

Caetano, R., & Mora, M. E. (1988). Acculturation and drinking among people of Mexican descent in Mexico and the United States. *Journal of Studies on Alcohol, 49,* 462–471.

Cameron, J. A., Alvarez, J. M., Ruble, D. N., & Fuligni, A. J. (2001). Children's lay theories about ingroups and outgroups: Reconceptualizing research on prejudice. *Personality and Social Psychology Review, 5*(2), 118–128.

Castillo, A. (1994). *Massacre of the dreamers: Essays on Xicanisma.* New York: Plume.

Coltrane, S., & Valdez, E. O. (1997). Reluctant compliance. In M. Romero & P. Sotelo (Eds.), *Challenging fronteras: Structuring Latina and Latino lives in the U.S.* (pp. 229–247). New York: Routledge.

Comas-Díaz, L. (1994). An integrative approach. In L. Comas-Díaz & B. Greene (Eds.), *Women of color: Integrating ethnic and gender identities in psychotherapy* (pp. 287–318). New York: Guilford Press.

Cooley, C. H. (1902). *Human nature and the social order.* New York: Scribner.

Cooper, M. L., Russell, M., Skinner, J. B., Frone, M. R., & Mudar, P. (1992). Stress and alcohol use: Moderating effects of gender, coping, and alcohol expectancies. *Journal of Abnormal Psychology, 101,* 139–152.

Cordova, T. (1997). Grassroots mobilization by Chicanas in the environmental and economic justice movement. *Voces: A Journal of Chicana/Latina Studies 1,* 32–56.

Cortés, C. E. (1997). Chicanas in film: History of an image. In C. E. Rodriguez (Ed.), *Latin looks: Images of Latinos and Latinos in the U.S. Media* (pp. 121–141). Boulder, CO: Westview Press.

Davis, S. K., & Chavez, V. (1995). Hispanic househusband. In A. M. Padilla (Ed.), *Hispanic psychology* (pp. 257–272). Thousand Oaks, CA: Sage.

Del Castillo, A. R. (1996). Gender and its discontinuities in male/female domestic relations: Mexicans in cross-cultural context. In D. R. Maciel & I. D. Ortiz (Eds.), *Chicanas/Chicanos at the crossroads: Social, economic, and political change* (pp. 207–230). Tucson: University of Arizona Press.

Díaz, R. M. (1998). *Latino gay men and HIV.* New York: Routledge.

Dore, M. M., & Dumois, A. O. (1990). Cultural differences in the meaning of adolescent pregnancy. *Families in Society, 71*(2), 93–101.

Driscoll, A. K., Biggs, M. A., Brindis, C. D., & Yankah, E. (2001). Adolescent Latino reproductive health: A review of the literature. *Hispanic Journal of Behavioral Sciences, 23,* 255–326.

Duck, J. M., Hogg, M. A., & Terry, D. J. (2000). The perceived impact of persuasive messages on "Us" and "Them." In D. J. Terry & M. A. Hogg (Eds.), *Attitudes, behavior, and the social context: The role of norms and group membership* (pp. 265–293). Mahwah, NJ: Lawrence Erlbaum Associates.

Espín, O. M. (1994). Feminist approaches. In L. Comas-Díaz and B. Greene (Eds.), *Women of color: Integrating ethnic and gender identities in psychotherapy* (pp. 265–286). New York: Guilford Press.

Facio, E. (1996). *Understanding older Chicanas.* Thousand Oaks, CA: Sage.

Feagan, J. R. (2000). *Racist America: Roots, current realities, and future reparations.* New York: Routledge.

Fiske, S. T., & Taylor, S. E. (1991). *Social cognition.* New York: McGraw-Hill.

Flores-Ortiz, Y. (1993). La Mujer y la violencia: A culturally based model for the understanding and treatment of domestic violence in Chicana/Latina communities. In *Mujeres activas en letras y cambio social (MALCS): Chicana critical issues* (pp. 169–182). Berkeley, CA: Third Woman Press.

Flores-Ortiz, Y. (1997). The broken covenant: Incest in the Latino family. *Voces: A Journal of Chicana/Latina Studies, 1*(2), 48–70.

Gándara, P. (1995). *Over the ivy walls: The educational mobility of low-income women.* Albany: State University of New York Press.

Garcia, A. M. (1989). The development of Chicana feminist discourse, 1970–1980. *Gender and Society, 3,* 217–238.

Gilbert, J. M., Mora, J., & Ferguson, L. R. (1994). Alcohol-related expectations among Mexican American women. *The International Journal of the Addictions, 29,* 1127–1147.

González, J. T. (1988). Dilemmas of the high achieving women: The double bind factor in male and female relationships. *Sex Roles, 18,* 367–379.

Hossfeld, K. J. (1994). Hiring immigrant women: Silicon Valley's "simple formula." In M. B. Zinn & B. T. Dill (Eds.), *Women of color in U.S. society* (pp. 65–94). Philadelphia: Temple University Press.

Hughes, D. (1997). Racist thinking and thinking about race: What children know but don't say. *Ethos, 25,* 117–125.

Humphrey, N. D. (1945). The stereotypes and the social types of Mexican-American youths. *The Journal of Social Psychology, 22,* 69–78.

Hurtado, A. (1995). Variations, combinations, and evolutions: Latino families in the United States. In R. E.

Zambrana (Ed.), *Understanding Latino families: Scholarship, policy, and practice* (pp. 40–61). Thousand Oaks, CA: Sage.

Jones, J. M. (1997). *Prejudice and Racism* (2nd ed.). New York: McGraw-Hill.

Jussim, L., & Fleming, C. (1996). Self-fulfilling prophecies and the maintenance of social stereotypes: The role of dyadic interactions and social forces. In C. N. Macrae, C. Stangor, & M. Hewstone (Eds.), *Stereotypes and stereotyping* (pp. 161–191). New York: Guilford Press.

Jussim, L. J., McCauley, C. R., & Lee, Y. T. (1995). Why study stereotype accuracy and inaccuracy? In Y. T. Lee, L. J. Jussim, & C. R. McCauley (Eds.), *Stereotype accuracy: Toward appreciating group differences* (pp. 3–28). Washington, DC: American Psychological Association.

Kanter, R. M. (1977). *Men and women of the corporation.* New York: Basic Books.

Landrine, H. (1995). Introduction: Cultural diversity, contextualism, and feminist psychology. In H. Landrine (Ed.), *Bringing cultural diversity to feminist psychology* (pp 1–20). Washington, DC: American Psychological Association.

Lee, Y. T., Jussim, L. J., & McCauley, C. R. (1995). *Stereotype accuracy: Toward appreciating group differences.* Washington, DC: American Psychological Association.

Marín, G., & Salazar, J. M. (1985). Determinants of hetero- and autostereotypes: Distance, level of contact and socioeconomic development in seven nations. *Journal of Cross-Cultural Psychology, 16,* 403–422.

Martinez, E. (1998). *De colores means all of us.* Cambridge, MA: South End Press.

McArthur, L. Z., & Baron, R. M. (1983). Toward an ecological theory of social perception. *Psychological Review, 90,* 215–238.

Mindiola, T., Niemann, Y. F., & Rodriguez, N. (in press). *Black-Brown relations and stereotypes.* Austin: University of Texas Press.

Mirandé, A. (1985). *The Chicano experience: An alternative perspective.* Notre Dame, IN: University of Notre Dame Press.

Mirandé, A., & Enríquez, E. (1979). *La Chicana: The Mexican-American woman.* Chicago: University of Chicago Press.

Mora, J. (1997). Learning to drink: Early drinking experiences of Chicana and Mexican Women. *Voces: A Journal of Chicana/Latina Studies, 1,* 89–111.

Niemann, Y. F. (1999). The making of a token. *Frontiers: A Journal of Women Studies, 20,* 111–134.

Niemann, Y. F. (2001). Stereotypes about Chicanas and Chicanos: Implications for counseling. *The Counseling Psychologist, 29,* 55–90.

Niemann, Y. F., & Dovidio, J. F. (1998). Relationship of solo status, academic rank, and perceived distinctiveness to job satisfaction of racial/ethnic minorities. *Journal of Applied Psychology, 83,* 55–71.

Niemann, Y. F., Jennings, L., Rozelle, R. M., Baxter, J. C., & Sullivan, E. (1994). Use of free response and cluster analysis to determine stereotypes of eight groups. *Personality and Social Psychology Bulletin, 20,* 379–390.

Niemann, Y. F., & Lai, F. (1999). The relationship between alcohol consumption and stereotype endorsement for Mexican Americans. Manuscript submitted for publication.

Niemann, Y. F., Pollak, K., Rogers, S., & O'Connor, E. (1998). The effects of physical context on stereotyping of Mexican American males. *Hispanic Journal of Behavioral Sciences, 20,* 349–362.

Niemann, Y. F., Romero, A., & Arbona, C. (2000). The effects of cultural orientation on the perception of conflict between relationship and education goals for Mexican American college students. *Hispanic Journal of Behavioral Sciences,* 46–63.

Niemann, Y. F., Romero, A., Arredondo, J., & Rodriguez, V. (1999). What does it mean to be "Mexican?": Social construction of an ethnic identity. *Hispanic Journal of Behavioral Sciences, 21,* 47–60.

Niemann, Y. F., & Secord, P. (1995). The social ecology of stereotyping. *The Journal for the Theory of Social Behavior, 25,* 1–14.

Nyamathi, A., & Vasquez, R. (1995). Impact of poverty, homelessness, and drugs on Hispanic women at risk for HIV infection. In A. M. Padilla (Ed.), *Hispanic psychology: Critical issues in theory and research* (pp. 213–230). Thousand Oaks, CA: Sage.

Oakes, P. J., Haslam, S. A., & Turner, J. C. (1994). *Stereotyping and social reality.* Oxford, UK: Blackwell.

Ortiz, V. (1995). The diversity of Latino families. In R. E. Zambrana (Ed.), *Understanding Latino families: Scholarship, policy, and practice* (pp. 18–39). Thousand Oaks, CA: Sage.

Pardo, M. (1990). Mexican American women grassroots community activists: Mothers of East Los Angeles. *Frontiers: A Journal of Women's Studies, 11,* 1–7.

Paz, O. (1985). *The labyrinth of solitude.* New York: Grove Press.

Perez, E. (1991). Gulf dreams. In C. Trujillo (Ed.), *Chicana lesbians: The girls our mothers warned us about* (pp. 96–108). Berkeley, CA: Third Woman Press.

Pesquera, B. M., & Segura, D. M. (1993). There is no going back: Chicanas and feminism. In *Mujerres activas en letras y cambio social (MALCS): Chicana critical issues* (pp. 95–116). Berkeley, CA: Third Woman Press.

Pinel, E. C. (in press). Getting there is only half the fun: Maintaining diversity in higher education. *Journal of Social Issues.*

Pollak, K., & Niemann, Y. F. (1998). Black and White tokens in academia: A difference of chronic vs. acute distinctiveness. *Journal of Applied Social Psychology, 11,* 954–972.

Porter, R. Y. (2000). Understanding and treating ethnic minority youth. In J. F. Aponte & J. Wohl (Eds.), *Psychological intervention and cultural diversity* (2nd. ed., pp. 167–182). Boston, MA: Allyn and Bacon.

Rennison, C. M., Welchans, S., & BJS Statisticians (2000). *Intimate partner violence: Bureau of Justice Statistics special report.* National Council on Justice Report No. 178247.

Rivera, J. (1994). Domestic violence against Latinas by Latino males: An analysis of race, national origin, and gender differentials. *Boston College Third World Law Journal, Summer,* 1–22.

Rodriguez, J. (1994). *Our Lady of Guadalupe: Story, icon, experience.* Austin: University of Texas Press.

Rodriguez, M. R. (1997). (En)Countering domestic violence, complicity, and definitions of Chicana womanhood. *Voces: A Journal of Chicana/Latina Studies, 1,* 104–141.

Rodriguez, N., Ramirez, M., & Korman, M. (1999). The transmission of family values across generations of Mexican, Mexican American and Anglo American families: Implications for mental health. In R. H. Sheets & E. R. Hollins (Eds.), *Racial and ethnic identity in school practices: Aspects of human development* (pp. 141–155). Mahwah, NJ: Lawrence Erlbaum Associates.

Romero, G., & Wyatt, G. (1999). The prevalence and circumstances of child sexual abuse among Latina women. *Hispanic Journal of Behavioral Sciences, 21,* 351–365.

Segura, D. A. (1994a). Inside the work worlds of Chicana and Mexican immigrant women. In C. Moraga & G. Anzaldua (Eds.), *This bridge called my back: Writings by radical women of color* (pp. 95–112). New York: Kitchen Table, Women of Color Press.

Segura, D. A. (1994b). Walking on eggshells: Chicanas in the labor force. *Hispanics in the Work Force* (pp. 173–193). Newbury Park, CA: Sage.

Stangor, C., & Shaller, M. (2000). Stereotypes as individual and collective representations. In C. Stangor (Ed.), *Stereotypes and prejudice* (pp. 64–82). Philadelphia: Psychology Press.

Steele, C. M. (1997). A threat in the air: How stereotypes shape intellectual identity and performance. *American Psychologist, 52,* 613–629.

Straus, M., & Smith, C. (1989). Violence in Hispanic families in the United States: Incidence rates and structural interpretations. In M. Straus & R. Gelles (Eds.). *Violence in American families: Risks and adaptations in 8,145 families* (pp. 351–367). New Brunswick, NJ: Transaction.

Thomas, M. E., Herring, C., & Horton, H. D. (1995). Racial and gender differences in returns from education. In G. E. Thomas (Ed.), *Race and ethnicity in America* (pp. 239–254). Washington, DC: Taylor and Francis.

Trager, H. G., & Yarrow, M. R. (1952). *They learn what they live: Prejudice in young children.* New York: Harper and Brothers.

Trujillo, C. (1997). Chicana lesbians: Fear and loathing in the Chicano community. In A. M. García (Ed.), *Chicana feminist thought: The basic historical writings* (pp. 281–286). New York: Routledge.

United States Bureau of the Census. (2000). *Statistical abstract of the United States.* Washington, DC: U.S. Government Printing Office.

Valenzuela, A. (1999). Checking up on my guy. *Frontiers: A Journal of Women Studies, 20,* 60–79.

Valle, I. (1994). *Fields of toil: A migrant family journey.* Pullman: Washington State University Press.

Vasquez, M. J. (1997). Confronting barriers to the participation of Mexican American women in higher education. In A. Darder, R. D. Torres, & H. Gutierrez (Eds.), *Latinos and education: A critical reader* (pp. 454–467). New York: Routledge.

Vasquéz, M. J. T. (1984). Power and status of the Chicana: A social-psychological perspective. In J. L. Martinez & R. H. Mendoza (Eds.), *Chicano psychology* (pp. 269–288). New York: Academic Press.

Vasquéz, M. J. T. (1995). Hispanic women. In L. Comas-Díaz & B. Greene (Eds.), *Women of color: Integrating ethnic and gender identities in psychotherapy* (pp. 114–138). New York: Guilford Press.

Vega, W. A. (1995). The study of Latino families: A point of departure. In R. E. Zambrana (Ed.), *Understanding Latino families: Scholarship, policy, and practice* (pp. 3–17). Thousand Oaks, CA: Sage.

Worchel, S. (1999). *Written in blood: Ethnic identity and the struggle for human harmony.* New York: Worth.

Zavella, P. (1997). Reflections on diversity among Chicanas. In M. Romero, P. Hondagneu-Sotelo, & V. Ortiz (Eds.), *Challenging fronteras* (pp. 187–194). New York: Routledge.

Problem Behaviors of Chicana/o and Latina/o Adolescents: An Analysis of Prevalence, Risk, and Protective Factors

Manuel Barrera, Jr.
Nancy A. Gonzales
Vera Lopez
A. Cristina Fernandez
Arizona State University

The headline of a front-page story in the October 14, 2001, issue of the *Arizona Republic* read: "5 Key Factors Threaten Arizona's Economy" (Wilson, 2001). One of the factors was said to be education of Latina/o youth. The article noted that Latina/os constituted 50% of the under-18 population in the state's two largest metropolitan areas (Phoenix and Tucson), but that only half of Latina/o youth finish high school. That newspaper article touched on three points that are relevant for the present chapter. First, children and adolescents represent a larger percentage of the Mexican American population than they do in other ethnic groups in the United States. Data from the 2000 national census are summarized in Table 5.1 for four states that have sizable Mexican American populations: Arizona, California, New Mexico, and Texas. The data show that between 33% and 38% of the Latina/o populations of those states are younger than 18 years of age, 13 to 17 percentage points higher than for non-Latina/o Whites and 5 to 7 percentage points higher than for non-Latina/o Blacks. Second, Mexican American youth experience significant problems, not only with school achievement, but in other situations as well. Finally, Mexican American youths' success in school, physical health, use of drugs, involvement in crime, childbearing, and subsequent quality of work and family lives should concern everyone. For some, this concern might be framed in economic terms. For others, the concern is motivated by considerations of equity in psychological health, the distribution of social justice, and human welfare.

Our focus in this chapter is on adolescence. The beginning of this developmental period is, of course, defined by changes in reproductive organs and secondary sex

TABLE 5.1
Percentage of Hispanics and Non-Hispanics Below 18 Years of Age
in Arizona, California, New Mexico, and Texas: Census 2000 Data

	Arizona	California	New Mexico	Texas
Hispanic or Latino	38.06	36.94	33.82	35.79
Non-Hispanic White	20.73	20.38	20.32	22.93
Non-Hispanic Black	31.14	29.97	28.67	31.00

characteristics, but it is also marked by distinct changes in problem behaviors that emerge or increase in prominence (Gullotta, Adams, & Markstrom, 2000; Peterson & Hamburg, 1986).

This chapter is organized into four major parts. The first reviews research on Mexican American adolescents' involvement in some major forms of adolescent problem behavior: antisocial behavior, substance use, academic failure, and sexual behavior. Unlike previous publications that have summarized epidemiological findings on the prevalence of these problem behaviors for Mexican American youth (Chavez & Roney, 1990) and ethnic minority youth more generally (Allen & Mitchell, 1998), we refer to factors that elevate the risk of problem behavior by Mexican American adolescents and factors that might protect them from those risk factors in the second and third parts, respectively. The chapter ends with a summary of the major conclusions and suggested topics for future research.

At key junctures in the chapter, we present the words of Mexican American adolescents or their parents that were shared during qualitative studies we conducted. These quotations are intended to ground the research findings in the actual life experiences of contemporary Mexican American youth, vividly illustrating many of the ideas contained in the review of empirical studies.

ANTISOCIAL BEHAVIOR

Delinquency among Latina/o youth is an important area of study because it is associated with school dropout, disrupted family bonds, substance abuse, unsafe sexual behavior, and stigmatizing police records that are often barriers to employment (Rodriguez & Zayas, 1990). With a pre-existing marginal status, Latina/o youth might be particularly susceptible to snares that make it more difficult for them to desist, resulting in many far-reaching and seemingly insurmountable consequences (Moffitt, Caspi, Dickson, Silva, & Stanton, 1996). For this reason, the study of delinquency among Latina/os needs more attention, particularly for Mexican Americans who constitute 64% of the Latina/o population.

Latina/o children who grow up in economically disadvantaged urban communities represent a population with an elevated risk for developing antisocial and criminal behaviors (Prinz & Miller, 1991). Rates of violence are highest among ethnic minority men living in the most disadvantaged urban neighborhoods (Fingerhut & Kleinman, 1990). This is especially true for Latino men (12%), who are more likely than White men (9%) and slightly less likely than African American men (13%) to have been arrested for a criminal offense.

Data from a number of sources indicate that Latino adolescent boys have a much higher incarceration rate than their White counterparts. Latino boys are also more likely than White boys to be in residential placement for juvenile offenses. In 1997, there were 515 Latino adolescent males in custody for every 100,000 Latino adolescent males in the general population (Office of Juvenile Justice and Delinquency Prevention Census of Juveniles in Residential Placement, n.d.), versus 204 White male adolescents for every 100,000. More pronounced disparities existed in some states than in others. For example, in seven states—Colorado, Connecticut, Iowa, Montana, Nebraska, Pennsylvania, South Dakota, Wisconsin, Wyoming, and Utah—over 700 Latino males were in custody for every 100,000 Latino youths in the general population. In contrast, for White juvenile arrestees in residential placement, state rates ranged from a low of 137 to a high of 454 for every 100,000 White youths.

Latino adolescent boys are at risk for engaging in certain types of group-initiated delinquency and violence. Gang involvement is one type of delinquency that is particularly prevalent among Latino youths. Indeed, the 1998 National Youth Gang Survey (Office of Juvenile Justice and Delinquency Prevention, 1998) revealed that Latinos were the predominant ethnic group, accounting for 46% of all gang members, followed by African Americans (34%) and Whites (12%). Because gang involvement is highly correlated with other types of problem behaviors (Adler, Ovando, & Hocevar, 1994; Curry & Spergel, 1992), the alarmingly high proportion of Latino adolescents who join gangs represents a significant public health problem.

Latinos are substantially overrepresented in the ranks of violent arrestees relative to their representation in the general population. For example, 24% (n = 4,752) of juvenile arrestees in residential placement for committing a violent crime (criminal homicide, violent sexual assault, robbery, or aggravated assault) are Latinos, compared to 47% (n = 9,069) for African Americans and 29% (n = 5,637) for Whites (Office of Juvenile Justice Delinquency Prevention Census of Juveniles in Residential Placement, n.d.). When these percentages are compared to those of Latinos (15%), African Americans (15%), and Whites (63%) in the general population of adolescents (United States Census, 2002), it is clear that both Latinos and African Americans are disproportionately represented.

In terms of property offenses committed by adolescents, official statistics generally suggest that rates for Latinos are lower than those for African American and White arrestees (OJJDP Census of Juveniles in Residential Placement, n.d.). For example, 19% (n = 3,756) of youths arrested for a property crime (burglary, theft, auto theft, or arson) are Latinos, compared to 36% (n = 7,245) who are African Americans and 45% (n = 9,114) who are Whites. However, it should be noted that the percentage of Latinos committed to residential placement for a property offense is higher than the percentage of Latinos in the general adolescent population (19% vs. 15%).

Several large national crime databases (e.g., FBI Supplementary Homicide Reports) do not include information on Latinos, focusing instead on the so-called racial categories of White and Black. Official statistics (e.g., OJJDP Census of Juveniles in Residential Placement, n.d.; OJJDP National Youth Gang Survey, 1997) that do include Latinos fail to delineate the different Latino subgroups (e.g., Mexican American). Furthermore, those databases generally do not provide much information on two other groups of Latina/o adolescent offenders: Latina girls and immigrant offenders. The need for data on these groups is particularly salient given recent statistics suggesting that crimes committed by girls (Chesney-Lind & Shelden, 1998) and Latina/o immigrants (Scalia, 1996) are on the rise.

SUBSTANCE USE

Drug experimentation during adolescence is not uncommon and does not inevitably result in drug abuse or dependence (Baumrind, 1987). Nevertheless, concern about adolescent drug use is justified because heavy use interferes with the developmental tasks of adolescence, increases the probability of accidents and death, and contributes to drug problems in adulthood (Newcomb, 1987). Unfortunately, it is difficult to make strong, simple statements about the prevalence of Mexican American adolescents' substance use or how it compares to substance use by adolescents from other ethnic groups. There have not been broad, household-based epidemiological studies of adolescent disorders comparable to the Epidemiological Catchment Area studies (Robins & Regier, 1991) or the national comorbidity survey (Kessler et al., 1994). What is available for the most part are estimates of prevalence from studies done in specific communities and school-based surveys that are limited in their utility for making population estimates. For example, Chavez and Roney (1990) reviewed studies that varied considerably in their conclusions regarding Mexican American adolescents' substance use relative to substance use by African Americans, European Americans, and other adolescents. This variability from study to study might have resulted from regional differences in substance use (Oetting & Beauvais, 1990). Substance use also tends to vary across time because of the fluctuating popularity of certain drugs. Moreover, some studies summarize data for broad categories of Latina/os and do not report specifically on Mexican-heritage youth (Delgado, 1990).

Despite these limitations, some summary statements have been made about Latina/o youths' substance use relative to other ethnic youth. Kandel (1995) summarized 14 epidemiological reports and concluded that Native American adolescents had the highest rates of lifetime use of most substances and that Asian American adolescents had the lowest. Of the three other major ethnic groups in the United States, the highest rates were found for European Americans and the lowest for African Americans. Substance use by Latina/o adolescents was between that found for African Americans and European Americans except for cocaine; Latina/o youth reported the highest rates of cocaine use in some studies (Kandel, 1995).

The Monitoring the Future (MTF) study is a series of in-school surveys of nationally representative samples of high school seniors that have been conducted since 1975. Since 1991, 8th-and 10th-grade students also have been surveyed. Racial and ethnic comparisons for African Americans, Latina/os, and European Americans were added to the MTF monographs in 1991. Unfortunately, sample sizes have been too small to permit separate estimates of substance use for Mexican Americans, Puerto Ricans, Cubans, and other Latina/o subgroups.

The most recent MTF results are cause for some alarm (Johnson, O'Malley, & Bachman, 2000). African Americans, European Americans, and Latina/os were compared using combined data from 1998 and 1999. European American 12th graders reported the greatest lifetime and annual prevalence of use of many substances including cigarettes, alcohol, inhalants, amphetamines, barbiturates, hallucinogens, and heroin. Latina/o seniors reported the highest lifetime and annual use of cocaine, crack, and steroids. Because Latina/os have higher high school dropout rates than African and European Americans, it is possible that substance use among Latina/os of high school age is even greater than the estimates provided by the seniors in MTF (cf. Swaim, Beauvais, Chavez, & Oetting, 1997). This possibility was supported by MTF data on 8th graders. Compared to the other two ethnic groups, Latina/o 8th graders reported the greatest lifetime, annual, and past-month use of virtually all of the substances assessed in the MTF (except amphetamines and smokeless tobacco). Some of the differences were substantial. For example, 30% of Latina/o 8th graders reported marijuana use sometime in their lives compared to 20% of European Americans and 24% of African Americans. Lifetime cocaine use was 10%, 4%, and 1.4% for Latina/os, European Americans, and African Americans respectively. Reports of lifetime crack use were also higher for Latina/os (6.8%) than for the other two groups (2.7% and 1% respectively). Unfortunately, these data were aggregated across Latina/o subgroups, thus, it is not certain whether the general patterns shown by Latina/o students represent specific patterns for Mexican Americans.

Perhaps the best epidemiological data on Mexican American youth were provided in a national probability sample of 2,530 8th-grade and 1,837 12th-grade Mexican American students and 1,547 8th-grade and 2,243 12th-grade non-Latina/o White students (Chavez & Swaim, 1992). Compared to non-Latina/o White 8th-grade students, Mexican American 8th-grade students reported more lifetime use of marijuana (24.2% vs. 15.8%), more cocaine use (6.3% vs. 3.7%), more heroin use (4.9% vs. 3.3%), more crack use (5.4% vs. 2.7%), more cigarette use (49.6% vs. 45.75), and more steroid use (2.9% vs. 0.8%). None of those same differences was found in the sample of 12th-grade students. The authors speculated that the higher dropout rates among Mexican American students led to an underestimate of substance use among Mexican Americans. An analysis of substance use among Mexican American adolescents showed that the lifetime prevalence of substance use in high school dropouts was 2.2 times higher than in in-school students (Swaim et al., 1997). The lifetime prevalence was 2.02 times higher for non-Latina/o White dropouts compared to non-Latina/o White students. Due to the extremely high dropout rates for Mexican Americans (46%, compared to 11% for White students in this study), in-school surveys substantially underestimate the substance use of Mexican American adolescents.

ACADEMIC FAILURE

The completion of high school is critical for future academic and career success for all young people. High school dropouts are more likely to be unemployed, to earn less than those who hold high school diplomas, to utilize welfare services, and to be incarcerated (Hauser, Simmons, & Pager, 2000; Kaufman, Kwon, Klein, & Chapman, 2000). Each year the National Center for Education Statistics (NCES) publishes a report on the status of high school dropouts in the United States. Over the past 28 years, academic failure among Latina/o youth, particularly Mexican Americans, has been remarkably high (Kaufman et al.; National Center for Education Statistics, 1992).

According to the most recent annual report by the NCES, 5% of all youth ages 15 to 24 dropped out of school in the 1998–1999 scholastic year (event dropout), 11.2% of all youth ages 16 to 24 were dropouts in 1999 (status dropout), and 14.1% of all youth ages 18 to 24 had not completed high school in 1999 (Kaufman et al., 2000). Among the ethnic groups accounted for in the NCES annual survey (non-Latina/o White, non-Latina/o Black, Latina/o, and Asian-Pacific Islander), Latina/os showed the greatest dropout. 7.8% of Latina/o youth ages 15 to 24 dropped out of high school in the 1998–1999 scholastic year compared to 4% of White students, 6.5% of Black students, and 5% of Asian-Pacific Islander students. Latina/o youth ages 18 to 24 were also more likely (36.6%) to have not completed high school in 1999 compared to White youth (8.8%), Black youth (16.5%), and Asian-Pacific Islander youth (6%).

The status dropout rate (percentage of dropouts ages 16 to 24) for Latina/o youth was 28.6% in 1999 compared to 7.3% for Whites, 12.6% for Blacks, and 4.3% for Asian-Pacific Islanders, and Latina/o status dropout rates have been consistently higher than those of Blacks for the last 28 years (Kaufman et al., 2000). Furthermore, although Latina/os make up 14.8% of the population of youths ages 16 to 24, they are overrepresented in the percentage of dropouts in 1999 (37.7%), second only to Whites (42.7%), who make up 65.6% of the youth population, and compared to Blacks (16.2%), who comprise 14.5% of the youth population.

The higher rates for Latina/o youth might be due, in part, to the high status dropout rate of Latina/o immigrant youth (Kaufman et al., 2000). Latina/o youth born outside of the United States had a status dropout rate of 44.2% compared to first generation Latina/o youth, whose status dropout rate was 16.1%, and second generation Latina/o youth, with a status dropout rate of 16%. Language and age at immigration may contribute to the higher percentage of dropouts among immigrant youth (Kaufman et al.). In 1995, 80% of Latina/o youth who had never enrolled in school came from households where English was reported to be not spoken well or not spoken at all. Moreover, because these rates include youth up to the age of 24, some Latina/o immigrants may have immigrated at an age older than the traditional high school age. Nevertheless, Latina/o youth in the United States of any generation remain at a disadvantage with respect to educational attainment.

In an attempt to gain a better understanding of the relationship between ethnicity and dropout over the last three decades, Hauser et al. (2000) analyzed a sample of 167,400 youths between the ages of 14 and 24 who were at risk for high school dropout. The risk for dropout was determined by the event dropout rate, that is, a student was enrolled in the previous academic year at the time of the first survey, but was not enrolled in the following academic year during the second survey.

In that survey, Latina/o youth at risk for dropout were 1.4 times more likely to drop out of school than Whites in the 10th grade, 1.75 times more likely in the 11th grade, and 2.4 times more likely in the 12th grade (Hauser et al., 2000). Furthermore, the odds of dropout for Latina/os compared to Whites has increased over the last three decades. During the 1970s, Latina/o youth were 1.8 times more likely than White youth to drop out of high school, and during the 1980s and 1990s they were approximately 2.3 times more likely to drop out of high school. However, Hauser et al. noted that, when family and socioeconomic background are statistically controlled, the differentials reverse, such that in the 10th grade Latina/o youth are 1.6 times less likely to drop out of school than White youth, and the odds decrease with each year in school. The same occurred when odds were examined over the past three decades.

Mexican Americans merit special attention because they make up approximately 64% of the Latina/o population (National Center for Education Statistics, 1992). In 1992, the NCES reported that the status dropout rate for Mexican Americans was 35.8%, similar to the overall rates for Latina/os (31.%) and Puerto Ricans (32.1%), but much higher than "other Latina/os" (19%) and Cubans (9.2%). Furthermore, Mexican Americans comprised approximately 74% of Latina/o dropouts. For those Mexican Americans born outside of the U.S., the dropout rate was 55% and they made up 48% of the total Latina/o dropouts.

TEEN PREGNANCY AND SEXUALLY TRANSMITTED DISEASES

According to the U.S. Department of Health and Human Services, half of Latina/o high school students in 1999 had been sexually active (National Center for Health Statistics, 2000). With sexual activity comes increased risk for sexually transmitted diseases and teen pregnancy. Singh and Darroch (1999) studied a sample of female adolescents from the 1995 National Survey of Family Growth and found that 56% of Latina women ages 15 to 19 had already had intercourse and 44.9% had had intercourse in the 3 months preceding the survey. Another survey of sexual behavior among high school students in the United States for the years 1990 to 1995 showed that over half of the sample of Latina/o students had had intercourse and Latino males were more likely to have had intercourse than females (Warren et al., 1998). The median age of first intercourse experience reported for Latina/o high school students was 16.2 years. Almost 40% of the Latina/o students had had intercourse in the 3 months prior to the survey, and 17.6% reported that they had had four or more partners. Latino high school males (23.6%) were more likely to have had four or more partners than Latina high school females (11.9%).

Latina/o rates of sexual activity tend to be slightly higher than White adolescents' rates and lower than Black adolescents' rates (Warren et al., 1998). For example, in 1995, 48.9% of White high school students and 73.4% of Black high school students had already had intercourse, compared to 57.6% of Latina/os. Moreover, the median age at first intercourse for Black males (13.6 years) was significantly lower than the median age for Latino males (15.9 years), which was slightly lower than the median age for White males (16.7 years).

Given the rates of sexual activity among Latina/o adolescents, contraceptive use becomes a significant concern for the prevention of sexually transmitted diseases and teen pregnancy. In one study, Latina female adolescents were less likely than White female adolescents to agree that their peers should use condoms during intercourse (Hodges, Leavy, Swift, & Gold, 1992), and in another study pregnant Mexican American adolescents were less likely than non-Latina White and non-Latina Black pregnant adolescents to have used contraceptives (Lindeman & Scott, 1982). However, Mexican American females ages 15 to 19 were more likely to use effective birth control than Puerto Rican, Cuban, or other Latina females (DuRant, Seymore, Pendergrast, & Beckman, 1990). Furthermore, approximately 44% of Latinas ages 15 to

19 reported that they had used a condom the last time they had intercourse, and Latino males (56.1%) were more likely to have done so than Latina females (33.4%; Warren et al., 1998). It appears that Latina females merit special attention when it comes to contraception use given their low endorsement and low use.

Fortunately, the rates of sexually transmitted diseases remain generally low for Latina/os, with the exception of rates of chlamydia for Latina females ages 10 to 19 (2,500 cases per 100,000) compared to those of Latino males (500 cases per 100,000; National Center for Health Statistics, 2000). Moreover, Latina/o adolescents have higher rates of AIDS and HIV than non-Latina/o White adolescents, although they are significantly lower than non-Latina/o Black adolescents.

Finally, teen pregnancy rates for Latinas remains one of the highest relative to other adolescents (National Center for Health Statistics, 2000). As a single problem behavior, teen pregnancy has considerable negative outcomes. Compared to adolescents who delay having children, adolescent mothers are less likely to finish high school or have consistent employment and are more likely to utilize welfare services and have unstable marriages (Alan Guttmacher Institute, 1994).

In 1999, mothers who were younger than 20 accounted for 16.7% of births to Latinas, 9.2% of births to non-Latina Whites, and 20.6% of births to non-Latina Blacks. Mexican-American adolescents, in particular, tend to have one of the highest birth rates among Latina subgroups and have a higher birth rate than non-Latina Whites (Centers for Disease Control, 1991). Recently, the National Center for Health Statistics (2001) issued a news release to announce that the U.S. teen birth rate had reached a record low in the year 2000, showing a decline of 22% from 1991. The Latina teen birth rate also had declined, but it had declined the least (12%) compared to Black teen birth rates, which came down 31% from 1991 to 2000.

STRUCTURE OF ADOLESCENT PROBLEM BEHAVIOR

> *Like when I was in sixth grade I didn't care about learning. I didn't care about going to school. That's why I really don't know my times tables because that's when they teach you. I don't care about learning or going to school. I just cared about having fun, hanging around. I started drinking alcohol, messing with girls. I never did care about school.*

Some have argued that diverse problem behaviors such as substance use, antisocial behaviors, academic difficulties, and precocious sexuality are sufficiently interrelated to justify their conceptualization as a construct of problem behaviors (Jessor et al., 1991; McGee & Newcomb, 1992; Petersen, 1993). Conceptualizing problem behaviors in this way does not preclude a developmental sequence of events that might begin in childhood with school failure, acting-out behaviors, and rejection by peers (Patterson, DeBaryshe, & Ramsey, 1989) or a sequencing of substance use that begins with cigarettes and alcohol and progresses to illicit drugs (Kandel, Yamaguchi, & Chen, 1992). By early adolescence, those problem behaviors appear to co-occur with sufficient frequency to warrant their consideration as a construct that might have common factors that maintain them.

Newcomb (1995) argued that the structure of the problem behavior construct has not been tested adequately with ethnic samples. He cited data that indicated that its structure might not be the same across diverse ethnic samples (Vega, Zimmerman, Warheit, Apospori, & Gil, 1993; Watts & Wright, 1990). Newcomb's reanalysis of some published correlational data showed that the relation between minor delinquency and use of illegal drugs (excluding marijuana) was stronger for Latina/os than for Caucasians. Similarly, correlations of delinquency with alcohol and illegal drugs were higher for Latina/os than for Caucasians. In light of those ethnic group differences, Newcomb argued that problem behaviors might have different patterns for various ethnic groups and that this feature was critical for designing interventions with ethnic minority adolescents. Apart from arguments made by Newcomb, there are reasons to suspect that Mexican American youth's academic problems might be due to language differences and unreceptive schools rather than the common elements of problem behavior. If that was the case, the problem behavior construct might not be as coherent for Mexican American adolescents as it is for European American adolescents.

The viability of a problem behavior construct for Latina/o adolescents was investigated in a study of 546 Latina/o (51% girls), 404 American Indian (47% girls), and 500 European American (51% girls) adolescents from the state of Oregon (Barrera, Biglan, Ary, & Li, 2001). Although Latina/o adolescents were not asked to specify nationality in this study, it should be noted that the vast majority of Latina/os in Oregon are of Mexican descent (78%). Three components of the problem behavior construct were assessed: antisocial behaviors, substance use, and poor academic performance. Measurement modeling was conducted to determine if the three components could be structured as a problem behavior construct and if the construct was equivalent for six subgroups made up of the three ethnic groups and two genders. Results showed that, for the most part, the three measures of antisocial behavior, substance use, and poor academic performance formed a problem behavior construct for Latina/o boys and girls, and that the construct was equivalent for the subgroups established on the basis of gender and ethnicity. In one exception, substance use loaded on the problem behavior construct for all groups, but the loadings were particularly strong for American Indian girls and were somewhat weaker for Latina girls. There are many circumstances in which a single type of problem behavior (e.g., substance use) should be studied, but the findings from Barrera, Bigland, Ary, & Li supported the utility of a problem behavior construct for Mexican American youth that recognizes the substantial co-occurrence of substance use, antisocial behavior, and academic problems. The concern that academic problems would not be related to the other problem behaviors for Mexican American adolescents was not supported by the findings.

RISK FACTORS AND PREDICTIVE MODELS

Descriptive epidemiology provides information about the prevalence of various adolescent problem behaviors. Other studies have moved beyond descriptions toward an understanding of factors that appear to contribute to Mexican American adolescents' problem behavior. Some studies have focused on specific risk factors (e.g., inadequate parenting) and individual problem behaviors (e.g., substance use), but others have used modeling procedures that show the interrelationships of several risk factors and, in some cases, several problem behaviors. Our review of research on risk factors gives special attention to prominent studies and those that have estimated models that included several risk factors.

Cumulative Risk For Substance Use

A well-known longitudinal study of Latina/o, Asian, Black, and White adolescents illustrated a distinct approach toward understanding the influences on one particular form of adolescent problem behavior—substance use (Newcomb & Bentler, 1988; Newcomb, Maddahian, & Bentler, 1986). Of the numerous papers that have been culled from this study, several adopted the strategy of combining risk factors into a cumulative risk index that reflected the combined experience of adverse characteristics such as low academic achievement, early alcohol use, low self-esteem, psychopathology, perceived peer drug use, perceived adult drug use, sensation seeking, lack of social conformity, poor family relationships, and lack of religiosity (Félix-Ortiz & Newcomb, 1992; Maddahian, Newcomb, & Bentler, 1988; Newcomb et al.). The presence of each risk factor was given a score of "1" and then added into a single risk index, which was then used as a predictor of various forms of substance use. The strategy was noteworthy for several reasons. On the one hand, the risk index was consistent with some causal models of adolescent problem behavior because the index contained variables such as perceived peer drug use and poor family relations that appeared in those models. On the other hand, the cumulative risk index ran counter to popular conceptions of problem behavior because several of the risk factors (low academic achievement, psychopathology, lack of social conformity) could be considered forms of problem behavior, that is, part of the same metaconstruct as substance use rather than factors that cause substance use.

Maddahian et al. (1988) provided an excellent illustration of how the risk index was used to study ethnic group differences and similarities in the risk factors themselves and in the risk factors' relations with substance use. This study used a sample of 145 Latina/o, 169 Black, 71 Asian, and 609 White adolescents in grades 10, 11, and 12. They first assessed ethnic group differences in exposure to risk. Among the many differences that were found, Latina/os were: (a) more religious than Asians and Whites, (b) much more likely to show a lack of law abidance than Asians and Blacks, (c) more likely to show sensation seeking than Blacks, and (d) much more likely to report peer and adult drug use than Asians. Overall, Latina/o youth had a cumulative risk index that was second only to that of Whites, but significantly higher than the index for Black adolescents.

Despite ethnic group differences in exposure to risk factors, there were remarkable ethnic group similarities in the relation of risk to frequency of substance use. Correlations were calculated between the cumulative risk index and five classes of substance use (cigarettes, alcohol, cannabis, nonprescription medications, and hard drugs) for each ethnic group. All 20 of those correlations were statistically significant except one (the correlation between risk and nonprescription drug use for Latina/os). There were significant ethnic group differences in the magnitude of correlations for one drug class, hard drugs, in which the correlation for Blacks was significantly lower than the correlations for Latina/os, Asians, and Whites. The correlation between risk and cannabis use was also somewhat lower for Blacks than it was for

Whites. There were no ethnic group differences at all when partial correlations were computed between risk factors assessed in a baseline year and frequency of substance use 1 year later (controlling for baseline frequency of substance use).

Those results illustrated that the cumulative risk index predicted frequency of substance use for Latina/o youth about as well as it did for the other youth. This comparability was obtained despite some ethnic differences in the prevalence of risk factors and the prevalence of substance use.

Family and Peer Relations as Predictors of Problem Behavior

I got in trouble a lot. . . . I never had any discipline. My mother was hardly ever around because she was working all the time. The only ones who were around would be my sisters and my sisters were not very good of an influence either because my mom wasn't around as much around them either. . . . She would work all day in a deli until 11 all day long and then when she came home at night time, sometimes she'd get dressed and go out. She'd come home, go to sleep, and then go back to work the next day.

We was just sitting back. We was getting high. He had never gotten high before and was acting all stupid. . . . He asked me if I wanted to go out and do some stuff. And I'm like, "What?" He was like, "Break in a house or break in a car or something." And I was like, "I ain't going to break in no house." He said, "Well if you don't come with me, I'm going to do it by myself." It was like one of those things, those guilt-trip type things. So it's like a little thing like a daddy taking his son to a baseball game or something for the first time or something like that. He wanted to go do it real bad so I went and did it with him. We got all the stuff. Came back to the house.

Growing evidence exists that family and peer group relations are associated with the onset and maintenance of problem behaviors (Steinberg, Dornbusch, & Brown, 1992). Much has been written about the lack of supportive parents and family members as a factor in the development of substance use and other externalizing behaviors (Barrera & Li, 1996). Moreover, affiliation with deviant peers is regarded as a strong, proximal influence on adolescents' problem behavior. Although they have not been studied extensively with Mexican American adolescents, it is difficult to imagine that family and peer relations that are prominent in research with majority youth would not be applicable to the understanding of Mexican American adolescents' problem behavior.

One model of family and peer influences on the development of adolescent problem behavior has been replicated in analyses of two longitudinal studies of adolescents (Ary, Duncan, Biglan, et al., 1999; Ary, Duncan, Duncan, & Hops, 1999). As shown in Fig. 5.1, there are three aspects of family relationships included in the hypothetical model: family conflict, positive family relations, and inadequate parental monitoring. In that model, family conflict is thought to have a detrimental effect on positive family relations. Positive family relations, in turn, can affect parental monitoring practices, which are thought to depend, in part, on open communication between parents and adolescents. Inadequate monitoring can contribute to adolescents' associations with deviant peers and diverse problem behaviors defined by the variables of antisocial behavior, poor academic performance, and substance use. In addition to inadequate parental monitoring, adolescents' associations with deviant

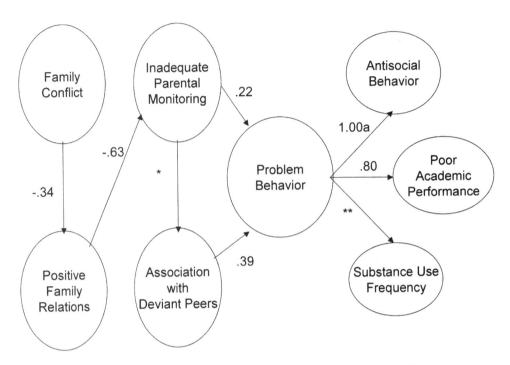

FIG. 5.1.   A higher-order factor model of adolescent problem behavior.   *There were group differences in the structural coefficients for this path: β = .846 for American Indian girls, β = .762 for American Indian boys, β = .562 for Caucasian and Hispanic boys, and β = .404 for Caucasian and Hispanic girls.   **There were group differences in the second-order factor loadings: V = .492 for Caucasian, Hispanic, and American Indian boys, and Caucasian girls; V = .352 for Hispanic girls, and V = .608 for American Indian girls.   ᵃSet to unity for model identification purposes.

peers were thought to affect levels of engagement in problem behaviors. Each link in that model has received some support in the literature. Ary, Duncan, Biglan, et al. and Ary, Duncan, Duncan, & Hops provided convincing evidence in support of the hypothesized model. Not only were the two studies longitudinal, but they measured constructs with reports from parents and adolescents. However, an important limitation of both studies was that they were based on samples consisting primarily of non-Latina/o Caucasian adolescents (91% and 92% respectively).

The same study that tested the viability of the problem behavior construct for Latina/o adolescents also used this construct in evaluating the fit of Ary et al.'s model of family and peer influences for Latina/o, American Indian, and European American adolescents (Barrera, Biglan, Ary, & Li, 2001). As expected, the model provided a good fit for Latina/o adolescents and was essentially equivalent to the models for American Indian and European American boys and girls. The pathway for inadequate parental monitoring to deviant peer associations showed some subgroup differences, which were due to extremely high relations between constructs for American Indian boys and girls, but moderate relations for Latina/o and European American boys and girls. Overall, the results suggested that family conflict, supportive family relationships, parental supervision, and association with deviant peers might be fundamental, nonspecific factors that affect adolescent problem behavior for Mexican Americans and other ethnic groups.

The Influence of Stress and Economic Conditions

> *The only problem is that I have a little problem getting him to the school. He wanted to change schools because last year he witnessed a kid—one of his friends—fought another kid and this other kid was, I guess, these two kids were fighting and some other kid picked up a bat and started hitting the kid in the head. Well, [my son] got really upset about that and he didn't want to go back to that school. And I told him I don't really have a choice, you know, you have to go there. I don't know. He doesn't like that school at all, because of that.*

> *My life was f—d up. Shit, living on food stamps. We didn't have no food, never had nothing nice like other people have. Shit, it was f—d. Life was just totally f—d up. Every since we were growing up we lived in shelters and all that shit. That shit was stressful. Scared. You didn't know what the f—k to do. You was just—man life was f—ked up. So whenever we found a chance to get away and have fun, we did crime. That was just something fun. It was something fun to do. We felt good. We felt accepted, happy.*

Stressful life events and family economic conditions are two variable domains that have high relevance for Mexican American youth. Unfortunately, the model estimated by Barrera, Biglan, Ary, and Li (2001) did not include those variables. Children and adolescents growing up in low-income families, particularly families living in poverty, are at much greater risk for negative outcomes in physical health, educational attainment, and mental health than their economically advantaged peers (Brooks-Gunn & Duncan, 1997). Unfortunately, children and adolescents are overrepresented among those living in poverty in the United States; 23% of young children lived in poverty in 1996, compared with 11% of adults (National Center for Children in Poverty, 1998).

Because of the prevalence of Mexican American youth who are at risk because of economic circumstances, it is important to identify the processes through which family economic status might affect children's development and well-being. A family's economic status can influence a child's development by threatening parents' psychological functioning and their parenting (Conger & Elder, 1994; Duncan & Brooks-Gunn, 1997). Similarly, a family's economic circumstances might place children in environments where local schools, neighborhoods, and peer groups expose them to adversity. A recent study with a predominantly Mexican American sample of adolescents evaluated a model that considered processes both within and outside the family that could explain how economic conditions lead to psychological distress (Barrera et al., 2002).

The model estimated by Barrera et al. (2002) contained two major pathways that originated from indicators of objective economic hardship (see Fig. 5.2). One of the pathways was directed through supportive parenting practices and the other included stress events that occurred outside the family in peer relationships, schools, and neighborhoods. Like the model estimated in Barrera, Biglan, Ary, and Li (2001), both of these pathways were channeled through a common construct, associations with deviant peers, which is the proximal link to adolescents' mental health. Associ-

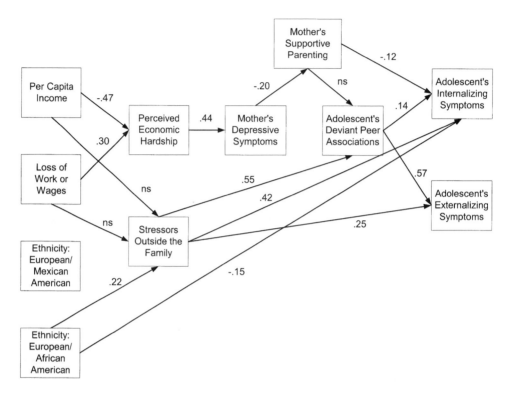

FIG. 5.2. A model of pathways from family economic conditions to adolescents' distress: supportive parenting, stressors outside the family, and deviant peers. Standardized path coefficients are shown. Ethnicity was coded so that European American families were coded 0 and African American and Mexican American families were coded 1. From Barrera, Biglan, Ary, & Li, *Journal of Early Adolescence, 21*(2), p. 145, © 2001. Reprinted by permission of Sage Publications, Inc.

ation with deviant peers is a major predictor of adolescent problem behavior and is, therefore, a critical construct in models that purport to explain pathways from economic hardship to adolescents' mental health and problem behavior (Ary, Duncan, Biglan, et al., 1999; Ary, Duncan, Duncan, & Hops, 1999; Barrera, Biglan, Ary, & Li, 2001; Chassin, Curran, Hussong, & Colder, 1996; Chassin, Pillow, Curran, Molina, & Barrera, 1993; Hawkins, Catalano, & Miller, 1992).

Participants in the study by Barrera et al. (2002) were 300 adolescents (138 boys and 162 girls) who ranged in age from 11 to 15 (mean age of 12.9 years) and their parents. They included 66 African American (AA), 59 European American (EA), and 175 Mexican American (MA) families. Parents and adolescents completed extensive structured interviews in the language of their choice.

Results showed that many, but not all, of the hypothesized paths in the model were supported by the data. As shown in Fig. 5.2, objective indicators of economic status (i.e., per capita income and loss of work or wages) were related in the expected direction to perceived economic hardship. Perceived economic hardship was, in turn, related to mothers' depressive symptoms, which were associated with less supportive parenting from mothers. Mothers' reports of supportive parenting then predicted adolescents' reports of internalizing behavior. Additional analyses showed that mothers' depressive symptoms and supportive parenting mediated the effect of perceived economic hardship on adolescents' internalizing symptoms.

The second hypothesized pathway, from objective indicators of economic status to stress outside the family, to association with deviant peers, and then to problem behaviors (i.e., internalizing and externalizing), was not fully supported. Contrary to hypotheses, objective indicators of economic status were not related to stress outside the family. Nonetheless, stress outside the family was related to internalizing and externalizing behavior through both direct and indirect paths. Tests of indirect effects indicated that association with deviant peers was a significant mediator between stress outside the family and both internalizing and externalizing behaviors.

It is important to note that this model fit the data extremely well when just the Mexican American participants were included (Hazel Prelow, personal communication, August 16, 2001). Thus, the model shown in Fig. 5.2 is consistent with the assertion that externalizing behaviors by Mexican American adolescents are associated with their affiliations with deviant peers and with stressors in the environment.

Parental Problem Drinking, Stress, and Parenting

> Adolescent: *My mom was going through divorce at that time and my father was an alcoholic so it was just kind of rough. . . . I guess at that time my mom was going to remarry. So I really wasn't too happy about that. I rebelled a lot towards that. And there was just a lot of anger at that time, at that age. I hated my stepfather for one. . . . I ditched school. I even smoked. I just didn't listen to my mom at all.*
>
> Interviewer: *So what role did your real dad play in that? You said that he was an alcoholic. Did he help raise you?*
>
> Adolescent: *Well he left when I was probably 11. Eleven or 12. So he wasn't around too much. When he came around he was drunk. So he wasn't around very much at all.*

Because alcohol abuse is a prevalent problem among Mexican American men, it merits special consideration as a factor that might influence the welfare of Mexican American adolescents (Barrera, Li, & Chassin, 1993). An additional hypothetical model includes the concepts of parental problem drinking, children's stressful life events, supportive parenting, and inconsistent discipline as predictors of children's conduct disorder and depression symptoms (Roosa, Tein, Groppenbacher, Michaels, & Dumka, 1993). That hypothetical model posited that parental problem drinking would increase children's exposure to negative family life events, which were thought to impair supportive parenting and the consistency of parental discipline. These parenting problems were hypothesized as mediators of the influence of stress on childhood depression and conduct disorder. The original sample included both Latina/o and non-Latina/o children in grades 4 to 6, however, models had to be estimated separately for the two subgroups because preliminary analyses showed the nonequivalence of data matrices. Results for the Latina/o subsample showed that stress and supportive parenting (but not parental problem drinking and inconsistent discipline) were significant predictors of conduct disorder and depression. Furthermore, supportive parenting mediated the relation of stress to child conduct disorder and depression.

The studies by Barrera et al. (2002) and Roosa et al. (1993) used different approaches to the assessment and modeling of supportive parenting and they produced differing results with respect to the role of supportive parenting in mediating the effects of life stress on externalizing problems. Roosa et al.'s results are consistent with many other studies that have found relations between parental support and externalizing problems of children and adolescents (Barrera & Li, 1996). Even though perceived adult drug use and parental problem drinking are thought to be risk factors for adolescent problem behavior (Chassin, Barrera, & Montgomery, 1997; Maddahian et al., 1988), Roosa et al. found a relation between parental problem drinking and mental health only for non-Latina/os. Other research has also found evidence that Latina/o adolescents are less vulnerable to the effects of parental alcoholism than European American adolescents (Barrera, Li, & Chassin, 1993, 1995). Although there are many similarities between Mexican American adolescents and adolescents of other ethnic groups with respect to predictors of problem behaviors (Barrera, Biglan, Ary, & Li, 2001; Flannery, Vazsonyi, & Rowe, 1996; Vazsonyi & Flannery, 1997), there is some evidence that certain risk factors (e.g., parental problem drinking) might not have the same predictive power.

PROTECTIVE FACTORS

It's just like you know how girls like they do things that they're not supposed to and they [my parents] think that I'm going to go off and do something like that, so they always want to know who I'm with and who's going if I'm [inaudible]. They're like always on your case because my dad always has a 1-hour talk before I go anywhere.

Empirical research on factors that moderate hypothesized pathways through which economic, family, and peer influences lead to problem behavior is almost nonexistent for Mexican Americans. However, theoretical perspectives regarding protective factors for Latina/os are offered frequently and have most often focused on the influence of supportive family bonds, youths' ties to their ethnic culture, and intrapersonal coping resources. Individual differences among Latina/o youth on these interrelated dimensions are thought to mitigate the negative effects of risks for problem behavior, including several of the most consistently supported pathways to problem behavior that were discussed in the previous section.

Family Support

Social support has long been considered an important factor in buffering the effects of negative life events throughout the lifespan (Barrera, 2000). Support from the family, particularly parental support, has also been central to theories about the development of a wide range of problem behaviors and to extant models of resiliency (Barrera & Li, 1996; Garmezy, 1993; Masten et al., 1999). For Mexican Americans, family support assumes added theoretical importance because it reflects cultural values about family loyalty, support, and solidarity that are paramount for this group (Keefe & Padilla, 1987). Research has shown that, although some aspects of familism change with acculturation, these values appear to be enduring for many Mexican American families (Sabogal, Marin, Otero Sabogal, Marin, & Perez-Stable, 1987).

Positive family relationships and supportive parenting were included as predictors in the empirical models presented earlier (see Figs. 5.1 and 5.2). According to these models, economic hardship and other familial and extrafamilial stressors lead to deteriorations in parents' ability to adequately support developing youths, leaving them more susceptible to associations with deviant peers. However, despite evidence to support these pathways, family conflict and economic hardship generally explain no more than a modest amount of the variance in positive family relationships or supportive parenting in these or in other similar models of Mexican Americans (e.g., Dumka, Roosa, & Jackson, 1997; Gonzales, Pitts, Hill, & Roosa, 2000). Thus, there is clearly a large percentage of families who maintain strong bonds and parents who provide ongoing support to developing youths despite such adverse conditions. Several scholars have proposed that, when family social support is maintained, it operates to decrease susceptibility of Latina/o youths to negative influences outside the family (Szapocznik, Kurtines, Santisteban, & Rio, 1990; Vega, Gil, Warheit, Zimmerman, & Apospori, 1993).

In addition to operating as a mediator in models to explain adolescent problem behavior, supportive family ties also may be important as a moderator of risks for problem behavior. Empirical evidence that supports this perspective has been provided in the general Latina/o literature. For example, Frauenglass, Routh, Pantin, and Mason (1997) investigated the interplay of family support and peer modeling on adolescent alcohol, tobacco, and marijuana use and gang involvement with a predominantly Latina/o sample of 8th-grade students in high-risk, impoverished Miami neighborhoods. They found that family social support reduced the influence of deviant peers on some of the problem behaviors reported by these adolescents, specifically tobacco and marijuana use. Similary, Wills, Vaccaro, and McNamara (1992) found that family social support buffered the effects of stress on Latina/o adolescents' alcohol and marijuana use and Warr (1993) found that the amount of time Latina/o youths spent with family members buffered the effects of deviant peers on substance use. Focusing on mechanisms of risk and protection within the family, Formoso, Gonzales, and Aiken (2000) found maternal and paternal support (attachment and monitoring) buffered the effects of family conflict on female adolescent delinquency for a multiethnic sample that included a large percentage of Mexican Americans.

Acculturation and Cultural Identification

Research has shown that Latina/o rates of problem behavior vary by acculturation and generation status, with U.S.-born and more acculturated youths displaying higher rates of externalizing behavior and involvement in delinquent activities (Fridrich & Flannery, 1995; Samaniego & Gonzales, 1999), decreased academic performance and higher dropout rates (Rumbaut, 1995), and greater involvement in risky sexual behavior (Ford & Norris, 1993), compared to immigrant or less acculturated youths (cf. Gonzales, Knight, Morgan-Lopez, Sirolli, & Saenz, 2002, for a review). A similar pattern has been reported for substance use (Brook, Whiteman, Balka, Win, & Gursen, 1998; Félix-Ortiz & Newcomb, 1995), although some of this work suggests that whereas increasing acculturation consistently leads to greater substance use for females, the pattern is less consistent for males (Amaro & Zuckerman, 1990; Polednak, 1997).

A variety of explanations have been offered to account for these trends. One set of explanations focuses on adolescents' increasing vulnerability to American peers as they become more acculturated and integrated into that culture. Brook et al. (1998), for example, suggested that, as acculturating youths become more similar to American peers, they adopt their substance-using habits and display substance use levels that are more comparable to European American samples. Research also has shown that more acculturated youths are more vulnerable to antisocial peer pressures (Fridrich & Flannery, 1995; Wall, Power, & Arbona, 1993). Wall et al. used antisocial hypothetical situations and an abridged version of an acculturation questionnaire to demonstrate an empirical link between acculturation and susceptibility to antisocial peer pressure with a sample of Mexican American early adolescents (grades 9 to 12). They suggested that parental control may be weakened as Mexican immigrant children acculturate because their parents are viewed as ineffective sources of knowledge and guidance; peers then become relatively more important behavioral models.

A second set of explanations focuses on increased stressors encountered by Latina/o youths in the process of acculturation, including discrimination and blocked opportunities, acculturation-related family disruptions and conflict, and language difficulties. The work of Vega and colleagues with Cuban and Puerto Rican adolescents (Gil, Vega, & Dimas, 1994; Vega, Khoury, Zimmerman, Gil, & Warheit, 1995) and Gonzales and colleagues with Mexican American adolescents (Samaniego & Gonzales, 1999), as well as others, has shown that these cultural conflicts are associated with higher rates of problem behavior, including delinquency (Biafora et al., 1993), substance use (Szapocznik et al., 1990), and academic problems (Okagaki, Frensch, & Dodson, 1996). This research has also shown that generational differences may be associated with differences in the types of acculturative stressors that Latina/o youths encounter and in their vulnerability to specific stressors associated with acculturation and minority status. For example, Vega et al. found that, whereas immigrant youths are more vulnerable to the effects of language conflicts, U.S.-born youths are more vulnerable to their perceptions of discrimination and blocked opportunities. They explained that adolescents born in the United States are more sensitive to the minority group definitions of self that likely emerge from their interactions in school and other settings outside the home.

A third set of explanations for the link between acculturation and problem behaviors has focused on the likelihood that more acculturated youths have less access to the traditional values, practices, and sense of shared ethnic identity that are protective for youths who maintain ties to their ethnic culture. Whereas acculturation is the process of learning about and retaining ties to the mainstream culture, enculturation is the process of learning about and maintaining ties to the ethnic culture (Gonzales, Knight, Birman, & Sirolli, in press). Extant theories about these dual processes suggest that, to the extent that individuals remain more enculturated, irrespective of how acculturated they become, they might be less vulnerable to stress caused by discrimination, poverty, unemployment, inadequate educational opportunities, a sense of powerlessness, and exposure to deviant peer models. The protective effects of enculturation might operate through traditional gender and parent roles, religious or spiritual orientation, maintenance of traditional family values that promote greater cohesiveness and support among family members, or ethnic solidarity and pride, all of which may shape adolescents' reactions and vulnerability to risks associated with problem behavior and substance use. Despite substantial focus on these processes in the theoretical literature, very few studies test them directly.

A few recent studies have shown that ethnic identity operates as a protective factor in relation to adolescents' risk for substance use. In a study of Puerto Rican adolescents living in East Harlem, Brook et al. (1998) found that being born in the United States was positively related to severity of drug use, preferring Spanish to English was inversely related to drug use, and ethnic identity was unrelated to late adolescents' drug stage. However, when ethnic identity was examined in interaction with other risk and protective factors for drug use, it was shown to protect against the effects of drug-related personal risks, family drug tolerance and modeling, peer deviant attitudes and modeling, and drug availability in predicting stage of drug use. The protective effect of viewing drugs as harmful also interacted with and was enhanced by ethnic identity factors, including a sense of attachment to one's ethnic group and identification with Puerto Rican friends, leading to a lower stage of drug use. Similar interactive effects were found in a study predicting drug and alcohol use among predominantly Mexican American adolescents in Los Angeles (Félix-Ortiz & Newcomb, 1995) and in a prospective study of risk factors predicting an increase in substance use from 7th to 8th grade among Latina/o youths in New York City (Scheier, Botvin, Diaz, & Ifill-Williams, 1997).

Several scholars have suggested that biculturalism, that is, integration with both the mainstream and ethnic cultures, might be the most adaptive form of acculturation for Latina/os and other visible minorities (e.g., Ramierez, 1984; Rogler, Cortes, & Malgady, 1991; Szapocznik & Kurtines, 1980). Bicultural individuals benefit from knowledge and participation in the host culture, while retaining the positive, protective factors of their traditional culture. In addition, biculturalism is advantageous because it allows personal flexibility to draw upon different sets of skills depending on the specific cultural demands of different situations (Birman, 1998). In support of this view, the research of Szapocznik et al. (1986) showed that interventions that promote biculturalism are effective in reducing substance abuse problems and problem behavior for Cuban American adolescents. Similarly, Rumberger and Larson (1998) found that bilingual Mexican American students have better grades and complete more credits than either limited-English proficiency students or English-only students. However, more research is needed to explore the complex dynamics of biculturalism and whether it affects Mexican American adolescents' risk for problem behavior.

The picture that emerges from research on cultural identity is quite mixed, with far more studies reporting null or inconsistent findings. Several scholars have argued that such inconsistencies reflect the fact that the link between enculturation or ethnic identity and problem behaviors such as substance use is far more complex than is typically supposed in the literature (Oetting, Donnermeyer, Trimble, & Beauvais, 1998; Schinke, Moncher, Palleja, Zayas, & Schilling, 1988). Previous studies have generally failed to account for the broader context and corresponding values to which youths may be enculturating. Some social environments, for example, many urban barrios, engender subcultures with attitudes and perceptions conducive to the development of delinquent subcultures (Rodriguez & Zayas, 1990). Consequently, Oetting and Beauvais (1990/1991) emphasized that, depending on the particular cultural or subcultural reference group, a strong cultural identification may operate to potentiate rather than protect against culturally prescribed behaviors. To illustrate with an example that also relates to the role of family support, MacNeil, Kaufman, Dressler, and LeCroy (1999) found that strong family ties were negatively associated with adolescent substance use. However, among adolescents whose family members used drugs or alcohol, adolescents who felt more accepted, valued, and cared for by significant others in their lives were more likely to use drugs or alcohol than those who felt less accepted, valued, or cared for. Oetting and Beauvais (1990/1991) proposed that, to understand the links between cultural identification and drug use, the following connections have to be assessed and examined interactively: process (patterns of identification), content (cultural and gender roles), peer relationships, and environmental factors.

INTRAPERSONAL RESOURCES FOR COPING WITH ADVERSITY

Research has identified intrapersonal resources that might protect youths who are exposed to risk factors for a variety of problem behaviors, including a variety of self-system processes (e.g, control-related beliefs, efficacy, self-esteem, attributional processes) that have been shown to influence child and adolescent adjustment (Bandura, 1989; Sandler, Kim-Bae, & McKinnon, 2000) as well as the specific skills and competencies used to cope with life stress (Compas, Malcarne, & Fondacaro, 1988). For example, research has shown that positive future expectations represent an important protective factor for highly stressed children (Werner & Smith, 1992; Wyman, Cowen, Work, & Kerley, 1993). Positive future expectations and visions of oneself in the future—called possible selves—are important motivators of present behavior (Markus & Nurius, 1986). Motivation to engage in behavior to attain possible selves increases when individuals have more concrete, elaborated, and positive visions of themselves in the future (e.g., me as a high school graduate) that are balanced by negative visions in the same domain (e.g., me as a high school dropout) (Oyserman & Markus, 1990). Research with disadvantaged inner-city samples has shown that when youths have balanced possible selves they tend to perform better in school and are less impulsive, more competent at social problem-solving, more likely to show school persistence, and less likely to be delinquent (Oyserman, Gant, & Ager, 1995; Oyserman & Saltz, 1993).

Theories about the role of possible selves and future expectations are particularly relevant to Mexican American youths. Many of these youths must seek out and sustain a sense of positive possibilities for the self within social contexts (e.g., low education, under- or unemployment, negative stereotypes) that do not afford construction of plausible futures in which conventional paths, such as school success, lead to occupational success in adulthood. It has been previously argued that many Mexican American and African American youths initially view association with delinquent peers as a means to create selves that they could become (Oyserman & Markus, 1990); delinquency may be a means to attain such possible selves as independent, daring, competent, or fun-loving and adventurous. The negative consequences of delinquency might not be taken into account initially, especially by youths who lack balanced possible selves.

Although research on possible selves and other self-system variables has rarely included Mexican American youths, there is some preliminary evidence to indicate the potential importance of such variables in models of problem behavior for Mexican American youth. MacNeil et al. (1999) tested a model of social influence on substance use that focused on adolescents' social networks and their attitudes about their own futures with a predominantly Mexican American sample of 11- to 15-year-olds. By far the most important predictors of adolescent substance use were the number of family members or friends who used drugs or alcohol. Adolescent beliefs about their future had a direct effect on their substance use and also a moderating effect whereby friends' use was significantly less predictive for adolescents who were optimistic about their future.

Research has identified cognitive and behavioral coping strategies that predict better mental health outcomes and provide protection against the negative effects of stress (Sandler, Tein, & West, 1994). A few recent studies have demonstrated the protective effects of coping for inner-city youths, including a substantial number of Mexican Americans (Gonzales, Tein, Sandler, & Friedman, 2001; Tolan, Guerra, & Montaini-Klovdahl, 1997). Gonzales et al. used a confirmatory factor-analytic approach to test a model for the assessment of coping with a multiethnic, inner-city sample. The four-factor model, initially validated with a nonurban sample (Ayers, Sandler, West, & Roosa, 1996), provided a good fit to the data for the assessment of coping across three ethnic groups and for both English-speaking and Spanish-speaking Mexican Americans. The four factors included: (a) active coping (cognitive decision making, direct problem solving, seeking understanding, and positive cognitive restructuring), (b) avoidance (cognitive avoidance and avoidant action), (c) distraction (distracting action and physical release of emotion), and (d) support seeking (emotion-focused support and problem-focused support). This study found evidence for the effects of active coping, support seeking, and distraction in predicting fewer conduct problems and higher grades, and some support for the stress-buffering effects of active coping and distraction. Active coping and distraction buffered the relation between family stress and conduct problems and between community stress and grades for girls. However, at high levels of these stressors, active coping had no effect on conduct problems or grades for boys. The findings also showed that avoidant coping was associated with increased conduct problems and lower grades under low to moderate levels of these stressors. However, at high levels of stressors, avoidance predicted decreased conduct problems and, for girls, better grades. The authors explained that many of the family and community stressors experienced by these inner-city adolescents were uncontrollable and that, at high levels of uncontrollable stressors, active coping might be less effective and avoidance more adaptive for inner-city youths.

Almost 20 years ago, the first author wrote a chapter (Barrera, Zautra, & Baca, 1984) for the second edition of *Chicano Psychology* (Martinez & Mendoza, 1984) on the stress and distress of Mexican Americans, based on sparse data on Mexican American adults and children and extrapolations from relevant studies on non-Latina/o samples. It contained much speculation and a hypothetical model of culture's influence on stress-distress processes. Enough progress has been made since then to allow us to write a data-based review of the much narrower topic of adolescent problem behavior. Despite the progress, however, the literature is seldom specific to Mexican-heritage adolescents and, thus, invites questions about the generalizability of findings based on Latina/o subsamples. Moreover, because of the prevalence of school dropout among Chicana/o youth, it will be particularly critical to conduct research with household-based samples rather than relying on school samples.

From the available data, it appears that problem behavior, particularly school dropout, among Mexican American youth is high relative to other ethnic groups. This kind of comparative research is often criticized because it runs the risk of conclusions that blame the culture. After all, if ethnic and racial groups constitute the basis of comparison, there is some real danger that differences will be attributed to the quasi-independent variable in these correlational design studies. Obviously, any attributions to cultural deficits as the cause of ethnic group differences are unjustified. Nevertheless, ethnic group comparisons do have some value as reference points for determining those topics that might have special merit for research and perhaps intervention.

With a few exceptions, the risk and protective factors that appear to contribute to Mexican American adolescents' problem behavior are the same as those related to the problem behaviors of other adolescents. Community stressors, family conflict, supportive parenting, parental supervision, associations with deviant peers, and coping are constructs that are familiar to researchers who study adolescents of any ethnic group in the United States. It is arguable that we know enough at this point to divert more resources into intervention research designed to change these risk and protective factors, in studies with experimental designs that are intended to prevent or reduce adolescent problem behaviors. Acculturation, the stress of immigration, and ethnic identity are topics that have some unique features for Mexican American adolescents, yet they also present considerable complexities. Future research could bring some clarity to their potential relations to adolescent problem behaviors. Finally, more research could be devoted to understanding the development of competencies and talents among Mexican American youth. It would be unfortunate if the present emphasis on adolescent problem behavior was interpreted as an indication that problem behaviors define the lives of Mexican American youth or that they should be the sole focus of our efforts.

REFERENCES

Adler, P., Ovando, C., & Hocevar, D. (1994). Familiar correlates of gang membership: An exploratory study of Mexican-American youth. *Hispanic Journal of Behavioral Sciences, 6,* 65–76.

Alan Guttmacher Institute. (1994). *Sex and America's teenagers.* New York: Alan Guttmacher Institute.

Allen, L., & Mitchell, C. (1998). Racial and ethnic differences in patterns of problematic and adaptive development: An epidemiological review. In V. C. McLoyd & L. Steinberg (Eds.), *Studying minority adolescents: Conceptual, methodological, and theoretical issues* (pp. 29–54). Mahwah, NJ: Lawrence Erlbaum Associates.

Amaro, H., & Zuckerman, B. S. (1990). Patterns and prevalence of drug use among adolescent mothers. In A. R. Stiffman & R. A. Feldman (Eds.), *Contraception, pregnancy, and parenting: Advances in adolescent mental health* (Vol. 4, pp. 203–221). London: Kingsley.

Ary, D. V., Duncan, T. E., Biglan, A., Metzler, C. W., Noell, J. W., & Smolkowski, K. (1999). Development of adolescent problem behavior. *Journal of Abnormal Child Psychology, 27,* 141–150.

Ary, D. V., Duncan, T. E., Duncan, S, C., & Hops, H. (1999). Adolescent problem behavior: The influence of parents and peers. *Behaviour Research and Therapy, 37,* 217–230.

Ayers, T. S., Sandler, I. N., West, S. G., & Roosa, M. W. (1996). A dispositional and situational assessment of children's coping: Testing alternative models of coping. *Journal of Personality, 64,* 923–958.

Bandura, A. (1989). Regulation of cognitive processes through perceived self-efficacy. *Developmental Psychology, 25,* 729–735.

Barrera, M., Jr. (2000). Social support research in community psychology. In J. Rappaport & E. Seidman (Eds.), *Handbook of community psychology* (pp. 215–245). New York: Plenum Press.

Barrera, M., Jr., Biglan, A., Ary, D., & Li, F. (2001). Modeling parental and peer influences on problem behavior of American Indian, Hispanic, and non-Hispanic Caucasian youth. *Journal of Early Adolescence, 21,* 133–156.

Barrera, M., Jr., & Li, S. A. (1996). The relation of family support to adolescents' psychological distress and problem behaviors. In G. R. Pierce, I. Sarason, & B. Sarason (Eds.), *The handbook of social support and family relationships* (pp. 313–343). New York: Plenum Press.

Barrera, M., Jr., Li, S. A., & Chassin, L. (1993). Ethnic group differences in vulnerability to parental alcoholism and life stress: A study of Hispanic and non-Hispanic Caucasian adolescents. *American Journal of Community Psychology, 21,* 15–35.

Barrera, M., Jr., Li, S. A., & Chassin, L. (1995). Effects of parental alcoholism and life stress on Hispanic and non-Hispanic Caucasian adolescents: A prospective study. *American Journal of Community Psychology, 23,* 479–507.

Barrera, M., Jr., Prelow, H. M., Dumka, L. E., Gonzales, N. A., Knight, G. P., Michaels, M. L., Roosa, M. W., & Tein, J. Y. (2002). Pathways from family economic conditions to adolescents' distress: Supportive parenting, stressors outside the family, and deviant peers. *Journal of Community Psychology, 30,* 135–152.

Barrera, M., Jr., Zautra, A., & Baca, L. M. (1984). Some research considerations in studying stress and distress of Mexican Americans. In J. L. Martinez & R. H. Mendoza (Eds.), *Chicano psychology* (2nd ed., pp. 223–247). New York: Academic Press.

Baumrind, D. (1987). A developmental perspective on adolescent risk taking in contemporary America. In C. E. Irwin, Jr. (Ed.), *Adolescent social behavior and health* (pp. 93–125). San Francisco: Jossey-Bass.

Biafora, F. A., Warheit, G. J., Zimmerman, R. S., Gil, A. G., Apospori, E., & Taylor, D. (1993). Racial mistrust and deviant behaviors among ethnically diverse Black adolescent boys. *Journal of Applied Social Psychology, 23,* 891–910.

Birman, D. (1998). Biculturalism and perceived competence of Latino immigrant adolescents. *American Journal of Community Psychology, 26,* 335–354.

Brook, J. S., Whiteman, M., Balka, E. B., Win, P. T., & Gursen, M. D. (1998). Drug use among Puerto Ricans: Ethnic identity as a protective factor. *Hispanic Journal of Behavioral Sciences, 20,* 241–254.

Brooks-Gunn, J., & Duncan, G. J. (1997). The effects of poverty on children. *The Future of Children, 7,* 56–71.

Centers for Disease Control. (1991, May). Childbearing patterns among selected racial/ethnic minority groups—United States, 1990. *Morbidity and Mortality Weekly Report, 42,* 398–403.

Chassin, L., Barrera, M., Jr., & Montgomery, H. (1997). Parent alcoholism as a risk factor. In S. Wolchik & I. N. Sandler (Eds.), *Handbook of children's coping with common life stressors: Linking theory, research, and interventions* (pp. 101–129). New York: Plenum Press.

Chassin, L., Curran, P. J., Hussong, A. M., & Colder, C. R. (1996). The relation of parent alcoholism to adolescent substance use: A longitudinal follow-up study. *Journal of Abnormal Psychology, 105,* 70–80.

Chassin, L., Pillow, D. R., Curran, P. J., Molina, B. S. G., & Barrera, M., Jr. (1993). Relation of parent alcoholism to early adolescent substance use: A test of three mediating mechanisms. *Journal of Abnormal Psychology, 102,* 3–19.

Chavez, E. L., & Swaim, R. C. (1992). An epidemiological comparison of Mexican-American and White non-Hispanic 8th- and 12th-grade students' substance use. *American Journal of Public Health, 82,* 445–447.

Chavez, J. M., & Roney, C. E. (1990). Psychocultural factors affecting the mental health status of Mexican American adolescents. In A. R. Stiffman & L. E. Davis (Eds.), *Ethnic issues in adolescent mental health* (pp. 73–91). Newbury Park, CA: Sage.

Chesney-Lind, M., & Shelden, R. (1998). *Girls, delinquency, and juvenile justice* (2nd ed.). Belmont, CA: Wadsworth.

Compas, B. E., Malcarne, V. L., & Fondacaro, R. M. (1988). Coping with stressful events in older children and young adolescents. *Journal of Consulting and Clinical Psychology, 56,* 405–411.

Conger, R. D., & Elder, G. H., Jr. (1994). *Families in troubled times: Adapting to change in rural America.* New York: de Gruyter.

Curry, D., & Spergel, I. (1992). Gang involvement and delinquency among Hispanic and African American males. *Journal of Research in Crime and Delinquency, 29,* 273–291.

Delgado, M. (1990). Hispanic adolescents and substance abuse: Implications for research, treatment, and prevention. In A. R. Stiffman & L. E. Davis (Eds.), *Ethnic issues in adolescent mental health* (pp. 303–320). Newbury Park, CA: Sage.

Dumka, L. E., Roosa, M. W., & Jackson, K. M. (1997). Risk, conflict, mother's parenting, and children's adjustment in low-income, Mexican immigrant, and Mexican American families. *Journal of Marriage and the Family, 59,* 309–323.

Duncan, G. J., & Brooks-Gunn, J. (Eds.). (1997). *Consequences of growing up poor.* New York: Russell Sage Foundation.

DuRant, R. H., Seymore, C., Pendergrast, R., & Beckman, R. (1990). Contraceptive behavior among sexually active Hispanic adolescents. *Journal of Adolescent Health Care, 11,* 490–496.

Félix-Ortiz, M., & Newcomb, M. D. (1992). Risk and protective factors for drug use among Latino and White adolescents. *Hispanic Journal of Behavioral Sciences, 14,* 291–309.

Félix-Ortiz, M., & Newcomb, M. D. (1995). Cultural identity and drug use among Latino and Latina adolescents. In G. J. Botvin (Ed.), *Drug abuse prevention with multi-ethnic youth* (pp. 147–165). Newbury Park, CA: Sage.

Fingerhut, L. A. & Kleinman, J. C. (1990). International and interstate comparisons of homicide among young males. *Journal of the American Medical Association, 263,* 3292–3295.

Flannery, D. J., Vazsonyi, A. T., & Rowe, D. C. (1996). Caucasian and Hispanic early adolescent substance use: Parenting, personality, and school adjustment. *Journal of Early Adolescence, 16,* 71–89.

Ford, K., & Norris, A. E. (1993). Urban Hispanic adolescents and young adults: Relationship of acculturation to sexual behavior. *Journal of Sex Research, 30,* 316–323.

Formoso, D., Gonzales, N. A., & Aiken, L. (2000). Family conflict and children's internalizing and externalizing: Protective factors. *American Journal of Community Psychology, 28,* 175–199.

Frauenglass, S., Routh, D. K., Pantin, H. M., & Mason, C. A. (1997) Family support decreases influence of deviant peers on Hispanic adolescents' substance use. *Journal of Clinical Child Psychology, 16,* 15–23.

Fridrich, A. H., & Flannery, D. J. (1995). The effects of ethnicity and acculturation on early adolescent delinquency. *Journal of Child and Family Studies, 4,* 69–87.

Gil, A. G., Vega, W. A., & Dimas, J. M. (1994). Acculturative stress and personal adjustment among Hispanic adolescent boys. *Journal of Community Psychology, 22,* 43–54.

Gonzales, N. A., Knight, G. P., Birman, D., & Sirolli, A. (in press). Acculturation and enculturation among Hispanic youths. In C. Schellenbach, K. Maton, B. Leadbetter, & A. Solarz (Eds.), *Investing in children, families, and communities: Strengths-based research and policy.* Washington, DC: American Psychological Association.

Gonzales, N. A., Knight, G. P., Morgan-Lopez, A., Saenz, D., & Sirolli, A. (2002). Acculturation and the mental health of Latino youths: An integration and critique of the literature. In J. M. Contreras, K. A. Kerns, & A. M. Neal-Barnett (Eds.), *Latino children and families in the United States* (pp. 45–74). Westport, CT: Greenwood.

Gonzales, N. A., Pitts, S. C., Hill, N. E., & Roosa, M. W. (2000). A mediational model of the impact of interparental conflict on child adjustment in a multiethnic, low-income sample. *Journal of Family Psychology, 14,* 365–379.

Gonzales, N. A., Tein, J., Sandler, I. N., & Friedman, R. J. (2001). On the limits of coping: Interactions between stress and coping for inner-city adolescents. *Journal of Adolescent Research, 16,* 372–395.

Gullotta, T. P., Adams, G. R., & Markstrom, C. A. (2000). *The adolescent experience* (4th ed,). San Diego: Academic Press.

Hauser, R. M., Simmons, S. J., & Pager, D. I. (2000, January). *High school dropout, race-ethnicity, and social background from the 1970s to the 1990s.* Paper presented at the forum of The Civil Rights Project at Harvard University's Graduate School of Education and Achieve, Inc., Cambridge, MA.

Hawkins, J. D., Catalano, R. F., & Miller, J. Y. (1992). Risk and protective factors for alcohol and other drug problems in adolescence and early adulthood: Implications for substance abuse prevention. *Psychological Bulletin, 112,* 64–105.

Hodges, B. C., Leavy, M., Swift, R., & Gold, R. S. (1992). Gender and ethnic differences in adolescents' attitudes toward condom use. *Journal of School Health, 62,* 103–106.

Jessor, R., Donovan, J. E., & Costa, F. M. (1991). *Beyond adolescence: Problem behavior and young adult development*. Cambridge, UK: Cambridge University Press.

Johnson, L. D., O'Malley, P. M., & Bachman, J. G. (2000). *Monitoring the future: National survey results on drug use, 1975–1999: Vol. 1. Secondary school students* (NIH Publication No. 00-4802). Bethesda, MD: National Institute on Drug Abuse.

Kandel, D. (1995). Ethnic differences in drug use: Patterns and paradoxes. In G. J. Botvin, S. Schinke, & M. A. Orlandi (Eds.), *Drug abuse prevention with multiethnic youth* (pp. 81–104). Thousand Oaks, CA: Sage.

Kandel, D., Yamaguchi, K., & Chen, K. (1992). Stages of progression in drug involvement from adolescence to adulthood: Further evidence for the gateway theory. *Journal of Studies on Alcohol, 53*, 447–458.

Kaufman, P., Kwon, J. Y., Klein, S., & Chapman, C. D. (2000). *Dropout rates in the United States: 1999* (NCES Publication No. 2001-022). Washington, DC: U.S. Government Printing Office.

Keefe, S. E., & Padilla, A. M. (1987). *Chicano ethnicity*. Albuquerque: University of New Mexico Press.

Kessler, R. C., McGonagle, K. A., Zhao, S., Nelson, C. B., Hughes, M., Eshleman, S., Wittchen, H. U., & Kendler, K. S. (1994). Lifetime and 12-month prevalence of DSM-III-R psychiatric disorders in the United States. *Archives of General Psychiatry, 51*, 8–19.

Lindeman, C., & Scott, W. (1982). The fertility related behavior of Mexican American adolescents. *Journal of Early Adolescence, 2*, 31–38.

MacNeil, G., Kaufman, A. V., Dressler, W. W., & LeCroy, C. W. (1999). Psychosocial moderators of substance use among middle school-aged adolescents. *Journal of Drug Education, 29*, 25–39.

Maddahian, E., Newcomb, M. D., & Bentler, P. M. (1988). Risk factors for substance use: Ethnic differences among adolescents. *Journal of Substance Abuse, 1*, 11–23.

Markus, H., & Nurius, N. (1986). Possible selves. *American Psychologist, 41*, 954–969.

Martinez, J. L., & Mendoza, R. H. (Eds.). (1984). *Chicano psychology* (2nd ed.). New York: Academic Press.

Masten, A. S., Hubbard, J. J., Gest, S., Tellegan, A, Garmezy, N., & Ramirez, M. (1999). Competence in the context of adversity: Pathways to resilience and maladaptation from childhood to late adolescence. *Development and Psychopathology, 11*, 143–169.

McGee, L., & Newcomb, M. D. (1992). General deviance syndrome: Expanded hierarchical evaluations at four ages from early adolescence to adulthood. *Journal of Consulting and Clinical Psychology, 60*, 766–776.

Moffitt, T., Caspi, A., Dickson, N., Silva, P., & Stanton, W. (1996). Childhood-onset versus adolescent-onset antisocial conduct problems in males: Natural history from ages 3 to 18 years, *Development and Psychopathology, 8*, 399–424.

National Center for Education Statistics. (1992, August). *Are Hispanic dropout rates related to migration?* (Issue Brief No. NCES-92-098). Washington, DC: Author.

National Center for Children in Poverty. (1998). Young children in poverty: A statistical update (March 1998 ed.). Retrieved April 22, 1999, from *http://cpmcnet.columbia.edu/dept/nccp/98uptext.html*

National Center for Health Statistics. (2000). *Health, United States, 2000 with adolescent health chartbook* (DHHS Publication No. PHS 2000-1232-1). Washington, DC: U.S. Government Printing Office.

National Center for Health Statistics. (2001, July). New CDC report shows teen birth rate hits record low: U.S. births top 4 million. *HHS News* [On-line]. Available: http://www.cdc.gov/nchs/releases/01news/newbirth.htm

Newcomb, M. D. (1987). Consequences of teenage drug use: The transition from adolescence to young adulthood. *Drugs and Society, 1*, 25–60.

Newcomb, M. D. (1995). Drug use etiology among ethnic minority adolescents: Risk and protective factors. In G. J. Botvin, S. Schinke, & M. A. Orlandi (Eds.), *Drug abuse prevention with multiethnic youth* (pp. 105–129). Thousand Oaks, CA: Sage.

Newcomb, M. D., & Bentler, P. M. (1988). *Consequences of adolescent drug use: Impact on the lives of young adults*. Newbury Park, CA: Sage.

Newcomb, M. D., Maddahian, E., & Bentler, P. M. (1986). Risk factors for drug use among adolescents: Concurrent and longitudinal analysis. *American Journal of Public Health, 76*, 525–531.

Oetting, E. R., & Beauvais, F. (1990). Adolescent drug use: Findings of national and local surveys. *Journal of Consulting and Clinical Psychology, 58*, 385–394.

Oetting, E. R., & Beauvais, F. (1990/1991). Orthogonal cultural identification theory: The cultural identification of minority adolescents. *The International Journal of the Addictions, 25*, 655–685.

Oetting, E. R., Donnermeyer, J. F., Trimble, J. E., & Beauvais, F. (1998). Primary socialization theory: Culture, ethnicity, and cultural identification. The links between culture and substance use. *Substance Use and Misuse, 33*, 2075–2107.

Office of Juvenile Justice and Delinquency Prevention (n.d.). Census of Juveniles in Residential Placement Databook 1997 and 1999. Retrieved January 14, 2002 from http://ojjdp.ncjrs.org/ojstatbb/cjrp/

Office of Juvenile Justice and Delinquency Prevention (1998, December). *1997 National Gang Youth Gang Survey Summary* (NCJ178891). Retrieved January 14, 2002 from http://www.ncjrs.org/html.ojjdp/97_ygs/contents.html

Office of Juvenile Justice and Delinquency Prevention (1999, December). *Minorities in the Juvenile Justice System 1999 National Report Series Juvenile Justice Bulletin* (NCJ179007). Retrieved January 14, 2002, from *http://www.ncjrs.org/html/ojjdp/9912_1/min2.html*

Okagaki, L., Frensch, P. A., & Dodson, N. E. (1996). Mexican American children's perceptions of self and school achievement. *Hispanic Journal of Behavioral Sciences, 18,* 469–484.

Oyserman, D., Gant, L., & Ager, J. (1995). A socially contextualized model of African American identity: Possible selves and school persistence. *Journal of Personality and Social Psychology, 69,* 1216–1232.

Oyserman, D., & Markus, H. (1990). Possible selves in balance: Implications for delinquency. *Journal of Social Issues, 2,* 141–157.

Oyserman, D., & Saltz, E. (1993). Competence, delinquency, and attempts to attain possible selves. *Journal of Personality and Social Psychology, 65,* 360–374.

Patterson, G. R., DeBaryshe, B. D., & Ramsey, E. (1989). A developmental perspective on antisocial behavior. *American Psychologist, 44,* 329–335.

Peterson, A. C. (1993). Creating adolescents: The role of context and process in developmental trajectories. *Journal of Research on Adolescence, 3,* 1–18.

Peterson, A. C., & Hamburg, B. A. (1986). Adolescence: A developmental approach to problems and psychopathology. *Behavior Therapy, 17,* 480–499.

Polednak, A. P. (1997). Gender and acculturation in relation to alcohol use among Hispanic (Latino) adults in two areas of the Northeastern United States. *Substance Use and Misuse, 32,* 1513–1524.

Prinz, R. & Miller, G. (1991). Issues in understanding and treating childhood conduct problems in disadvantaged populations. *Journal of Clinical Child Psychology, 20,* 379–385.

Ramirez, M., II. (1984). Assessing and understanding biculturalism-multiculturalism. In J. L. Martinez and R. H. Mendoza (Eds.), *Chicano psychology* (2nd ed., pp. 77–94). New York: Academic Press.

Robins, L. N., & Regier, D. A. (1991). *Psychiatric disorders in America: The Epidemiologic Catchment Area study* (pp. 81–115). New York: Free Press.

Rodriguez, O., & Zayas, L. H. (1990). Hispanic adolescents and antisocial behavior: Sociocultural factors and treatment implications. In A. R. Stiffman & L. E. Davis (Eds.), *Ethnic issues in adolescent mental health* (pp. 147–171). Thousand Oaks, CA: Sage.

Rogler, L. H., Cortes, D. E., Malgady, R. G. (1991). Acculturation and mental health status among Hispanics: Convergence and new directions for research. *American Psychologist, 46,* 585–597.

Roosa, M. W., Tein, J. Y., Groppenbacher, N., Michaels, M., & Dumka, L. (1993). Mothers' parenting behavior and child mental health in families with a problem drinking parent. *Journal of Marriage and the Family, 55,* 107–118.

Rumbaut, R. G. (1995). The new Californians: Comparative research findings on the educational progress of immigrant children. In R. G. Rumbaut & W. A. Cornelius, (Eds.), *California's immigrant children: Theory, research and implications for educational policy* (pp. 17–69). San Diego, CA: Center for U.S.-Mexican Studies.

Rumberger, R. W., & Larson, K. A. (1998). Toward explaining differences in educational achievement among Mexican American language-minority students. *Sociology of Education, 17,* 69–93.

Sabogal, F., Marin, G., Otero-Sabogal, R., Marin, B. V., & Perez-Stable, E. J. (1987). Hispanic familism and acculturation: What changes and what doesn't? *Hispanic Journal of Behavioral Sciences, 9,* 397–412.

Samaniego, R. Y., & Gonzales, N. A. (1999). Multiple mediators of the effects of acculturation status on delinquency for Mexican American adolescents. *American Journal of Community Psychology, 27,* 189–210.

Sandler, I. N., Kim-Bae, L. S., & MacKinnon, D. (2000). Coping and negative appraisal as mediators between control beliefs and psychological symptoms in children of divorce. *Journal of Clinical Child Psychology, 29,* 336–347.

Sandler, I. N., Tein, J., & West, S. (1994). Coping, stress, and the psychological symptoms of children of divorce: A cross-sectional and longitudinal study. *Child Development, 65,* 1744–1763.

Scalia, J. (1996). Noncitizens in the federal criminal justice system, 1984–94. Bureau of Justice Statistics Special Report (NCJ 160934). Retrieved December 31, 2003 from http://www.ojp.usdoj.gov/bjs/pub/pdf/nifcjs.pdf

Scheier, L. M., Botvin, G. J., Diaz, T., & Ifill-Williams, M. (1997). Ethnic identity as a moderator of psychosocial risk and adolescent alcohol and marijuana use: Concurrent and longitudinal analyses. *Journal of Child and Adolescent Substance Abuse, 6,* 21–47.

Schinke, S. P., Moncher, M. S., Palleja, J., Zayas, L. H., & Schilling, R. F. (1988). Hispanic youth, substance abuse and stress: Implications for prevention research. *International Journal of the Addictions, 23,* 809–826.

Singh, S., & Darroch, J. E. (1999). Trends in sexual activity among adolescent American women: 1982–1995. *Family Planning Perspectives, 31,* 212–219.

Swaim, R. C., Beauvais, F., Chavez, E. L., & Oetting, E. R. (1997). The effect of school dropout rates on estimates of adolescent substance use among three racial/ethnic groups. *American Journal of Public Health, 87,* 51–55.

Steinberg, L., Dornbusch, S. M., & Brown, B. B. (1992). Ethnic differences in adolescent achievement: An ecological perspective. *American Psychologist, 47,* 723–729.

Szapocznik, J., & Kurtines, W. M. (1980). Acculturation, biculturalism and adjustment among Cuban Americans. In A. M. Padilla (Ed.), *Acculturation: Theory, models, and some new findings* (pp. 139–159). Boulder, CO: Westview Press.

Szapocznik, J., Kurtines, W., Santisteban, D. A., & Rio, A. T. (1990). Interplay of advances between theory, research, and application in treatment interventions aimed at behavior problem children and adolescents. *Journal of Consulting and Clinical Psychology, 58,* 696–703.

Szapocznik, J., Rio, A., Perez-Vidal, A., Kurtines, W., Hervis, O., & Santisteban, D. (1986). Bicultural Effectiveness Training: An experimental test of an intervention modality for families experiencing intergenerational/intercultural conflict. *Hispanic Journal of Behavioral Sciences, 8,* 303–330.

Tolan, P. H., Guerra, N. G., & Montaini-Klovdahl, L. R. (1997). Staying out of harm's way: Coping and the development of inner-city children. In S. A. Wolchik & I. N. Sandler (Eds.), *Handbook of children's coping: Linking theory, research, and interventions* (pp. 453–479). New York: Plenum Press.

U.S. Census Bureau (2002, January). United States Census 2000 population by race and Hispanic or Latino Origin for the United States: 1990 and 2000 (PHC-T-1). Retrieved February 10, 2003 from http://www.census.gov/population/www.cen2000/phc-t1.html

Vazsonyi, A. T., & Flannery, D. J. (1997). Early adolescent delinquent behaviors: Associations with family and school domains. *Journal of Early Adolescence, 17,* 271–293.

Vega, W. A., Gil, A. G., Warheit, G. J., Zimmerman, R. S., & Apospori, E. (1993). Acculturation and delinquent behavior among Cuban American adolescents: Toward an empirical model. *American Journal of Community Psychology, 21,* 113–125.

Vega, W. A., Khoury, E. L., Zimmerman, R. S., Gil, A. G., & Warheit, G. J. (1995). Cultural conflicts and problem behaviors of Latino adolescents in home and school environments. *Journal of Community Psychology, 23,* 167–179.

Vega, W. A., Zimmerman, R. S., Warheit, G. J., Apospori, E., & Gil, A. G. (1993). Risk factors for early adolescent drug use in four ethnic and racial groups. *American Journal of Public Health, 83,* 185–189.

Wall, J. A., Power, T. G., & Arbona, C. (1993). Susceptibility to antisocial peer pressure and its relation to acculturation in Mexican American adolescents. *Journal of Adolescent Research, 8,* 403–418.

Warr, M. (1993). Parents, peers, and delinquency. *Social Forces, 72,* 247–264.

Warren, C. W., Santelli, J. S., Everett, S. A., Kann, L., Collins, J. L., Cassell, C., Morris, L., & Kolbe, L. J. (1998). Sexual behavior among U.S. high school students, 1990–1995. *Family Planning Perspectives, 30,* 170–172, 200.

Watts, W. D., & Wright, L. S. (1990). The relationship of alcohol, tobacco, marijuana, and other illegal drug use to delinquency among Mexican-American, Black, and White adolescent males. *Adolescence, 25,* 171–181.

Werner, E. E., & Smith, R. S. (1992). *Overcoming the odds: High risk children from birth to adulthood.* Ithaca, NY: Cornell University Press.

Wills, T. A., Vaccaro, D., & McNamara, G. (1992). The role of life events, family support, and competence in adolescent substance use: A test of vulnerability and protective factors. *American Journal of Community Psychology, 20,* 349–374.

Wilson, S. (2001, October 14). 5 key factors threaten Arizona's economy. *The Arizona Republic,* p. A1.

Wyman, P. A., Cowen, E. L., Work, W. C., & Kerley, J. H. (1993). The role of children's future expectations in self-system functioning and adjustment to life stress: A prospective study of urban at-risk children. *Development and Psychopathology, 5,* 649–661.

Folk Healing and Curanderismo Within the Contemporary Chicana/o Community: Current Status

Martin Harris
Vanguard University of Southern California

Roberto J. Velásquez
San Diego State University

Jerre White
Teresa Renteria
Vanguard University of Southern California

> *Culture creates characteristic types of conflicts that are handled in both healthy and unhealthy ways depending on the individual, his personal history, his constitution or inherited equipment, and his life experiences.*
>
> —Kiev (1968, p. x)

The study of alternative methods of healing has a long tradition in the psychological, psychiatric, medical, and anthropological literature. Researchers all over the world have studied different peoples and cultures to determine the origins, definitions, and treatments of illness, whether psychological, medical, or culture bound (Jilek, 1994; Koss-Chioino, 1995; Lefley, Sandoval, & Charles, 1998; Ness & Wintrob, 1981; Tseng & Streltzer, 2001; Westermeyer, 1985; Wing, 1998). For example, researchers have attempted to identify world views, indigenous belief systems, culture- or religion-based attributions about illness, and systems of classification of illness that are unique to specific cultural groups. In many cases, they have attempted to determine whether such healing practices parallel Western methods of understanding and treating illness, the salient curative factors that contribute to resilience and mental health, and the "power" and "magic" of belief systems in protecting persons from illness. Researchers have also attempted to explain why such beliefs are maintained in light of medical and psychiatric advances and how such beliefs affect the utilization of medical and psychiatric services.

A systematic review of the literature indicates that research on healing practices, the role of healers and shamans in indigenous communities, and the use of alternative forms of medicine continues to grow (Harris, 1998; Harris & Harris, 1994). A glimpse at international publications indicates that recent studies have examined healing practices in Japan (Etsuko, 1991), China (Li & Phillips, 1990), Indonesia (Krippner, 1984), Southeast Asia (Heinze, 1985), Italy (Giovetti, 1984), and Peru (Dobkin, 1968), just to name a few geographic locales.

In the United States, researchers have examined the folk beliefs of African Americans (e.g., Parks, 1997), Greek immigrants (e.g., Tripp-Reimer, 1983), and Latina/os (e.g., Baez & Hernandez, 2001; Cervantes & Ramirez, 1992; De la Cancela & Martinez, 1983; Falicov, 1999; Lefley, 1981; Ruiz, 1977; Ruiz & Langrod, 1976; Schwartz, 1985). More specifically within the Latina/o community, investigators have focused on Puerto Ricans and espiritismo (e.g., Delgado, 1988; Fernandez, 1987; Perez y Mena, 1977; Suarez, Raffaelli, & O'Leary, 1996), Cubans and santeria (e.g., Alonso & Jeffrey, 1988; Garcia, 1980; Martinez & Wetli, 1982; Santi, 1997), and Chicana/os and curanderismo (e.g., Edgerton, Karno, & Fernandez, 1970; Kiev, 1968; Slessinger & Richards, 1981; Trotter, 1982).

Curanderismo is the most widely studied of all belief systems in the social science literature (e.g., Alegria, Guerra, Martinez, & Meyer, 1977; Applewhite, 1995; Del Castillo, 1999; Edgerton et al., 1970; Gafner & Duckett, 1992; Gangotena-Gonzalez, 1980; Gilestra, 1981; Guajardo, 1999; Hockmeyer, 1991; Kiev, 1968; Krajewski-Jaime, 1991; Kramer, 1996; Krassner, 1986; Kreisman, 1975; Lauren, 1987; Lawrence, Bozzetti, & Kane, 1976; Rivera, 1988; Slessinger & Richards, 1981; Trotter, 1982; Velez-Ibanez, & Parra, 1999; Weclew, 1975). This makes sense given the fact that persons of Mexican descent compose the largest subgroup of all Latina/os in the United States, especially in the Southwest. It is often said that a Chicana/o is more likely to know where the nearest curandera/o's practice is located than a medical doctor's.

Curanderismo or faith healing is a Mexican American folk-healing practice. The curendero/a or healer is typically a person from the community who shares his or her clients' experiences, geographic location, socioeconomic status, class, language, religion, and beliefs regarding the causes of pathology (Trotter & Chavira, 1984). This shared world view between patient and healer explains why Mexican Americans seek help from the curandera/os.

Curendera/os are believed to have supernatural power, or access to such power. Curative activities include confession, atonement, absolution, and restoration of balance, wholeness, and harmony through self-control, involvement of family and community in treatment, and communication through the supernatural. Healing methods may also include the use of medicinal herbs and prayer. Curendera/os deal with physical ailments such as diabetes and social problems including marital conflicts. They also attempt to influence people's fortunes in love, business, or home life, and guard against misfortune or illness caused by hexes.

Curandera/os are well respected and common in many Mexican communities. Their services are particularly solicited when ailments of the body and mind are regarded as "too sacred" for contemporary remedies. When a family's attempt to heal a troubled member fails or becomes overwhelming, they may seek a curandera/o's guided intervention (Ieefe et al., 1979). This line of treatment may supercede that typically offered by a physician, psychiatrist, psychologist, pastor, priest, or other mental health care worker. Spiritual healing, massages, tea, and prayer are often prescribed by curandera/os for emotional conditions or cultural syndromes such as *susto* (extreme fright or fear), *mal puesto* (hexes), *mal de ojo* (the evil eye), and *envidia* (extreme jealousy). In their study on curenderismo, Alegria et al. (1977) interviewed several curanderos in order to explore the reasons people utilize these folk healers. They found a unique contrast to traditional practices when it came to the practicing environment, *el hospital invisible* (the invisible hospital), located in their private home: "The setting for the *curanderos* practice is invariably their homes. There is a waiting area as well as a room for private consultation. The curers all practice in the community they serve. In this respect they are completely integrated with their clients" (Algeria et al., p. 1356).

The present chapter has five goals: first, to discuss the extant to which folk beliefs are brought to therapy by Chicana/os; second, to examine the etiological treatment of mental disorders; third, to discuss the etiological pathways of cultural syndromes; fourth, to consider key unifying concepts in folk healing from a Chicana/o-Mexicana/o perspective; and, finally, to present some case studies that illustrate some of the issues in Chicana/o psychology.

THE PRESENCE OF FOLK HEALING
AND CURANDERISMO-BASED CONCEPTS
IN PSYCHOTHERAPY WITH CHICANA/OS

Our own experience in working with Chicana/os in therapy suggests that many clients bring their beliefs, attitudes, and ideas about psychological illness, pathology, or dysfunction into therapy. Initially, they may attempt to present the origins or cause of their illness or condition using a more traditional medical model, only to quickly fall back on more indigenously based beliefs. Many clients talk about these beliefs at the beginning of therapy, whereas others are more likely talk about such issues once they have gained trust in the therapist.

The following are some of our impressions and observations about the extent to which such curanderismo or indigenously based beliefs are brought into therapy by Chicana/os:

1. Chicana/os of all ages are likely to bring curanderismo-based concepts and ideas to therapy. There is a stereotypical belief that only the elders or *viejitos* in the Chicana/o community practice folk healing and that the young are not interested in such practices. However, our experience suggests that both young and elder clients are likely to bring up ideas or beliefs that are not consistent with Western concepts of mental illness or mental health and that are usually based on indigenous ideas about how one can become mentally ill, with causes ranging from hexing to possession (Bird & Canino, 1981). One client, who was only 9 years old, said that her behavior problems may have resulted from being hexed by a relative.

2. Many clients may have consulted with indigenous healers or psychics prior to visiting a psychologist and may indicate that they "consulted" with a healer because they believe that they had a spiritual rather than a mental health problem. Their visit to a healer may have included the use of specific herbs, teas, foods, or roots as part of

treatment (Brandon, 1991). Some clients may not ever admit that they have previously visited a curandera/o for fear that they may be ridiculed, yet they may have experienced a *limpia* (cleansing ritual) or sweat from a curandera/o.

3. Chicana/o clients' knowledge base of folk healing and curanderismo concepts may be limited or highly comprehensive. For example, many Chicana/o clients may have learned some concepts from their parents, who learned them from their parents, and so on. A fourth- or fifth-generation Chicana/o may not possess a thorough knowledge of the many beliefs and rituals of curanderismo, but may possess specific beliefs most salient to their family of origin and acquired through the socialization process. One adult male client indicated that, "while I don't mess around with the spirits, I do believe that the spirits are both good and bad."

4. Chicana/o clients are likely to talk about religious deities within psychotherapy, including God, the Virgen de Guadalupe, and the saints, especially as defined through the Catholic religion. They are likely to refer to these deities as either sources of causation of a particular problem or mental illness or as potential sources of healing. Many are likely to use such references as adjuncts to traditional psychotherapy, whereas others seek advice from the therapists regarding how to work with these deities.

5. It appears that, for many Chicana/os, the use of Spanish in therapy facilitates talking about religious, spiritual, or curanderismo-based concepts or ideas. This suggests that language and its nuances moderate the extent to which a client is likely to talk, or not talk, about such issues in therapy. Moreover, it appears that, when Chicana/o or Mexicana/o clients use English in therapy, they are more likely to refer to Westernized medical views about illness than when they use Spanish.

6. Many Chicana/o clients are likely to use specific healing rituals in their daily lives, sometimes without even knowing it. For example, it is very common for Chicana/os to make the sign of the cross every morning prior to leaving home, while passing a church, or before taking a trip (e.g., by airplane or car). For many Chicana/os, these rituals are done automatically without much thought. The lighting of candles, praying the rosary, making offerings to saints, constructing special altars to honor deceased relatives, and so on, are other examples of healing rituals that Chicana/os practice. One elder client admitted to growing marijuana in her back yard because she believed that mixing the marijuana into rubbing alcohol helped ease her rheumatism and increased her energy level.

7. Chicana/o clients are likely to have specific culture-based theories about illness. For example, there exists a theory within the culture about cold and heat in relation to illness. Many clients continue to believe that a cold is caught by stepping on a cold floor after taking one's shoes off (i.e., feet are hot and the cold enters through the palm of the foot and makes its way to the head), going outdoors with wet hair (i.e., after a shower), or being exposed to a draft of cold air. Recently, one client attributed his symptoms of schizophrenia to hot air entering his brain. In addition, these clients are likely to identify specific syndromes such as *nervios, ataque de nervios, mal de ojo, empacho, espanto, susto,* or *hechisamiento.*

8. Treatments or methods of ridding oneself of mental illness are also based on indigenous and religious beliefs for Chicana/os. Very few Chicana/os, even after two or three generations in this country, do not practice some aspect of curanderismo,

whether it is the use of specific teas, herbs, or foods for the treatment of physical, mental, or spiritual illness.

THE ROLE OF THE CURANDERO, FAMILIA, FAITH, AND LA VIRGEN DE GUADALUPE IN THE HEALING PROCESS IN CHICANA/OS

El Curandero/La Curandera

Curandera/os are considered very important and special persons within many Chicana/o or Mexicana/o communities throughout the United States. They are revered and respected for their role as healers, spiritual advisors, wise persons, and counselors. Their history as healers can be traced to the period prior to the conquest of Mexico by the Spaniards.

Like priests, psychologists, or physicians, they must undergo lengthy training and education that includes understanding both indigenous and religious beliefs and practices or rituals (usually steeped in both Catholicism and Indian religions). In many towns and villages in Mexico, curandera/os continue to play an important role in the health care system, especially if a medical doctor is not available or accessible because of geographic barriers. Often, they represent the initial pathway into medical treatment, because many curandera/os work side by side with physicians, practice some elements of medicine, including recommending or prescribing certain medications, usually over the counter, or injecting vitamins. In this country, Chicana/os may seek the services of a curandera/o prior to seeing a physician or psychologist because of a limited income, no access to care, or a strong belief in curanderismo or after traditional treatments have not worked for either medical (e.g., cancer, diabetes) or psychological problems (e.g., depression, a broken heart). They may also seek treatment with a curandera/o because their physician or psychologist has not established a more profound relationship with them (as is often seen in Mexico) or because "the doctor didn't give me anything today" ("*el doctor no me hizo or no me dio nada*"). For example, in Mexico, a successful doctor's visit includes a prescription for medication or a vaccination.

Chicano families often seek a curandera/o's consultation when a particular member becomes highly distressed, loses faith (*perdida de fe*), experiences a dramatic change in personality (*cambio de caracter o genio*), is using drugs or alcohol (*se ha hecho un marijuano*), or is believed to have been hexed (*ser embrujado*). Wives often seek out a curandera/o when their husbands have undergone a change in life (*cambio de vida*) or are having affairs or being a womanizer or *mujeriego*. Obviously, Chicana/os and Mexicana/os also seek out treatment for culturally based syndromes, which are likely to originate from the intersection of culture and religion. This includes *susto* (extreme fright or fear), *mal puesto* (hexes), *mal de ojo* (the evil eye), and *envidia* (extreme jealousy).

In recent years, some of the best images of curandera/os have been portrayed in film, as in the movie *La Bamba*, the life story of the Chicano music pioneer Richie Valens. Valens' brother, a strong believer in curanderismo, takes Richie to visit an old curandero in Mexico. With gray hair, thick dark leathery skin, and Indian features,

TABLE 6.1
Cultural Etiological Beliefs

Etiology of Psychopathology	Example of Psychopathology
Natural	The curandera/o (faith healer) disorder of *empacho* (digestion problems), which is believed to be caused by a food that has not digested properly
Emotional	*Susto* (extreme fear), believed to be caused by a severe *envidia* (fright) that may have been caused by extreme desire or jealousy
Supernatural or Spiritual	Someone influenced by God as punishment for a particular behavior

the curandero sits with Richie and shares his wisdom about life by using metaphors or *dichos*. The curandero also rips the skin off a snake in a ritualistic sacrificial manner and states that life is like a snake. Richie is struck by the power of this exchange. He is given a talisman with special powers in order to protect him from bad spirits and negative energy and, more importantly, to help him with his fear of dying in an airplane accident.

In the movie "Mi Familia," a young woman named Maria, whose infant child nearly drowns in a river, visits a curandera in order to heal the child, who is near death. During a ceremony, mainly conducted in an Indian dialect, the curandera uses the power of candles, prayer, and oils to perform a healing ritual known as a *limpia*. In the movie "El Norte," a young woman named Rosa, who suffers from an unknown illness (which is later identified as typhus, transmitted through a rat bite while crossing the border to come to this country) seeks out a curandera who uses a variety of rituals and techniques to heal her. In addition to the use of prayer and the lighting of candles, the curandera also uses intense and intense massage and "bone cracking" as a means of breaking the fever Rosa is experiencing. In Mexico and in barrios in the United States, it is very common that persons go to a masseuse or *sobador* for bone readjustments.

In their study on curanderismo entitled "El hospital invisible," Alegria et al. (1977) interviewed several curanderos in order to explore the reasons people utilize their services. The curanderos indicated that clients came to them for many reasons, including broken hearts, medical illness, depression, alcoholism, bad luck, poverty, drug addiction, and divorce. Table 6.1 presents three key reasons that are linked to illness in the Chicana/o community.

La Familia or The Family

The Mexican family has long been considered a valuable mental health resource for those suffering from psychological stress, maladaptive behaviors, or emotional problems. Jaco (1959), in a classic study on curanderismo in southern Texas, found that the Mexican family provided considerable emotional support to family members in times of mental health crisis. Jaco further found that one of the key roles that the Mexican family plays is to provide comfort, love, and social support to the afflicted member.

Within the supportive family system, the mother or *madre* is the primary provider of psychological support and often serves as a buffer to distress. Mothers often work closely with other female family members, and sometimes non-family members, in order to provide a network of maternal-type support to family members who are suffering through difficult times. They are there to console, offer wisdom to, and support the person who is going through a difficult moment. They are also there to act as an archetypical image of the competent, loving, and loyal mother who is strong in every sense of the word and always sensitive and nonjudgmental.

The mother, being the foundation of religious and spiritual faith, is also the one likely to carry on indigenously based beliefs within a family. Thus, the mother serves as a locally based curandera within her own home, using remedies, plants, and recipes handed down from her mother and grandmother. It is often the mother who is most connected with the surrounding community and church and who is attuned to the alternative methods of healing that are available within the neighborhood. Thus, the mother may actually consult a curandera/o as others would a medical doctor in times of need.

Faith in Treatment

Although traditional psychotherapy looks at a variety of issues affecting the client, most approaches do not include faith and spiritual issues as an integral part of therapy. This can be especially problematic for the Chicana/o client whose culture is often significantly intertwined with faith-related issues. Of particular significance are the Catholic church and, in particular, the Virgin Mary. Successful treatment of Mexican American clients without consideration of their faith may be problematic.

La Virgen de Guadalupe

Many Mexican Americans highly esteem the Virgin Mary, or Virgen de Guadalupe, and consider her their "spiritual mother," thus looking to for help and spiritual guidance. Unlike folk medicine, the Virgin is not considered a direct healer, but rather seems to be regarded as a helper, guide, protector, and conduit to God (Lee, 1947; Rodriguez, 1994; Watson, 1964). Watson suggested that Mary is equated to God and believed to be the intercessor between God and humans. Watson noted that "Mary, Mother of God and spiritual Mother of men, [is] ever at the side of Jesus interceding for her children" (p. 72) and that "Christ is the fountain [and] Mary the aqueduct" (p. 73). For many Chicana/os and Mexicans, the image and concept of Our Lady of Guadalupe is more tangible, real, and accessible than God.

These descriptions indicate that the Virgin Mary is not only looked to for help, but is also expected to pray for, intercede for, and protect her people and her children. It is essential to understand the role clients assign to the Virgin Mary and how they perceive their relationship to her. According to Rodriguez (1994), exploring the Virgin Mary's history and impact on a Chicana/o client may improve one's understanding of the client's faith development, familial role, cultural traditions, and cultural expectations.

We present here a story illustrating faith in the Virgen de Guadalupe and the consequences of Western influence on traditional beliefs. There was a young Mexican Indian who suffered a great deal at the loss of his wife. Every morning at 4:00 A.M., before working in the fields, the Indian came to the pueblo's church wearing tattered clothes and a straw hat, with his feet wrapped in thin leather sandals he had made himself. He walked to the front of the church and knelt at the feet of a statue of the Virgin Mary. He removed his hat and began to pray. He asked the Virgin to bless the soul of his lost wife, for relief of his sadness and pain in his body and for the protection of his children. He prayed in his native tongue and often with nonsense syllables. Upon completion of this hour-long prayer, he felt the presence of the Virgin Mary and, as he finished his prayer, the statue of the Virgin smiled at the young man.

TABLE 6.2
Symptom Profiles for Common Curandera/o Syndromes

Condition	Syndrome
Mal de ojo (the evil eye)	One may interpret the behavior of a look (the evil eye), glance, or stare of a stranger or enemy as an attempt to inoculate them with this illness. Headaches, crying, irritability, restlessness, and stomach ailments are common symptoms.
Envidia (extreme jealousy)	*Envidia* translates as a desire or jealousy resulting from an intense anger toward, dislike of, or jealousy of another. Symptoms often mimic a number of anxiety syndromes and may resemble a common illness such as a severe cold or fever.
Susto (extreme fright or fear)	*Susto* (typically the result of extreme fright or fear) is a traumatic experience. Symptoms mimic post-traumatic stress disorder: feeling keyed up or on edge, bodily complaints, restlessness, fatigue, major change in appetite, anhedonia, bodily complaints, withdrawal, and depression.
Mal puesto (hexing)	Hexes may be placed by someone who is familiar with witchcraft. Symptoms may include somatic complaints, gastrointestinal problems, paranoia, and anxiety.

TABLE 6.3
Common Treatment Interventions

Curandero		Western	
Syndrome	Treatment	Similar Syndrome	Treatment
Nervios	Herbal tea, spiritual healing	General anxiety	Medication, psychotherapy
Ataque de nervios	Herbal tea, spiritual healing	Panic attack disorder	Medication, psychotherapy
Empacho	Herbal tea, spiritual healing, abdominal massage	Stomach ailment	Medication, diet, exercise
Mal puesto	Spiritual healing	Paranoia	Medication, psychotherapy
Susto	Spiritual healing, herbal tea	Panic attack, phobic disorder, extreme fear	Medication, psychotherapy
Mal de ojo	Spiritual healing	Paranoia	Medication, psychotherapy
Tos	Herbal tea, spiritual healing	Cold, cough	Medication

One day the priest of the church noticed this unique phenomenon. He was astounded at the way this peasant approached the Virgin, prayed seemingly nonsensically, and was given a response. The priest, who had been born, raised, and theologically trained in Spain, felt he must study this bizarre ritual. He watched over the course of the next few days and noticed as the exact same procedure repeated itself. He became confused and then enraged. He had never seen the statue of the Virgin respond with a smile. He decided to teach the young Indian man how to pray. The next day the priest approached the man, introduced himself as head of the church, and began to teach him how to utilize the rosary and several prayers including the Hail Mary and the Lord's Prayer. The young Indian was thrilled at these new prayer skills. Upon his return to the church he began to use all he had learned. Alas, the Virgin never smiled again.

Chicana/o clients may place much trust in and give much power to their faith and La Virgen de Guadalupe during times of need and suffering. Consequently, a psychotherapist's attempt to teach clients the "right" way to deal with their problems may fail. When this occurs, a likely unfortunate outcome is that the individual seeking help will now have fewer options for comfort and treatment than they had prior to seeking professional help.

CULTURAL SYNDROMES

The most common types of conditions treated by a curandera/o include mal de ojo, envidia, susto, and mal puesto. Table 6.2 outlines the symptom profile for each. As noted, these conditions or syndromes may appear to be other psychopathology as listed in the *Diagnostic and Statistical Manual of Mental Disorders* (American Psychological Association, 2000), but are actually caused by culturally associated situations.

In addition to the differences in etiological pathways and symptom profiles of curandera/o versus Western syndromes, treatment interventions also vary. Table 6.3 lists some of the common interventions used by curandera/os. The curandera/o's treatments often include herbal tea treatments, which have long been used to treat a variety of maladies ranging from the common cold to several types of cancer, as well as to treat psychological or emotional symptoms. In fact, the curandera/os have developed a number of herbal treatment options to cover a variety of anxiety-type disorders. Table 6.3 also illustrates common curandera/o syndromes and the Western disorders each syndrome mimics (Cuellar et al., 1983).

CASE STUDIES ON CURANDERISMO

Two case examples are included in order to illustrate the connection of cultural and emotional issues that may impact both the diagnostic process and treatment of Chicana/o clients. The first is about Esperanza, a 16-year-old female living in the Yucatan peninsula in Mexico, who was seeking the assistance of a curandero. The second is about Lorenzo, a 12-year-old boy who was born in Michoacan, Mexico, and at the age of 5 was sent to live with relatives in the United States.

Both cases illustrate the need for diverse and complex approaches to emotional crises that may include utilizing a curandera/o. Both adolescents were of Mexican ancestry and accustomed to the curandera/o tradition, trust and belief in the power of the healer.

Case #1: Esperanza.   Esperanza is a 16-year-old Mexican female from the Yucatan peninsula. She is single, attractive, standing about 5 feet tall with a medium build. Her long black hair is woven into a single thick braid, which she carries over her shoulder. Her family comes from a long history of Mayan Indians and both her parents and maternal grandparents raised her. Her father is a *campesino* (field-worker) and her mother stays at home. Esperanza is the youngest of 10 children (six brothers and four sisters) and all of her siblings work in the fields. Esperanza went to public schools until the fifth grade, when her parents decided that she had been educated enough, believing that "too much education would ruin her for a good man."

Esperanza, bright and energetic, longed to continue her education. She continued friendships with schoolmates, borrowed their books, and spent hours reading discarded books from the library and bookshops. Esperanza wanted to experience more, but felt that her life situation was doomed by history, racism, and pressure from her traditional family. Esperanza dreamed of something more than the seemingly timeless cycle of life that was experienced by the Mayan people.

At 16 years of age, she began to experience a host of problems. She felt her heart race at tremendous speed, occasionally lost consciousness, vomited profusely, and had considerable trouble breathing. At first her parents were not aware of these symptoms, because Esperanza hid them, not wanting to worry them with what she called "mild fainting spells." However, as the situation progressed and she began to have these attacks more frequently, the family became alarmed. Esperanza's mother took her to a local clinic staffed with occasional medical personnel, nurses, and a priest. The clinical evaluation revealed no medical problem and the family was referred to a psychologist in the city. The family, wanting to avoid the hint that there was something "crazy" going on with their daughter, chose to seek the advice, wisdom, and treatment of one of the town's curanderos, Don Wicho.

Don Wicho was a gentleman in his early seventies, with wrinkled hands and gray and white hair. His office was his back yard, with no books, waiting rooms, medicine, or magazines. He had one chair resting under a tree that looked older than Don Wicho himself. He also had one candle that he carried under his left arm, a rosary in his mouth, and a few olive branches in his right hand. Don Wicho sat Esperanza down, asking no questions, and for 20 minutes prayed with his candle lit. He occasionally waved the branches over her face and body as she sat motionless in her chair, arms extended outward.

Upon completion of the "intervention," Don Wicho informed the parents that the situation involved a boy and that Esperanza should consider marriage if the parents approved. On her next visit to Don Wicho (a day later) Esperanza confessed to the curandero that she was pregnant and felt she could not tell her parents about the pregnancy. She was reluctant to admit to herself that she would have to continue her role in the Indian cycle of life. However, she added that she loved her boyfriend very much and knew she must get married. Don Wicho prescribed some tea to help her with her nausea and told her to pray for her developing child and for her upcoming marriage. In addition, he provided a special healing intervention to assist in her plans to move away from her family and start her new home. The symptoms and treatment for Esperanza were complicated by a host of medical, psychological, and cultural twists. Esperanza's belief in the healer aided her recovery.

Case #2: Lorenzo. Lorenzo was born in Mexico. When he was 4 years old, his parents experienced financial and emotional troubles and it was rumored that they were going to break up. At that time his parents sent him to the United States to be raised by his maternal aunt and uncle, first-generation Mexicans who had migrated to the United States illegally during the 1950s and lived in a rural agricultural community in the Southwest.

Lorenzo adjusted to his new environment and to the cultural norms of an American child. He loved video games, fast food, and sports. Everything seemed to be going well for him and he had many friends, both Mexican American and Anglo. He was very popular at school and was very close to his aunt and uncle. The occasional problems his biological family in Mexico experienced distressed him, but he continued to do well socially and academically.

All was well until the summer before he was to begin junior high school. He was now 12 years old and began to worry about the next level of his education and the challenges it would present. He wondered if he would be able to fit in, if the other students would accept him, and if he could compete academically. These worries began to generalize to worries about his aunt and uncle. He began to worry that they might reject him if he did not do well academically or socially and to wonder if they would be there for him or if they would abandon him. These worries eventually resulted in nightmares about abandonment by his aunt and uncle. He would wake up with night sweats, his heart racing, experiencing intense fear and anxiety. During these episodes Lorenzo wished to be consoled and reassured by his aunt and uncle that they would not leave him. These worries eventually began to affect his social life and mood. He became less interested in sports, his friends, and his appearance. The aunt, feeling she was untrained to help her nephew, called upon a local curandera, Angelita, to assist with the situation.

Angelita was a chubby woman about 60 years old with black and gray hair. She was soft-spoken and calm and came to the home to assess the situation. She was welcomed with *cafe con leche* (coffee and cream) and *pan dulce* (Mexican sweet bread). Angelita brought with her a special concoction of herbs, teas, and a rosary. She had Lorenzo undress down to his shorts and lie on the living room floor, crushed some leaves over his body, and for about 12 minutes prayed with the rosary and called on the saints and angels to protect the child and to remove his fears. Later, she prepared a special tea from crushed leaves that she carried in a small plastic sandwich bag. She told the aunt to prepare this tea twice a day for Lorenzo until the bag was empty. Angelita was paid a small donation for her services.

The boy's fears returned that night and continued for several days. The aunt, worried about the child's well-being, consulted with a priest and a doctor who recommended she take the boy to a psychologist, which she reluctantly did. The psychologist began by having Lorenzo explain his fears, subsequently tracing them to the problems with his biological family in Mexico. After the course of about 2 months of visits, by exploring the origins of the child's fear and reassuring him, the psychologist was able to successfully treat Lorenzo.

Over the past 30 years, researchers who have examined the psychological treatment of Chicana/os have unanimously concluded that folk healing plays an important role in their community. The majority of these researchers have suggested that psychologists be sensitive to the indigenous beliefs about mental illness, taking them into consideration in assessment and treatment and perhaps even using indigenously based rituals or interventions in psychotherapy. Researchers have further noted that psychologists should undergo training in indigenous healing practices as a means of linking traditional psychotherapeutic approaches to those unique to particular cultural groups like Chicana/os.

To date, it remains unclear to what extent Chicana/o and non-Chicana/o psychologists take into consideration indigenously based concepts of mental illness in the assessment or treatment of this population. A review of the research indicates that there are no studies that have surveyed the use of folk healing practices in the treatment of Chicana/os. Moreover, and in spite of the presence of culture-bound syndromes in the *DSM-IV-R* (2000), there exist no epidemiological studies that consider these syndromes in any segment of the Chicana/o population. If fact, culture-bound syndromes such as *nervios* (nerves) and *mal de ojo* (evil eye) are placed in a section of the *DSM-IV-R* that is considered an appendix or add-on. Clinicians are not given any guidance on how to incorporate such diagnoses, from a technical point, on Axes I or II of the *DSM-IV-R*. Moreover, culture-bound syndromes are not reimbursable psychiatric disorders. Thus, there is minimal incentive to actually diagnose clients with such syndromes. In many ways, it appears that culture-bound syndromes and acculturation problem, which is a "V" code, have only been included in the *DSM-IV-R* to placate those who have criticized its cross-cultural validity and to internationalize the sale of the manual.

Psychologists, psychiatrists, and other mental health care providers need to understand the phenomenology associated with the application of various or individual forms of psychotherapy. In other words, considering each client's strengths, weaknesses, and specific problems is a prerequisite to choosing treatment for them. For example, based on research and practice, we understand that a cognitive-behavioral approach often serves to alleviate anxiety or depressive symptoms (Colon, 1988) and we understand to some degree the psychotropic side effects of medication. We also know that there are times when a psychoanalytic approach might not be appropriate for some individuals. Nevertheless, we often continue to maintain a singular approach when it comes to understanding and classifying the origins of mental illness, symptom profiles, and diagnostic categories. It is understood that there is not a monothetic approach to treating depression, anxiety, schizophrenia, or other emotional disorders.

Past research has attempted to understand and explain the reasons and motives behind the underutilization patterns exhibited by Chicana/os in the field of psychology. These researchers have suggested that many may have no need for traditional psychotherapy and may instead make use of alternative treatments, have family buffers that often replace or decrease the need for treatment, and make significant use of curanderos. All of these are viable explanations for why Chicana/os may not seek traditional forms of psychological care.

REFERENCES

Alegria, D., Guerra, E., Martinez, C., & Meyer, G. G. (1977). El hospital invisible: A study of curanderismo. *Archives of General Psychiatry, 34,* 1354–1357.

Alonso, L., & Jeffrey, W. D. (1988). Mental illness complicated by the Santeria belief in spirit possession. *Hospital and Community Psychiatry, 39,* 1188–1191.

American Psychiatric Association. (2000). *Diagnostic and statistical manual of mental disorders* (4th ed., Rev.). Washington, DC: Author.

Applewhite, S. L. (1995). Curanderismo: Demystifying the health beliefs and practices of elderly Mexican Americans. *Health and Social Work, 20,* 247–253.

Baez, A., & Hernandez, D. (2001). Complementary spiritual beliefs in the Latino community: The interface with psychotherapy. *American Journal of Orthopsychiatry, 71,* 408–415.

Bird, H., & Canino, I. (1981). The sociopsychiatry of Espiritismo. *Journal of the American Academy of Child Psychiatry, 20,* 725–740.

Brandon, G. (1991). The uses of plants in healing in an Afro-Cuban religion, Santeria. *Journal of Black Studies, 22,* 55–76.

Cervantes, J. M., & Ramirez, O. (1992). Spirituality and family dynamics in psychotherapy with Latino children. In L. A. Vargas & J. D. Koss-Chioino (Eds.), *Working with culture: Psychotherapeutic interventions with ethnic minority children and adolescents* (pp. 103–128). San Francisco, CA: Jossey-Bass.

Colon, E. (1998). Alcohol use among Latino males: Implications for the development of culturally competent prevention and treatment services. In M. Delgado (Ed.), *Alcohol use/abuse among Latinos: Issues and examples of culturally competent services* (pp. 147–159). New York: Haworth Press.

Cuéllar, I., Martinez, R., & Gonzalez, R. (1983). Clinical psychiatric case presentation: Culturally responsive diagnostic formulation and treatment in a Hispanic female. *Hispanic Journal of Behavioral Sciences, 5,* 93–103.

De la Cancela, V., & Martinez, I. Z. (1983). An analysis of culturalism in Latino mental health: Folk medicine as a case in point. *Hispanic Journal of Behavioral Sciences, 5,* 251–274.

Del Castillo, R. R. (1999). Effective management strategies when incorporating curanderismo into a mainstream mental health system. *Dissertation Abstracts International, 60,* 1524B.

Delgado, M. (1988). Groups in Puerto Rican spriritism: Implications for clinicians. In C. Jacobs & D. D. Bowles (Eds.), *Ethnicity and race: Critical concepts in social work* (pp. 34–47). Silver Spring, MD: National Association of Social Workers.

Dobkin, M. (1968). Folk curing with a psychedelic cactus in the north coast of Peru. *International Journal of Social Psychiatry, 15,* 23–32.

Edgerton, R. B., Karno, M., & Fernandez, I. (1970). Curanderismo in the metropolis: The diminished role of folk psychiatry among Los Angeles Mexican-Americans. *American Journal of Psychotherapy, 24,* 124–134.

Etsuko, M. (1991). The interpretations of fox possession: Illness as metaphor. *Culture, Medicine, and Psychiatry, 15,* 453–477.

Falicov, C. J. (1999). Religion and spiritual folk traditions in immigrant families: Therapeutic resources with Latinos. In F. Walsh (Ed.), *Spiritual resources in family therapy* (pp. 104–120). New York: Guilford Press.

Fernandez, V. E. (1987). The effects of belief of spiritism and/or Santeria on psychiatric diagnosis of Puerto Ricans in New York City. *Dissertation Abstracts International, 47,* 3106B.

Gafner, G., & Duckett, S. (1992). Treating the sequelae of a curse in elderly Mexican-Americans. *Clinical Gerontologist, 11,* 145–153.

Gangotena-Gonzalez, M. (1980). Rhetorical visions of medicine compared and contrasted: Curanderismo and allopathic family practice as held by Mexican-American and Anglo patients and practitioners. *Dissertation Abstracts International, 41,* 1835A.

Garcia, M. A. (1980). The effects of Spiritualism and Santeria as a cultural determinant in New York Puerto Rican women, as reflected by their use of projection. *Dissertation Abstracts International, 40,* 3927B.

Gilestra, D. M. (1981). Santeria and psychotherapy. *Comprehensive Psychotherapy, 3,* 69–80.

Giovetti, P. (1984). Folk healers in Italy. *PSI Research, 3,* 131–135.

Guajardo, K. A. (1999). Spirituality and curanderismo in Mexican-American culture: A psychospiritual model of conjoint treatment. *Dissertation Abstracts International, 60,* 2340B.

Harris, J., & Harris, M. L. (1994). Mental health care utilization by American minorities: Factors for consideration in cross-cultural therapy, research and practice. *Psychotherapy Bulletin, 29,* 391–400.

Harris, M. L, (1998). *Curandersimo and the DSM-IV: Diagnostic and treatment implications for the Mexican American client* (Tech. Rep. No. 45). East Lansing: Michigan State University.

Heiman, E. M., Burruel, G., & Chavez, N. (1975). Factors determining effective psychiatric outpatient treatment for Mexican Americans. *Hospital and Community Psychiatry, 25,* 515–517.

Hockmeyer, A. L. (1991). The social construction of a curandera: A model for bicultural adaptation. *Dissertation Abstracts International, 51,* 6105–6106B.

Jaco, E. G. (1959). *Mental health of the Spanish American in Texas, culture and mental health: Cross culture studies.* New York: Macmillan.

Jilek, W. G. (1994). Traditional healing in the prevention and treatment of alcohol and drug abuse. *Transcultural Psychiatric Research Review, 31,* 219–258.

Keefe, S. E., Padilla, A. M., & Carlos, M. L. (1979). The Mexican American extended family as an emotional support system. *Human Organization, 38,* 144–152.

Kiev, A. (1968). *Curanderismo: Mexican-American folk psychiatry.* New York: Free Press.

Koss-Chioino, J. D. (1995). Traditional and folk approaches among ethnic minorities. In J. F. Aponte & R. Y. Rivers (Eds.), *Psychological interventions and cultural diversity* (pp. 145–163). Needham Heights, MA: Allyn and Bacon.

Krajewski-Jaime, E. R. (1991). Folk-healing among Mexican-American families as a consideration in the delivery of child welfare and child health care services. *Child Welfare, 70,* 157–167.

Kramer, M. (1996). Hispanic folk healing as culturally responsive psychotherapy. *Dissertation Abstracts International, 56,* 5772B.

Krassner, M. (1986). Effective features of therapy from the healer's perspective: A study of curanderismo. *Smith College Studies in Social Work, 56,* 157–183.

Kreisman, J. J. (1975). The curandero's apprentice: A therapeutic integration of folk and medical healing. *American Journal of Psychiatry, 132,* 81–83.

Krippner, S. (1984). Folk healing in Indonesia and around the world. *PSI Research, 3,* 149–157.

Lauren, S. E. (1987). Ritual as therapy: Psychotherapeutic healing rituals in curanderismo as exemplified by the work of Diana Velazquez, curandera. *Dissertation Abstracts International, 47,* 4430A.

Lawrence, T. F., Bozzetti, L., & Kane, T. J. (1976). Curanderas: A unique role for Mexican women. *Psychiatric Annals, 6,* 65–73.

Lee, G. (1947). *Our Lady of Guadalupe: Patroness of the Americas.* New York: Catholic Book.

Lefley, H. P. (1981). Psychotherapy and cultural adaptation in the Caribbean. *International Journal of Group Tensions, 11,* 3–16.

Lefley, H. P., Sandoval, M. C., & Charles, C. (1998). Traditional healing systems in a multicultural setting. In S. O. Okpaku (Ed.), *Clinical methods in transcultural psychiatry* (pp. 88–110). Washington, DC: American Psychiatric Press.

Li, S., & Phillips, M. R. (1990). Witch doctors and mental illness in mainland China: A preliminary study. *American Journal of Psychiatry, 147,* 221–224.

Martinez, R., & Wetli, C. V. (1982). Santeria: A magico-religious system of Afro-Cuban origin. *American Journal of Social Psychiatry, 2,* 32–38.

Ness, R. C., & Wintrob, R. M. (1981). Folk healing: A description and synthesis. *American Journal of Psychiatry, 138,* 1477–1481.

Parks, F. M. (1997). Attribution models of helping and coping: A transgenerational theory of African-American traditional healing. *Dissertation Abstracts International, 57,* 3624A.

Perez y Mena, A. I. (1977). Spiritualism as an adaptive mechanism among Puerto Ricans in the United States. *Cornell Journal of Social Relations, 12,* 125–136.

Rivera, G. (1988). Hispanic folk medicine utilization in urban Colorado. *Sociology and Social Research, 72,* 237–241.

Rodriguez, J. (1994). *Our Lady of Guadalupe: Faith and empowerment among Mexican American women.* Austin: University of Texas Press.

Ruiz, P. (1977). Culture and mental health: A Hispanic perspective. *Journal of Contemporary Psychotherapy, 9,* 24–27.

Ruiz, P., & Langrod, J. (1976). Psychiatry and folk healing: A dichotomy? *American Journal of Psychiatry, 133,* 95–97.

Santi, A. (1997). Santeria compared to psychology as a mental health care system. *Dissertation Abstracts International, 58,* 1545B.

Schwartz, D. (1985). Caribbean folk beliefs and Western psychiatry. *Journal of Psychosocial Nursing and Mental Health Services, 23,* 26–30.

Slessinger, D. P., & Richards, M. (1981). Folk and clinical medical utilization patterns among Mejicano migrant farm workers. *Hispanic Journal of Behavioral Sciences, 3,* 59–73.

Suarez, M., Raffaelli, M., & O'Leary, A. (1996). Use of folk healing practices by HIV-infected Hispanics living in the United States. *AIDS Care, 8,* 683–690.

Tripp-Reimer, T. (1983). Retention of folk-healing practice (matiasma) among four generations of urban Greek immigrants. *Nursing Research, 32,* 97–101.

Trotter, R. T. (1982). Contrasting models of the healer's role: South Texas case examples. *Hispanic Journal of Behavioral Sciences, 4,* 315–327.

Trotter, R. T., & Chavira, J. A. (1984). *Curanderismo: Mexican American folk healing* (2nd ed.). Athens: University of Georgia Press.

Tseng, W. S., & Streltzer, J. (2001). *Culture and psychotherapy: A guide to clinical practice.* Washington, DC: American Psychiatric Press.

Velez-Ibanez, C. G., & Parra, C. G. (1999). Trauma issues and social modalities concerning mental health concepts and practices among Mexicans of the Southwest United States with reference to other Latino groups. In K. Nader & N. Dubrow (Eds.), *Honoring differences: Cultural issues in the treatment of trauma and loss* (pp. 390–405). Philadelphia, PA: Brunner/Mazel.

Watson, S. (1964). *The cult of Our Lady of Guadalupe.* Collegeville, MN: Liturgical Press.

Weclew, R. V. (1975). The nature, prevalence, and level of awareness of "curanderismo" and some of its implications for community mental health. *Community Mental Health Journal, 11,* 145–154.

Westermeyer, J. (1985). Psychiatric diagnosis across cultural boundaries. *American Journal of Psychiatry, 142,* 798–805.

Wing, D. M. (1998). A comparison of traditional folk healing concepts with contemporary healing concepts. *Journal of Community Health Nursing, 15,* 143–154.

II

Psychological Assessment of Chicana/os

Integrating a Cultural Perspective in Psychological Test Development

Steven R. López
University of California, Los Angeles

Amy Weisman
University of Miami

The purpose of this chapter is to review and evaluate critically the development of psychological tests for Mexican Americans and Latinos residing in the United States. To accomplish this objective, we first present an anthropologically informed definition of culture, one that respects the dynamic and social nature of culture (Lopez & Guarnaccia, 2000). The implication of this contemporary definition is that test developers, researchers, and examiners respect the changeable nature of culture and look to the social world to ascribe meaning to research findings and test results. We then review selected advances in test development as they relate to Latina/os in general and Mexican Americans in particular. Our main interest is to identify how culture is considered and to evaluate such considerations. We limit the scope of this chapter to the assessment of cognitive-intellectual functioning and psychodiagnosis because they represent central aspects of psychological assessment and are among the most widely studied. Based on the critical evaluation, we then recommend ways in which test development can better incorporate a cultural perspective.

AN ANTHROPOLOGICALLY INFORMED DEFINITION OF CULTURE

We draw on Kleinman's (1995) theoretical notion of experience as the basis of our definition of culture. Experience is viewed as the "felt flow" of the intersubjective space between individuals (their minds and bodies) and their social world. In this theoretical space, the individual and his or her social world are interconnected and inseparable. For practical purposes this intersubjective medium is what is at stake or what matters for individuals and groups. Kleinman pointed out that "preservation of life, aspiration, prestige, and the like" (p. 97) is relevant for all, but it is that which is at stake in peoples' daily lives that is tied closely to culture. He argued that the cultural scientist's central concern then is to interpret what matters for specific individuals in specific situations.

The notion that culture is associated with what is at stake for people in specific local worlds advances the cross-cultural psychology definition of culture as values, beliefs, and practices (Berry, Poortinga, Segall, & Dasen, 1992; Betancourt & López, 1993) in significant, interrelated ways. First, the scientist or examiner must look to the community of interest to determine what is at stake. Anthropological investigators do not typically apply existing measures of values, beliefs, or norms, nor do they infer what is at stake given the ethnic group under study. Instead, they observe the social world within specific settings to discern what matters. Second, researchers applying this anthropologically informed definition are not necessarily tied to studying specific ethnic or so-called cultural groups. Instead, researchers are free to determine what aspects of the community are relevant to identifying what is at stake; these could be other social categories such as age or gender, as well as particular experiences of a group of individuals with a shared history. Third, it is important to consider interconnected systems within social contexts—the historical, the political, and the economic circumstances in particular settings. Such considerations are likely to contribute to a rich analysis of the sociocultural context and avoid cultural glosses that reflect superficial analyses. For example, spirituality may be as much a function of individuals' adjustment to longstanding economic and social difficulties as it is a set of values and beliefs passed from generation to generation. In all, the definition of culture associated with what is at stake for individuals and groups in local contexts represents an open construct that is capable of capturing culture's richness and complexity.

Culture conceived as an open construct is not without limitations. Some may view this definition as too abstract and diffuse to be of value to standardized testing (see Segall, 1984, for a similar critique). We acknowledge the challenge in bringing interpretative anthropology and classical test theory into the same conceptual and applied space. However, we believe that there are ways in which psychological assessment, particularly test development, can move toward integrating a cultural perspective, particularly one that respects the rich and dynamic qualities of culture.

TEST DEVELOPMENT

The consideration of what is at stake for individuals in their local worlds is probably best addressed within the clinical domain as examiners collect and interpret data. Test developers, however, can take steps to facilitate the consideration of what matters most for specific groups. We examine the ways test developers take into account or fail to take into account ethnicity and culture in the development of selected cognitive-intellectual and psychodiagnostic tests used in the assessment of Mexican Americans and other Latina/o groups within the United States. (For related reviews, see Cervantes & Acosta, 1992; Dahlstrom, Lachar, & Dahlstrom, 1986; Geisinger, 1992; and McShane & Cook, 1985.) The current analysis is based largely on the review of test manuals and technical manuals of selected tests as they reflect the actual test development. The only exception is the Minnesota Multiphasic Personality Inventory-2 (MMPI-2) with Mexican norms. Research articles are used for the review of that test, as the manual was not available.

Within the cognitive-intellectual domains, we consider: (a) the widely used English-language Wechsler scales for adults and children, (b) their Spanish-language versions with Spanish-language norms, (c) the Woodcock Johnson Cognitive Ability Test and its Spanish-language version (Batería-R; Woodcock & Muñoz-Sandoval, 1996), and (d) selected nonverbal tests, specifically an adult test, the General Ability Measure for Adults (GAMA; Naglieri & Bardos, 1997), and a children's test, the Universal Nonverbal Intelligence Test (UNIT; Bracken & McCallum, 1998). Within psychodiagnostic assessment, we consider the MMPI-2 and the Millon Clinical Multiaxial Inventory–III (MCMI-III). This selective range of tests provides an indication of how some test developers are attending to ethnic and cultural factors in the psychological assessment of Latina/os in general and Mexican Americans in particular. Table 7.1 summarizes the characteristics of each test.

Cognitive Intelligence Measures

English-Language Wechsler Scales. Test developers of the Wechsler Adult Intelligence Scale (WAIS) have taken steps to enhance the assessment of Latina/os since the test's original publication (Wechsler, 1955). The test manual of the original WAIS indicated that the standardization sample included a proportionate representation of the "non-White" United States population, however, the actual size and composition of this subsample was not reported. The actual distribution of the non-White subsample was reported for the first time with the Wechsler Adult Intelligence Scale-Revised (WAIS-R; Wechsler, 1981). In particular, the percentage of non-Whites within specific age groups by region, occupational group, and gender were compared with expected percentages from 1970 and later census data. No breakdown of Latina/os was provided, however. With regard to language, the manual stated that individuals whose primary language was something other than English were included in the standardization sample "only if they were able to speak and understand English" (Wechsler, 1981, p. 18). With the publication of the WAIS-III (Wechsler, 1997), specific racial or ethnic groups were recognized for the first time, specifically African Americans and Hispanics. Data were presented on each of these groups by age group, educational level, and sex. Overall, Hispanic representation within the standardization sample ($N = 181$; 7.4%[1]) falls short of the estimated percentage of Hispanics 16 years or older among the same age population within the United States overall in 1995 (9.3%; U.S. Census Bureau, 1998). However, among age groups ranging from 16 to 29, representation in the standardization sample ranged from 11 to 13%, nearly identical to Hispanic's representation within the nation for the same age ranges (11.7 to 13.7%) as reported in Wechsler (1997).

Another first for the WAIS in its third edition was the reporting of both subjective and objective efforts to identify and eliminate items that might be biased for specific racial or ethnic groups. Among the steps taken were content reviews by "bias experts" and statistical analysis based on (a) the WAIS-R standardization sample, (b) a nationwide "tryout" study that included an oversampling of 162 African American

---

[1]Extrapolated from percentage data in Tables 2.9 and 2.12 (Psychological Corporation, 1997).

TABLE 7.1

Characteristics of Selected Intelligence and Psychodiagnostic Tests Used in Assessing Chicanos/Latinos

Test	Year Published	Publisher	Country/ Locale of Norming Sample	% Latinos Norming Sample	Reliabilities Reported for Latinos			Validities Reported for Latinos				Comments
					Split-Half	SEM	Temporal Stability	Test & Scale Intercorrelations	With Other Tests	Factor Analyses	Differential Item Functioning	
Intelligence												
English Language												
WAIS-III	1999	Psych Corp	U.S.	7.4%								Uses U.S., English-language norms from WISC-R
WISC-III	1998	Psych Corp	U.S.	11.0%								Based on public school sample only
Spanish Language												
EIWN-R	1983	Psych Corp	U.S.	not reported								
WISC-RM	1984	Manual Moderno	Mexico City	100.0%	X	X		X				
EIWN-RPR	1992	Psych Corp	Puerto Rico	100.0%	X	X	X	X	X			Uses U.S., English-language norms
WAIS-III Español	2001	Manual Moderno	U.S.	7.4%			X					Outdated norms
EIWA	1967	Psych Corp	Pureto Rico	100.0%	X	X		X				
Batería-R	1996	Riverside	U.S.	9.3%	X	X						Equated norms based on U.S. standardization sample
Nonverbal												
GAMA	1997	NCS	U.S.	7.8%		.						Instructions verbally administered
UNIT	1998	Riverside	U.S.	13.0%	X	X			X	X	X	Completely noverbal; included special studies with bilingual and LEP students

Test	Year Published	Publisher	Country/ Locale of Norming Sample	% Latinos Norming Sample	Reliabilities Reported for Latinos			Validities Reported for Latinos				Comments
					Split-Half	SEM	Temporal Stability	Test & Scale Intercorrelations	With Other Tests	Factor Analyses	Differential Item Functioning	
Psychodiagnosis												
English Language												
MMPI-2	1989	NCS	U.S.	2.8%								
MCMI-III	1997	NCS	U.S.	2–2.8%								
Spanish Language												
MMPI-2 U.S. Hispanics	in press	U. Minnesota	Puerto Rico, Miami, Los Angeles	100.0%			X					
MMPI-2 Mexico	2001		Mexico	100.0%			X			X		Also examined differences between college student and patient samples

and Hispanic examinees, and (c) the standardization sample of the WAIS-III plus an oversampling of 200 African American and Hispanic participants. Test items that were found to be biased or potentially biased by these subjective and objective analyses were reported as not included in the test. Reliability and validity data were not reported by ethnicity or race, however.

An important change in the WAIS-III is that the scale score for each subtest is based on the scores of a nonimpaired reference group by specific age group. In other words, to determine how a given individual's performance compares to others, the examiner compares that score to others from the same age group. This differs from the earlier Wechsler adult tests of intelligence for which only one age group—from 20 to 34—served as the reference group for all age groups. The problem with this single reference group is that older persons who may be functioning within the normal range for their age group appear to be impaired when compared to the 20- to 34-year-old reference group (Ryan, Paolo, & Brungardt, 1990). To avoid this problem, the scale scores in the WAIS-III now adjust for the age of the examinee. The importance of this change is that the test developers are directly considering for the first time in adult assessment a contextual factor—age and development—in determining a person's level of functioning. This advancement has implications for the consideration of other factors for which specific subgroup norms may be helpful.

The development of the Wechsler Intelligence Scale for Children (WISC) follows the same general pattern as that of its adult assessment counterpart. The original WISC manual (Wechsler, 1949) made no mention of race or ethnicity in the sampling design or standardization sample, whereas the WISC-III (Wechsler, 1991) addressed race and ethnicity in a very similar way to the WAIS-III with regard to item bias and sampling. Latina/os represented 11% of the standardization sample, which compares favorably to their percentage within the 1988 U.S. population of children ages 6 through 16—10.8% (Wechsler, 1991). In addition, only English-speaking children comprised the sample.

In summary, the recent English-language Wechsler tests of cognitive-intellectual abilities take into account ethnicity through their sampling and assessment of item bias. However, the tests' reliability and validity for Latina/os and for limited English-speaking individuals were not reported in the technical manuals.

Spanish-Language Wechsler Scales.   There are a number of Spanish translations and adaptations of the Wechsler scales. The earliest translation that we know of is the Escala de Inteligencia Wechsler para Niños (EIWN; Wechsler, 1951), which was developed by Pablo Roca for the assessment of children on the island of Puerto Rico. Three studies with small convenience samples (Ns = 18, 41, and 69) were carried out to begin to examine test properties, primarily the level of difficulty of subtest items and the sample's mean level of functioning. Examiners who used this Spanish translation applied the U.S. English-language norms, as no norms were associated with the Spanish-language translation and adaptation (Herrans, 1985).

Several years later, at least three Spanish-language versions of the WISC-R (Wechsler, 1974) were developed: Escala Wechsler para Niños-Revisada (EIWN-R; Wechsler, 1983), Escala de Inteligence Revisada para el Nivel Escolar (WISC-RM; Wechsler, 1984, adapted and normed in Mexico by Margarita Gómez-Palacio, Eligio Padilla, and Samuel Roll), and la Escala de Inteligencia Wechsler para Niños-Revisada en Puerto Rico (EIWN-RPR; Wechsler, 1992, adapted and normed by Laura Herrans and

135

Juana Rodriguez). The Psychological Corporation published both the EIWN-R and EIWN-RPR. They are both still listed and available for purchase on the Psychological Corporation's product catalog as of July 8, 2003. The WISC-RM is published and distributed by Editorial el Manual Moderno, a publishing company in Mexico dedicated, in part, to psychological tests and literature.

According to Herrans and Rodriguez (in Wechsler, 1992), the EIWN-R was a literal translation of the WISC-R carried out in Dade County, Florida, comprised largely of Cuban Americans. Except for the English-to-Spanish translation, there was no adaptation of the instrument for Spanish-speaking children and there were no norms developed for its use.[2] Herrans and Rodriguez reported that the only changes made to the instrument were changes in the scoring criteria used to identify acceptable responses, for example, in the vocabulary and comprehension subtests. Prewitt-Diaz and Rodriguez (1986), however, noted that two of the original WISC-R vocabulary words were deleted, thus, the content of the Spanish and English versions are nearly identical. Given that the norms were the same for the EIWN-R and the WISC-R, which limits their applicability to the assessment of Spanish-speaking children, we have chosen to focus on the two Spanish-language versions of the WISC-R that have Spanish-language norms—the WISC-RM and the EIWN-RPR.

Like the EIWN-R, the WISC-RM is also a Spanish-language translation in which few changes were made. Only the information, vocabulary, and comprehension subtests differ from the WISC-R and these changes included the deletion of nine, seven, and five items from each respective subtest and the inclusion of seven, six, and five new or significantly modified items. For other subtests, the content is the same, but slight alterations were made to the order of a few items. In addition to these changes, the WISC-RM was standardized on a sample of students from public schools in Mexico City during 1980 to 1981 (Padilla, Roll, & Gómez-Palacio, 1982). The sample was comprised of 1,100 students ages 6 through 16. Thus, the WISC-RM is a close literal translation of the WISC-R and it has its own norms.

With regard to the psychometric properties of the WISC-RM, some reliability estimates and only one limited test of validity were reported in the test manual.[3] The reliability of the subtests was assessed using the split-half method with Spearman-Brown corrections. The average correlation across the 11 age ranges for each subtest ranged from .65 to .82. For the three IQ scales (verbal, performance, and full scale), their average reliability across the age ranges were .90, .89, and .94, respectively.[4] The standard error of measurement (*SEM*) was also reported. Averaging across the age ranges, the *SEM* for the subtests ranged from 1.29 (block design) to 1.77 (comprehension). For the scales the standard errors of measurement were 4.64 (verbal), 5.06 (performance), and 3.79 (full scale).[5] In terms of the test's validity, the intercorrelations of the subtests and the three IQ scales were reported for each age group. In addition, the

---

[2]Limited assessments of the EIWN-R's reliability and validity have been conducted (Prewitt-Diaz & Rodriguez, 1986; Rodriguez & Prewitt-Diaz, 1990).

[3]A factor analysis has since been conducted on a sample of 300 Mexican children from Baja California (Rousey, 1990).

[4]For the three IQ scales (verbal, performance, and full scale), reliability coefficients were computed according to a formula based on a composite of several tests (Guilford, 1954).

[5]Note that the standard error of measurement is inversely related to the reliability coefficient; that is, the greater the reliability, the lower the standard error of measurement. Furthermore, the differences between the subtests and the scales are a function of different standard deviations (3 for the subscales and 15 for the scales). Thus, the lower scores of the subtests do not mean that they are necessarily more reliable.

average intercorrelations of the subtests and the three IQ scales were reported across all age groups. A general pattern of the average intercorrelations indicated that the verbal subtests correlated more highly with the overall verbal subtest score (.45 to .71) than with the overall performance subtest score (.31 to .52). A more attenuated pattern was observed in the relations between the overall performance subtest score with each of the performance subtests (.34 and .58) and each of the verbal subtests (.38 to .49).[6]

The third Spanish-language version, the EIWN-RPR, is like the WISC-RM in that it was translated and renormed. In this case, the standardization sample was based on 2,200 Puerto Rican island children whose ages ranged from 6 through 16 and who were enrolled in both public and private schools from 1986 to 1987 and 1989 to 1990. In addition to the renorming, changes were made to the test content in all subtests except digit span, object assembly, coding, and mazes, which were identical to those of the WISC-R. According to Herrans and Rodriguez (1992), changes were made to ensure that the test content was congruent with the life experiences of Puerto Rican children. Of the subtests that were modified, the percentage of changes ranged from 15% of the picture completion items to 47% of the similarities items (Wechsler, 1992). More than one third of the subtest items were changed for only three subtests. Thus, the EIWN-RPR is the version of the WISC-R that was most adapted for use with a Spanish-language group. Moreover, it has specific norms for Puerto Rican children.

The psychometric properties of the EIWN-RPR were assessed using the same tests as those for its Mexican counterpart, plus tests of temporal stability and concurrent validity. With regard to internal consistency, the average correlation across the 11 age ranges for each subtest ranged from .62 to .84. For the three IQ scales (verbal, performance, and full scale), the average reliability across the age ranges was .92, .88, and .94, respectively. Averaging across the age ranges, the standard error of measurement for the subtests ranged from 1.20 (block design) to 1.94 (object assembly). For the scales, the standard errors of measurement were 4.26 (verbal), 5.23 (performance), and 3.77 (full scale). To assess the test's temporal stability, the test was administered a second time within a 2-week period to a subsample ($n = 150$) of five age groups.[7] The corrected stability correlation coefficients ranged from .53 (mazes) to .91 (vocabulary) for the subtests and were .91, .77, and .90 for the three main scales of verbal, performance, and full scale.

To assess the EIWN-RPR's validity, the intercorrelations of the subtests and the three IQ scales were first reported for each age group and then for the average intercorrelations across all age groups. The verbal subtests correlated more highly with the overall verbal subtest score (.51 to .73) than with the overall performance subtest score (.39 to .46). A less differentiated pattern was observed in the relations between the overall performance subtest score with each of the performance subtests (.23 and .57) and each of the verbal subtests (.25 to .43). In addition to examining the inter-

---

[6]When correlations were computed for subtests with scales that included that particular subtest (e.g., vocabulary with verbal IQ), then the correlation was corrected following procedures outlined in McNemar (1955). In addition, for the correlational analyses, the verbal and the performance scale scores did not include the digit span or mazes, respectively.

[7]The test-retest stability coefficients were corrected for the variability of the standardization sample, which provides an estimate of the score stability within the population.

correlations, small groups ranging from 31 to 48 subjects were administered the EIWN-RPR and other intelligence tests, including the Raven Progressive Matrices, the Test Rapido de Barranquilla (BARSIT), and the Escala de Inteligencia Wechsler para Adultos (EIWA). The participants' total scores on each of these tests were significantly associated with their total score on the EIWN-RPR: BARSIT, $r = .56$; Raven's $r = .58$; EIWA, $r = .84$. In addition, a significant correlation ($r = .50$) was observed between the Full Scale IQ of the EIWN-RPR and the academic record of nearly all the examinees from the standardization sample (1,956 of 2,200).

With regard to assessing Spanish-speaking adults, we know of two test versions, the Escala de Inteligencia para Adultos, or WAIS-III Español (Wechsler, 2001), and the Escala de Inteligencia Wechsler para Adultos (EIWA; Wechsler, 1967). Like the EIWN-R, the WAIS-III Español is a literal translation of the WAIS-III with no new norms or reported psychometric properties. It is published and distributed by Editorial el Manual Moderno. The EIWA, on the other hand, is similar to the EIWN-RPR, as it has its own norms based on an adaptation and standardization carried out on the island of Puerto Rico. The Psychological Corporation publishes and continues to distribute this test as it is the only Spanish-language intelligence test that was normed on a specific Latina/o community (country) of origin outside the mainland, with potential relevance to Latina/os residing in the United States.

The reliability of the EIWA was estimated primarily by calculating split-half correlations[8] and the standard errors of measurement for three age groups 16 to 19, 25 to 34, and 45 to 54 taken from the standardization sample. For the 25 to 34 age group ($N = 224$), for example, the subtests' reliabilities ranged from .66 (digit span) to .95 (vocabulary) and the three scales were .97 (verbal), .96 (performance), and .98 (full scale). Considering the same age group, the standard errors of measurement for the subtests ranged from .66 (vocabulary) to 1.71 (digit span) and for the scales they were 2.64 (verbal), 2.85 (performance), and 2.01 (full scale).

Intercorrelations of the subtests and the scales comprised the only assessment of the EIWA's validity. Again, data were reported for the three age groups used in the reliability assessment. Based on the 25 to 34 age group, for example, the correlations of the six verbal subtests with the verbal scale ranged from .72 to .85 and from .68 to .78 with the performance scale, which was made up of the five subtests. In contrast, the associations of the performance subtests with the performance scale ranged from .75 to .82 and from .64 to .77 for the verbal scale. No tests of concurrent or predictive validity were reported.

In summary, there are two types of Spanish-language versions of the Wechsler tests. One type includes a Spanish translation with minimal adaptation and the use of the U.S. English language norms, whereas the second type includes a Spanish translation with more significant adaptation and new Spanish-language norms based on examinees from Puerto Rico or Mexico. The Spanish-language normed tests report the most comprehensive assessment of the test's psychometric properties for Spanish-speaking individuals. However, these data are based on children and adults living outside the United States mainland. No data were reported regarding the tests'

---

[8]The exception to calculating the subtests' reliability via split-half correlation pertained to the digit span, which was assessed by correlating the scores from the forward and reverse recall procedures, and to the digit symbol, which was assessed by correlating the scores of the first and second administration (test-retest).

reliability and validity in the assessment of Spanish-speaking children and adults residing on the mainland.

Woodcock Johnson Psycho-Educational Battery. The Woodcock Johnson Psycho-Educational Battery–Revised (WJ-R) is described as a "wide-range, comprehensive set of individually administered tests for measuring cognitive abilities, scholastic aptitudes, and achievement" (Woodcock & Mather, 1989/1990, p. 1).[9] The WJ-R is comprised of 21 subtests to measure cognitive ability (7 subtests in the standard battery and 14 supplemental subtests) and 18 subtests to measure achievement (9 subtests in the standard battery and 5 subtests and 4 derivative measures for the supplementary battery). In addition, two subtests from the cognitive battery and two subtests from the achievement battery are used to comprise a separate language survey (Woodcock & Muñoz-Sandoval, 1993). Together, the WJ-R battery provides a comprehensive assessment of cognitive ability and achievement skills and serves as the foundation on which its Spanish-language version, the Batería-R, is based.

The cognitive abilities tests of the Batería-R are referred to as the "Pruebas de habilidad cognitiva–Revisada" (Batería-R COG, Woodcock & Muñoz-Sandoval, 1996b) and the achievement tests are referred to as the "Pruebas de aprovechamiento–Revisada" (Batería-R ACH, Woodcock & Muñoz, 1996a). All subtests in the Batería-R were adapted from the parallel English-language subtests in the WJ-R. Some subtests have identical item content and task requirements for the two language versions (e.g., spatial relations). Other tests with significant verbal content have different item content in the two language forms (e.g., oral vocabulary). The authors of the Batería-R based the Spanish-language norms on the U.S. English-speaking normative sample (Woodcock & Muñoz-Sandoval, 1996b). They argued that drawing a set of norms from Spanish-speaking individuals residing in the United States would be difficult because this community is in flux and because professionals would not likely accept such a group as a representative norming sample for assessment purposes (Woodcock & Muñoz-Sandoval, 1996b, p. 23). Moreover, the authors noted that U.S. English-speaking individuals are "identifiable," "relatively stable over time," and represent the "standard reference for norms on tests" in the United States.

Because the norms of the Batería-R were based on the U.S. English-speaking norms, it is important to consider the English-language standardization sample, a U.S. national sample of 6,359 persons, ages 24 months to 95 years. It used a stratified sampling design that controlled for four community variables (e.g., census region and community size) and six examinee characteristics (e.g., race, Hispanic origin, and educational level). The examiner's manual indicates that subjects were randomly selected within this stratified sampling design, although the manner in which this was carried out was not delineated. A total of 9.3% of the standardization sample was Hispanic, which compares favorably to the group's representation across all ages in the 1980 U.S. census (6.4%). Individual subject weighting was used in the data analysis so that the distribution of the subsamples as they relate to the 10 sampling variables approximated the 1980 U.S. census data.

---

[9]The Woodcock Johnson-III (WJ-III) is now available, but because its Spanish-language companion has yet to be published, we do not consider the WJ-III in this chapter.

For those Spanish-language subtests with content identical to their English-language counterparts, no new norms were derived. The U.S. English-language norms were applied without modification. For those tests in which the subtest content differed, equated U.S. norms were developed that are very similar, though not identical, to the U.S. English-language norms. An important step in developing the equated norms was to calibrate the Spanish-language items with largely monolingual Spanish-speaking individuals. The calibration analyses addressed the assessment of item difficulty rather than the development of specific Spanish-language norms. This sample was comprised of approximately 2,000 native Spanish-speaking persons who primarily resided in Mexico and the United States; others lived in Costa Rica, Peru, Puerto Rico, and Spain. Those from the United States reported having been born in 21 different Latin American countries, including the United States and Spain. Thus, for the calibration analyses, test developers sampled monolingual Spanish-speaking individuals from a large number of Spanish-speaking countries and the United States.

The reliability assessment of the Batería-R was based on the calibration sample data. The test's internal consistency reliability coefficients (split-half correlations corrected for length by the Spearman-Brown formula) and standard error of measurement were reported. The median internal consistency coefficients across a number of ages and for selected subtests ranged from .83 (incomplete words) to .92 (verbal analogies). The median standard error of measurement for the same selected ages and subtests ranged from 4.9 (verbal analogies) to 8.1 (memory for words).

Two limited concurrent validity studies were reported in the supplemental manual examining the relationship between the oral language cluster measures from the Batería-R to other language measures. One study of about 70 kindergarten students designated as limited English proficient (LEP) found correlations ranging from .44 to .85. The second study with about 120 LEP second graders found a wider range of associations, from .15 to .88.[10] The authors did not indicate why they chose to focus specifically on language measures rather than other measures of cognitive-intelligence abilities. Based on this limited assessment of reliability and validity, the authors reported that "the reliability and validity characteristics of the Batería-R COG meet basic technical requirements for both individual placement and programming decisions" (Woodcock & Muñoz-Sandoval, 1996b, p. 29).

In summary, the Batería-R COG distinguishes itself by being a Spanish-language version of a cognitive-intelligence performance test using equated norms based on the U.S. English-language norms. There were no reports of the test's validity in the assessment of cognitive-intellectual functioning.

Nonverbal Tests of Cognitive Ability. The General Ability Measure for Adults (GAMA; Naglieri & Bardos, 1997) is a standardized, norm-referenced test developed to measure intellectual abilities of adults using nonverbal stimuli. Some researchers have argued that tests requiring English-language skills and knowledge learned in school are limited in assessment ability (e.g., Prewett, 1995), particularly among

---

[10]The supplemental manual reported that the developers tested the associations between the Batería-R oral-language test and the Woodcock-Munoz Language Survey–Spanish oral-language test in these two studies. However, given that the two oral-language tests are noted as having common content, we did not include them in the range of correlations.

persons with diverse educational, cultural, and linguistic backgrounds. One of the objectives of this test then is to address that concern by using abstract designs as the test's content. The test is brief (66 total items), can be administered individually or in groups, and is comprised of four subtests: matching, analogies, sequences, and construction. The test contains a general set of written instructions that are to be read aloud for each subtest as well as written instructions for each of the 66 items. The reading level is noted to be at the third-grade level. A Spanish-language version of the test is available.

The test was standardized on a sample of 2,360 people from 18 to 96 years of age. The sample included nine age groups stratified by race or ethnicity, gender, five educational levels, and four geographical regions. The racial and ethnic groups were African American, American Indian, Asian or Pacific Islander, Hispanic, and White. The stratification by the main demographic variables approximated the 1990 U.S. census. This generally appeared to be the case with regard to the age and educational level of Hispanics who comprised 7.8% of the sample and who in 1990 comprised 7.9% of residents 18 years and older in the United States (U.S. Census, 2001a). In addition to being represented in the standardization sample, race and ethnicity were also considered in the composition of the tryout sample of 604 persons. The manual reports that differential item functioning (DIF) for Whites and non-Whites was assessed based on the tryout data and, where possible, the items with a significant DIF were eliminated. Three such items were identified as having a significant differential item function for Whites and non-Whites. With regard to language background, nearly 7% reported that they spoke more than one language. Thus, it appears that the sample was over 93% English speaking only, with the remaining sample having some unknown level of proficiency in another language.

Overall, the test authors report a range of reliability and validity assessments, although none were conducted specifically with Hispanics. Given that this is a nonverbal test of intelligence it is most important to consider how it relates to other tests of intellectual ability that include verbal content. In one study, the GAMA was administered concurrently with the WAIS-R and the Kaufman Brief Intelligence Test (K-BIT; Kaufman & Kaufman, 1990) and found to have a similar pattern of mean scores and significant correlations with these other tests' full IQ scores (.75, .70), verbal scores (.65, .54), and performance scores (.74, .72). These data support the validity of the GAMA as a general measure of intellectual ability. The sample of this study was comprised of 194 individuals of whom 88% were identified as White; no Hispanics were noted as being included in this sample.

The Universal Nonverbal Intelligence Test (UNIT; Bracken & McCallum, 1998) represents a recently developed, individually administered nonverbal measure for children and adolescents from ages 5 through 17. Like the GAMA, the UNIT is principally designed to address issues of fairness in the cognitive-intellectual abilities of youth, particularly those "who may be disadvantaged by traditional verbal and language-loaded measures" (Bracken & McCallum, p. 1). Among these groups are children and adolescents from diverse cultural, linguistic, educational, and hearing-impairment backgrounds. In addition, the UNIT is intended to measure a broad range of abilities, not relying on a single ability dimension (e.g., problem solving). Another key characteristic of the UNIT is that it is completely nonverbal, from test content to test administration.

The test is comprised of six subtests, three measures of memory and three measures of reasoning. In addition, the instrument is designed to tap symbolic processes, those thought to be associated with language, and nonsymbolic processes, those thought to be less associated with language. The test can be administered as an abbreviated or screening battery (two subtests), a standard battery for placement decision making (four subtests), or an extended battery for additional diagnostic information (six subtests).

The UNIT is norm referenced and has been standardized with a sample of 2,100 children and adolescents. An additional 1,765 youth participated in studies that assessed reliability, validity, and fairness. The sample was stratified according to the usual demographics including race and ethnicity, sex, geographical region, community setting (rural, urban, or suburban), and parental educational attainment (four levels). With regard to Hispanics, 13% comprised the normative sample, which is consistent with the census reports for 1995 for children in the 5 to 17 age range (13.1%, U.S. Census Bureau, 1996). In addition to these usual demographic variables, the test designers included in the standardization sample students receiving special education services, such as services for learning disabilities (5.6%), bilingual education (1.8%), and English as a Second Language (ESL; 2.0%).

Given the main objective of the UNIT, to provide a fair assessment of persons from diverse backgrounds, considerable attention was given to fairness. The authors first presented the steps they took to reduce any potential cultural bias. Included among the steps was the subjective review by ethnic minority psychologists and hearing-impaired individuals for items that were potentially biased or for any materials that might be perceived as offensive. Another step was the assessment of differential item functioning of all items within and between ethnic groups, level of English-language proficiency, and other key sample characteristics. In analyses with Hispanics, only one item was identified as possibly having a different meaning for Hispanics as opposed to the overall normative sample. However, after careful review of the data and the content, bias experts and the authors concluded that the evidence did not support the hypothesis that the item was biased and it was therefore retained.

To further assess the test's fairness, the reliability and validity of these tests were examined separately for specific demographic groups, including Hispanics ($Ns = 120$ to 156). In terms of the subtests' reliability for Hispanics, correlations using the split-half method with Spearman Brown corrections ranged from .75 (mazes) to .94 (cube design). The internal consistency of the scales for the standard battery, for example, ranged from .91 (symbolic) to .95 (full scale). The standard error of measurement for the subtests ranged from .57 (cube design) to 1.12 (object memory) and for the scales of the standard battery from 2.46 (nonsymbolic scale) to 4.06 (symbolic scale). The age range and source of the sample for the reliability assessment were not reported.

In terms of validity, the authors reported the correlation of the UNIT with the Batería-R (Broad Cognitive Ability Early Development) for two native Spanish-speaking samples, from bilingual education classrooms ($n = 27$) and ESL classrooms ($n = 26$). For the bilingual classroom students, the correlations of the scale scores for the standard battery of the UNIT and the cognitive ability scores of the Batería-R ranged from .10 (nonsymbolic scale) to .38 (symbolic scale). The same correlations for the ESL sample were noticeably lower, from .04 (reasoning scale) to .23 (memory scale). Moreover, confirmatory factor analyses for Hispanics drawn from the standardization sample (n = 215) showed that the models tested had an adequate fit to the data.

In addition to carrying out tests of reliability and validity, the authors of the UNIT tested whether the scale means differed for three pairs of groups, all relevant in the assessment of Hispanics. These comparisons included matched samples of Hispanics and non-Hispanics, Bilingual or ESL students and English-speaking examinees, and Ecuadorians and a subsample from the standardization sample. For the standard battery, effect sizes of the scales' mean differences for these comparisons ranged as follows: Hispanics and non-Hispanics (.04 to .20), bilingual/ESL and English speaking (.06 to .36), and the Ecuadorian and standardization subsample (.04 to .73).

In summary, the selected nonverbal tests of cognitive-intellectual functioning range from considering ethnicity much like the English-language Wechsler tests, with attention to sampling and tests of bias, as was the case with the GAMA, to examining the test's technical properties specifically for U.S. Latina/os, as reported in the UNIT's test manual. In addition, for the UNIT, studies of the test's reliability and validity were reported for limited-English-speaking children in the United States and for a non-U.S. sample of Latina/o children from Ecuador.

Psychodiagnostic Measures

MMPI and MMPI-II. The second edition of the Minnesota Multiphasic Personality Inventory (MMPI-II; Hathaway & McKinley, 1991) is the most widely used objective psychodiagnostic measure in the world (Greene, 1991) and among U.S. Latina/os (Velasquez, Ayala, & Mendoza, 1998). This self-report instrument contains 567 items that comprise 10 clinical scales and 3 basic validity scales. Many additional scales are also routinely scored to supplement the clinical scales, including scales to address areas such as substance abuse (MacAndrew Alcoholism Scale) and response consistency (e.g., Variable Response Inconsistency). The normative sample of this instrument is large (n = 1,138 men; n = 1,462 women) and was selected from seven geographic regions within the United States. Overall demographic characteristics of the sample parallel the 1980 census data in areas such as age, gender, and some ethnic group representation (Whites, Blacks, and American Indians). However, the normative sample deviates from the 1980 census (U.S. Census Bureau, 2001b) in the underrepresentation of Hispanics (2.8% in sample, 6.4% in U.S.) and persons with a high school education or less. In addition, there was an overrepresentation of persons with at least some college education.

Other than reporting the ethnic breakdown of the sample, the only other analyses of Hispanics reported in the test manual were included in a table of the mean raw scores from the normative sample for Hispanics and Caucasians by gender (see Appendix H, tables H-1 and H-2). The data indicated that Hispanic men's (n = 35) average raw score was slightly higher than that of Caucasian men (n = 933) on two of the three traditional validity scales and 7 of 10 clinical scales (Graham, 2000). Hispanic women (n = 38) in the normative sample were found to score higher than their Caucasian counterparts (n = 1,184) on all but one validity scale and two clinical scales. The meaningfulness of these group differences is limited by many factors, including the small sample size of Hispanics, the lack of statistical analyses, and in general small mean differences. In fact for men, none of the scale mean differences were greater than the standard deviation for any of the scales for either Hispanics or Whites.[11]

To our knowledge, the MMPI was first translated into Spanish in 1949 for use in Cuba by Bernal and Fernandez (cited in Butcher, Cabiya, Lucio Maquero, & Velasquez, in press). Since then, several Spanish-language translations have been developed, including the Nuñez translation for Mexico and the García and Azán translation in 1984. García and Azán (1993) also translated the MMPI-2, which has been widely used in the U.S. and in Puerto Rico. Until recently, there were no norms developed for the Spanish-language MMPI-2. Butcher, Azán-Chaviano, Cabiya, and Scott (in press) normed the Spanish-language version of the MMPI-2 with a sample from three U.S. cities, Los Angeles (N = 205 with 165 valid-usable profiles), Miami (N = 200 with 165 valid-usable profiles), and San Juan (N = 200 with 151 valid-usable profiles). Study participants were primarily of Mexican, Cuban, and Puerto Rican descent but persons from other Latin American countries were included in the sample if they met criteria. Participants were selected based on the following guidelines: (a) 18 years or older, (b) able to read Spanish at a 6th-grade level or higher, and (c) of "normal" mental health (i.e., not mental health clients). An additional criterion was that no site was to include more than 10% college or graduate students in the sample. The average level of education for the Hispanic sample was 13.56 years for males and 13.41 years for females. With respect to gender, 52.9% of the sample was female. Most of the sample (52%) was married or never married (35.1%) and few participants were divorced (7.8%), widowed (3%), or separated (2.1%). The authors reported adequate test-retest reliability for all of the clinical scales, ranging from .61 to .91. A manual supplement will soon be available from the University of Minnesota Press with the U.S. Hispanic set of norms.

In addition to the U. S. Hispanic set of norms, Lucio and colleagues developed a Spanish-language translation (Lucio, Reyes-Lagunes, & Scott, 1994) and a set of norms for Mexico (Lucio, Ampudia, Durán, León, & Butcher, 2001). In their initial line of investigation they compared the responses of Mexico City college students from la Universidad Nacional Autonoma de Mexico (UNAM; N = 2,174) to those of U.S. college students (N = 1,312). The authors found few significant differences (SD > .5) between the two samples on the validity and clinical scales (Lucio et al., 1994). In a second study examining the validity, clinical, and content scales, the investigators found that the responses of UNAM college students (N = 2,246) differed greatly from a diagnostically heterogeneous sample of patients (N = 233) from three psychiatric hospitals in Mexico City (Lucio, Palacios, Durán, & Butcher, 1999). In addition, they carried out a factor analysis of the patients' responses to the validity and clinical scales separately for men and women.[12]

In an effort to extend the norms beyond a college student sample, Lucio et al. (2001) developed adult norms based on a sample of 1,744 (860 men and 884 women) from different parts of Mexico that represent the "economically active urban population" (p. 1461). The standardization sample included persons between the ages of 19 and 80

---

[11] See Velásquez et al. (1998) for a review of the available studies of the MMPI-2 with Latina/os.

[12] In two other studies, the authors report on the internal consistency and temporal stability of the Spanish-language MMPI-2 with Mexican college student samples (Ampudia, Durán, & Lucio, 1995; Lucio, Pérez-Farías, & Ampudia, 1997). We could not evaluate these findings as we were unable to obtain copies of these two Spanish-language research reports.

years (M = 31). In addition, over one third of the sample had at least a college-level education (38% for men and 44% for women). Lucio et al. reported that the internal consistency of the validity and clinical scales ranged from .62 to .87 for males and .59 to .86 for females. In addition, they examined the differences between the Mexican and U.S. norms. Significant nationality differences (effect sizes greater than .40) were observed for three scales for men (L, Hs, Mf) and seven scales for women (L, F, Hs, D, Mf, Sc, Ma).[13] The authors concluded that, although there is considerable similarity between the norms of the two countries, it is "preferable to use the Mexican norms" in the assessment of Mexicans because such norms take into account cultural factors.

Millon Clinical Multiaxial Inventory–III. The MCMI-III is another widely used self-report inventory that focuses on the assessment of personality disorders associated with the *Diagnostic and Statistical Manual of Mental Disorders* (American Psychiatric Association, 1994) as well as other clinical syndromes related to Millon's theory of personality. This instrument contains 175 true-false items that provide scores on a variety of scales. Fourteen scales measure clinical personality patterns (Axis II), three scales measure severe personality pathology (Axis II), seven scales measure clinical syndrome (Axis I), and three scales measure severe clinical syndrome scales (Axis I). There are also three modifying indices and a validity scale. The three modifying indices—disclosure, desirability, and debasement—assess response tendencies that are associated with particular personality patterns or Axis I conditions. This instrument is intended for use with adults who can read at the 8th-grade level or higher and for those who are seeking mental health services. A strength of the MCMI-III is its strong theoretical framework, but few validation studies have been conducted to verify the accuracy of the theoretical deductions.

Like the standardization sample of the MMPI-2, Hispanics were not well represented in the standardization sample of the MCMI-III: they made up only 2.8% of the development sample and 2% of the cross-validation sample of the MCMI-III (Millon, 1997), compared to 9.2% of the 18 and older U.S. 1995 population (U.S. Census, 1998). No breakdown was given in terms of subgroups (e.g., Cuban Hispanics vs. Puerto Rican Hispanics), due to the fact that the overall number was modest (T. Millon, personal communication, February 6, 2002). Millon (personal communication, February 6, 2002) also conveyed that, although the test developers had intended to collect separate minority group norms, this idea was dropped in the MCMI-III because several scholars reacted negatively, suggesting that "group separations" such as White and Black with such a small sample could produce pernicious and false comparisons. The MCMI-III is available commercially in both English and Spanish. However, no published data are yet available on differences between Hispanics and Whites on the MCMI-III (Strack, 1999).

EVALUATION

Perhaps the single critical question with regard to norm-referenced tests is: What is the appropriate norm for Mexican Americans? Given our definition of culture, which

---

[13]The full names of the noted scales are: L = Lie: F = Frequency; Hs = Hypochondriasis; D = Depression; Mf = Masculinity-Femininity; Sc = Schizophrenia; Ma = Hypomania.

acknowledges its shifting and changing nature and which emphasizes the importance of specific local contexts, multiple norms are essential for the psychological assessment of persons of Mexican origin living in the United States. Among the most important contributions by test developers in the assessment of Mexican Americans is the development of Spanish-language tests based on standardization samples from Mexico. Spanish language tests developed in other locales (e.g., Puerto Rico) have also been helpful. Those persons of Mexican origin who are likely to be at the greatest risk for error in psychological assessment are those whose predominant language is Spanish or who are recent immigrants to the United States (Figueroa, 1989). Having Spanish-language tests normed within a Spanish-speaking locale adds greatly to the available English-language tests and nonverbal tests that can be used in assessing Mexican Americans and other Latina/os.

The EIWN-RPR is, in our view, one of the best Spanish-language normed tests developed thus far. Thoughtful adjustments were made to the test content, scoring, and administration to take into account the specific background of Puerto Rican island children. In addition, the adjustments do not result in significant deviations from the original WISC-R. It is not clear, however, if the test can be effectively used with mainland Puerto Ricans and other Latina/o children in the United States. The careful translation and adaptation suggests that it is a promising measure for other Latina/o children, however.

The Mexican adaptation of the WISC-R is limited by having only sampled children from public school settings. As a result, it may tend to overestimate children's level of functioning (Fletcher, 1989). The very recent developments of U.S. Hispanic norms and Mexican norms for the Spanish-language MMPI-II are also encouraging. However, the investigation of the MMPI-II scale's relations with other clinical measures is needed to examine further its construct validity.

A second development in testing that has important implications for the assessment of Mexican Americans is the further development of nonverbal tests of cognitive-intellectual functioning with contemporary norms. Like the Spanish-language versions of tests, these tests can contribute to assessing those Latina/o adults and children most at risk for error in their assessment. The UNIT is exemplary in the multiple ways the authors considered ethnicity and related examinee variables in the test's development. For example, of the tests reviewed in this chapter for which U.S. national norms were obtained, the UNIT was the only test that reported reliability and validity data for Latina/o and limited English-proficient persons. Nonverbal tests can be most beneficial in the assessment of limited English-speaking Latina/os, but also in other circumstances (e.g., with deaf individuals).

In addition to the strides made in developing Spanish-language normed tests and nonverbal tests, there have been key developments in how tests are standardized in the United States. For example, most test developers now include in their standardization sample a representative proportion of the major racial and ethnic groups. The selected cognitive-intellectual tests for the most part met this standard, whereas the psychodiagnostic tests fell short. A second, relatively new development is the assessment of potentially biased test items. Consultants from racial and ethnic minority groups were asked to carry out subjective reviews to identify potentially biased or insensitive items. In addition, objective statistical analyses, specifically, analyses of differential item functioning, are now part of test development protocols. In the best of circumstances, persons from the major racial and ethnic groups are oversampled and then analyses based on item response theory are carried out for the specific groups. With regard to Latina/os, this type of analysis was only carried out in the development of the UNIT. The other cognitive-intellectual tests grouped the ethnic minority groups together to assess for DIF. The test developers of the psychodiagnostic tests did not report such analysis, although studies have since been published to begin examining the DIF of the MMPI (Waller, Thompson, & Wenk, 2000).

Other developments include the analyses and reporting of test reliability and validity not only by the entire sample or selected subsamples (e.g., age cohorts), but also by racial and ethnic groups. Reliability and validity analyses by race and ethnicity, including separate analyses of Latina/os, were reported only in the UNIT. The reliability analysis for the Batería-R, however, was limited to the Spanish-language calibration sample and the validity assessment only concerned language skills.

Tests that are developed in Spanish but then equated with U.S. English-language norms, as is the case for the Batería-R, have some strengths and limitations. The strength of this approach is that the examiner can compare individuals' level of functioning in Spanish to that of their English-language peers in the United States. In other words, given equated norms, a certain level of functioning in Spanish corresponds to a certain level of functioning in English. Another advantage is that the examiner can administer both language versions of the test to assess how a given individual performs in both languages using a nearly identical metric. It may be that the individual has a higher or lower level of functioning in one language than in another. Using the same metric, one can discern the relative strengths or weaknesses in one language compared to the other. When using distinct norms for each language version of the same or similar test, it is difficult to know the relative level of functioning given that the metric may change with the two distinct sets of norms (one from Puerto Rico and the other from the United States, for example). Thus, having one metric apply to two language versions of a given test has clear advantages.

The limitation, however, is significant; it is not clear how a given Spanish-speaking person is functioning relative to others from that country or place of origin. For example, if a Spanish-language-dominant person performs in English at a level consistent with mild mental retardation, then the examiner may want to assess the person's level of functioning in Spanish as one way to ascertain the role of language and possible sociocultural factors in the evaluation. It may be that the low level of functioning is the result of limited English-language skills. If the person performs within the mild mental retardation range in Spanish compared to others having been raised in Mexico, for example, then this would suggest that linguistic and sociocultural factors do not likely contribute to the identified level of functioning. The examinee is functioning within the mild mental retardation range in both English and Spanish, compared to a U.S. sample and a Mexican sample as well. However, if the Spanish-language assessment reveals that the person is performing within the average range in her native language compared to others raised in a similar environment, then it is more likely that language and sociocultural factors contributed to the English language-based assessment that suggested mild mental retardation. Assessing the person's level of functioning in English and Spanish and comparing that functioning to U.S. and Mexican norms provides a unique vantage point to examine whether linguistic and sociocultural factors play a role. If the Spanish-language test is equated to approximate English-language norms, as is the case with the Batería-R, then the Spanish-language test will not be able to address the question of how language and other possible sociocultural factors may play a role in the examinee's observed functioning.

The assumption underlying the equated norms is that the U.S. English-language norm is the most relevant norm in carrying out cognitive-intellectual assessment. An anthropologically informed perspective would argue for the availability of multiple norms to advance an understanding of a given individual relative to specific local contexts. This is not unlike the decision to apply age-appropriate norms for the WAIS-III rather than one set of norms across the adult ages, as was done in prior versions of the WAIS.

The most striking limitation of tests for Mexican Americans and other Latinos residing in the United States concerns the development of norm-referenced Spanish-language tests (U.S. Department of Health and Human Services, 2001, p. 145). The available Spanish-language tests of cognitive-intellectual ability of adults, for example, are limited by either significantly outdated norms or limited reports of reliability and validity. Among the most frequently used options for psychologists who administer Spanish-language verbal tests of cognitive intellectual functioning to adults residing in the United States include the EIWA with norms that are over 35 years old, the WAIS-III Español with no reported reliability or validity for Spanish-speaking individuals, and the Batería-R COG with very limited assessments of its reliability and validity. Up-to-date, psychometrically valid instruments in Spanish are clearly needed.

FUTURE DIRECTIONS

To build on the reported developments and to address the noted limitations, we recommend that test developers consider a number of issues (see also Suzuki & Valencia, 1997). We believe that the general idea of the Batería-R as a family of tests built around a basic test provides a fruitful design for the development of tests for Mexican Americans and other Latina/os residing in the United States. Such a test would have the English-language version with U.S. norms as well as the Spanish-language version with Mexico, Puerto Rico, or both sets of norms. With both English- and Spanish-language sets of norms available from specific countries or locales of origin, an examiner could then administer a cognitive ability test and examine how that child or adult functions relative to U.S., Mexican, or other Spanish-speaking children or adults. Many alternatives would be available to the examiner, providing a rich assessment protocol.

Let us consider such a test in the assessment of a 13-year-old Mexican immigrant youth who has lived in the United States for 5 years and is having academic difficulties. Let us assume that she is Spanish dominant but also speaks English. The examiner could evaluate her in Spanish first. Her performance could then be compared to that of Mexican children her age. This comparison is useful because it provides a metric that is close to her sociocultural background.

In addition to comparing her functioning with Spanish-speaking Mexicans, this hypothetical test could also be used to assess her functioning with English-speaking youth from the United States. The English-language version could be administered as well. The relative functioning of this adolescent girl in the two languages compared to the two normative samples would provide a wealth of information. Questions of whether her academic difficulties are a function of language, culture, or low cognitive ability can be better addressed by having data from both linguistic and cultural perspectives. For example, if she was found to have some deficits in English and not in Spanish then this would suggest that her academic difficulties may be related to her transitioning to English. On the other hand, if she was found to be low functioning in a given area in both English and Spanish, then this would suggest a deficit in that specific area.

The potential contribution of a multiple-normed test is great, but there are two interrelated challenges in developing such an instrument. One concerns the degree of overlap in test content. Should the two language versions of the same subtests have identical content whenever possible? For example, should the content be the same or different for short-term recall of digits? The advantage of similar or identical content is that a similar metric can be developed. The disadvantage is related to the second challenge, which concerns order effects. If the content is similar or identical in the two language versions, then the level of functioning as assessed with whichever test is administered second is likely to be elevated due to order effects. On the other hand, if the content is different, then it is less clear that the two language versions reflect the same metric. These challenges are not insurmountable. For example, a large item pool could be developed, equated, and drawn from if more than one test version is administered.

In addition to developing Spanish- and English-language test versions, multiple Spanish-language versions could be adapted and standardized with other Spanish-language populations (e.g., Mexicans and Puerto Ricans), if so desired. This could be applied to tests of psychodiagnostics as well as of cognitive-intellectual functioning. Multiple norms could be developed for nonverbal tests as well. The main idea is to have more than one norm for a given test. From an anthropological point of view, this test prototype attempts to understand a given person's functioning within his or her given context. For some individuals, this may mean the U.S. English-language norm, for others the Mexican Spanish-language norm, and still for others both sets of norms will be useful in trying to understand their behavior within their specific setting or settings.

In addition to developing a multiple-language and multiple-normed test, test developers can take steps to improve the way they consider ethnicity and culture in the development of single-norm tests, particularly in developing English-language or nonverbal tests. It would be particularly helpful if test developers oversampled Latina/os and other major ethnic groups. This would not only help in carrying out subsequent DIF analyses for specific ethnic groups, but would also enable test developers to examine within-group variance. Analyses by ethnicity, especially of English-speaking-only Latina/os, provide little opportunity to examine the role of language and immigration, among other potentially important variables. The tests that are shown to be reliable and valid with Spanish-dominant and immigrant subgroups are the tests that are more likely to be used with those subgroups that are the most difficult to assess.

For tests with multiple language versions and multiple norms, it is most important that the psychometric properties be assessed for all versions of the test. One can not assume that the reliability and validity of the original English-language version applies to Spanish-language versions, even if they have been carefully translated, calibrated, or even equated. Also, Spanish-language tests and their norms should be revised periodically to maintain their relevance in our changing world (Lopez & Taussig, 1991). In all, the highest standards of test development should be applied to all tests, regardless of whether they are the original English-language versions or adapted Spanish-language versions.

For many Mexican Americans in the United States who were born in the United States and whose dominant language is English, available psychological tests can be applied effectively. In fact, the lack of systematic test bias with this segment of Mexican Americans (see Sattler, 2001, for a review) suggests that traditional assessment approaches are likely to be valid. For Spanish-dominant Mexican Americans, particularly those who are recent immigrants, U.S. English-language standardized tests have significant limitations. In this chapter, we found advances in a number of areas of selected cognitive ability and psychodiagnostic tests. However, there is still much to accomplish before we have an adequate set of assessment tools that consider the complex and dynamic nature of culture. The development of multiple-normed tests, norms that reflect U.S. English-language norms and Mexican Spanish-language norms, is of greatest value in assessing persons of Mexican origin, especially those who are Spanish-language dominant and are recent immigrants. Moreover, the availability of well-established nonverbal tests can be of great help (Figueroa, 1990). Given the rapidly increasing number of Mexican Americans throughout the United States (U.S. Census, 2001a), it is imperative that the proper assessment tools be developed and made available to address the complexities of language, culture, and psychological functioning.

REFERENCES

American Psychiatric Association. (1994). Diagnostic and statistical manual of mental disorders (4th ed.). Washington, D.C.: Author.

Ampudia, A., Durán, C., & Lucio, E. (1995). Confiabilidad de las escalas suplementarias del MMPI-2 en población mexicana. *Revista Iberoamerican de Diagnóstico y Evaluación Psicológica, 2,* 25–49.

Berry, J. W., Poortinga, Y. H., Segall, M. H., & Dasen, P. R. (1992). *Cross-cultural psychology: Research and applications.* New York: Cambridge University Press.

Betancourt, H., & López, S. R. (1993). The study of culture, ethnicity, and race in American psychology. *American Psychologist, 48,* 629–637.

Bracken, B. A., & McCallum, R. S. (1998). *Universal Nonverbal Intelligence Test: Examiner's manual.* Chicago: Riverside.

Butcher, J. N., Cabiya, J. J., Lucio Maquero, E., & Velasquez, R. J. (in press). *MMPI-2: Assessment of Hispanic Americans in the United States.* Minneapolis: University of Minnesota Press.

Butcher, J. N., Azán-Chaviano, A. A., Cabiya, J. J., & Scott, R. L. (2001). *Manual Supplement: Hispanic version of the MMPI-2 for the United States.* Unpublished manuscript.

Cervantes, R. C., & Acosta, F. X. (1992). Psychological testing for Hispanic Americans. *Applied and Preventive Psychology, 1,* 209–219.

Dahlstrom, W. G., Lachar, D., & Dahlstrom, L. E. (1986). *MMPI patterns of American minorities.* Minneapolis: University of Minnesota Press.

Figueroa, R. A. (1989). Psychological testing of linguistic-minority students: Knowledge gaps and regulations. *Exceptional Children, 56,* 145–152.

Figueroa, R. A. (1990). Assessment of linguistic minority group children. In C. R. Reynolds & R. W. Kamphaus (Eds.), *Handbook of psychological and educational assessment of children* (pp. 671–696). New York: Guilford Press.

Fletcher, T. (1989). A comparison of the Mexican version of the Wechsler Intelligence Scale for Children—Revised and the Woodcock Psycho-Educational Battery in Spanish. *Journal of Psychoeducational Assessment, 7,* 56–65.

Garcia, R. E., & Azán, A. A. (1993). *Inventario Multifasico de la Personalidad-2 Minnesota: Versión Hispana.* Minneapolis: University of Minnesota Press.

Geisinger, K. F. (1992). (Ed.). *Psychological testing of Hispanics.* Washington, DC: American Psychological Association.

Graham, J. R. (2000). *MMPI-2: Assessing personality and psychopathology* (3r ed.). New York: Oxford University Press.

Greene, R. L. (1991). *The MMPI-2/MMPI: An interpretive guide.* Boston: Allyn and Bacon.

Guilford, J. P. (1954). *Psychometric methods* (2nd ed.). New York: McGraw-Hill.

Hathaway, S. R., & McKinley, J. C. (1991). *Manual for administration and scoring MMPI-2.* Minneapolis: University of Minnesota Press.

Herrans, L. L. (1985). *Psicología y medición: El desarrollo de pruebas psicológicas en Puerto Rico.* Mexico, DF, Mexico: Limusa.

Herrans, L. L., & Rodríguez, J. M. (1992). *Proyecto EIWN-R de Puerto Rico: Informe final.* San Juan: Departamento de Salud, Secretaría Auxiliar de Salud Mental.

Kaufman, A. S., & Kaufman, N. L. (1990). *Kaufman Brief Intelligence Test Manual.* Circle Pines, MN: American Guidance Service.

Kleinman, A. (1995). *Writing at the margin: Discourse between anthropology and medicine.* Berkeley: University of California Press.

López, S. R., & Guarnaccia, P. J. (2000). Cultural psychopathology: Uncovering the social world of mental illness. *Annual Review of Psychology, 51,* 571–598.

López, S. R., & Taussig, I. M. (1991). Cognitive-intellectual functioning of impaired and nonimpaired Spanish-speaking elderly: Implications for culturally sensitive assessment. *Psychological Assessment: Journal of Consulting and Clinical Psychology, 3,* 448–454.

Lucio, E., Ampudia, A., Durán, C., León, I., & Butcher, J. N. (2001). Comparison of the Mexican and American norms on the MMPI-2. *Journal of Clinical Psychology, 57,* 1459–1468

Lucio, E., Palacios, H., Durán, C., & Butcher, J. N. (1999). MMPI-2 with Mexican psychiatric inpatients: Basic and content scales. *Journal of Clinical Psychology, 55,* 1541–1552.

Lucio, E., Pérez-Farías, J. M., & Ampudia, A. (1997). Un estudio de confiabilidad test-retest del MMPI-2 en grupo de estudiantes Mexicanos. *Revista Mexicana de Psicología, 14,* 55–62.

Lucio, E., Reyes-Lagunes, I., & Scott, R. L. (1994). MMPI-2 for Mexico: Translation and adaptation. *Journal of Personality Assessment, 63,* 105–116.

McNemar, Q. (1955). *Psychological statistics.* New York: Wiley.

McShane, D., & Cook, V. J. (1985). Transcultural intellectual assessment: Performance by Hispanics on the Wechsler scales. In B. B. Wolman (Ed.), *Handbook of intelligence: Theories, measurements, and applications* (pp. 737–785). New York: Wiley.

Millon, T. (1997). *Millon Clinical Multiaxial Inventory-III.* Minneapolis, MN: National Computer Systems.

Naglieri, J. A., & Bardos, A. N. (1997). *GAMA: General ability measure for adults.* Minneapolis: National Computer Systems, Inc.

Padilla, E. R., Roll, S., & Gómez-Palacio, M. (1982). The performance of Mexican children and adolescents on the WISC-R. *Interamerican Journal of Psychology, 16,* 122–128.

Prewett, P. (1995). A comparison of two screening tests (the Matrix Analogies Test—Short Form and the Kaufman Brief Intelligence Test) with the WISC-III. *Psychological Assessment, 7,* 69–72.

Prewitt-Diaz, J. O., & Rodriguez, M. D. (1986). Reliability of an experimental version in Spanish of the WISC-R with Puerto Rican children 9–5 to 13–1 years of age. *Psychological Reports, 58,* 271–275.

Psychological Corporation (1997). *WAIS-III WMS-III: Technical manual.* San Antonio, TX: Author.

Rodriguez, V. L., & Prewitt-Diaz, J. O. (1990). Correlations among GPA and scores on the Spanish version of the WIS-R and the Woodcock-Johnson achievement subtests for 10- to 12-year old Puerto Rican children. *Psychological Reports, 66,* 563–566.

Rousey, A. (1990). Factor structure of the WISC-R Mexicano. *Educational and Psychological Measurement, 50,* 351–357.

Ryan, J. J., Paolo, A. M., & Brungardt, T. M. (1990). Standardization of the Wechsler Adult Intelligence Scale—Revised for persons 75 years and older. *Psychological Assessment, 2,* 404–411.

Sattler, J. M. (2001). *Assessment of children: Cognitive applications* (4th ed.). San Diego: Jerome M. Sattler Publisher.

Segall, M. H. (1984). More than we need to know about culture, but are afraid not to ask. *Journal of Cross-Cultural Psychology, 15,* 153–162.

Strack, S. (1999). Millon's normal personality styles and dimensions. *Journal of Personality Assessment, 72,* 426–436.

Suzuki, L. A., & Valencia, R. R. (1997). Race-ethnicity and measured intelligence: Educational implications. *American Psychologist, 52,* 1103–1114.

U.S. Census Bureau (1996). *Statistical abstract of the United States: 1995.* Washington, DC: Author.

U.S. Census Bureau (1998). *Selected social characteristics of all persons and Hispanic persons, by type of origin: March 1995.* [On-line]. Available: www.census.gov/population/socdemo/hispanic/cps95/sumtab-1.txt

U.S. Census Bureau (2001a). *Mapping census 2000: The geography of U.S. diversity: Hispanic or Latino origin.* [On-line]. Available: www.census.gov/population/cen2000/atlas/his_lat.pdf

U.S. Census Bureau (2001b). *Statistical abstract of the United States: 2000.* Washington, DC: Author.

U.S. Department of Health and Human Services. (2001). *Mental health: Culture, race and ethnicity a supplement to mental health: A report of the surgeon general.* Rockville, MD: U.S. Department of Health and Human Services, Public Health Service, Office of the Surgeon General.

Velásquez, R. J., Ayala, G. X., & Mendoza, S. A. (1998). *Psychodiagnostic assessment of U.S. Latinos with the MMPI, MMPI-2, and MMPI-A: A comprehensive resource manual.* East Lansing: Julian Samora Research Institute, Michigan State University.

Waller, N. G., Thompson, J. S., & Wenk, E. (2000). Using IRT to separate measurement bias from true group differences on homogeneous and heterogeneous scales: An illustration with the MMPI. *Psychological Methods, 5,* 125–146.

Wechsler, D. (1949). *Wechsler Intelligence Scale for Children.* New York: The Psychological Corporation.

Wechsler, D. (1951). *Escala de Inteligencia Wechsler para Niños.* New York: The Psychological Corporation.

Wechsler, D. (1955). *Wechsler Adult Intelligence Scale.* New York: The Psychological Corporation.

Wechsler, D. (1967). *Escala de Inteligencia Wechsler para Adultos.* New York: The Psychological Corporation.

Wechsler, D. (1974). *Wechsler Intelligence Scale for Children-Revised.* New York: The Psychological Corporation.

Wechsler, D. (1981). *Wechsler Adult Intelligence Scale-Revised.* New York: The Psychological Corporation.

Wechsler, D. (1983). *Escala de Inteligencia Wechsler para Niños Revisada: Edición de investigación.* New York: The Psychological Corporation.

Wechsler, D. (1984). *Escala de Inteligencia para Nivel Escolar Wechsler: WISC-RM.* Mexico, DF, Mexico: El Manual Moderno.

Wechsler, D. (1991). *Wechsler Intelligence Scale for Children* (3rd ed.). San Antonio, TX: The Psychological Corporation.

Wechsler, D. (1992). *Escala de Inteligencia Wechsler para Niños–Revisada (EIWN-R de Puerto Rico).* San Antonio, TX: The Psychological Corporation.

Wechsler, D. (1997). *Wechsler Adult Intelligence Scale* (3rd ed.). San Antonio, TX: The Psychological Corporation.

Wechsler, D. (2001). *Escala de Inteligencia para Adultos: WAIS-III Español.* México, DF, Mexico: El Manual Moderno.

Woodcock, R. W., & Mather, N. (1989/1990). WJ-R Tests of Cognitive Ability-Standard and Supplemental Batteries: Examiner's manual. In R. W. Woodcock & M. B. Johnson (Eds.), *Woodcock-Johnson Psycho-Educational Battery–Revised.* Chicago: Riverside.

Woodcock, R. W., & Muñoz-Sandoval, A. F. (1993). *Woodcock-Muñoz Language Survey.* Chicago: Riverside.

Woodcock, R. W., & Muñoz-Sandoval, A. F. (1996a). *Batería Woodcock-Muñoz: Pruebas de aprovechamiento–Revisada, supplemental manual.* Chicago: Riverside.

Woodcock, R. W., & Muñoz-Sandoval, A. F. (1996b). *Batería Woodcock-Muñoz: Pruebas de habilidad cognitiva–Revisada, supplemental manual.* Chicago: Riverside.

Culturally Competent Assessment of Chicana/os With the Minnesota Multiphasic Personality Inventory-2

Roberto J. Velásquez
San Diego State University

Maria Garrido
University of Rhode Island

Jeanett Castellanos
University of California, Irvine

Maria Patricia Burton
San Diego State University

The Minnesota Multiphasic Personality Inventory-2 (MMPI-2) is the most widely used instrument in research on Latina/os in the United States including Chicana/os or Mexican Americans (Velásquez, Ayala, & Mendoza, 1998), surpassing use of the Rorschach Thematic Apperception Test (TAT), Millon Clinical Multiaxial Inventory-III (MCMI-III), and Personality Assessment Inventory (PAI). Whereas there exists only a handful of studies with instruments such as the Rorschach or PAI (even when considering the unpublished literature), there is a burgeoning body of research with the MMPI-2 (Corrales et al., 1998; Velásquez, Ayala, & Mendoza). This even extends to the MMPI-A, which is the adolescent version of the MMPI-2 (Garrido, 2000). There are more studies on Latina/os with the MMPI-2 than with other instruments, such as the Rorschach, because the MMPI-2 is an objective measure that is less likely to be influenced by the test administrator and is relatively easy to administer and score (Velásquez et al., 1997).

In clinical practice, as in research settings, the MMPI-2 is also one of the most widely used instruments in assessing Chicana/os and members of other Latina/o groups (Rangel & Velásquez, 2000; Rangel, Velásquez, & Castellanos, 2000). For example, in clinical or psychiatric settings, the MMPI-2 is frequently applied to Chicana/os in order to identify and describe psychopathology, confirm psychiatric diagnoses, and aid in treatment planning (Velásquez, Ayala, & Mendoza, 1998). Recently, a Chicano psychologist noted that "the MMPI-2 offers more than other instruments when evaluating Chicana/o clients because of its many scales and subscales, which offers more hypotheses to test from a cultural perspective" (McNeill, 2003). In non-clinical settings, the MMPI-2 is frequently applied to Chicana/os who are candidates for employment, involved in child custody litigation (e.g., fitness for parenting), incarcerated in correctional facilities, or are applicants for disability benefits or worker's compensation (Velásquez, Ayala, et al., 2000).

The present chapter has five goals. First, we wish to highlight some basic facts about the current status of the MMPI-2 (and MMPI-A) as it relates to Chicana/os. For example, Chicana/o men and women were included in the norms of the MMPI-2 as part of the restandarization of the original MMPI (Butcher, Dahlstrom, Graham, Tellegen, & Kaemmer, 1989). Second, we highlight some key trends in research conducted on Latina/os, including Chicana/os. For example, studies have examined the linguistic comparability of the Spanish and English versions of the MMPI-2 (e.g., Velásquez, Chavira, et al., 2000). Third, we present a series of interpretive tips based on both research and our clinical experience when applying the MMPI-2 to Chicana/os and members of other Latina/o groups. For example, the Masculinity-Femininity (Mf) scale appears to be useful in understanding the world view of Chicana/os as it relates to sex roles, attitudes, and behaviors, and does not necessarily reflect machismo or marianismo (Anderson, 1999; Anderson, Fernandez, Callahan, & Velásquez, 2001; Anderson & Velásquez, 2002; Anderson, Velásquez, & Callahan, 2000). Fourth, we present several case studies to illustrate the use of the MMPI-2 with Chicana/os. For example, we present the case of Sandra, who was first evaluated with the English-language MMPI-2 and then the Spanish MMPI-2. Major differences are noted as a function of language, which ultimately affected both diagnosis and treatment. Finally, we present additional case studies in order to illustrate how the MMPI-2 findings can be used with Chicana/o clients to test hypotheses that may be reflective of culture in the manifestation of emotional problems.

SOME BASIC FACTS ABOUT THE MMPI-2 AS IT RELATES TO CHICANA/OS AND OTHER LATINA/OS

The MMPI-2 and MMPI-A are very popular instruments among psychologists who evaluate Chicana/os and members of other Latina/o groups for several key reasons.

First, Latina/os are included in the norms of the English-language version of the MMPI-2 (Butcher et al., 1989). In fact, the sample of Latina/os ($n = 73$) was collected in San Diego, California and is made up of primarily persons of Mexican descent. At the same time, it is important to note that there has been some controversy about the fact that the sample is not as reflective of the diversity in the greater Latina/o population (Grillo, 1994); or, that the norms misrepresent the Latino population. For example, data was not collected in other parts of the country such as Miami, which has a large population of Cuban Americans. On the other hand, English-speaking Latina/o adolescents from different parts of the United States were included in the norms for the MMPI-A (Butcher et al., 1992).

Second, there are numerous Spanish translations of the MMPI-2 available for use with Latina/os. In addition to an official translation of the MMPI-2 for use in the

United States, there exist adaptions for use in Puerto Rico and throughout Latin America (Butcher, 1996). For example, Lucio and colleagues (1994, 2000, 2001, 2002) conducted extensive research on the official Mexican version of the MMPI-2, including the development of Mexican norms for both the MMPI-2 and MMPI-A.

Third, norms were recently devised for the Spanish version of the MMPI-2 for the United States and Puerto Rico (Butcher, 2002; Butcher, Azan-Chaviano, Cabiya, & Scott, 2002). Data were gathered on a representative sample of Latina/os ($n = 484$), including persons of Mexican descent, in the three major cities of Los Angeles, Miami, and San Juan, Puerto Rico. In general, the norms approximate those of the original MMPI-2 normative sample.

Fourth, as for the MMPI-2, there exist numerous Spanish-language adaptations of the MMPI-A. In addition to the official version that was developed for use in the United States and Puerto Rico, there are adaptations for other Latin American countries, including Mexico (Butcher, 1996). In addition, there is an experimental bilingual version of the MMPI-2, in which items are presented in both languages.

Fifth, normative groups exist for the Spanish translation of the MMPI-A. Samples of adolescents from San Juan, Miami, Florida, and Los Angeles were included in the norms (Butcher et al., 1998).

Sixth, technical manuals with extensive psychometric data on both the MMPI-2 and MMPI-A for Latina/os have been developed. Currently, there exist two manual supplements, one for the MMPI-A (Butcher et al., 1998) and one for the MMPI-2 (Butcher, Cabiya, Lucio, & Velásquez, in press).

Finally, additional resources on research on Latina/os are available, including Butcher's (1996) "International Adaptations of the MMPI-2" and Velásquez, Ayala, and Mendoza's (1998) *Psychodiagnostic Assessment of U.S. Latinos with MMPI, MMPI-2, and MMPI-A: A Comprehensive Resource Manual*. Soon to be published is an edited book by Velásquez and Garrido (in press) entitled *The Handbook of Latino MMPI-2/ MMPI-A Research and Application* that summarizes all research conducted with Chicana/os and other Latina/o groups with the MMPI-2 and MMPI-A and includes chapters on new research in Puerto Rico, Mexico, Venezuela, and Cuba.

TRENDS IN RESEARCH ON CHICANA/OS WITH THE MMPI-2

Although it is beyond the scope of this chapter to review every single study that has been conducted with Chicana/os and members of other Latina/o groups, it is important to highlight some of the most salient trends in research. (For a comprehensive review of the literature, see Velásquez, Ayala, & Mendoza, 1998; Velásquez & Garrido, in press. For research on other ethnic or cultural groups, see Velásquez, Ayala et al., 2000.) Following are some of the key trends in research on Chicana/os and Latina/os.

First, Chicana/os or Mexican Americans are the most widely studied Latina/o subgroup with the MMPI-2 and MMPI-A (Gomez et al., 2000; Bumbiner, 1998; Velásquez, Ayala, & Mendoza, 1998). The only other group that has received significant attention are Puerto Ricans in Puerto Rico (e.g., Alamo, Cabiya, & Pedrosa, 1995; Cabiya, 1994; Cabiya, Colberg, Perez, & Pedrosa, 2001; Fournier, 2001; Pena, Cabiya, & Echevarria, 1995, 1996).

Second, research studies continue to compare the MMPI-2 performance of Chi-cana/os to that of other groups, most notably Euro Americans (Velásquez, Ayala, & Mendoza, 1998). Comparisons are usually conducted on the basic validity and clini-cal scales and are less likely to involve the content, supplementary, or Harris-Lingoes subscales (Callahan, 1997; Callahan, Velásquez, & Saccuzzo, 1995; Cook, 1996; Frank, Velásquez, Reimann, & Salazar, 1997; Garrido, Velásquez, Parsons, Reimann, & Salazar, 1997; Ladd, 1996; Maiocco, 1996; Whitworth & McBlaine, 1993; Whitworth & Unterbrink, 1994). Our analysis of these studies resulted in one robust finding: Chicana/os are likely to score higher than Euro Americans on the L (Lie) scale (Calla-han; Garrido, Velásquez, Parsons, Reimann, & Salazar, 1997; Haskell, 1996; Hernan-dez, 1994; Whitworth & McBlaine; Whitworth & Unterbrink), leading us to conclude that Chicana/os may respond differentially on the L scale because of a tendency toward cultural defensiveness, or presenting themselves in the best light to strangers and not airing their dirty laundry in public.

Third, there is a growing body of research that considers intracultural variation on the MMPI-2 (Velásquez, Ayala, & Mendoza, 1998; Velásquez, Ayala et al., 2000). These studies are likely to consider comparisons by gender, psychiatric diagnosis, degree of acculturation, and geographic location (e.g., Anderson et al., 1993; Cabiya et al., 2000; Colon, 1993; Donovan, Castellanos, Velásquez, & Orozco, 2002; Erdman et al., 2000; Fantoni-Salvador & Rogers, 1997; Flores, Chavira, Perez, Engel, & Velásquez, 1996; Garrido et al., 1998; Greenwood et al., 1998; Hudak, 2001; Jella, 2001a, 2001b; Lapham et al., 1997; Maness et al., 2001; Mendoza-Newman, Greene, & Velásquez, 2000; Negy, Leal-Puente, Trainor, & Carlson, 1997; Netto, Aguila-Puentes, Burns, Sellars, & Garcia, 1998). For example, Fantoni-Salvador and Rogers found that Puerto Rican psychiatric patients obtained higher scores on the psychotic- and anxi-ety-related scales when compared to Mexican Americans.

Fourth, researchers have examined the role of acculturation on the MMPI-2 per-formance of Chicana/os exclusively (Callahan, 1997, 2000; Canul, 1993; Canul & Cross, 1994; Chavira, Velásquez, Montemayor, & Villarino, 1995; Chavira, Malcarne, Velásquez, Liu, & Fabian, 1996; Hernandez, 1994; Lessenger, 1997; Mason, 1997; Quintana, 1997), that is, no studies have been conducted on other Latina/o sub-groups, including Puerto Ricans or Cuban Americans. Although findings on the effects of acculturation remain equivocal or inconsistent, it does appear that accul-turation can affect the MMPI-2 performance of Chicana/os. Canul, for example, found that Mexican Americans who were pro-White and anti-Mexican in their ethnic identity orientations tended to score higher on the L scale, whereas those with a pos-itive view toward their own group and a negative view toward the White majority were more likely to obtain lower K (defensiveness) scores. Quintana and Lessenger, using the Acculturation Rating Scale for Mexican Americans-II (ARSMA-II; Cuéllar, Arnold, & Maldonado, 1995) found no relationship between acculturation and the MMPI-2 scales. Unfortunately, none of these studies considered the full range of con-tent, supplementary, or Harris-Lingoes subscales.

Fifth, research has examined the equivalence of linguistic translations to the Eng-lish version of the MMPI-2 (Chavira, Montemayor, Velásquez, & Villarino, 1995; Chavira, Velásquez et al., 1995; Karle, 1994; Pena, 1996; Saavedra, 2000; Velásquez, Callahan, Reimann, & Carbonell, 1998; Velásquez, Chavira et al., 2000; Velásquez, Gutierrez, Jimenez, & McClendon, 1999). The results of these investigations suggest high linguistic equivalence between Spanish adaptations and the original English-language MMPI-2, and the potential for use with monolingual and bilingual Latina/os in the United States. Cabiya (1994) reported on the adaptation of the Chilean version for use in Puerto Rico. Although 22 items had to be modified for the new adaptation, the overall results indicated strong equivalence. Karle and Velásquez, Chavira et al. found good comparability between the U.S. Hispanic Spanish adaptation and the English version. They also found high comparability, as defined by the lack of scale differences, and high test-retest reliability coefficients between two Spanish-language adaptations, the U.S. Hispanic and official Mexican adaptations.

Finally, as previously noted, the majority of the studies conducted with Chicana/os and other Latina/o groups tended to focus on the validity and clinical scales of the MMPI-2. However, a few investigations have considered additional subscales or indices. Colon (1993), in a study in Puerto Rico, found that male psychiatric patients obtained higher scores than male college students on all content scales except the anger (ANG) scale. A similar finding was obtained with female patients, who had higher scores on all scales except depression (DEP) and social discomfort (SOD). Flores et al. (1996) found that age of onset of alcohol use was negatively correlated with the obsessiveness (OBS), posttraumatic stress disorder (PK), ANG, and Cynicism (CYN) scales for Mexican immigrants. Hernandez (1994) found that more traditional Mexican American males obtained higher scores than those assimilated to Anglo values on the fears (FRS) subscale. Mason (1997) found a strong positive relationship between the addiction admission scale (AAS) and greater acculturation toward mainstream values in a group of Latino veterans with posttraumatic stress disorder (PTSD). In our clinical experience, we have found that the additional MMPI-2 scales often yield more information or clinical hypotheses than the validity or clinical scales alone when assessing ethnic minority clients.

Although major strides have been made in research on Chicana/os with the MMPI-2 and MMPI-A, there clearly remain many voids in the literature. Following are some areas that require significant inquiry.

First, much of the research on Chicana/o and other Latina/o groups still needs to be published. Although we cite many studies in this chapter, including dissertations, theses, and conference papers, many remain inaccessible to practitioners and researchers.

Second, there remains a need to conduct studies in the Chicana/o community with persons who fit the general demographic portrait of the population. The majority of the studies conducted on Chicana/os up to this point tend to focus on college students. Unfortunately, at this time, this subpopulation is not reflective of the greater Chicana/o population, which continues to struggle for higher educational attainment (Grillo, 1994).

Third, there is a need for investigations that consider not only the distribution of code types (i.e., configural analyses) for Chicana/os, but also the meaning of these code types through empirical clinical correlates (Ladd, 1994, 1996). The MMPI-2's success is largely based on the empirical correlates associated with scale elevations and profile configurations.

Fourth, further studies are needed on the role of language in the expression of psychopathology through the MMPI-2 for Chicana/os and other Latina/o groups. Although research has focused on examining the comparability of the English and

Spanish translations of the MMPI-2 with bilingual college students, there remains a significant need to examine the performance of psychiatric patients who are bilingual because they are likely to perform differently on two linguistic versions, given the nuances of language and the idioms of distress that are unique to a culture and its language.

Fifth, culture-bound syndromes like *nervios, susto,* and *mal de ojo* as measured by the MMPI-2 need to be investigated. To date, studies that have examined the MMPI-2 performance of Chicana/os have employed traditional psychiatric disorders defined by the *Diagnostic and Statistical Manual of Mental Disorders* (American Psychiatric Association, 2000).

Sixth, there remains a need for computerized interpretation reports to incorporate empirically based and culturally relevant interpretive statements that focus on different ethnic or cultural groups including Chicana/os. For example, it is now feasible for interpretive systems to include statements such as: "The results of the validity scales suggest that Chicana/os (or Latina/os) with this particular scale score (e.g., L) or configuration (code type) are likely to perform in this manner because of the need to present oneself as socially competent." These types of statements, tied to research, would advance the field substantially.

Finally, research conducted in Latin America (Arias, Mendoza, Atlis, & Butcher, 2002; Boscan et al., 2000; Boscan et al., 2002; Hernandez & Lucio, 2002; Lucio et al., 2001; Lucio et al., 2002; Maness, Gomez, Velásquez, Silkowski, & Savino, 2000; Scott & Pampa, 2000) must be linked with research conducted in the United States with Chicana/os (and other Latina/o groups). Recently, Cabiya et al. (2000) described MMPI-2 data from Mexico, Puerto Rico, and the United States; the sample from the United States consisted of Latina/os. They found virtually no differences between the three groups on any of the MMPI-2 validity and clinical scales. The upcoming book by Velásquez and Garrido (in press) not only considers research on Latina/os in the United States and Puerto Rico, but also attempts to establish a linkage by including research from Mexico, Cuba, Venzuela, Colombia, and Peru.

SOME CULTURALLY, CLINICALLY, AND EMPIRICALLY BASED TIPS FOR INTERPRETING SOME SCALES OF THE MMPI-2

Based on our knowledge of Chicana/o and Mexican culture, our extensive work with Chicana/o clients in a variety of settings, and the results of studies conducted with Chicana/os and other Latina/o groups, we now propose some tips for interpreting some of the scales from the MMPI-2.

Lie (L) Scale

The Lie (L) scale of the MMPI-2 is considered to tap into characteristics of persons who are likely to be lying or attempting to deceive or to appear virtuous. Research on Chicana/os indicates that this scale may be elevated in many settings (above 65T) because of an attempt to not air out one's dirty laundry in public. Chicana/os and other Latina/os are socialized to not discuss problems with persons outside of their family. At the same time, Chicana/os are also taught to present the best possible image of themselves, even when under duress or in emotional pain. In other words, one should always appear socially competent.

Infrequency (F) Scale

The Infrequencey (F) scale is considered to be an indicator of general psychological functioning, severity of psychopathology, or both. The F scale can also be used to evaluate the extent to which a person is attempting to fake mental illness, presenting a cry for help, and a client's understanding or comprehension of the MMPI-2 items. In some instances, extremely high elevations among Chicana/o clients are also likely to suggest a lack of understanding due to problems in reading and comprehension, whether in English or Spanish. In some cases, Chicana/o clients whose first language is Spanish have insisted on being evaluated in English. High F scale scores (over 100T) produced by these clients are more likely to suggest that the clients overestimated their proficiency in English and that the MMPI-2 should be readministered in Spanish. Other reasons for high elevations for Chicana/o and other Latina/o clients on the F scale include panic, anxiety, depression, and feelings of being overwhelmed due to personal problems or acculturative stress. Recently, a client obtained a very high score on the F scale (120T) as well as on the Hypochondriasis (Hs), Depression (D), Hysteria (Hy), Paranoia (Pa), Psychasthenia (Pt), and Schizophrenia scales. By all technical standards, such a high F score would automatically invalidate the MMPI-2 protocol, but the client was overwhelmed by circumstances around him and felt out of control. This performance is very common in Chicana/os who have significantly delayed seeking treatment.

Defensiveness (K) Scale

The Defensiveness (K) scale taps into a more defensive or guarded approach toward the MMPI-2. Persons who score over 60T are generally considered to be approaching the MMPI-2 in a defensive, guarded, and suspicious manner. Yet, it is not unusual for Chicana/os to score high on this scale, because they may feel as though their integrity is being judged or they may feel mistrust toward the assessment process. Moreover, many Chicana/os are socialized by their families and within their communities to always be on guard, to be protective of themselves and their family, not trust others, and to be careful about others wanting to take advantage of them. Historically, Chicana/os have been placed in many situations, within many institutions, in which they have to prove themselves to others. Recently, one highly educated Mexican American executive was administered the MMPI-2 as part of an independent evaluation for employment fitness. During the feedback session, the client was asked if he felt defensive and guarded during the evaluation. The client noted that he has always felt as if he has to prove himself to others, especially to White peers, and that he had developed over time an "adaptive defensive and paranoid posture which helps me by everyday."

Masculinity-Femininity (Mf) Scale

The Masculinity-Femininity (Mf) scale taps into attitudes and values toward the same and opposite genders, sex roles, and preferred activities (i.e., masculine versus feminine oriented). Persons who obtain very low scores on the MMPI-2, whether female or male, are likely to be viewed as more traditional, socially rigid, less open to androgynous or nongendered ideals, and more likely to perceive themselves as traditionally masculine or feminine. In research studies, it has been consistently found that Chicano men are more likely to have below-average scores (less than 50T) on the Mf scale, whereas Chicanas are likely to have greater variation (Anderson, 1999; Anderson et al., 2001; Anderson et al., 2000). With regard to Chicano men, it appears that education, socioeconomic status, and upward mobility are less likely to affect their performance on the Mf scale, indicating a tendency toward a more traditional view of themselves. On the other hand, it appears that Chicanas who obtain lowered scores are more likely to view themselves in a traditional manner, yet have other views that are less defined by gender and culture. Chicanas and other Latinas who have been studied in university settings have been found to obtain scores on the Mf scale within the 60 to 65T score range. It has been hypothesized that these Latinas are less likely to be psychologically attached to more traditional views of themselves because they are in academic settings and have left their home environment. They are also more likely to be confronting acculturative stress in academic settings, and having to take on characteristics (e.g., independence, competitiveness, etc.) that ensure success in those settings. Researchers and practitioners are advised to not simply conclude that a Chicana/o's low performance on the Mf scale is a reflection of machismo or marianismo, or that males are hypermasculine and aggressive and females are passive, submissive, and dependent. Furthermore, the Mf scale can usually be clarified by inspecting the Gender Masculine (GM) and Gender Feminine (GF) subscales.

Social Introversion (Si) Scale

High scores on the Social Introverion (Si) scale suggest isolative and withdrawing behaviors, the possibility of psychological decompensation under stress, and feeling uncomfortable or anxious in social or interpersonal situations. High scores for Chicana/os may reflect feelings of alienation, disconnectedness from mainstream culture, social mistrust, and a lack of connectedness to their own culture. We have observed that clients who are less connected with their culture through their identity, socialization patterns, and use of Spanish are more likely to score high on the Si scale. Moreover, they are likely to feel marginalized. On the other hand, it is not unusual for Chicana/os to obtain very low scores on the Si scale, suggesting that they are very socially involved. Chicana/os can be very connected to their families, friends, and community to the point of feeling more than just comfortable around others. In fact, in many families of Mexican descent, children are socialized to be around large groups of people in many social situations and family rituals (e.g., weddings, funerals, *quinceneras*). At the same time, the culture highly values persons who are socially competent because many interactions in the culture stress a sense of familism.

Health Concerns (HEA) Scale

The Health Concerns (HEA) scale is considered an adjunct subscale to the Hs and Hy scales. Usually, those who obtain high scores on the Hs and Hy scales are also likely to have a high score (over 65T) on the HEA. The scale is assumed to tap into somatic and physical concerns and is often related to actual medical problems that the client may have. In many ways, high scores on this subscale for Chicana/os are not surprising, given the fact that they, like other Latina/os, are likely to express many of their psychological problems through physical or somatic symptoms. For example, many Chicana/os are more likely to seek medical treatment from their family practitioner for psychological problems that are expressed physically and are more likely to report that they are physically ill, not suffering from emotional problems. Common physical symptoms reported by many Chicana/os who say they have *nervios* (which they view as a medical condition) include headaches, dizziness, acid reflux, fainting spells, diarrhea, and general physical pain.

Cynicism (CYN) Scale

The Cynicism (CYN) scale was devised to examine a client's general attitude toward society. Persons who score high on this scale are more likely to display high levels of cynicism, pessimism, mistrust, paranoia, and possibly even anger. Usually, the cynicism is highly generalized and not directed at one specific target. This scale is also very important when taken into consideration with the Negative Treatment Indicator (TRT) scale because both are likely to suggest a poor prognosis in treatment. We have observed that Chicana/os and African Americans are likely to score high on the TRT, suggesting a general negative attitude toward society that is defined by mistrust, anger, and the belief that they are unlikely to be assisted by institutions such as medicine, mental health, and the police. We have found that Chicana/o clients who live in very marginal situations, including poverty, and who report being victimized by prejudicial or racist acts are likely to elevate this scale. It is often best to begin discussing the CYN scale in a therapeutic feedback session in order to promote trust, which is crucial in the successful treatment of Chicana/os.

In addition to the scales just described, we also present a series of questions that must be posed by the practitioner (and researcher) prior to administering the MMPI-2 or MMPI-A to Chicana/os. These questions are likely to enhance the validity and realism of the MMPI-2 for Chicana/o clients:

1. Is the MMPI-2 the most appropriate measure for my client? Although we consider the MMPI-2 to be the best first measure to apply to Chicana/o clients in order to obtain an overall measure of psychological functioning prior to treatment, it is important to determine whether the MMPI-2 (or MMPI-A) is the most suitable measure for a particular client. For example, if the client is an immigrant from Mexico, has very little formal education, and has limited reading comprehension, then the MMPI-2 should not be administered.

2. Are there any potential barriers to obtaining a valid MMPI-2 measure? Although we cannot evaluate all possible issues or barriers that might affect the MMPI-2 performance of a Chicana/o client prior to administration of the measure, we can begin to identify some factors that are likely to affect the validity of the measure. For example, if the client has had a history of bad experiences with the mental health or legal systems, then it would not be surprising to see the client be defensive or guarded, not take the evaluation seriously, and respond in a haphazard or random

manner on the MMPI-2. One client reported that he was not willing to take the MMPI-2 because "it had been used by my social worker to take my children away from me, to lose my family and my job." On the other hand, a client who was originally evaluated by a non-Chicana/o psychologist reported that this was her chance (or second opportunity) to be honest because the first psychologist "was a gringo, did not speak Spanish, and did not appear to be interested in helping me. I'm glad that you are Latina because at least you can understand my culture, yet I don't want you to write me a good report simply because you are Latina."

3. Is my client currently experiencing significant acculturative stress? Chicana/os, and other Latina/os, who are experiencing heightened levels of acculturative stress on an acute basis are more likely to produce profiles that are invalid or questionably valid. We have found that clients who report *nervios* (nerves), *mal de ojo* (evil eye), and *ataques de nervios* (nervous attacks), and who may need stabilization with psychotropic medications, are more likely to generate extremely high F scale scores and floating profiles (i.e., all scales are extremely elevated) that appear to be consistent with their perceived lack of control, psychological weakness or *debilidad*, fears or *miedos*, and feelings of intense and overwhelming anxiety. In many outpatient settings, Chicana/os are likely to endorse a very high number of pathological items as true because at the present moment, they are in crisis. In fact, a large part of psychotherapy with Chicana/os is crisis-oriented.

4. Has my client been previously evaluated with the MMPI-2 (or MMPI-A) and was it a positive or negative experience? As noted previously, it is always important to ask Chicana/o clients about their past history in treatment and participation in a psychological evaluation. Clients who report negative experiences with the MMPI-2 are less likely to take the measure seriously. Persons who have had good experiences with the MMI-2 are likely to report that they received feedback from their psychologist that may have been painful, but that did promote insight and change in behaviors, feelings, or attitudes. Moreover, we have found that Chicana/o clients who report that "feedback" was positive because it confirmed their problems to themselves are more likely to fully participate in therapy.

5. Should I administer the MMPI-2 in English or Spanish, or should I administer both linguistic versions? This is a very critical question to ask given the fact that Chicana/os and other Latina/o groups are likely to be monolingual English or Spanish speaking, bilingual with one language being dominant, fully proficient in both languages, or some combination thereof. Typically, prior to administering the MMPI-2 to Chicana/o clients, we ask them which language is most frequently accessed when they have to talk about their feelings, either good or bad, painful or happy, or which language is preferred for talking about their feelings or problems with others. With Latina/o clients who are proficient in both English and Spanish, we always make the assumption that the clients' use of either language is dependent on many situations or factors including whether the client is at work or home, with Chicana/o and non-Chicana/o friends, and so on. We also assume that many clients may begin therapy in one language, then switch to the other, and then use both interchangeably. For example, the case of Sandra, which is discussed later in this chapter, illustrates our assumption quite well. She chose to begin therapy in English, continued for several sessions in English, but then switched to Spanish when she could not locate a particular word or idiom to describe her psychological pain. From that point on, therapy continued only

in Spanish. In many situations, we have seen psychologists misapply the MMPI-2 to Chicana/o and other Latina/o clients because they did not consider the important role of language. This behavior on the part of the professional, which we consider unethical, is likely to result in poor, substandard, or inappropriate treatment for the client.

CLINICAL CASE STUDIES

Following are three case studies illustrating some of the potential problems of not considering cultural or linguistic factors in the interpretation of the MMPI-2. Solutions for each are proposed.

Case #1: Sandra

Sandra was a 24-year-old female college student who was born and raised in Mexico until the age of 13, when her family moved to the United States. She identified herself as "Mexicana." Sandra entered therapy in English, but quickly switched to Spanish because she felt more comfortable self-disclosing in her native language. Her therapist identified herself as Mexican American and Spanish speaking. Sandra was administered the MMPI-2 a total of three times. At intake she was administered the MMPI-2 in English and obtained a valid profile suggesting severe psychopathology and perhaps a psychotic disorder. This was evidenced in her profile configuration, which included elevations on the Sc, Pt, and Pa scales, an 8-7-6 code type. An additional elevation on the Si scale also suggested the potential for severe withdrawal and isolation. If these results were allowed to stand alone, the likely diagnosis (e.g., schizophrenia) would have suggested the possibility of hospitalization and the use of psychotropic medications. However, this was an unlikely diagnosis given the clinical observations by the therapist. Given the fact that she had language switched after the third session, the decision was made to readminister the MMPI-2 in Spanish. This time she obtained a profile more suggestive of interpersonal problems and not psychosis, as demonstrated by her code type with elevations on the Pt, Sc, and Psychopathic Deviate (Pd) scales, a 7-8-4 code type. Her Si scale was significantly lower and suggestive not of isolation, but of social involvement. Many of the content scale scores dropped by at least 10 T-score points (or one standard deviation), including Bizarre Mentation (BIZ), Antisocial Practices (ASP), and Social Discomfort (SOD), also affecting the diagnostic impression.

She was readministered the MMPI-2 in Spanish about 8 months later as part of her treatment. Although there was a drop in some scores, her code type remained essentially the same, supporting the hypothesis that Sandra's problems were more long-standing and interpersonally related. Clearly, she did not appear to be in need of hospitalization or medication, but instead required long-term interpersonally oriented psychotherapy.

Case #2: Maria

Maria was a 39-year-old self-identified Mexican American woman who was referred for individual counseling by her couple's therapist. Maria was born and raised in Mexico until the age of 16, when she and her family moved to the United States.

Maria's primary complaint was her inability to understand herself and her husband of 12 years as she described feelings of depression, anxiety, hopelessness, and frustration. Maria endured emotional and physical abuse from her husband for many years, but continued to feel an obligation to stay with him and care for him and their children.

At intake, Maria was administered the MMPI-2 in English because she preferred to speak English. Her profile appeared to be valid and suggested that Maria likely had a serious thought disorder with paranoid features, possibly paranoid schizophrenia. After several therapy sessions, the therapist's clinical observations (combined with history) did not substantiate the client's profile and the MMPI-2 was readministered in Spanish. In both the Spanish and English versions, Maria reported a significant amount of distress, yet it appeared that she expressed her concerns more openly in Spanish, due to a lower K scale on the Spanish version.

The Spanish version also yielded decreased scores on eight clinical scales: Between the two versions, four of the scale scores differed by at least one standard deviation. The greatest difference was evident in the Pa scale, by which there was a decrease of two standard deviations. In addition, the D and Pd scales decreased by 15 and 13 points, respectively, on the Spanish version. Despite such drastic decreases in several of the clinical scales, Maria's profile remained elevated on six clinical scales. In addition to decreases on clinical scales, four content scales dropped to the subclinical level in the Spanish version. These differences were evidenced on the LSE, Work Interference (WRK), FAM, and TRT scales, suggesting that Maria's MMPI-2 performance in English reflected greater pathology. These differences provide further evidence for identifying the client's comfort zone with respect to language for self-disclosure in psychotherapy.

Case #3: Mr. and Mrs. Gonzalez

Mr. and Mrs. Gonzalez were evaluated for couple's therapy they had been married for 20 years. She was born in the United States and he was born in a small village in Mexico. She had a college degree in business, whereas he had an eighth-grade education from Mexico. The primary concern voiced by Mrs. Gonzalez was that, "since being married, we have discovered that we are very different, because of our culture and where we were born." She stated that "it is like being married to someone from another race. We always seem to argue about our values, including my goal to achieve a career as a teacher. He would prefer to have me stay at home. Also, he complains about me identifying as Chicana while he continues to identify himself as Mexicano."

As part of the evaluation, both were administered the MMPI-2, Mr. Gonzalez in Spanish and Mrs. Gonzalez in English. Their MMPI-2 performance reflected both similarities and differences. For example, both had highly elevated L scales, suggestive of a need to appear socially competent and free of major problems and consistent with research findings and clinical data. On the other hand, there were major differences on the Mf scale, which appeared to reflect differences in cultural values, sex role ideologies, and, perhaps more importantly, acculturation. Mr. Gonzalez appeared to possess a more traditional masculine, rough, and aggressive world view, whereas Mrs. Gonzalez appeared to possess a more nontraditional perspective. This included being competitive, socially active, and highly independent. In addition, it appeared that Mrs. Gonzalez' issues included a mood component, whereas Mr. Gonzalez appeared to minimize any problems. In this case, it was very important to work with the couple around issues of communication, sex role expectations, and long-term family goals. It is important to note that one year later Mrs. Gonzalez filed for divorce and became a teacher.

PROVIDING FEEDBACK TO CHICANA/OS WITH THE MMPI-2

Case #1: Patricia

Patricia was a 42-year-old Chicana who had been married for 22 years. She is a third-generation American and was born in Arizona. She had a 24-year-old son who is in the military and a daughter who was 17 years old and finishing high school. She indicated that she came to therapy because she continues to have cravings for alcohol although she was sober at the time. She stated that her husband had been sober for 5 years and that she had been hospitalized 3 years earlier when "I had been drinking all day. I threw a tantrum. My husband called the police. The police set me up at a crisis center for 2 weeks. I did really good. After many months sober, I started drinking again. I was arrested for petty theft and went to jail for 3 months. I got out, did well. It's been 2 years since I got out of jail."

Patricia indicated that she was very afraid of her marriage ending and her family abandoning her because of her alcoholism, especially if she relapsed. She indicated that she had recently experienced a panic attack and had to be taken to a hospital emergency room. She stated that this attack was related to her desire to want to drink and said that "I know the next time I drink, I'll kill myself." She was placed on several medications including Serzone, Respirdol, and Celexa.

Patricia was administered the MMPI-2 in English after the third session, when rapport and trust had been firmly established. Prior to giving feedback to her, which occurred during the fourth session, she was asked about her general reactions to the MMPI-2. She replied: ". . . not difficult to do. I was surprised about the questions, about my parents. However, it touched some tender subjects because I had a very emotional time as a child. I was trying to be open and honest."

A review of the MMPI-2 validity scales indicated that the profile was valid and interpretable, with the L scale at 47T, F at 55T, and K at 56T. A review of the clinical scales indicated significant elevations on the Hs (71T), D (88T), Hy (87T), Pd (87T), Pt (63T), and Sc (82T) scales. Prior to reviewing the clinical scales with Patricia, and to better understand the meaning of the scales, three key subscales, elevated within the clinical range, were presented and discussed with her. She was told that her performance on the MMPI-2 indicated significant fear and worry (FRS scale). She responded, "Yes, fear of losing my husband, my mind will think that way. Tomorrow I can die. I'm trying to get into the moment." She was also told that the results reflected significant family problems or issues (FAM scale). She replied, "What I can see happening is going to prison. Killing myself, that would be first but not now. I was the one pushing it that way. I said some damaging things, verbal abuse, to my

husband and kids." A review of the Harris-Lingoes subscales indicated many elevations on the various subscales, but one was consistent with her family problems and
being the identified patient (i.e., Authority Problem-Pd2). She responded, "My son,
always telling me to do things right. Telling me I'm wrong. He definitely, he has
issues too. He made me very angry because he was being the father figure and I was
being the daughter. My daughter has oftentimes been the mother-wife in this family,
especially when I went on my drinking binges and she had to take care of me."
As part of the feedback, including goals for treatment, she was also told that her
MMPI-2 indicated that she was at risk for having racing thoughts likely to make her
anxious and panicky in the future (Psychomotor Acceleration-Ma2), for having
explosive behaviors (Explosive Behavior-ANG1), and for performing acts to alienate
herself from her family, including saying hurtful things to her children and husband
(Familial Alienation-FAM2). Today, she remains sober and in supportive-oriented
psychotherapy.

Case #2: Rogelio

Rogelio was a 50-year-old Chicano male who was evaluated after the first meeting
with him. During the intake, he stated that he wanted to receive help for his problems with his family. He stated that he had been recently separated from his wife
because he had been verbally abusive and disrespectful toward her. He stated: "I'm
depressed. I had problems with my wife. I got jealous. I accused her of being with
others. I haven't discovered anything. We were separated 2 weeks ago, maybe
more." He also indicated that his family had been hurt by his behaviors: "My children are affected. They are hurt by my actions and because I attacked my wife." In
addition to depression, he indicated the following symptoms: agitation, irritability,
racing thoughts, crying, guilt, poor sleep, and poor concentration." He noted that he
had also been diagnosed with Parkinson's disease about 3 years earlier.

Rogelio's MMPI-2 was found to be valid and interpretable for the first 370 items,
which include the basic validity and clinical scales. He obtained a score of 52T on the
L scale, 82T on the F scale, and 43T on the K scale. The reason why the latter half
of the MMPI-2 (items 371 to 567) could not be interpreted is that he obtained an Infre-
quency-Back (Fb) score of 116T, which suggested major difficulties or invalidity in
responding to the items, difficulties apparently related to his many symptoms,
including physical problems due to Parkinson's (e.g., poor concentration, low
energy, etc.). He also stated that "the MMPI-2 has a lot of questions. I did not lose
interest. I am not accustomed to reading. I would stop for a while so my mind could
rest." His score on the F scale suggested moderate to severe impairment, which
appeared to be consistent with his self-report of being overwhelmed by his problems. His scores on the clinical scales also reflected severe pathology and distress
including elevations on the Hs (81T), D (85T), Hy (84T), Pd (79T), Pa (105T), Pt (89T),
Sc (94T), and Si (66T). At the same time, it is important to note that, in contrast to
these scales, his Mf scale was relatively low (50T).

Rogelio was asked to respond to the Pa scale, which was the most elevated. He
stated that he had been paranoid because "I had my doubts about my wife. I know I
was wrong, but when she is not in the house I'm doubtful." He was also asked about
having unusual or strange thoughts related to being paranoid, as related to the Sc

scale. He stated that his paranoia about his wife being unfaithful had led him to believe that "I could feel humidity in her private parts and thus confirming my beliefs about her being with other men and unfaithful." He further indicated that "my wife would reject me sexually. We made love because I wanted to check if she was with someone else." When the BIZ scale was reviewed with Rogelio and he was asked to share other bizarre or unusual thoughts, he responded, "I was paranoid because my sister-in-law's boyfriend looked at my wife differently. I didn't like the way he looked at her. He would undress her with his looks." Rogelio was seen with his family in therapy for 6 subsequent sessions. He and his wife filed for divorce. He now lives with a brother.

Case #3: Juan

Juan was a 27-year-old male who was asked by his mother to come to therapy. His mother indicated that her son was currently living with a girlfriend who was pregnant by him. She also noted that "Juan is very good looking, self-centered, poorly motivated, aggressive, macho, and angry." She suspected that he may have been abusing drugs or alcohol, or both, although he denied this to her. She also noted that Juan had been very angry since childhood because she and Juan's father were divorced and she had married Juan's padrino or godfather (he was also married and left his wife for her). She stated that Juan might benefit from therapy, especially because he was about to become a father.

Juan was administered the MMPI-2 after the intake because he appeared to be very charming yet defensive, guarded, and manipulative. He also presented himself as a "victim" and narcissistic. He indicated that he did not need therapy because he was happy in his current situation, as his girlfriend was pregnant, yet he had a bruise on his face that suggested that he might have been in a recent fight. When asked about the bruise, he stated that he had recently fought his girlfriend's ex-boyfriend because he found him at their apartment being verbally abusive toward her. Yet, Juan had also been abusive toward her on several occasions and had called her a *puta* or whore.

A review of Juan's MMPI-2 indicated that the profile was valid and interpretable. His validity scales reflected a rather open approach or demeanor, with the L and K scales at 39T and the F scale at 51T. His performance on the clinical scales indicated only two elevations, on the Pd and Pa, yielding a 6-4 code type. In addition, his Mf scale was low relative to the Pd and Pa scales, at 50T. The only two elevated content scales were the BIZ (70T) and ANG (74T), indicating both unusual beliefs and significant anger and hostility. In spite of denying any type of substance use, the three substance-related scales were elevated: MacAndrew Alcoholism Scale-Revised (MAC-R; 73T), Addiction Acknowledgment Scale (AAS; 70T), and Addiction Potential Scale (APS; 73T). On the PSY-5 scales, Juan obtained elevations on the Aggression (AGGR; 74T) and Negativity (NEGE; 64T) scales supporting the presence of both high aggression and negativity. A review of the Harris-Lingoes subscales indicates elevations on Pd1 (Familial Discord), Pa1 (Persecutory Ideas), and Ma4 (Ego Inflation) scales. On the content component scales, Juan obtained elevations on the DEP1 (Lack of Drive), ANG1, ANG2 (Irritability), ASP2 (Antisocial Behavior), and TRT1 (Low Motivation) scales.

Collectively, the results of the MMPI-2 are consistent with his mother's description of him. The results also point toward an individual who is likely to hold very traditional hypermasculine beliefs and ideas about sex roles, including his girlfriend's, and to be inflexible and resistant to treatment. The results of the MMPI-2 were shared with Juan at the subsequent therapy session. Juan became very defensive and guarded when asked to talk about issues such as substance use, his rigid views toward women, and his negativity. Although admitting to using various illegal substances on a regular basis, he minimized the effects on his personality and well-being. When told that the MMPI-2 results indicated that he was likely to be more traditional with regard to expectations regarding his girlfriend's behavior, he responded, "I don't think so. That's why I chose to hook up with a *gringa* [White woman]. *Gringas* want a man who is tough, in control, and if need be, aggressive." It appears that the feedback was very threatening to Juan, as he did not return to therapy.

Case #4: Marisol

Marisol was a 37-year-old married Chicana who asked to be seen in therapy upon the completion of treatment of her 6-year-old son, who had been treated for shyness, low participation in school, and low self-esteem. Marisol noted that she was beginning to have doubts about her marriage and husband and was finding herself daydreaming about other men. She also indicated that she no longer found her husband attractive because he was obese and had sexual problems. She stated that she was becoming very anxious and worried about obsessing all of the time. She noted that she was feeling as though she was "stuck" in the marriage.

Marisol was administered the MMPI-2. A review of the validity scales indicated that the profile was questionably valid because she obtained elevations on the L (76T) and K (67T) scales, with a very low score on the F (51T) scale. This configuration reflected an attempt to look good, or free of pathology. Marisol obtained elevations on four of the clinical scales: Hs (84T), D (75T), Hy (82T), and Pt (70T). She also obtained elevations on the R (75T) and Ma1 (Amorality- 70T). This performance suggested the need for intensive cognitive therapy as she tended to think a lot, ruminate, worry, and become depressed. She confessed to having had an affair with another man and enjoying it sexually. Yet, she admitted to developing a series of somatic symptoms, especially when she laid in bed next to her husband. She also reported a lot of guilt and repression. She was treated for six months with Paxel to relieve her depressive and physical symptoms. She then entered couples therapy with her husband.

Case #5: Mercedes

Mercedes was a 43-year-old female who was born in Guanajuato, Mexico, and was living in San Diego, California. She identified herself as "Mexicana" and said that she sought treatment because she was feeling overwhelmed working 32 hours a week in a welfare-to-work program and had no time to be with her five children, including twins. In addition, she was attending a community college to obtain a certificate in child development. Mercedes had been separated from her husband for 4 months and on three previous occasions. Mercedes reported a history of domestic violence, with her husband exhibiting both verbally and physically abusive behavior. At intake, she reported symptoms of depression, insomnia, apathy, and *nervios.*

Mercedes chose to take the MMPI-2 in Spanish after the first therapy session. Prior to giving her feedback (at the second session), she was asked about her general reactions to the MMPI-2. In Spanish, she responded, "There were certain questions that I did not know how to answer. Other questions about whether I wanted to kill myself, other things. I have thought about being dead, but not killing myself. Then, there were some questions that I did not understand and so I put a question mark next to the question. At times, I got a headache from answering these questions and I could not concentrate."

A review of the MMPI-2 validity scales indicated that in spite of Mercedes' concerns, she responded in a valid and interpretable manner. Her validity configuration, with the F scale at 75T, the L scale at 66T, and the K scale at 37T, indicated that, although she did admit to many problems, she also attempted to present herself in the best light. A review of the clinical scales indicates only two elevations, on the Hs (73T) and Mf (69T) scales. When asked to talk about reasons why the Hs would be elevated, she stated that she had been stressed for a long time because "my pregnancies were always very difficult and because of my physical health." This was later substantiated on the HEA (77T) scale. She reported that she had a variety of illnesses, including diabetes, high blood pressure, high cholesterol, migraine headaches, and sinus problems. Given her level of education, her Mf scale was not surprisingly high (69T) until she began to talk about her work history, which included work in factories, cleaning homes, and waiting tables.

The primary objective of this chapter was to present a culturally competent approach to the application of the MMPI-2 to Chicana/os. We accomplished this task by highlighting the many recently established facts about the MMPI-2 (and MMPI-A) as it relates to Chicana/os and other Latina/o groups. We also highlighted some key trends in research, discussed areas that require further research, presented some tips for interpreting some important scales from the MMPI-2, and discussed several case studies with an emphasis on culturally competent interpretation and the provision of therapeutic feedback. Throughout our discussion, we highlighted many studies, published and unpublished, that support our comments, observations, and recommendations. However, we feel compelled to share some additional comments about the application of the MMPI-2 to Chicana/os:

- It is important to note that, although we fully support the use of the MMPI-2 and MMPI-A with Chicana/os, we nonetheless recognize that the MMPI-2 is an imperfect instrument. We acknowledge that, at times, the MMPI-2 may simply not be appropriate for a particular Chicana/o client and recommend using other clinical methods, including structured clinical interviews. Still, we always try to use the MMPI-2 as the starting point in our work with Chicana/os; even an invalid profile of a client may yield some important clinical information that can be used in further assessment and treatment.

- Although there exists a large body of research on Chicana/os and other Latina/o groups with the original MMPI, in both English and Spanish, we view this body of research with great caution. For example, Chicana/os were never included in the original test norms, linguistic translations of the MMPI were poorly designed, and the samples were ill defined. Furthermore, in many studies that compared Chicana/o psychiatric patients to Euro Americans, no controls were exercised over the severity of the Chicana/o patients' mental illness. Thus, Chicana/os were frequently found to appear more pathological on the MMPI because they were more severely impaired than the Euro Americans. Methodological reviews of this body of research suggest many problems that bring into question the integrity and validity of that literature. We view this past research as related to, but quite different from, the new literature on the MMPI-2 and MMPI-A.

• We consider the MMPI-2 to be a good instrument for testing out hypotheses about Chicana/o clients' problems, maladaptive behaviors, and interpersonal issues. We always use the results to test hypotheses about the etiology of our clients' problems, yet we recognize that the MMPI-2 will not yield the origins of problems. Thus, we use the results of the MMPI-2 to identify dysfunctional patterns of behavior that can be treated in psychotherapy.

• We reject the notion discussed by other researchers that the MMPI-2 is simply an "etic" measure and therefore biased against Chicana/os. The MMPI-2 was designed to identify and describe psychopathology via symptom patterns. In our collective experience of treating Chicana/o and other Latina/o clients, we have observed that many of their symptoms are no different from those of non-Chicana/os. What does appear to be different are the attributions or explanations made by Chicana/os with regard to the origin and symbolic meaning of these symptoms as evidenced in case studies. This is where we believe culture is most critical and where we, as assessment psychologists, are most challenged to integrate culture.

• Although we may have given the impression in this chapter that the only instrument that we use with Chicana/os is the MMPI-2, the reality is that we use other important measures, such as instruments designed to evaluate intelligence and neuropsychological functioning. We adhere to the use of multiple methods of assessment in order to gain a thorough assessment portrait of the Chicana/o client, yet we also believe that redundancy, by using too many measures, can be problematic.

In closing, we hope that the reader has gained an understanding of why it is important to always conduct psychological evaluations that reflect good standards of practice, respect, and openness to cultural and linguistic diversity, and to engage clients in a format that is grounded in cultural collaboration.

REFERENCES

Alamo, R. R., Cabiya, J. J., & Pedrosa, O. (1995, March). *Utility of the MMPI-2 in the identification of emotional indicators in a sample of Puerto Ricans who experienced armed assault.* Paper presented at the Annual Symposium on Recent Developments in the Use of the MMPI-2, St. Petersburg, FL.

American Psychiatric Association. (2000). *Diagnostic and Statistical Manual of Mental Disorders.*

Anderson, T. R., Thompson, J. P., & Boeringa, J. A. (1993, August). *MMPI-2 and Mississippi scale profiles of Hispanic veterans with post-traumatic stress disorder.* Paper presented at the 101st Annual Meeting of the American Psychological Association, New Orleans, LA.

Anderson, U. (1999). Validation of the MMPI-2 Masculinity-Femininity scale with Latino men and women: Preliminary findings. *The SDSU McNair Journal, 6,* 70–77.

Anderson, U., Fernandez, S., Callahan, W. J., & Velásquez, R. J. (2001, May). *Validation of the MMPI-2 Masculinity-Femininity scale with Latino men and women*. Paper presented at the Annual Symposium on Recent Developments in the Use of the MMPI-2, Minneapolis, MN.

Anderson, U., & Velasquez, R. J. (2000, June). *Machismo and marianismo: Are they a reflection of low MMPI-2 Mf scores*. Paper presented at the Annual Symposium on Recent Developments in the Use of the MMPI-2, Minneapolis, MN.

Anderson, U., Velásquez, R. J., & Callahan, W. J. (2000, August). *Sex roles, cultural differences and Mf scores of Latinos*. Paper presented at the Annual Meeting of the American Psychological Association, Washington, DC.

Arias, G., Mendoza, K., Atlis, M., & Butcher, J. N. (2002, May). *MMPI-2 use in Cuba: An illustration and future directions*. Paper presented at the Annual Symposium on Recent Developments in the Use of the MMPI-2, Minneapolis, MN.

Boscan, D. C., Penn, N. E., Velásquez, R. J., Reimann, J., Gomez, N., Guzman, M., Berry, E. M., Infantes, L. D., Jaramillo, L. F., & De Romero, M. C. (2000). MMPI-2 profiles of Colombian, Mexican, and Venezuelan university students. *Psychological Reports, 87*, 107–110.

Boscan, D. C., Penn, N. E., Velásquez, R. J., Savino, A., Maness, P., Guzman, M., & Reimann, J. (2002). MMPI-2 performance of Mexican male university students and prison inmates. *Journal of Clinical Psychology, 58*, 465–470.

Butcher, J. N. (1996). *International adaptations of the MMPI-2*. Minneapolis: University of Minnesota Press.

Butcher, J. N. (2002, February). *Workshop on the new norms for the Hispanic version of the MMPI-2 for Spanish speaking people in the United States*. Paper presented at the MMPI-2 Workshops and Symposia, Irvine, CA.

Butcher, J. N., Azan-Chaviano, A., Cabiya, J. J., & Scott, R. (2002, May). *New norms for the Hispanic version (Garcia-Azan) of the MMPI-2*. Paper presented at the Annual Symposium on Recent Developments in the Use of the MMPI-2, Minneapolis, MN.

Butcher, J. N., Cabiya, J., Lucio Maquero, E., Pena, L., Reuben, D. L., & Scott, R. (1998). *MMPI-A: Inventario Multifasico de la Personalidad- para Minnesota, Adolescentes*. Minneapolis: University of Minnesota Press.

Butcher, J. N., Cabiya, J., Lucio Maquero, E., & Velásquez, R. J. (in press). *MMPI-2: Assessment of Hispanic Americans in the United States*. Minneapolis: University of Minnesota Press.

Butcher, J. N., Dahlstrom, W. G., Graham, J. R., Tellegen, A., & Kaemmer, B. (1989). *Manual for the restandardized Minnesota Multiphasic Personality Inventory: MMPI-2: An administrative and interpretive guide*. Minneapolis: University of Minnesota Press.

Butcher, J. N., Williams, C. L., Graham, J. R., Archer, R. P., Tellegen, A., Ben-Porath, Y. S., & Kaemmer, B. (1992). *Minnesota Multiphasic Personality Inventory-Adolescent: Manual for administration, scoring, and interpretation*. Minneapolis: University of Minnesota Press.

Cabiya, J. J. (1994, May). *Application of the Hispanic MMPI-2 in Puerto Rico*. Paper presented at the Annual Symposium on Recent Developments in the Use of the MMPI-2, Minneapolis, MN.

Cabiya, J. J., Colberg, E., Perez, S., & Pedrosa, O. (2001, March). *MMPI-2 clinical profiles of female victims of domestic violence and sexual abuse*. Paper presented at the Annual Symposium on Recent Developments in the Use of the MMPI-2, Tampa, FL.

Cabiya, J. J., Lucio, E., Chavira, D. A., Castellanos, J., Gomez, F. C., & Velásquez, R. J. (2000). MMPI-2 scores of Puerto Rican, Mexican, and U.S. Latino college students: A research note. *Psychological Reports, 87*, 266–268.

Callahan, W. J. (1997). Symptom reports and acculturation of White and Mexican-Americans in psychiatric, college, and community settings. *Dissertation Abstracts International, 58*(8-B), 4439.

Callahan, W. J. (2000). *Mexican-American acculturation and MMPI-2 performance*. Paper presented at the Annual Meeting of the American Psychological Association, Washington, DC.

Callahan, W J., Velásquez, R. J., & Saccuzzo, D. P. (1995, August). *MMPI-2 performance of university students by ethnicity and gender*. Paper presented at the 103rd Annual Meeting of the American Psychological Association, New York, NY.

Canul, G. D. (1993). The influence of acculturation and racial identity attitudes on Mexican Americans' MMPI-2 performance. *Dissertation Abstracts International, 54*, 6442B.

Canul, G. D., & Cross, H. J. (1994). The influence of acculturation and racial identity attitudes on Mexican Americans' MMPI-2 performance. *Journal of Clinical Psychology, 50*, 736–745.

Chavira, D. A., Montemayor, V., Velásquez, R. J., & Villarino, J. (1995, August). *A Comparison of two Spanish translations of the MMPI-2 with Mexican Americans*. Paper presented at the 103rd Annual Meeting of the American Psychological Association, New York, NY.

Chavira, D. A., Malcarne, V., Velásquez, R. J., Liu, P. J., & Fabian, G. (1996, August). *Influence of ethnic experience on Spanish MMPI-2 performance.* Paper presented at the 103rd Annual Meeting of the American Psychological Association, Toronto, Canada.

Chavira, D. A., Velásquez, R. J., Montemayor, V., & Villarino, J. (1995, March). *U.S. Latinos' performance on the Spanish language MMPI-2 and acculturation.* Paper presented at the Annual Symposium on Recent Developments in the Use of the MMPI-2, St. Petersburg, FL.

Colon, C. C. (1993). *Relationship between the MMPI-2 content scales and psychiatric symptoms with Puerto Rican college students and psychiatric patients.* Unpublished doctoral dissertation, Caribbean Center for Advanced Studies, San Juan, Puerto Rico.

Cook, W. A. (1996). Item validity of the MMPI-2 for a Hispanic and White clinical sample. *Dissertation Abstracts International, 56B,* 5761.

Corrales, M. L., Cabiya, J. J., Gomez, F., Ayala, G. X., Mendoza, S., & Velásquez, R. J. (1998). MMPI-2 and MMPI-A research with U.S. Latinos: A bibliography. *Psychological Reports, 83,* 1027–1033.

Cuéllar, I., Arnold, B., & Maldonado, R. (1995). Acculturation Rating Scale for Mexican Americans II: A revision of the original ARSMA scale. *Hispanic Journal of Behavioral Sciences, 17,* 275–304.

Donovan, N., Castellanos, J., Velásquez, R. J., & Orozco, V. (2002, May). *The relationship between hypochondriasis, health concerns, cynicism, acculturation, and health locus of control for Chicanos.* Paper presented at the Annual Symposium on Recent Developments in the Use of the MMPI-2, Minneapolis, MN.

Erdman, K., Velásquez, R. J., & Flores, L. (2000, May). *Applying the BSI and MMPI-2 in the assessment of Spanish-speaking DUI offenders.* Paper presented at the Annual Symposium on Recent Developments in the Use of the MMPI-2, Minneapolis, MN.

Fantoni-Salvador, P., & Rogers, R. (1997). Spanish versions of the MMPI-2 and PAI: An investigation of concurrent validity with Hispanic patients. *Assessment, 4,* 29–39.

Flores, L., Chavira, D. A., Perez, J., Engel, B., & Velásquez, R. J. (1996, June). *MMPI-2 codetypes of Spanish-speaking Hispanic DUI offenders: Preliminary findings.* Paper presented at the Annual Symposium on Recent Developments in the Use of the MMPI-2, Minneapolis, MN.

Fournier, M. (2001, March). *Validation of the emotional scale using MMPI-2: A prelimary exploration of aggression predictive factors for the psychiatric population of Puerto Rico.* Paper presented at the Annual Symposium on Recent Developments in the Use of the MMPI-2, Tampa, FL.

Frank, J. G., Velásquez, R. J., Reimann, J., & Salazar, J. (1997, June). *MMPI-2 profiles of Latino, Black, and White rapists and child molesters on parole.* Paper presented at the Annual Symposium on Recent Developments in the Use of the MMPI-2, Minneapolis, MN.

Garrido, M. (2000, May). *MMPI-A use with Latinos: A review of the literature and case study.* Paper presented at the Annual Symposium on Recent Developments in the Use of the MMPI-2, Minneapolis, MN.

Garrido, M., Gionta, D., Diehl, S., & Boscia, M. (1998, March). *The Megargee MMPI-2 system of inmate classification: A study of its applicability with ethnically diverse prison inmates.* Paper presented at the Annual Symposium on Recent Developments in the Use of the MMPI-2, Clearwater, FL.

Garrido, M., Velásquez, R. J., Parsons, J. P., Reimann, J., & Salazar, J. (1997, June). *MMPI-2 performance of Hispanic and White abusive and neglectful parents.* Paper presented at the Annual Symposium on Recent Developments in the Use of the MMPI-2, Minneapolis, MN.

Gomez, F. C., Johnson, R., Davis, Q., & Velásquez, R. J. (2000). MMPI-A performance of African and Mexican American adolescent first-time offenders. *Psychological Reports, 87,* 309–314.

Greenwood, K., Velásquez, R. J., Suarez, R., Rodriguez-Reimann, D., Johnson, A., Flores-Gonzalez, R., & Ledeboer, M. E. (1998, March). *MMPI-2/MMPI-A profiles of Latino mother and daughter dyads in an outpatient community mental health center.* Paper presented at the Annual Symposium on Recent Developments in the Use of the MMPI-2, Clearwater, FL.

Grillo, J. (1994, August). *Underrepresentation of Hispanic Americans in the MMPI-2 normative group.* Paper presented at the 102nd Annual Meeting of the American Psychological Association, Los Angeles, CA.

Gumbiner, J. (1998). MMPI-A profiles of Hispanic adolescents. *Psychological Reports, 82,* 659–672.

Haskell, A. (1996). Mexican American and Anglo American endorsement of items on the MMPI-2 Scale 2, the Center for Epidemiological Studies Depression Scale, and the Cohen-Hoberman Inventory for Physical Symptoms. *Dissertation Abstracts International, 57,* 4708B.

Hernandez, J. (1994). *The MMPI-2 performance as a function of acculturation.* Unpublished master's thesis, Sam Houston State University, Huntsville, TX.

Hernandez, Q., & Lucio, E. (2002, May). *Personality and IQ of high-performance Mexican adolescent students.*

Paper presented at the Annual Symposium on Recent Developments in the Use of the MMPI-2, Minneapolis, MN.

Hudak, K. V. B. (2001). An investigation of variables related to attrition of Hispanic men from a domestic violence treatment program. *Dissertation Abstracts International, 61,* 6137B.

Jana, Y. A. (2001). The effectiveness of the MMPI-2 in detecting malingered schizophrenia in adult female inmates in Puerto Rico who receive coaching on diagnostic-specific criteria. *Dissertation Abstracts International, 62,* 1084B.

Jella, S. H., Penn, N., Boscan, D., Maness, P., & Velásquez, R. J. (2001a, May). *MMPI-2 profiles of Mexican DUI offenders and college students.* Paper presented at the Annual Symposium on Recent Developments in the Use of the MMPI-2, Tampa, FL.

Jella, S. H., Penn, N., Boscan, D., Maness, P., & Velásquez, R. J. (2001b, August). *MMPI-2 profiles of Mexican born DUI offenders and non-offenders.* Paper presented at the Annual Meeting of the American Psychological Association, San Francisco, CA.

Karle, H. R. (1994). *Comparability of the English and Spanish versions of the MMPI-2: A study of Latino bilingual-bicultural students.* Unpublished master's thesis, San Diego State University, San Diego, CA.

Ladd, J. S. (1994). Codetype agreement between MMPI-2 and estimated MMPI profiles in chemically dependent inpatients. *Psychological Reports, 75,* 367–370.

Ladd, J. S. (1996). MMPI-2 critical items norms in chemically dependent inpatients. *Journal of Clinical Psychology, 52,* 367–372.

Lapham, S. C., Skipper, B. J., & Simpson, G. L. (1997). A prospective study of the utility of standardized instruments in predicting recidivism among first DWI offenders. *Journal of Studies on Alcohol, 58,* 524–530.

Lessenger, L. H. (1997). Acculturation and MMPI-2 scale scores of Mexican-American substance abuse patients. *Psychological Reports, 80,* 1181–1182.

Lucio, E., Ampudia, A., Duran, C., Leon, I., & Butcher, J. N. (2001). Comparison of the Mexican and American norms of the MMPI-2. *Journal of Clinical Psychology, 57,* 1459–1468.

Lucio, E., Cordova, G. V., & Hernandez, Q. (2002, May). *Discriminative sensitivity of the Koss-Butcher and Lachar-Wrobel critical item sets in alcoholic patients.* Paper presented at the Annual Symposium on Recent Developments in the Use of the MMPI-2, Minneapolis, MN.

Lucio, E., Palacios, H., Duran, C., & Butcher, J. N. (2000). MMPI-2 with Mexican psychiatric inpatients: Basic and content scales. *Journal of Clinical Psychology, 55,* 1541–1552.

Lucio, E., & Reyes-Lagunes, I. (1994). MMPI-2 for Mexico: Translation and adaptation. *Journal of Personality Assessment, 63,* 105–116.

Maiocco, M. (1996). The relationship between ethnicity and somatization in workers' compensation claimants (African-American, Hispanic). *Dissertation Abstracts International, 57,* 2199B.

Maness, P., Gomez, N., Velásquez, R. J., Silkowski, S., & Savino, A. (2000, May). *Gender differences on the MMPI-2 for Colombian university students.* Paper presented at the Annual Symposium on Recent Developments in the Use of the MMPI-2, Minneapolis, MN.

Maness, P. J., Silkowski, S., Velásquez, R. J., & Meadows, A. (2001, March). *MMPI-2 and sexual offenders: An ethnic comparison.* Paper presented at the Annual Symposium on Recent Developments in the Use of the MMPI-2, Tampa, FL.

Mason, K. (1997). Ethnic identity and the MMPI-2 profiles of Hispanic male veterans diagnosed with PTSD. *Dissertation Abstracts International, 58*(4-B), 2129.

Mendoza-Newman, M. C., Greene, R. L., & Velásquez, R. J. (2000, August). *Acculturation, SES, and the MMPI-A of Hispanic adolescents.* Paper presented at the Annual Meeting of the American Psychological Association, Washington, DC.

Negy, C., Leal-Puente, L., Trainor, D. J., & Carlson, R. (1997). Mexican American adolescents' performance on the MMPI-A. *Journal of Personality Assessment, 69,* 205–214.

Netto, D. S., Aguila-Puentes, G., Burns, W. J., Sellars, A. H., & Garcia, B. (1998, August). *Brain injury and the MMPI-2: Neurocorrection for Hispanics.* Paper presented at the 106th Annual Meeting of the American Psychological Association, San Francisco, CA.

Pena, C., Cabiya, J. J., & Echevarria, N. (1995, March). *Changes in mean MMPI-2 T scores of violent offenders in a social learning treatment program.* Paper presented at the Annual Symposium on Recent Developments in the Use of the MMPI-2, St. Petersburg, FL.

Pena, C., Cabiya, J. J., & Echevarria, N. (1996, November). *MMPI-2 scores of a representative sample of state prison inmates in Puerto Rico.* Paper presented at the 43rd Convention of the Puerto Rican Psychological Association, Mayaguez, Puerto Rico.

Pena, L. (1996, June). *Spanish MMPI-A and Cuban Americans: Profiles of adolescents using the Spanish version of the MMPI-A.* Paper presented at the Annual Symposium on Recent Developments in the Use of the MMPI-2, Minneapolis, MN.

Quintana, J. P. (1997). Acculturation of Hispanic-American college students and its relationship to MMPI-2 scores. *Dissertation Abstracts International, 57,* 7265.

Rangel, S. J., & Velásquez, R. J. (2000, May). *Utilization of the MMPI-2 by Latino psychologists: Preliminary results of a national survey.* Paper presented at the Annual Symposium on Recent Developments in the Use of the MMPI-2, Minneapolis, MN.

Rangel, S. J., Velásquez, R. J., & Castellanos, J. (2000, August). *Utilization and opinions of the MMPI-2 by Latino psychologists.* Paper presented at the Annual Meeting of the American Psychological Association, Washington, DC.

Saavedra, L. T. (2000). The translation and validation of the SCT-75 for assessing malingering among Hispanics involved in personal injury litigation. *Dissertation Abstracts International, 61,* 2814B.

Scott, R. L., Butcher, J. N., Young, T. L., & Gomez, N. (2002). The Hispanic MMPI-A across five countries. *Journal of Clinical Psychology, 58,* 407–417.

Scott, R. L., & Pampa, W. M. (2000). The MMPI-2 in Peru: A normative study. *Journal of Personality Assessment, 74,* 95–105.

Velásquez, R. J., Ayala, G. X., & Mendoza, S. A. (1998). *Psychodiagnostic assessment of U.S. Latinos with the MMPI, MMPI-2, and MMPI-A: A comprehensive resource manual.* East Lansing: Julian Samora Research Institute, Michigan State University.

Velásquez, R. J., Ayala, G. X., Mendoza, S., Nezami, E., Castillo-Canez, I., Pace, T., Choney, S. K., Gomez, F. C., & Miles, L. E. (2000). *Culturally competent use of the Minnesota Multiphasic Personality Inventory-2 with minorities.* In I. Cuéllar & F. A. Paniagua (Eds.), *Handbook of multicultural mental health* (pp. 389–417). San Diego, CA: Academic Press.

Velásquez, R. J., Callahan, W. J., Reimann, J., & Carbonell, S. (1998, August). *Performance of bilingual Latinos on an English-Spanish MMPI-2.* Paper presented at the 106th Annual Meeting of the American Psychological Association, San Francisco, CA.

Velásquez, R. J., Chavira, D. A., Karle, H., Callahan, W. J., Garcia, J. A., & Castellanos, J. (2000). Assessing Spanish-speaking Latinos with translations of the MMPI-2: Initial data. *Cultural Diversity and Ethnic Minority Psychology, 6,* 65–72.

Velásquez, R. J., Maness, P. J., & Anderson, U. (2002). Culturally competent assessment of Latino clients: The MMPI-2. In J. N. Butcher (Ed.), *Clinical personality assessment* (2nd ed., pp. 154–170). New York: Oxford University Press.

Velásquez, R. J., Gonzales, M., Butcher, J. N., Castillo-Canez, I., Apodaca, J. X., & Chavira, D. (1997). Use of the MMPI-2 with Chicanos: Strategies for counselors. *Journal of Multicultural Counseling and Development, 25,* 107–120.

Velásquez, R. J., Gutierrez, N. M., Jimenez, R., & McClendon, V. (1999, April). *Development of a bilingual MMPI-2 for Mexican Americans: Initial psychometric data.* Paper presented at the Annual Symposium on Recent Developments in the Use of the MMPI-2, Huntington Beach, CA.

Velásquez, R. J., & Garrido, M. (in press). *Handbook of Latino MMPI-2/MMPI-A research and application.*

Whitworth, R. H., & McBlaine, D. D. (1993). Comparison of the MMPI and MMPI-2 administered to Anglo- and Hispanic-American university students. *Journal of Personality Assessment, 61,* 19–27.

Whitworth, R. H., & Unterbrink, C. (1994). Comparison of MMPI-2 clinical and content scales administered to Hispanic- and Anglo-Americans. *Hispanic Journal of Behavioral Sciences, 16,* 255–264.

III

Conceptualizing Effective Intervention:
La Mujer y El Hombre

Psychotherapy of Chicano Men

Roberto J. Velásquez
Maria Patricia Burton
San Diego State University

> *El hombre es el arquitecto de su propio destino*
> *(Man is the architect of his own destiny)*
> —Mexican Saying

The treatment of Chicano or Mexican American men in psychotherapy remains one of the most challenging of all endeavors for the psychologist or therapist (Valdes, Barón, & Ponce, 1987). Unlike Chicana women, whose presence in psychotherapy has been increasing over the years, Chicano men are less likely to voluntarily seek out treatment for emotional or psychological problems (Altarriba & Bauer, 1998; Falicov, 1998; Fragoso & Kashubeck, 2000; Valdes et al.). This is especially evident in the community. When Chicano men are in therapy, they are likely to be there because: (a) they have been mandated to go to therapy by the courts, (b) they have been brought to therapy by the spouse, children, or parents, or (c) they are older and have been referred by a medical professional.

For example, Pablo was a 32-year-old single Chicano male diagnosed with schizophrenia, who lived at home and was consistently brought to psychotherapy by his mother. He also had a history of problems with the law and was required to attend treatment by his probation officer. Francisco was a 56-year-old Mexican immigrant male who was brought to therapy by his three adult children after many years of alcoholism and of being verbally abusive and disrespectful to his ex-wife. Toward the end of this marriage, the alcohol had affected him so much that he was highly delusional and accused his wife of having countless affairs. Manuel was a 70-year-old three times divorced Mexican American male, who was referred by his physician to therapy. The common themes that he discussed in therapy were his past sexual exploits, medical illnesses, and his fear of growing old. Jorge, a 50-year-old married Chicano male, was brought to therapy by his daughter, Ana, because he would not allow her to pursue a university education. Instead, Jorge was insistent that Ana only pursue a *carrera corta,* or junior college education, because her role in life was to be a good mother and wife and to give him grandchildren.

For Chicanos, the idea of entering psychotherapy can be very intimidating, scary, *extrano* or unusual, threatening, and emasculating. It also brings with it images of having to admit defeat, imperfection, personal problems, weakness, jealousy or *envidia,* vulnerability, insecurity, and that they cannot take it as a man or *aguantar* (tolerate). Moreover, Chicano men who enter psychotherapy might have to pay a heavy price within their family and social circle, and thus avoid treatment. This price may include having to uncover their masculine persona to others, including the psychologist, displaying an emotional or feminine side that includes crying, and appearing "less than a man" because they are unable to solve their own problems. Admittedly, even to the first author, who maintains a practice largely composed of Chicanas and Mexicanas, and who is accustomed to working with women, it is sometimes more difficult to work with Chicano men because they rarely seek out treatment, thus keeping this psychologist rusty, or out of practice.

On the other hand, Chicana women are much easier to work with because they are much more knowledgeable and sophisticated with regard to seeking out mental health services (North, 1996; Sheets, 1997). They are usually the ones in charge of day-to-day activities including paying the bills, attending PTA meetings, understanding their insurance coverage, and caring for their children. Chicana women are also more likely to be involved in other activities that bring them into contact with pathways into psychotherapy (Medina & Reyes, 1976; Palacios & Franco, 1986). For example, many Chicanas who are involved in activities related to the education of their children, or who serve as community change agents, like *promotoras* or *educatoras* (health educators) are more likely to be involved in discussions or *platicas* that support or reinforce help-seeking behaviors. Moreover, Chicana and Mexicana women, more than Chicano and Mexicano men, are likely to prescribe to prevention activities related to both medical and mental health, that is, they are more likely to involve themselves in health promotion activities, whereas men are less likely to follow suit.

In other instances, Chicana clients have had previous experiences with psychotherapy, and are sold on the idea that therapy can be highly beneficial, life changing, and healing. They are also more likely to appreciate the process of psychotherapy, which includes wrestling with all of the emotions related to a particular problem or issue (Constantine & Barón, 1997). Even those Chicanas who have not had previous experience in psychotherapy usually seem prepared to jump into therapy because they have processed their issues with others in ways that resemble the therapeutic process itself (Schneider, Laury, & Hughes, 1980). In many instances, they have had discussions and cathartic experiences with *comadres,* their grandmother or *abuelita,* godmother or *madrina,* or a best friend (Ramos-Sanchez, 2001). These experiences have allowed them to cry, grieve, and reframe problems. This is usually not the case with Chicano men, who usually walk into therapy full of anger or rage, anxious, defensive or guarded, or ready to explode because they have repressed their feelings for a long time.

Another challenge to the treatment of men in psychotherapy is breaking through the many psychological layers largely defined by Chicano-Mexicano pride or *orgullo.* Chicano men, like many other Latino men, have a lot invested in their ego, which is defined by many traditional beliefs about what the Chicano man is supposed to be like in this world (Medina, Marshall, & Fried, 1988). For example, from early childhood, the Chicano male child is socialized to be strong, *orgulloso* or prideful, sexually potent, ultra responsible and protective, especially with regard to children and family, loyal to the extended family and friends including *compadres,* aloof and distant yet selectively loving, and hard working (Casas, Turner, & Ruiz de Esparza, 2001; Casas, Wagenheim, Branchero, & Mendoza-Romero, 1995; Fragoso & Kashubeck, 2000; Gutierrez, 1991; Manrique-Reichard, 1996; Panitz, McConchie, Sauber, & Fonseca, 1983; Torres, 1998; Valdes et al., 1987). Recently, the first author was treating a 10-year-old Chicano boy who talked about how important it was for him to be "macho," especially when confronted by other boys in the neighborhood.

An excellent example of this type of male figure is seen in the role of the father in the movie "Mi Familia/My Family," a man who was rather stoic and distant, strong and rigid, and self-sacrificing while expecting ultimate loyalty from his wife and children. The Chicano male child is also socialized to defend the family name at all costs, especially the image of the mother figure. He is also taught to integrate male-dominated interests through behaviors including drinking alcohol, being highly protective of his *ruca, heina,* or woman, being highly *trucha* or hypersensitive to the world, being involved or having an interest in sports including boxing, and taking pride in his "'hood" or *barrio,* and defending it if necessary.

Thus, psychotherapy with the Chicano male requires an understanding of the many psychological layers that have been shaped and reinforced through parental socialization and peer relationships, that are salient to the culture, and that are transmitted through an ethos or collective unconscious (Mirande, 1980). More times than not, Chicano men who do seek out psychotherapy are likely to drop out or stop attending because these layers are not fully understood by the psychologist, or because they are automatically pathologized, especially in light of more modern (or postmodern) Euro American images of men, which suggest less of an emphasis on masculinity and traditional sex roles, and more attention to an androgynous orientation (Ponterotto, 1987).

Their are six aims in the present chapter. First, we present reasons why Chicano men do not typically seek out psychotherapy, from their view that attending psychotherapy is unmanly to a staunch belief that they can "do it on their own" as they have other things in life. Second, we discuss reasons why Chicano men do enter psychotherapy. At this time, the utilization of psychotherapy by Chicano-Mexicano men remains very low and those who do seek out therapy are usually court ordered or are brought to therapy by family. Third, we present a list of therapeutic options that many Chicano men consider, including going to a local bar. Within the male subculture, for better or worse, there is a built-in support system that includes seeking consultation from a *compadre* or a bartender. Fourth, we illustrate some idioms of distress that are used by Chicano men, including feeling that they have been hexed. Fifth, we present some basic assumptions about Chicano men in therapy. These assumptions can be used as hypotheses when conducting psychotherapy and may serve to penetrate the thick armor often displayed by Chicano-Mexicano male clients. Finally, we present some recommendations for treating Chicanos in psychotherapy. These recommendations are rather practical and intended to quickly affect the Chicano-Mexicano client.

From the onset, it is important to note that all of the observations that are reported are taken largely from the first author's 20-year experience of providing services in a working-class Chicano-Mexicano community. Consequently, the recommendations given here vary across communities according to educational, generational, socio-economic, and acculturation levels.

REASONS WHY CHICANO MEN DO NOT SEEK PSYCHOTHERAPEUTIC TREATMENT

We here present a list of reasons why Chicano men do not seek psychological treatment from a psychologist or therapist:

• "Psychotherapy is for jotos or maricones (homosexuals), or viejas (old women)." Many Chicano men, borrowing from traditional images of Mexican manhood and homophobia, are likely to view psychotherapy as something for persons who are weak or *debil,* for women because they are assumed to be the weaker sex, or for homosexual men. For many men, going to a psychologist is tantamount to being unable to have control over their life and others, including their wife and children, or no longer being capable of controlling their emotions in a manner reflective of manhood (Ponterotto, 1987), that is, being strong, quiet, stoic, detached, and aloof. For example, many Chicano-Mexicano men refuse to be tested for prostate cancer because they believe that the rectal examination will somehow strip them of their manhood or make them at risk for becoming homosexual. In the same way, many Chicano men are likely to reject psychotherapy because it is not something that "real men" do in order to solve their problems. From early childhood, the message given to many Chicano-Mexicano men by their parents, including their mothers, is to be strong and not weak—"to take it as a man."

• "Psychotherapy is only for people who are mentally ill or locos (crazy)." Many Chicano men believe that psychotherapy is only for persons who have a severe mental illness, such as schizophrenia: *para personas que estan chifladas, que les falta un tornillo, o locos* (for people who are crazy, they are missing a screw or crazy)." Chicano men often do not see interpersonal problems, including issues with their spouse or children, as mental illness. Instead, they view these problems as originating from their children or spouse, that is, they are likely to view themselves as the victims of others' problems or *locura.* Moreover, many Chicano men are likely to reject the notion that psychotherapy is appropriate for problems related to alcohol dependence or domestic violence, because they are likely to attribute the origin of these problems to external factors, stating that "my wife caused me to hit her," "I drink because it is the only way to cope with my family's problems," or "my family drove me to drink." Furthermore, many men report that their problems are physically based even in the face of evidence that indicates somatization or hypochondriasis.

• "Psychotherapy is simply chatting with another person." Many Chicano men refuse to go to psychotherapy because they view it as nothing more than chatting or having a *platica,* which they could easily do with a best friend over a beer. Many Chicano men indicate to the psychologist that they cannot understand how someone can address a problem by simply talking to another person (Garcia & Zea, 1996). Others take it one step further and ask to see a physician because "a physician can at least prescribe a medication to me, what can you do?"

• "Psychotherapy will simply open up problems that cannot be resolved." Many Chicano men who are a little more sophisticated with regard to psychotherapy, possibly because a family member has received treatment, are likely to take the stance that "psychotherapy will open up a lot of issues that can never be resolved" and are more likely to feel like they are "up against the wall" and need to be protective of themselves. They are also likely to challenge the psychologist to soften the interventions, which can be translated to mean "I will not talk about anything painful in my life" or the metamessage, "Leave me alone because, as a man, I must not be psychologically vulnerable or fragile."

REASONS WHY CHICANO MEN SEEK PSYCHOTHERAPEUTIC TREATMENT

As previously noted, Chicano men, like men from other Latino subgroups, are less likely to seek psychotherapy on their own or because of internal motivations. More often than not, they show up to therapy for external reasons, including the following:

• They have been court ordered to attend psychotherapy. Many Chicano men are court mandated to attend psychotherapy for various reasons, including being on probation or parole, being violent toward their spouse or children, or being abusive or neglectful toward their children. Usually, under these circumstances, Chicanos come into treatment with a rather defensive, guarded, or suspicious demeanor or they come to treatment angry at their spouse or at the psychologist because they have previously been in therapy.

• They have been placed on medication by their family physician. Usually, older men, over 45 years of age, come to therapy because they have been referred by their family physician or because they have been placed on psychotropic medications. In other cases, the physician has exhausted all types of examinations and found nothing wrong with the patient and would now prefer to have a mental health professional, such as a psychologist, follow up by conducting an assessment and psychotherapy.

• They have been "dragged in" by family members. Over the years, the first author has been privy to many situations in which the spouse and children of a Chicano male client "drag" or "fool" (as perceived by the client) the client into therapy. Usually, this act is orchestrated by the family out of desperation because the client is so out of control, problematic, or perhaps in danger of dying or destroying the family. In many circumstances, the father is affected by severe alcoholism or drug dependence. In other cases, the family has exhausted all possible sources of assistance and has now taken one final and desperate step toward fixing the problem because their beliefs about maintaining the family are so strong and because they have reached the boiling point, or *hasta el colmo*. In most of these situations, the client is very upset and angry, reports feeling deceived and humiliated by family members, and denies that any type of problems exist. Moreover, the client likelys swear to God or the Virgen de Guadalupe that he will stop drinking or taking drugs, or creating other problems. Unfortunately, the client is never seen or heard from again, the family continues to tolerate such problems.

- They have been threatened by their spouse or girlfriend to attend psychotherapy. Usually, these clients report that they are in therapy because they have been threatened or given an ultimatum by their girlfriend or spouse that if they do not attend psychotherapy, the relationship is likely to end. Thus, these clients are likely to want quick solutions to their problems in order to prove to their girlfriend or spouse that they really care about the relationship. They are likely to appear tense and anxious and demand advice or *consejos* that will help correct any problems as soon as possible. These clients are likely to be anxiously compliant to all aspects of therapy, including homework assignments, but are not likely to make any major changes in their personality functioning or world view. When seen by a female psychologist, these clients are likely to be very charming, endearing, and even flirtatious, which is what originally got them into trouble with their girlfriend or spouse. They are also likely to be more domineering and manipulative, perhaps never intending to really deal with their issues.

- They have a specific problem that they would like to solve as soon as possible. Many Chicano men who enter psychotherapy make it very clear at the beginning that they are ready to enter therapy and to be finished within a month, that is, they are demanding and have underestimated the purpose of psychotherapy. Instead, they view psychotherapy as an automobile tune up, in a rather mechanical fashion.

ALTERNATIVES TO PSYCHOTHERAPY FOR CHICANO MEN

Many Chicano-Mexicano men utilize other types of resources that may appear to be therapeutic to them, including consulting with compadres, friends, and coworkers (Prieto, McNeill, Walls, & Gómez, 2001; Young, 2001; Zinn, 1982). Other examples follow:

- For many Chicano men, a viable option to psychotherapy is the neighborhood bar or cantina. In bars, Chicanos can not only use alcohol as a means of self-medication, but also use the services of the bartender or *cantinero,* who uses one of the most important skills employed by the psychologist, listening. The bartender, like the psychologist, can listen to the client without being judgmental or, if judgmental, always takes the side of the Chicano male. The cantinero can also offer advice in a nonthreatening manner to the client, while affirming his values and masculinity. Moreover, many Chicano men see the cantina as a place where they can "check things out about relationships" with other women, especially if female bartenders are present.

- The act of *compadrismo,* to establish a relationship with another person or couple by having the person or couple baptize one's child, sets into motion a special type of relationship not seen in many other cultures. As a result of this ritual, steeped deeply in Catholicism and indigenous beliefs, the compadre gains a special status in which he serves as the Chicano male's confidante, as well as a friend, drinking partner, impromptu counselor, and even confessor. At the same time, the compadre is given the right to offer unsolicited feedback or consultation. As a result of this special relationship, many Chicano men prefer to seek out their compadres rather than psychologists or therapists. However, Chicano men always expect the compadre to take their side to the point of maintaining confidentiality and loyalty and sanctioning behaviors that may be dysfunctional or maladaptive (e.g., adultery, drug abuse).

• One of the roles often assigned to oldest sons in Chicano-Mexicano families is that of caretaker and role model for younger siblings. Another important role can be that of friend or confidante to his father, including drinking and socializing with the father, taking responsibility for him if he is inebriated, and rescuing him from difficult emotional situations. Although this bond between the father and son can be quite special, it can also cause many problems for the rest of the family. For example, the wife can be left out in the cold with regard to key information about her husband. Recently, one Chicana client reported to the first author that she was terribly distraught and angry, not because she had found out that her husband was living with another woman for a year, but because her oldest son knew about it and did not say anything to her. On the other hand, the husband indicated that his son had done the right thing in keeping quiet and respecting him as his father and that he was very proud of him.

• For many Chicano men, being involved in the church can be very therapeutic from both a spiritual and psychological point of view. That is, many men find a sense of repose in being involved in a variety of activities, from helping to maintain buildings, to working at church fiestas, to being members of special societies such as the Adoracion Nocturna (Society for the Adoration of the Sacred Heart) or the Knights of Columbus. At the same time, they may also establish a confidential relationship with the priest of the parish in which the Chicano-Mexicano feels supported, even if he has been sinful or hurtful toward others, especially family. This involvement in the church gives many Chicano men a sense of psychological security and establishes a brotherhood (or hemanidad) among other men who "have not been perfect in their own lives." Membership or involvement in other organizations or clubs can be therapeutic for Chicano men, but whether it helps in truly dealing with their psychological issues remains unclear.

• Many Chicano-Mexicano men seek out guidance from a girlfriend or *amante*, especially if they are married or involved in a committed relationship. They often indicate that "running things by a woman" like their amante helps them become more balanced, less stressed, and more clear headed. They also state that the amante takes the place of the wife for a brief moment and offers advice that can settle problems with their wife or children. For example, one male client stated that, "if it wasn't for Maria, my girlfriend, I would never have taken care of a problem with my wife. Maria suggested that I take my wife flowers, take her out to dinner, and buy her a new dress. I followed her advice and everything turned out okay. That is why Maria is, and will always be, my best friend." Another client, living in a border town, stated that, "I love my wife and family, but my other woman is just as important. That is why I disappear every Sunday morning for a few hours. I cross the border into Mexico, have my *menudo*, visit with her and my other children, listen to her wisdom, and then come home happier. I will never give this up, she's my psychologist, my therapist."

CHICANOS' IDIOMS OF DISTRESS
IN PSYCHOTHERAPY

The following idioms are frequently used by Chicano-Mexicano men who enter psychotherapy. Instead of being more direct, like their female counterparts, Chicanos often mask their problems by using certain code words that, if not understood by the psychologist, can cause problems in psychotherapy.

- The term *embrujado* means to be hexed by someone else, perhaps through some type of medium or *curandero*. Chicano men may report that the origin of their problems has to do with being embrujado or someone casting a spell on them. Symptoms typically reported when one is embrujado include generalized pain, tension, insomnia, poor appetite, cold sweats, and nightmares. It is very important to determine whether this is a real part of the client's belief system or a ploy to excuse themselves for problems they have caused. (Many persons with a long history of alcohol dependence are also likely to demonstrate such symptoms.)
- The term *encabronado* means to be highly angry or upset. Usually, Chicano men use the term to describe a very heightened level of anger directed at someone else. Men who report being encabronado usually report feeling ready to explode, strike, or even kill someone else, display a disregard for the consequences of their behavior, and are quite paranoid about others' intentions, including the psychologist.
- *Flojo* is used to describe a state of tiredness, apathy, or lack of energy. Many Chicano men who use this term may be talking about two possible conditions: (a) their girlfriend or spouse is indicating to them that they are lazy, or (b) they are reporting a state of being that may be related to feeling bad because they have always worked or been *muy trabajador* (hard working) or because they have suddenly lost the energy needed to work. Clients often use this word as a symptom of depression.
- Many Chicano men use the term *latoso*, which refers to being a "pain in the neck," when they have begun to develop physical or emotional problems that require other family members to take care of them. For example, it is not unusual for elder Chicanos to state that they wish they were dead because they would no longer be a burden to their family.
- *Loco de remate* is usually used by Chicano men to describe a fairly severe state of psychological functioning. Usually, someone who is loco de remate may have symptoms of madness, craziness, or psychosis. It also implies a lack of emotional control, odd or bizarre behaviors, or chronic craziness. Male clients often come in to therapy and state that they have been told by friends or family that they are loco de remate.
- The term *corajudo* usually implies someone who easily angers or who has sudden and unpredictable shifts in mood or affect. or who is moody. Persons who are described as being corajudo are argumentative and lose their temper easily with others. Some Chicano men who describe themselves as corajudo end up having signs and symptoms related to a bipolar condition.
- This term *hocicon* describes someone who is prone to be verbally oppositional, defiant, and disrespectful. Chicano men may use this term to describe how others view them.

- *Enfermo mental* implies mental illness in a very general sense and can be used by Chicano men when describing their general mental health status, which may be generally impaired, but lacking a specific type of condition or illness.
- *Volviendose loco* is used to describe the process of actually becoming crazy or mentally ill. Chicano men who use this term are likely to be expressing a decrease in their mental status and perhaps even decompensation. Usually, persons who feel as they though they are becoming crazy feel disconnected, alienated, and estranged from others. They begin to report unusual incidents that may include increased paranoia, hypervigilance, and the inability to access their feelings.
- One of the most difficult challenges in the treatment of Chicano-Mexicano men involves those who have problems with alcohol, but who deny it in a very passionate manner (Zimmerman & Sodowsky, 1993). Chicano men become very defensive and guarded about admitting that they have an addiction to alcohol and, instead of admitting to this addiction, they are more likely to indicate that they are a *borrachal*, which is a drinker (but not implying addiction, psychological weakness, etc.). Thus, many men are more likely to admit to being a borrachal, but not to being *vicioso* or addicted.
- *Chiflado* is a term used by many men to describe the condition of being emotionally gone or *ido* and reflects severe psychopathology that most likely requires professional intervention. To be chiflado is to have "lost one's marbles," to be mentally ill.
- The term *menso* is used to indicate low intellectual functioning, or acting and behaving as if one is stupid. Chicano men who use this term may be indicating that they are experiencing losses in cognitive functioning, including memory impairment and recall. If the client constantly uses this term, there should be a strong concern about intellectual decompensation.
- The term *safado* is used in the streets and usually means to be a little crazy, partially crazy, or out of control. One can become safado with drugs or alcohol, but one can also cure this condition by abstaining from one's vices.

BASIC ASSUMPTIONS ABOUT CHICANO MEN IN PSYCHOTHERAPY

Every psychologist or therapist possesses a series of assumptions about a particular clinical target group, largely extracted and refined from the research literature and clinical practice, that serve as guiding principles for the understanding of that group. Following are some of the assumptions about Chicano-Mexicano men that can be tested as hypotheses (It is important to note that these should never be considered as stereotypes of Chicano or Mexicano men; Niemann, 2001):

- Many Chicano men are likely to present themselves as being victimized by others, including family. Usually, this type of client comes to therapy feeling as though they have been taken advantage of by others (Soto-Fulp, Del Campo, & Del Campo, 1994). They also feel that they have no control over their problems until others change to suit their needs. Thus, they are likely to be very difficult to work with because they first need to see others change before they are is willing to make a move toward any type of self-change, with the condition that "I will possibly change a little, but the other person(s) needs to change more than me because they hurt me first, by victimizing me." Chicano men who come to psychotherapy as victims are also likely to view their self-defeating or problematic behaviors (e.g., heavy alcohol use) as acceptable because they are responses to others taking advantage of them or oppressing them (Falicov, 1998). Riding (2000, p. 8), on Mexican males' insecurity and machismo, stated that:

> Insecurity is best understood by [their] constant fear of betrayal by women. A contemporary anthropological explanation remains appealingly neat: Mexico's mestizaje began with the mating of Spanish men and Indian women, thus immediately injecting into the male-female relationship the concepts of betrayal by women and conquest, domination, force and even rape by men. Just as the conquerors could never fully trust the conquered, today's macho must therefore brace himself against betrayal. Combining the Spaniard's obsession with honor and the Indian's humiliation at seeing his woman taken by force, Mexico's peculiarly perverse form of machismo thus emerges: the Spaniard's defense of honor becomes the Mexican's defense of his fragile masculinity.

• Many Chicano men are more likely to ask for psychotherapy with a male therapist. It is not unusual for Chicano men to specifically request that they be seen by a male psychologist or therapist, especially if the professional is a member of their ethnic group (Abreu & Gabarin, 2000; Gilsdorf, 1978; Ponce & Atkinson, 1989; Sanchez & Atkinson, 1983). Usually, these men feel that: (a) it is easier to talk to a man than a woman, (b) a male therapist is more likely to understand their plight as a Chicano or Mexicano male, (c) they are less likely to be challenged, questioned, or "emotionally beat up" by a male therapist, and (d) they can strike up a relationship that is more like a friendship than psychotherapy. It is also possible to take a more psychoanalytic approach and view the Chicano male as highly defensive and guarded, and fearful that a female therapist is likely to behave like a punishing, anxiety- and guilt-provoking mother figure who may overwhelm the client, thus exposing his vulnerabilities as a man. Yet another way of viewing this client is to not take an analytic approach, but to allow the client to enter this type of therapy relationship, allow trust to develop, and then push the client to examine the many issues that he is likely to be denying, minimizing, or avoiding.

• Many Chicano men are more likely to present the origins of their problems as family or externally based. A major problem observed in many Chicano men who are in psychotherapy is their difficulty in viewing the etiology of their problems as stemming from within; accepting responsibility for having caused themselves or others problems is something very difficult for them (Falicov, 1998). To many Chicano men, their problems, whether substance dependence, aggressive behaviors, or depression, are caused by external factors beyond their control. For example, one Chicano client who was recently seen in therapy agreed that he was possessive and jealous of his wife to the point of being highly paranoid. In fact, he stated that he frequently imagined his wife being with other men and that, despite feeling this way, his wife was the cause of this problem because of the way she dressed. Another example is of a Mexicano client who had no problems admitting to being an alcoholic for many years and to being less than a responsible father, yet argued that his family led him to become an alcoholic because this was the only convenient outlet available to him.

• Many Chicano men are more likely to present themselves as defensive, guarded, or suspicious at the onset of psychotherapy. It is not unusual for many Chicano-Mexicano men to be highly suspicious of psychotherapy. They are often raised to believe that sharing one's inner feelings is not what real men do and those who do share their feelings are likely to be perceived as either dysfunctional or gay (Zinn, 1982). Thus, many men are likely to beat around the bush, make small talk, or be highly indirect when talking about their problems. For the psychologist, the challenge is to translate this type of communication pattern into one that is not threatening, but equally challenging and forceful. This is not an easy intervention and requires that the Chicano client not be in the testing mode with the psychologist (i.e., the client testing the psychologist in order to decrease authority and credibility).

• Chicano men are less likely to self-disclose at the beginning of psychotherapy. Instead, they are likely to measure their words (*medir sus palabras*), being very careful about what they say. In some situations, we have observed that such clients have a right to disclose less because they have been "burned" by other psychologists. For example, some Chicano clients are likely to begin therapy by being very cynical about trust ever developing because, in the past, other professionals broke confidentiality and shared valuable information with others, including family members.

• Many Chicano men are less likely to admit to substance use as a coping mechanism at the beginning of psychotherapy or they are likely to underreport their substance use. We have observed that Chicana women are more likely to be honest about their use of illicit substances than their male counterparts at the onset of psychotherapy. Chicana women are more likely to talk about their complete history of substance abuse, to disclose the accurate amount of time that they have been sober or free of drugs, and to take responsibility for their substance abuse. Indeed, it is not surprising for a psychologist to find out 6 months into therapy that a client has been using drugs or alcohol. Many Chicano men believe that using substances, such as alcohol or marijuana, is a suitable method of treating high levels of distress (Zimmerman & Sodowsky, 1993). It is our opinion that Chicano men who hide or minimize their substance use are less likely to be successful in psychotherapy than those who do acknowledge this problem.

• Chicano men are more likely to be protective of their parents and their upbringing. Whether this type of behavior is viewed as an action to protect their mother's reputation and image or to remain loyal to the family of origin, especially parents, Chicano men are more likely to view their upbringing in a positive light even if there is evidence to the contrary (Goldwert, 1985); they are less likely to report any type of history of physical, sexual, or emotional abuse or neglect. They are more likely to place their parents, especially if deceased, on a psychological pedestal, forgiving them for any problems that they may have caused. Thus, it is also not unusual for Chicano men to move back in with their parents, no matter what their age, after a divorce. To the Chicano male, home symbolizes everything comforting and innocent, and sanctuary from life's problems.

• Chicano men are less likely to view psychotherapy as therapy and more likely to view it as consultation. As has been alluded to previously, Chicano men are likely to view psychotherapy as a type of professional consultation that is directed at correcting some behaviors and attitudes, but not all. Thus, the Chicano client who prefers short sessions, say, of less than 30 minutes, or who occasionally misses a therapy session, is more likely to believe that he is simply gaining consultation on how to better behave. In our opinion, it is better not to argue about whether psychotherapy is, or is not, a consultation with the client. Instead, if the client is more likely to participate because the term *consultation* is used over *psychotherapy,* then so be it. Becoming hung up on semantics is likely to play into many Chicano clients' psychopathology, especially if they are being very intellectual.

• Many Chicano men are less likely to believe in democratic principles as they relate to their own families. In other words, many Chicano men are likely to view themselves as the head of their household, fully in charge, and deserving of full and complete loyalty from their spouse and children. They are also more likely to subscribe to autocratic principles and traditional viewpoints on the roles of men and women, especially as they relate to their children, and to seek complete submission from the spouse. Thus, the use of Adlerian or other family therapy principles that advocate for a greater sense of family equality are likely to be rejected by many Chicano men in favor of a hierarchical structure, where they view themselves as being on top. For example, one Mexicano client was very adamant that his daughter, who was recruited by many major universities out of high school, only attend a community college and obtain a short program of study or *carrera corta,* because her role was to prepare herself to be a wife and mother, not a lawyer (what the daughter wanted to be). Another Chicano client argued that it was well within his responsibility, as a father, to sponsor or *padronizar* his son's first sexual encounter at 15 years of age, with a prostitute. He noted that his father had initiated him and that he had not been negatively affected by this experience. He rationalized this type of behavior as being a part of his role as a father and role model. In the end, the son resisted this practice, but his father labeled him as a *maricon* or homosexual.

RECOMMENDATIONS FOR TREATING CHICANO MEN IN PSYCHOTHERAPY

• Establish a therapeutic alliance as soon as possible. Given that many Chicano men are entering therapy with doubts, fears, insecurities, and cynicism, it is important to hook the client as soon as possible. This can be accomplished by having shortened sessions at the beginning of therapy, especially because, for many male clients, an hour seems like an eternity. The therapist may want to conduct a formal psychological evaluation at the beginning. Many clients have voiced positive feelings about undergoing a psychological evaluation. One noted that "while I was taking the MMPI-2, I really thought about my problems in ways I had not before, and this prepared me for therapy."

• Engage the client in clarifying or defining his role as a father, husband, worker, and so on, and tie this in to his view of himself as a man (Mayo, 1997). Furthermore, if the client considers himself to be macho, challenge him to define this concept from his own world view, using his own adjectives, because the meaning of *macho* continues to evolve (Andrade, 1992; Gutmann, 1994; Mirande, 1980). It is interesting to note that, once men are challenged to define or clarify the concept of machismo, they often find that they may not be as macho as they feel they are or as they project to others, including their spouse or children. Recently, one 36-year-old Chicano male, in front of his wife, began to sob in therapy when he talked about how hard he had tried to gain his father's attention as a child. He stated that, as a result of being abandoned by his father, he had decided to never be "emotional" and "loving" to others.

• Always be formal when working with Chicano-Mexicano clients, especially if they are older. We have found that Chicana/o clients in general, whether male or female, are very respectful of the psychologist, as they are of teachers, priests, or medical doctors. The informality that is seen in mainstream Euro American clients is rarely seen in Chicana/os. Thus, the psychologist should always attempt to exert a sense of *respeto* or respect about their world view, which, chauvinistic or not, is their anchor point for viewing much of their reality (Aranda, 1990; Morales, 1999; Zuniga, 1997).

• Blend individual sessions with family sessions in order to better understand the individual psychology of the client and its foundations (Falicov, 1998). After 20 years of conducting psychotherapy with Chicano-Mexicano clients, it is clear that family of origin is critical. Thus, having sessions that include key family members from time to time is an acceptable practice, and one that educates the psychologist.

• Be clear with the client about what psychotherapy is and is not, and point out that there are risks in continuing therapy, including evolving into a better man. As previously noted, many Chicano-Mexicano men come to therapy afraid, nervous, and tense. Most of their images of psychotherapy are negative and inaccurate. Thus, it is important to engage the Chicano-Mexicano client immediately and to have him clarify what his impressions are about therapy. Usually, once things are clarified, the client is more likely to participate and not drop out.

• Clarify the role of religion in the client's life, attitudes, and values (Zea, Mason, & Murguia, 2000). For many Chicano-Mexicano men, religion remains a very important resource. It is important to understand the role of religion in the daily life of the client and to use certain elements of it in therapy. For example, a client may report that he has lost faith in everything except God. This belief may be used to buttress new cognitive schema that are being introduced by the psychologist (e.g., "I am a good person after all").

• Identify the internal dialogue or cognitive schema that the Chicano-Mexicano client has about his issues, problems, or concerns. Cognitive therapy appears to be an excellent option in working with many Chicano-Mexicano men, especially those who tend to overly rationalize and intellectualize. For example, one client's internal dialogue, since early childhood, included the following self-statements: "I must be very strong and never allow anyone to know me," "I must be the protector of my family, no matter what, and even if it kills me," and "I must always present myself as competent and capable to others, even if I'm not."

• Identify the extent to which the Chicano-Mexicano client is open to or flexible about seeing his problems differently. Clients are often so accustomed to seeing things in one, usually dysfunctional, way. They may argue with the psychologist about how they do not have the capacity to be less rigid. In working with many Chicano-Mexicano men, it is crucial that interventions target cognitive, emotional, and behavioral rigidity.

• Identify the level of defensiveness, guardedness, or suspiciousness that the Chicano-Mexicano client is exhibiting, especially in relation to sex roles (Ingoldsby,

1991). One nonthreatening way to address defensiveness and guardedness is to first evaluate the client and then give him therapeutic feedback based on the test results. For example, a Mexicano client refused to talk about himself for the first three sessions of therapy. He was then evaluated with several instruments, including the MMPI-2. His score on the masculinity–femininity scale was very low, suggesting a very traditional male role. The client was given feedback as an intervention and, as a result, he opened up and was able to talk about why his personality was the way it was. Eventually, the client talked about the difficulties of being a male in his social circle.

- Identify or be sensitive to the idioms of distress that the Chicano-Mexicano client is using to communicate his psychological pain. As previously noted, many Chicano-Mexicano men may not be direct with the therapist and may use coded language such as idioms or metaphors to describe their problems. The psychologist needs to be very alert to the use of such language.

- Use *dichos* or sayings as a means of initiating insight into the client's problems. Built within the Spanish language are two clear factors. First, unlike English, the locus of responsibility in Spanish is external. That is, the structure of the language is such that one can speak in a manner that attributes responsibility for one's problems to external factors. Second, *dichos* or cultural sayings (metaphors) are very popular within Latino culture and form part of the everyday vernacular.

- Consider the client's level of acculturation, although at this time it remains unclear to what extent acculturation is a moderator variable in psychotherapy (Mayo, 1997). In our experience, acculturation becomes less of a clinical issue when working with Chicano-Mexicano men as one penetrates their many levels of psychological armor. That is, many Chicano-Mexicano men, in spite of being highly acculturated to mainstream American culture or being bicultural, are likely to possess traditional views about the opposite sex. The psychologist must clearly understand this issue. One young male Chicano adult recently noted in a session that he preferred to date White women because they were more traditional than Chicanas.

The primary aim of this chapter was to present some clinical insights and treatment recommendations for Chicano men who seek psychological treatment. In order to accomplish this task, it was very important to present the reasons why Chicano men do and do not seek out psychotherapy, to discuss other therapeutic options that are available for them, to illustrate some idioms of distress that are used by Chicano men who are seeking treatment, to present some basic hypotheses about Chicano men in therapy, and to present some recommendations for treating Chicanos.

As was noted at the beginning of the chapter, there remains a lack of research on the psychotherapy of Chicano and Mexicano, as well as other Latino, men. A review of the traditional psychological literature yielded very few references. Although this literature was used as a backdrop for the preparation of this chapter, much of it was based on the first author's clinical experience of over 20 years. Clearly, there was a need to not only cite the key relevant studies, but also to take a tell-it-like-it-is stance in discussing many of the issues and problems that Chicano men bring to psychotherapy. Unlike many articles that tend to be rather careful about disclosure of cultural issues, an attempt was made to make this chapter hard hitting and maybe a little controversial in order to stimulate more research. The reader will notice that one term, *machismo*, was not discussed until the end of the chapter. This was done on purpose because the term continues to be used in a rather loose and general fashion within society, maybe to the point of clouding its meaning. Moreover, although many Chicano men value masculinity, they are not necessarily macho.

REFERENCES

Abreu, J. M., & Gabarin, G. (2000). Social desirability and Mexican American counselor preferences: Statistical control for a potential confound. *Journal of Counseling Psychology, 47,* 165–176.

Altarriba, J., & Bauer, L. M. (1998). Counseling the Hispanic client: Cuban Americans, Mexican Americans, and Puerto Ricans. *Journal of Counseling and Development, 76,* 389–396.

Andrade, A. R. (1992). Machismo: A universal malady. *Journal of American Culture, 15,* 33–41.

Aranda, M. P. (1990). Culture-friendly services for Latino elders. *Generations, 14,* 55–57.

Casas, J. M., Turner, J. A., & Ruiz de Esparza, C. A. (2001). Machismo revisited in a time of crisis: Implications for understanding and counseling Hispanic men. In G. R. Brooks & G. E. Good (Eds.), *The new handbook of psychotherapy and counseling with men: A comprehensive guide to settings, problems, and treatment approaches* (pp. 754–779). San Francisco: Jossey-Bass.

Casas, J. M., Wagenheim, B. R., Banchero, R., & Mendoza-Romero, J. (1995). Hispanic masculinity: Myth or psychological schema meriting clinical consideration. *Hispanic Journal of Behavioral Sciences, 16,* 315–331.

Constantine, M., & Barón, A. (1997). Assessing and counseling Chicano(a) college students: A conceptual and practical framework. In C. C. Lee (Ed.), *Multicultural issues in counseling: New approaches* (2nd ed., pp. 295–314). Alexandria, VA: American Counseling Association.

Falicov, C. J. (1998). *Latino families in therapy: A guide to multicultural practice.* New York: Guilford Press.

Fragoso, J. M., & Kashubeck, S. (2000). Machismo, gender role conflict, and mental health in Mexican American men. *Psychology of Men and Masculinity, 1,* 87–97.

Garcia, J. G., & Zea, M. C. (1996). *Psychological interventions and research with Latino populations.* Needham Heights, MA: Allyn and Bacon.

Gilsdorf, D. L. (1978). Counselor preference of Mexican-American, Black, and White community college students. *Journal of Non-White Concerns in Personnel and Guidance, 6,* 162–168.

Goldwert, M. (1985). Mexican machismo: The flight from femininity. *Psychoanalytic Review, 72,* 161–169.

Gutierrez, F. J. (1991). Exploring the macho mystique: Counseling Latino men. In D. Moore & F. Leafgren (Eds.), *Problem solving strategies and interventions for men in conflict* (pp. 139–151). Alexandria, VA: American Counseling Association.

Gutmann, M. C. (1994). The meanings of macho: Changing Mexican male identities. *Masculinities, 2,* 21–33.

Ingoldsby, B. B. (1991). The Latin American family: Familism vs. machismo. *Journal of Comparative Family Studies, 22,* 57–62.

Manrique-Reichard, M. E. (1996). Perception of machismo or hypermasculinity among Anglo-American and Mexican-American young adult males. *Dissertation Abstracts International, 57,* 2949B.

Mayo, Y. (1997). Machismo, fatherhood and the Latino family: Understanding the concept. *Journal of Multicultural Social Work, 5,* 49–61.

Medina, C., & Reyes, M. R. (1976). Dilemmas of Chicana counselors. *Social Work, 21,* 515–517.

Medina, S., Marshall, C. A., & Fried, J. J. (1988). Serving the descendants of Aztlan: A rehabilitation counselor education challenge. *Journal of Applied Rehabilitation Counseling, 19,* 40–44.

Mirande, A. (1980). *Hombres y machos: Masculinity and Latino culture.* Boulder, CO: Westview.

Morales, P. (1999). The impact of cultural differences in psychotherapy with older clients: Sensitive issues and strategies. In M. Duffy (Ed.), *Handbook of counseling and psychotherapy with older adults* (pp. 132–153). New York: Wiley.

Niemann, Y. F. (2001). Stereotypes about Chicanas and Chicanos: Implications for counseling. *The Counseling Psychologist, 29,* 55–90.

North, M. W. (1996). Mexican American women clients' expectations about counseling. *Dissertation Abstracts International, 56,* 3006A.

Palacios, M., & Franco, J. N. (1986). Counseling Mexican American women. *Journal of Multicultural Counseling and Development, 14,* 124–131.

Panitz, D. R., McConchie, R. D., Sauber, S. R., & Fonseca, J. (1983). The role of machismo and the Hispanic family in the etiology and treatment of alcoholism in Hispanic American males. *American Journal of Family Therapy, 11,* 31–44.

Ponce, F. Q., & Atkinson, D. R. (1989). Mexican-American acculturation, counselor ethnicity, counseling style, and perceived counselor credibility. *Journal of Counseling Psychology, 36,* 203–208.

Ponterotto, J. G. (1987). Counseling Mexican Americans: A multimodal approach. *Journal of Counseling and Development, 65,* 308–312.

Prieto, L. R., McNeill, B. W., Walls, R. G., & Gómez, S. P. (2001). Chicanas/os and mental health services: An overview of utilization, counselor preference, and assessment issues. *The Counseling Psychologist, 29,* 18–54.

Ramos-Sanchez, L. (2001). The relationship between acculturation, specific cultural values, gender, and Mexican Americans' help-seeking intentions. *Dissertation Abstracts International, 62,* 1595B.

Riding, A. (2000). *Distant neighbors: A portrait of the Mexicans.* New York: Vintage Books.

Sanchez, A. R., & Atkinson, D. R. (1983). Mexican-American cultural commitment, preference for counselor ethnicity, and willingness to use counseling. *Journal of Counseling Psychology, 30,* 215–220.

Schneider, L. J., Laury, P. D., & Hughes, H. H. (1980). Ethnic group perceptions of mental health service providers. *Journal of Counseling Psychology, 27,* 589–596.

Sheets, L. T. (1997). Mexican-American women in family therapy: A descriptive phenomenological study. *Dissertation Abstracts International, 58,* 1604A.

Soto-Fulp, S., Del Campo, R. L., & Del Campo, D. S. (1994). Mexican-American families and acculturation: Implications for family counseling. In C. H. Huber (Ed.), *Transitioning from individual to family counseling* (pp. 49–61). Alexandria, VA: American Counseling Association.

Torres, J. B. (1998). Masculinity and gender roles among Puerto Rican men: Machismo on the U.S. mainland. *American Journal of Orthopsychiatry, 68,* 16–26.

Valdes, L. F., Barón, A., & Ponce, F. Q. (1987). Counseling Hispanic men. In M. Scher & M. Stevens (Eds.), *Handbook of counseling and psychotherapy with men* (pp. 203–217). Thousand Oaks, CA: Sage.

Young, K. S. (2001). Barriers to counseling: Mexicans and other Hispanics compared with non-Hispanic Whites. *Dissertation Abstracts International, 61,* 3784A.

Zea, M. C., Mason, M. A., & Murguia, A. (2000). Psychotherapy with members of Latino/Latina religions and spiritual traditions. In P. S. Richards & A. E. Bergin (Eds.), *Handbook of psychotherapy and religious diversity* (pp. 397–419). Washington, DC: American Psychological Association.

Zimmerman, J. E., & Sodowsky, G. R. (1993). Influences of acculturation on Mexican-American drinking practices: Implications for counseling. *Journal of Multicultural Counseling and Development, 21,* 22–35.

Zinn, M. B. (1982). Chicano men and masculinity. *Journal of Ethnic Studies, 10,* 29–44.

Zuniga, M. E. (1997). Counseling Mexican American seniors: An overview. *Journal of Multicultural Counseling and Development, 25,* 142–155.

Psychotherapy With Gay Chicanos

Richard A. Rodriguez
University of Colorado at Boulder

> *Listen carefully, this is an important point. This system is something that we use against ourselves—our brothers and our sisters. It is called* internalized oppression. *I have heard it many times: Well, he's not a real Chicano; he doesn't even speak the language. She's a sell-out; her old man is White. We even do it to ourselves: Man, I don't know if they will accept me—I don't even know my history; or my skin* es tan güero *(too light), or too dark. Our men have used it against our women. And, our women have used it against each other. And homophobia continues to rage in our communities. Whether we recognize it or not, it infects our self-expression, and that of our* niños y niñas *(sons and daughters). The list goes on and on.*
>
> —Rocha-Singh (1995, p. 6)

An increasing body of work focusing on lesbians and gay men of color now exists in the literature (e.g., Greene, 1994, 1997; Morales, 1990; Rodriguez, 1998). One primary theme in this research is the process of identity formation—the intersection of race or ethnicity, gender, and sexual orientation. Models of identity stages, states, and developmental tasks have been described for African American gay men (Jones & Hill, 1996; Loiacano, 1989), Asian American gay men and lesbians (Chan, 1997; Liu & Chan, 1996), Latina lesbians (Alquijay, 1997; Espín, 1997), gay Latino men (Morales, 1996; Rodriguez, 1996), and Native American "two-spirit" persons (Tafoya, 1996). The "pull" is a common theme whereby a person feels that he or she must choose between one aspect of identity over others, resulting in significant levels of confusion, anxiety, and depression. Another primary theme in the literature suggests that lesbians and gay men of color need to find validation in multiple communities (e.g., ethnic or racial and gay or lesbian) and to psychologically integrate all aspects of their identities.

Focusing in on the literature related to gay and lesbian Latina/os, studies on identity development, sexual behavior, and HIV prevalence and prevention (e.g., Carballo-Diéguez & Dolezal, 1995; Díaz, 1998; Díaz, Morales, Bein, Dilán, & Rodriguez, 1999), general counseling issues (e.g., González & Espín, 1996; Morales, 1996), and clinical considerations in therapy of gay and lesbian Latina/os (e.g., Carballo-Diéguez, 1989; Parés-Avila & Montano-López, 1994) have been recently conducted.

The majority of these studies focus on Latina/os in general and some provide specific subgroup characteristics within their samples (i.e., Mexican American, Cuban, Puerto Rican). For example, Carrier (1985) and Carrier and Magaña (1991) examined the sexual behavior of men of Mexican descent who have sex with men (MSM), whereas Arias (1998) focused on the identity development of Latina/o gay youth and Dilán (1999) investigated the relationship between gay Latino men and their fathers. However, very few studies or literary accounts of people's lives focus on the unique issues faced by self-identified gay Chicanos and Chicana lesbians (Rodriguez, 1991; Trujillo, 1991, 1997).

Keefe and Padilla (1987) defined *ethnic identification* as "self-identification among group members as well as their attitude toward and affiliation with one ethnic group and culture as opposed to another" (p. 8). They further noted that ethnic identification implies taking on a label and adopting a certain set of ideologies, experiences, and world views. Although there are many similarities between Latina/o subgroups, a wide variety of differences exist as well. Unfortunately, many studies that examine Latina/o gays and lesbians fail to identify the specific subgoup studied. Today, the identity politics of Chicana/o identity and *Latinidad* (Latina/o identity) requires the researcher to discuss the definitions and meanings of the terms used to describe a specific Latina/o subgroup to avoid overgeneralizations.

For the purpose of this chapter, the working definition of a gay Chicano man includes the following elements: (a) a man who was born in the United States and has one or both parents of Mexican descent; (b) a man who self-designates himself as gay, queer, or *joto;* and (c) in this self-definition there is some level of awareness and affiliation with political ideologies rooted in the civil rights movement of the 1960s, which focused on racism, social justice, the politics of identity, and the social advancement of Chicana/os (Muñoz, 1989). However, this definition is not meant to be definitive for all, given the politics of identity and the ever-evolving nature of American culture.

This chapter focuses on clinical issues in psychotherapy with gay Chicano men, with an emphasis on a model of identity development. In a qualitative study (Rodriguez, 1991), I interviewed 15 adult gay Chicano men from three southern California counties (Los Angeles, Orange, and San Diego). Transcripts of the interviews were analyzed, yielding 38 discrete themes, grouped under three general headings: Chicano identity development, gay identity development, and the integration of Chicano and gay aspects of identity. A theory was proposed, based on themes from participants' statements. In particular, this theory described the process of identity development as well as the blocks, supports, and strategies utilized for identity maintenance in the absence of gay Chicano role models. Results from this study serve as the basis for this chapter of theoretical research on gay Chicano men.

The chapter is organized into three key sections: identity development, identity management, and the therapeutic process involved in therapy with Chicano gay men. Quotes from participants in the Rodriguez (1991) study are used to introduce and further highlight the important clinical issues. Anecdotes from my clinical experience further add to the discussion. Finally, a hypothetical intake interview is presented to illustrate the application of the concepts and issues to be considered in psychotherapy with gay Chicano men.

IDENTITY DEVELOPMENT

Identity Development of Gay Chicano Men

"My parents . . . we used to celebrate the Mexican holidays . . . the Santos [saints], Dia de los Reyes [Epiphany], you know." (Miguel)

"My parents raised us very Anglicized, you know—very mainstream culture. And so I didn't feel like I grew up Chicano at all. . . . It wasn't until later that I started identifying that way. . . . My parents just preferred not to really talk to me about that part of my identity or their identity." (John)

In the Rodriguez (1991) study, the family was viewed as the primary source of learning about Chicana/o culture, attitudes, and beliefs, and normative behavior and was cited as the source of emotional, financial, and moral support within the Chicana/o community. Out of a total of 15 participants, 6 reported that Spanish was the primary language used in the home, 6 reported that English was the primary language, and 3 reported growing up bilingual. Those raised in Mexican barrios related speaking Spanish to family and peers, eating Mexican food, and celebrating Mexican traditions. Several respondents reported being raised in Anglicized homes where only English was spoken; social contacts were with Anglo friends and only American traditions were celebrated.

Growing up without a solid sense of Chicano identity is often a significant issue raised in therapy by clients, irrespective of their sexual orientation. There is often embarrassment, shame, anger, and blame (of self or parents or both) attached to the lack of proficiency in Spanish or the lack of knowledge of Mexican traditions. Morales's (1990) model of identity formation for ethnic minority gays and lesbians describes an early state in which there is a denial of such conflicts. A common statement by a person in this state is: "Being Chicano isn't an issue for me." Exploration of how the client views him- or herself with respect to ethnic identity and its evolution within the person would be an appropriate approach. Identity development is an ongoing, dynamic process and working with the client to discover that he or she can reclaim lost or missing aspects of his ethnic identity is a reassuring and educational intervention.

Not Being "Brown Enough"

"Basically in high school they used to call me a coconut (brown on the outside, White on the inside), you know, because I used to hang around with the White Americans." (Fernando)

Many Chicanos feel discredited by members of their own culture based on not being "brown enough" (e.g., physical appearance, lack of cultural knowledge, English-speaking preferences, or socializing primarily with a non-Chicano peer group) or on their Mexican relatives being *pocho,* or not a part of Mexican or American culture. Frustration, confusion, and feeling misunderstood by others exacerbates preexisting issues of feeling different and not fitting in. As a result, persons who do not conform to cultural norms or who become highly acculturated are especially susceptible to this type of stressor. Being gay is often viewed as a "White man's disease" (Tremble, Schneider, & Appathurai, 1989) by minority communities. A stereotype within Chicana/o culture is that homosexuality is the result of hanging around with *gabachos* (Whites).

Normalizing these feelings and discussing the existence of diversity within the Chicana/o culture is an excellent intervention for men dealing with this issue. At the same time one acknowledges the value in diversity, it is also important to provide avenues for exploration of unknown aspects of identity. I have identified three pathways to developing an identity: (a) developing a Chicana/o identity first and later working on a gay identity, (b) developing a gay identity first and later working on a Chicana/o identity, and (c) simultaneously developing a Chicana/o and gay identity. A clinical example follows.

A supportive and loving White family adopted a former client at a young age. At the outset of therapy, we focused on internalized homophobia (i.e., self-hate for being gay) and the coming out process. Although his parents had attempted to raise him with a nonracist world view, a significant piece was missing for him—what it meant to be Chicano. Psychotherapy subsequently focused on internalized racism, homophobia, and the construction of a positive gay Chicano identity.

Religion and Spirituality

> *"But as far as church, I've always gone to church. . . . We used to go to mass at Delhi church, and that's about as Mexican as you can get, I guess . . . in Spanish." (David)*

All participants in Rodriguez (1991) were raised Catholics. Moreover, many Chicana/o clients feel like one of the participants who emphatically stated, "You can't separate Catholicism from being Chicano—they're one and the same thing." Several particpants noted feeling guilt about their homosexual feelings and behavior. They reported praying to God on a nightly basis to be able to "change." Some felt that God had rejected them, whereas others coped by rejecting organized religion or God. One participant, Fernando, said, "So I hoped it [gay feelings] would go away. . . . I remember just praying for it to go away . . . and it wouldn't."

When asked about their source of strength, a majority of the participants reported that their "faith in God" enabled them to persevere. One participant, Larry, stated:

> At the ripe old age of 21 [when I came out], I could look back at everything that had happened: My sisters all knew, my family knew, I had all kinds of friends. And I thought, "Oh, this is great." And I could look back and say, "You know what—there is a God. Because if there wasn't a God, then I wouldn't be so happy." I prayed and I prayed and I prayed. He didn't change me. He helped me accept myself for who I am. So to this day I still believe in God. You know, he's a different God. He's not an angry God or mean— he's a beautiful God.

In another case, a former client underscored the importance of a relationship with God in understanding his homosexuality. The client was a devout Catholic and had left the seminary after 2 years when he came out. There was a point in his therapy where we both acknowledged that there was someone to whom he had not yet come out—God. Our work at that point focused on his being out, open, and honest in his relationship with God.

In addition to traditional psychotherapy, clients can benefit greatly from bibliotherapy. There are many support-oriented books and information sites on the internet discussing the reconciliation of homosexuality and the Catholic church. There is also a national organization for gay Catholics, Dignity, which can be found in many cities.

Whether it be religion, spirituality, folk beliefs, or other practices, it is important to include a client's sense of spirituality in the overall assessment of his level of identity development. A client may or may not currently practice these beliefs, but may see them as key influences on his perceptions of himself in relation to family, culture, society, and the universe. For some clients, a therapist supporting consultation with a spiritual healer may make the difference between feeling misunderstood, judged, and pathologized, and increasing the client's overall self-acceptance.

Gender Role Socialization

> "It was like drilled into my head so many times. . . . My father wanted to buy me a Texaco truck . . . and I wanted a doll . . . and he got so angry with me—he used to tell me this story—many, many times. He got so angry with me that he didn't get me anything. [chuckling]." (Pablo)

Memories of learning what was culturally and socially appropriate behavior for boys during their formative years are very clear. There is little doubt about what is appropriate behavior for Chicano boys and punishment or ostracism is quickly meted out if norms are violated. I gave a lecture on gender role expectations and characteristics in a Chicano Studies class at the University of California, Berkeley, and observed that students' perceptions fell along the stereotypical lines of men being intelligent, hard working, and competitive and women being cooperative, caring, and nurturing. However, when the students were asked to privately describe themselves, both Chicanos and Chicanas responded with a combination of masculine and feminine traits. When asked about the consequences of publicly going outside the boundaries of these expectations, most students quickly responded that it would imply that the men were gay and the women were lesbian. The pressures to conform are further reflected in the following participant's (David) comment: "Some of us play baseball. Some don't. Some of us like flowery clothes. Some don't. I don't understand what's wrong with being different."

In the Spanish language, everything appears to be connected to gender and gender role expectations. People, things, and ideas—*el hombre* (man), *la mesa* (table), and *la idea* (idea)—are all grammatically masculine or feminine (Morales, 1996). Because language is a central component of culture, should the destruction or deconstruction of gender roles be viewed as an attempt to destruct or deconstruct Chicana/o culture? Clients, students, and community members to whom I have given presentations have frequently asked that question. I do not believe that there is anything inherently wrong with gender role expectations, but people who do not follow the norm and are chastised, rejected, and ostracized often suffer detrimental effects on their self-esteem and identity. When freedom of choice is allowed (i.e., it is okay to be different), diversity of opinion and expression can lead to positive identity development.

As a result, it is important to examine how the meaning of behavior influences the definition of sexual identity. Several authors have described differences in the definition of "homosexual behavior" and "being homosexual." According to Carrier (1985), "Heterosexuality is considered superior to homosexuality in Mexico. A Mexican male's gender identity, however, is not necessarily threatened by his homosexual behavior as long as he is masculine and plays the insertor role" (p. 84). The man literally on top does not have his masculinity questioned. The man on the bottom is often viewed as the passive, less powerful, and feminine-oriented partner. Sexism interacts with these interpretations. Researchers (Carballo-Diéguez, 1989, 1995; Carrier, 1985) have noted this point and advised that one may obtain a different response from Chicano men when asking, "Have you ever engaged in sexual behavior with another man?" rather than "Are you gay?" Identification as gay or bisexual may actually have little or nothing to do with a man's private sexual behavior (Díaz, 1998). Parés-Avila and Montano-López (1994) noted:

> This interpretation is questionable because there is no evidence that the active homosexual role is accepted among Latinos. Rather, the active partner's identification with a heterosexual lifestyle despite his bisexual behavior may reflect the active partner's mechanism for coping with homophobia in his community of origin. (p. 348)

A Chicano's homosexual behavior may be known within the family, but there is often a tendency within to deny it. At times, the behavior is met with a silent tolerance as long as the man continues to display his expected cultural role as a provider, husband, and father. Carballo-Diéguez (1989) noted how lying or hiding a significant aspect of one's identity in order to maintain the support and respect of the family could negatively impact one's self-esteem and mental health status.

The phrase about men being *feo, fuerte, y formal* (ugly, strong, and formal) rings loud and clear for most men. Processing the feelings of difference, nonconformity, pressures to conform to the normative heterosexual behavior, anxiety, and guilt are critical when a client is presenting with these issues. In a world where racism affects the emotional and physical well-being of Chicana/os, a gay man feels a pull to conform to his family's and community's norms. Nonconformity poses the risk of rejection and ultimately the permanent loss of a support system to deal with the interaction of societal racism and homophobia.

Machismo

"I learned what it means to be macho—to not cry, to be strong, you know, be the boss. In other words, getting into a lot of good fights ... stick up for anything. It doesn't have to be even if you're right." (José)

Machismo has been viewed as a set of standards, norms, and responsibilities for Latino men with respect to the family (Morales, 1996). One observation in Rodriguez (1991) was that the respondents tended to use the term *macho* as a way to talk about their father's or male parental figure's negative behavior and treatment of them as children. Unfortunately, this definition is perpetuated by popular culture and often leaves out significant aspects of the original definition, including protection and defense of the family.

The effects of negative views of machismo on the self-esteem and behavior of gay Chicano men often become a clinical issue. Internalized homophobia and racism are frequently the result of years of listening to or observing what happens to men who violate the norms of machismo. Homophobic comments and actions become indelibly etched into the minds of young boys struggling with conflicting feelings of sexual attraction to other boys or men. The author attended a *Dia de la Independencia* (Independence Day) community celebration in southern California during the early 1990s where a Mexican radio personality was on stage. He made some homophobic jokes, each one followed by the comment: "*Eso es el problema* [This is the problem]. *¡Que viva Mexico!*" As I listened, I wondered about the kids in the crowd who may have been struggling with their sexual feelings and the impact of those jokes on their sense of identity.

Growing up, these feelings can become internalized as a negative aspect of Chicana/o culture and may result in a preference for non-Chicano dating partners. A client may state, "I would never date a man who would treat me like the men in my family did!" Also, the race or ethnicity of a dating partner further serves to send the message that "I'm not brown enough," especially when other gay Chicanos hassle them for not dating other Chicanos. This situation can become another mechanism for developing internalized self-hatred.

IDENTITY MANAGEMENT

Disclosure or Coming Out

> "My mom, well, she said one day, 'Are you, kind of like this?' [wiggles wrist back and forth]. I said, 'Well, whatever you want me to be.' My father, I just couldn't tell him. I've never told him. My mom told me that she told him and that he said, 'Okay.' She told me, 'As long as you're happy.'"

> "But it never became real until my lover moved in with me and my parents found out. . . . That was 4 years ago and my father did not take it well at all. He hasn't really spoken to me ever since. . . . He said shit to me like, 'I regret having anything to do with your birth. . . . I regret that you were born.'" (Sammy)

Coming out to family is considered to be a significant event in gay identity development in various stage theories (Cass, 1979, 1996; Coleman, 1982). Literal subscription to these models has often produced an interpretation that not coming out is linked to an early stage of identity development. Pressures come from internal sources (i.e., "I should be out to the ones I love") and external sources ("You're not helping your [gay] community if you're in the closet"). For some, the fear of coming out may indeed be a developmental issue.

These models, however, appear to reflect primarily the developmental patterns of White gay men and lesbians. Cass's (1996) chapter on homosexual identity development acknowledged that the theory she proposed is more of a "Western phenomenon" and noted that the coming out process is very different for lesbians and gay men of color. Kanuha (1999) cautioned therapists about automatically pathologizing "passing" as straight as an identity developmental issue. She noted that passing could be the absolutely perfect adaptive coping mechanism to a real threat (e.g., job loss, rejection by family, and the loss of protection that the culture provides against the effects of racism).

In addition, from a Mexican cultural perspective, coming out can be seen as a violation of one of the primary cultural values of being indirect, aloof, and secretive in order to avoid conflict. Coming out is subsequently regarded as an overt confrontation that entails forcing the issue on others and potentially causing the family shame. A gay Chicano's statement about not coming out at a given point in time as a protection for his family completely fits within the perspective of *familismo* (familism). Strong expectations exist on the reliance on the family for both daily needs and crisis situations, creating a strong sense of obligation to the family (Marín, 1989).

Given the previous issues, how does a therapist work with a gay Chicano with regard to coming out? Empathizing with a man struggling to maintain strong Chicano family-focused values and beliefs and understanding the importance of protecting the family against shame (*¿Que dirán?* or What will people say?) is very crucial. Maintaining a nonjudgmental attitude toward coming out decisions also helps alleviate tension, anxiety, and loneliness ("I'm the only one who feels this way") as a client weighs the potential benefits and risks of coming out to family. The client has the power, control, and right to make his own decision regarding coming out. Considering the following query is critical: To what extent is the fear of or resistance to coming out a developmental one and to what extent are cultural values or a real or perceived threat operating in the decision-making process?

Multiple Identities, Multiple Sources of Oppression, and Acculturation

> Chicano community: *"They're homophobic; they don't want any gay people. I reject anything that's homophobic."*
>
> Gay community: *"I find myself extremely involved in social, religious activities. . . . I belong to so many groups."*
>
> Gay Chicano community: *"Being a part of GLLU [Gay and Lesbian Latinos Unidos] . . . it's the one thing that has really changed my life in a lot of ways . . . because it educates you a lot in the Latino and gay community."*

Of importance is an examination of the multiple communities in which a person socializes. This is an ongoing process—the messages from the various communities with whom one affiliates influence attitudes, values, language, and beliefs about what identity means. Morales (1990) noted that gays and lesbians of color are faced with managing life in three worlds: the ethnic community, the gay and lesbian community, and the predominantly White, heterosexual community. Each setting tends to carry with it an emotional either-or, zero-sum pull that creates both internal conflict and conflict with the community. Racism exists in the lesbian and gay community just as it does in the heterosexual community. Similarly, homophobia exists in communities of color as in the general White community.

The level of acculturation (learning and adopting the characteristics, attitudes, values, and beliefs of another culture, usually the majority) must be considered when developing clinical interventions for clients. Acculturation and the client's ties to ethnic-specific values and belief systems may very well mediate the pull of conflicting loyalties.

Lesbians and gay men of color frequently report feeling alone, isolated, and alienated, never being a part of any one group (Morales, 1990; Rodriguez, 1998). Many gay Chicano men feel conflicting loyalties, given that they have both a visible and invisible minority status and are often marginalized within each culture.

In their study of Chicana/o ethnicity, Keefe and Padilla (1987) reported that one factor, cultural loyalty, was a function of real or perceived threat. If Chicanos felt that the American aspect of identity was being threatened, they would tend to lean toward that aspect for a period of time. When they feel threatened with regard to their Mexican identity, they would probably tend to lean toward that aspect.

In 1992, the Governor of California vetoed Assembly Bill 101, which would have added sexual orientation to the nondiscrimination policy of the state. Angry protests and demonstrations occurred all over the state, with identifiable Chicana/o gay and lesbian organizations' participation. It can be inferred that these individuals were, perhaps, strongly and proudly expressing their lesbian and gay identities due to threat and oppression. Likewise, in 1995, the State of California passed Proposition 187, an anti-immigrant initiative and in subsequent years passed Propositions 209 and 226, the former against affirmative action and the latter against bilingual education. Again, gay and lesbian Chicana/o organizations were present during the demonstrations and were thus likely to be expressing their ethnic identity because of perceived threat and oppression. Capitalizing on the concept noted earlier, the phrase that I have found useful with gay Chicano clients dealing with "the pull" is: It's okay—and definitely healthy—to lean.

The gay Chicanos that I have studied frequently report that the crystallization of their identity is largely due to their *familia*:

> But I've made my own family bonds . . . because I didn't get the support from my blood family—I went out and found some very close friends, extremely close, where we know each other. And we've learned to accept each other for the people we are . . . and we're very supportive of each other. We made our own family and I'm part of that family."

This is *familia* for many gay Chicanos, in the sense of an addition of supportive people and not a blanket replacement or rejection of the family of origin. *Hermanos y hermanas* (brothers and sisters) are familiar terms in the community and include people from all races and ethnicities: men, women, gay, lesbian, transgender, and heterosexual. What matters is that they acknowledge, accept, and value the person for who they are. Cherrie Moraga (as cited in Trujillo, 1991) coined the phrase "to make familia from scratch." People in the familia become significant sources of support, community affiliation, and affirmation of identity. Supporting a client's definition of familia and reinforcing the importance of connection with a community can be one of the most therapeutic interventions in the maintenance of a positive gay Chicano identity.

In an interview with a Chicana lesbian author, Ana Castillo, Marta Navarro (1991) asked what consequences her characters would have to face if coming out were an option. Castillo replied:

In a homophobic world, "coming out," or establishing a relationship that is seen by and large by a religion and then by law as perverted, is taking away everything, it's suicidal. If you're barely surviving, and then you're going to take the risk to lose the respect, and the love, and the sense of place that you have with your own family, you have nothing. All that risk for a love affair? . . . White middle class people have a sense of place in this country, and have the luxury to go and tell their parents, "I think I'm gay." They're still gonna get the job at the bank, or wherever it is. They still see themselves reflected in the mass media, where we are not only invisible, but when acknowledged, we are acknowledged very negatively. So why add one more stigma to yourself? Why take one more horrible risk to be further disenfranchised from society? You have no place to go. (Marta Navarro, pp. 122–123).

Trujillo (1991) echoed this point:

Chicana lesbians have very little choice, because their quest for self-identification comes with the territory. This is why "coming out" can be a major source of pain for Chicana lesbians, since the basic fear of rejection by family and community is paramount. For our own survival, Chicana lesbians must continually embark on the creation or modification of our own *familia,* since this institution, as traditionally constructed, may be non-supportive of the Chicana lesbian experience. (p. 189)

Professional organizations are establishing gay Chicana/o-focused caucuses or subcommittees. As Coronado (2001) noted, within The National Association of Chicana and Chicano Studies (NACCS):

The *Joto* Caucus is probably the only place where people interested in researching Chicano queer sexuality can come together and not only share our ideas but also develop an intellectual community. . . . We may be gaining experience as emerging scholars, but, more than anything, the caucus has created a space for us to grow as a community of scholars and as friends. (p. 7)

Socializing with other gay Chicanos and Chicana lesbians also provides a significant source of social support, in that all aspects of their identities are represented. Given this, therapists' knowledge of community groups and organizations is a vital adjunct to psychotherapy. The National Latina/o Lesbian, Gay, Bisexual, and Transgender Organization (LLEGO) is the only national nonprofit organization devoted to Latina/o lesbian, gay, bisexual, and transgender (LGBT) communities on local, regional, national, and international levels, addressing the need to overcome social, health, and political barriers due to sexual orientation, gender identity, and ethnic background. LLEGO is made up of approximately 172 Network of Allies (*Afiliados* and *Aliados*), LGBT Latina/o community-based organizations, and those who serve the Latina/o LGBT communities.

The names of community- and university-based organizations provide a clear sense of the importance and meaning of community: Hogar Latino, Gay and Lesbian Latinos Unidos, La Familia, Ellas en Accíon, AGUILAS, El Ambiente, Hermanos de luna y sol. From a cognitive therapy perspective, both social and professional groups provide positive role models to counter the internalized negative view of a gay Chicano man, how he acts, and what his values and beliefs are. This can be invaluable in changing his view of himself and other gay Chicano men.

HIV and AIDS

HIV and AIDS have had a significant impact on identity and community for gay Chicano and Latino men. (A full discussion of this issue is beyond the scope of this chapter, but see Díaz, 1998.) Beyond the statistics and units of service data required for federal, state, and city-funded grants, there are several human service issues to be considered with regard to Chicanos and HIV and AIDS. As Díaz noted, Latino gay men have an almost fatalistic expectation that they will seroconvert: "We know we are going to get it [HIV] sooner or later . . ." (p. 3). Díaz concluded, based on a review of the literature, that many gay Latino men engage in high-risk sexual behavior in spite of substantial knowledge of HIV transmission, high perceived risk, and strong intentions to practice safer sex.

Prevention programs remain at the forefront of risk reduction. Of particular importance are the strategies and methodology utilized in delivering the message of safer sex, risk reduction, and relapse prevention. In a study of 427 high school students, ranging in age from 12 to 20 years and attending Family Life Education classes in Alameda, California, Faryna and Morales (2000) found that ethnicity appeared more significant in predicting risk behaviors than gender, self-efficacy, knowledge, attitudes, and beliefs. They concluded that HIV prevention programs need to take into account issues of acculturation, ethnic identity development, and ethnic communication in their development and implementation.

Times have changed since the beginning of the AIDS epidemic. In the early 1980s, AIDS was seen as an automatic death sentence and AIDS-phobia abounded in all communities. For gay Chicano men, fearing rejection from family based on sexual orientation was compounded when HIV became more prevalent in the community. Many experienced this rejection, but others reconnected with familia and community. Today, many gay Chicano men who have access to appropriate medical care are on medication protocols and consider HIV a manageable disease. There are mental health and social support groups for these men, with services available in both English and Spanish.

Social class is relevant here because there are many who lack access to medical or mental health care. Poverty, racism, and sociopolitical alienation appear to be likely causes of fatalistic views of being powerless, eventually leading to seroconversion (Díaz, 1998). Díaz observed:

> A consistent theme across the focus groups and individual interviews is the notion that somewhere out there is a group of powerful others that are responsible for multiple negative outcomes in the lives of Latino gay and bisexual men, including the spread of HIV. (p. 119)

The interaction of poverty, racism, and homophobia can create a powerful negative belief statement about one's ability to control his or her life. For some, HIV can be the realization of their greatest fears of being gay—the homophobic message that HIV is "God's revenge." Helping a client differentiate between behavior and identity can be extremely helpful in addressing internalized homophobia. A focus on familia for social support is useful—both family of origin and family of choice. Community support groups that gather together for traditional holidays like *La Navidad*

(Christmas) and *Dia de los Muertos* (Day of the Dead) provide the necessary social support that can be missing for gay Latino men. Validating the experience of the fragmentation of social support, given homophobia and HIV-phobia, and providing alternatives and community resources is critical.

It is a daunting task to adequately cover all of the aspects of the impact of HIV on the gay Chicana/o community. Part of the complexity of this task lies in attempting to identify differences in dealing with HIV in other communities. The overriding difference here is the interaction effects of racism, homophobia, and sexism—the backdrop of multiple sources of oppression—of which therapists must be cognizant when working with gay Chicano men with HIV.

Gay, Queer, *Joto:* What's in a Name?

> And the worst thing about it is, in Spanish, I find that there's no good word; at least I don't know of any good word for "gay." Here, gay is applied as not the fag, not the effeminate, and less scientific than homosexual. It has a comfortable medium. And in Spanish, I don't find that. It's homosexual or maricón, you know, derogatory. And so that made it hard to come out to my parents." (Francisco)

The power that words possess cannot be underestimated. Content, meaning, and affect are all mediated by the idioms one uses. The language of one culture may not easily translate into the culture of another. It is noted that there is no positive equivalent in the Spanish language for the term *gay* (Carballo-Diéguez, 1989; Rodriguez, 1996). Bilingual-bicultural gay men often feel frustrated because they believe the Spanish term *homosexual* carries a negative connotation and seek a term that depicts a more balanced picture of who they are. At the same time, in various parts of Mexico, the word *gay* is the term most often used by gay men to describe their own identity (Carballo-Diéguez, 1995).

Carballo-Diéguez (1985) noted that men who openly identified as gay were more likely to be highly acculturated and largely influenced by American or Western culture. Early research on gay and lesbian identity development sampled from a primarily Caucasian population (Cass, 1996). The cultural identifying words *homosexual, gay,* and *queer* continue to create controversy in the White gay community. *Queer* has been used by many to add an affiliation with a political activist ideology in terms of "taking back" the previously derogatory meaning of the term. In an episode of the "The Simpsons" television program, Homer confronted a gay character for his positive use of the term *queer.* Homer's position was: "And that's another thing. . . . You can't use that word. . . . That's the word that WE use to put YOU down."

I have noted a similar use of the word *joto.* It has traditionally been regarded as pejorative, similar to *maricón.* However, there are private, public, professional positive uses of the term in today's culture. A fund-raiser for the gay Latina/o social group AGUILAS in San Francisco used the game *lotería* with the title of the event: *Loteria Para la Joteria.* In 1993, NACCS recognized the National Association of Latino Gay Academics and Activists, later renamed as the Joto Caucus. The Lesbiana caucus, established in 1990, was a major supporter of this action (Coronado, 2001).

Part of the power that is felt by men who prefer the term *joto* is about being able to name one's self, rather than being labeled by others. It becomes an issue of empowerment. It is important to listen to the terms that clients use. Some men do not identify as gay or anything else and might simply state that they are in love with or are attracted to men. It is also important to pay attention to regional differences with respect to terminology. In an area where the term *joto* is the norm, it would not be uncommon to hear it used within the community. However, from my observation, this is very much a gay Chicano perspective that also interacts with regional differences. I would not expect homosexual men in Mexico to respond positively to hearing the term *joto* used so openly in public as it has not been embraced by community standards.

Chicana lesbian poet Natashia López (1991) addressed the issue of words and inclusion of multiple aspects of identity in her poem "Trying to be Dyke and Chicana." In the first stanza, she wrote:

> Dyk-ana
> Dyk-icana
> what do I call myself
> people want a name
> a label a product
> what's the first ingredient
> the dominant ingredient (p. 84)

In her discussion of identity and difference, Trujillo (1997) reminded us of age cohort differences with respect to identity:

> Perhaps due somewhat to the widening of the recognition of difference and lessening feelings of the need for conformity, identity seems to be becoming more fluid in the gay and lesbian community. When I came out 15 years ago, the lesbian communities I lived in worked intensely to try to convince me to act, look, and think within certain modalities. . . . Although I can now publicly admit that I never did as I was told, I certainly would not acknowledge it back then. (p. 275)

In my study of significant events in the identity development of 251 gay men in Utah (Rodriguez, 1989), I found statistically significant differences on 8 of the 11 variables investigated, based on a median split by age (half the sample being 18 to 30, half being 31 to 63). A major conclusion was that men who came out in the 1950s and 1960s experienced a different social, psychological, and political climate from those who came out in the 1970s and 1980s. Although it is critical to examine the development and management of a positive gay Chicano identity as defined by the client today, we must also acknowledge the change in meaning, fluidity, and perhaps overall definition, given the changes in the social, psychological, and political climate.

THE THERAPEUTIC PROCESS

Culturally Competent Services

As Sue and Sue (1999) noted, counselor-client cultural differences alone do not create barriers to counseling. A therapist's sensitivity to and knowledge of critical aspects of multicultural issues in therapy influence his or her ability to work effectively with a gay Chicano. Providing services to this population is a clinical specialty. Any therapist of any sexual orientation and any race or ethnicity can effectively work with this population as long as he or she has the requisite training and experience.

The American Psychological Association's (APA) Division 44 Committee on Lesbian, Gay, and Bisexual Concerns Joint Task Force (Division 44/CLGBC Joint Task Force) has published its *Guidelines for Psychotherapy with Lesbian, Gay, and Bisexual Clients* (2000). The APA's Council of Representatives formally adopted the guidelines in February 2000. There are 16 guidelines covering attitudes toward homosexuality and bisexuality, relationships and families, issues of diversity, and education. A few are reproduced here:

> Guideline 1: Psychologists understand that homosexuality and bisexuality are not indicative of mental illness.
>
> Guideline 2: Psychologists are encouraged to recognize how their attitudes and knowledge about lesbian, gay, and bisexual issues may be relevant to assessment and treatment and seek consultation or make appropriate referrals when indicated.
>
> Guideline 3: Psychologists strive to understand the ways in which social stigmatization (i.e., prejudice, discrimination, and violence) poses risks to the mental health and well being of lesbian, gay, and bisexual clients.
>
> . . .
>
> Guideline 9: Psychologists are encouraged to recognize the particular life issues or challenges that are related to multiple and often conflicting cultural norms, values, and beliefs that lesbian, gay, and bisexual members of racial and ethnic minorities face. (p. 1445)

Chicana/o clients often seek or are provided with referrals to Latino mental health agencies or private practitioners. Given the homophobia that exists in all ethnic and cultural communities, gay Chicano men may be wary of this type of traditional referral for fear that mental health practitioners view homosexuality as pathological. Likewise, gay clients seek or are provided with referrals to gay and lesbian mental health agencies or private practitioners. Given the racism that exists in the gay and lesbian and heterosexual communities, gay Chicano men are often wary of White gay and lesbian therapists.

Questions arise with respect to racism, prejudice, and cultural competence. Is the therapist homophobic? Will my problems be blamed on my sexual orientation? Will the therapist force me to come out to my family? Will the therapist understand me? How White is the agency? Are there any therapists of color—any Chicana/o therapists who are out? Do the therapists know anything about Chicana/o culture?

The guidelines from Division 44/CLGBC Joint Task Force (2000) serve as a useful reference, documenting the mental health needs of lesbian, gay, and bisexual clients as well as discussing the standards of care in providing services to this population: "The specific goals of these guidelines are to provide practitioners with (a) a frame of reference for the treatment of lesbian, gay, and bisexual clients and (b) basic information and further references in the areas of assessment, intervention, identity, relationships, and the education and training of psychologists" (p. 1440).

Language Usage

Espín (1997) described narrative research in the lives of lesbian immigrants. In focus groups with women describing their lives and changing identities through the process of immigration, she noted that the women were using English instead of Spanish. Espín, herself, is a native Spanish speaker and Spanish was the primary language for many women in the focus groups. Upon further inquiry, she found that English provided a safe, emotional distance from discussing issues of sexuality, which are not culturally sanctioned as open discussion. Espín observed:

> Apparently language, both the native tongue and English, is used to provide relational safety. It serves as an instrument that either enhances intimacy or provides distance in relationships and self-definition. I can hypothesize that the stronger the cognitive psychological identity development in the native language, the greater the comfort experienced when using it in intimate and sexual relationships and encounters. (p. 211)

As a bilingual-bicultural therapist, it is important to note not only the content, but also the language associated with the content. In training programs on cross-cultural therapy, I was always taught that, when clients hit a "hot" topic, they utilize their primary language because strong emotion is involved. However, given this context, the modulation of the language that the therapist uses can guide specific interventions. I have used this with clients as we talked about coming out to family. Role playing and shifting between English and Spanish with the client served as a positive therapeutic experience. With another client, I used a Gestalt intervention, playing the role of a supportive parent in dealing with the shame of childhood sexual abuse: *"Dime lo que pasó, mijo"* ["Tell me what happened, my son"]—an intervention in Spanish—influenced the client's expression of supressed emotions. Finally, with some clients I have used language modulation with respect to internalized racism and homophobia. From a cognitive-therapeutic perspective, helping clients associate positive thoughts with statements such as *Yo soy Chicano* (I am Chicano) and *Yo soy gay* (I am gay) can counter previously held negative beliefs associated with internalized self-hate.

An Intake With Tony

The following is a description of an intake session with a gay Chicano client and illustrates the application of the concepts covered earlier in the chapter. The perspective is that of examining critical issues and clinical considerations, acknowledging that there is no one right way to approach the client.

The setting is a counseling center at a predominantly White university on the west coast. The center primarily focuses on short-term psychotherapy. There are five professional staff and five predoctoral and post-Master's interns. Sonia is a bilingual-bicultural heterosexual Chicana psychologist who has been at the university for 6 years. She is well connected to the Chicana/o-Latina/o community on campus.

Tony was a 23-year-old first-year graduate student in ethnic studies. His family lived 500 miles away from the university. He had completed his undergraduate work at a small college near his home and then decided to branch out. He has two older brothers and one younger sister and was the first in his family to attend college. His parents are proud working-class people who want the best for their son, which is why they did not protest his leaving the area. Tony had a scholarship from a hometown regional Chicano foundation and a teaching assistantship from his department.

He lived in graduate student housing with another student, Chris, from the business school.

On the initial information sheet, Tony cited the following as his primary reason for coming to the center: "I've had a hard time focusing on my studies. I'm not as interested in my classes." He had never been in therapy before and was somewhat apprehensive as Sonia led him to her office. Sitting down, Tony very quickly scanned Sonia's office—the sarape on the wall, the posters and hangings related to Mexican and Chicana/o cultural traditions, the bookshelf filled with books on race, ethnicity, and cross-cultural psychotherapy.

Sonia: *¿Habla español?* Do you speak Spanish?
Tony: *Sí.* [Yes.]
Sonia: *¿Prefiere hablar en español, ingles, o Spanglish* [Do you prefer to speak in Spanish, English, or Spanglish] or however it comes out?
Tony: [Smiling] However it comes out is fine with me.

Sonia continued her standard intake procedures, checking in with Tony as they got along as to how he felt about the process. She probed into the meaning of his problems concentrating on his studies, depressive symptoms, medical history, family, and social relations. She found out that Tony came from a close-knit family described as "very Mexican." He identified himself as Chicano and said that during his undergraduate days he participated in Movimiento Estudiantil Chicana/os de Atzlán (MEChA), a Chicano-oriented student organization. With respect to relationships with each of his family members, he stated that he was "close" to his parents and somewhat distant from his siblings: "They really don't know me very well."

Sonia: How about your social support network? Whom do you hang with?
Tony: I haven't really made many friends yet. My roommate is okay, *pero el no me entiende* [but he doesn't understand me]. I feel kinda out of place. I don't know . . .
Sonia: I know; this is not a very diverse campus.
Tony: Yeah, in many ways.
        [Not wanting to assume anything, Sonia chooses gender-neutral terms as she proceeds with the intake.]
Sonia: How about dating? Are you seeing anyone?
Tony: I was . . . but it ended . . . recently . . . a couple of weeks ago.
Sonia: How long were the two of you together?
Tony: A year and a half. We've been doing the long-distance thing and it's just not working out.
Sonia: Tell me about your partner.
Tony: [Hesitantly] Well—we met in college. He—he was my first relationship. . . . I'm gay."

At this point, Sonia's response to Tony's disclosure was critical. He, in turn, focused on his perception of Sonia's Chicana identity and asked himself several questions. Does Sonia believe that homosexuality is a mental disorder? Is she a "traditional" Roman Catholic, believing that homosexuality is a sin? Will Sonia believe that I am *vendido* (a sellout) to White culture? Maybe she understands, maybe there's nothing to worry about.

There are many interventions that Sonia could have made at this point. The critical ideas for her to get across to Tony were: (a) that his feelings are normal, (b) that she is empathic and understanding of his situation, and (c) that she is nonjudgmental and accepting of him as a person. Fears of being rejected, judged, and pathologized can be alleviated through empathy, acceptance, and normalization of the client's experience. Both verbal interventions and environmental cues can accomplish these goals. Along with the books on race, ethnicity, and culture in a therapist's office, books on gay and lesbian psychotherapy can be reassuring to clients. For example, Sonia has a variety of books on her office shelf, including *Ethnic and Cultural Diversity Among Lesbians and Gay Men* (Greene, 1997), *Textbook of Homosexuality and Mental Health* (Stein & Cabaj, 1996), and *Lesbians and Gays in Couples and Families* (Laird & Green, 1996). A sticker taped to the wall, containing a pink triangle with the word "ally" printed in the middle, can also send a message of acceptance of lesbian and gay issues. Gay and lesbian clients are sensitive to examining signs of understanding, education or training, and acceptance in the environment.

Exploring family support systems and the client's relationships with each of his family members is critical. How out is he? Who knows? Who does not know? If he is not out to family members, to what extent is this a stage of gay identity development and to what extent is he appropriately following cultural values or real or perceived threat? What would happen to him or the family's honor within the larger extended family and the community in which they live? When he is leaving a family holiday gathering and his *abuelita* (grandmother) says, *"Te portas bien y deja las muchachas en paz"* (Be good and leave the girls alone), what cultural norms are operating as Tony considers his response? Saying "Don't worry" might lead his parents to think, *"Sin verguenza"* (How shameless). On the other hand, not responding or continuing to pass as straight may produce increased stress and anxiety for Tony. He may not be able to "be himself" with his *familia*. Normalizing his feelings and helping Tony to strategize responses in family situations could be very helpful.

> Sonia: At what age do you first recall being attracted to another man?
> Tony: As long as I can remember. I know I felt different from other guys. I would listen to my older brothers talking about girls and what they did—it wasn't like that for me. But I know that something was going on when I was around guys. But I knew I couldn't talk about it with them—I knew what they called those guys—*joto, maricón*. And I knew what happened to those guys.

With this and subsequent queries such as "What was it like growing up gay in the Chicano community? What was it like being Chicano in the gay community?" Sonia demonstrated knowledge of gay identity development theory. As with all theories, however, individual differences exist and Sonia needed to be able to demonstrate flexibility in validating Tony's experiences:

> Sonia: Who's *familia* for you? How connected are you with the Chicano community? The gay community? The gay Chicano community?

Assessment of Tony's level of identity development was a critical issue. With respect to social support network, how ready was Tony at this point to identify more publicly with gay Chicana/os? He was at a predominantly White university where it was possible that there was no La Familia student group. How did he feel about being Chicano in a predominantly White gay and lesbian community? What community cultural groups and resources might exist with whom Tony could identify?

Terminology can also be important at this point. Using the terms that Tony used to describe his identity (*Chicano, gay, familia*) showed respect and understanding for his identification and comfort level. *Joto, queer,* or *Hispanic* would not be appropriate terms for Sonia to use if Tony himself had not first used the words to describe himself.

> Sonia: Religious or spiritual affiliations?
> Tony: I was raised Catholic. I was an altar boy and the whole thing. I wanted to change these feelings. Nothing worked. I know the church's stance on homosexuality. I never went back, it's screwed.

Sonia's acknowledgment of the differentiation between organized religion and spirituality allowed for exploration of the meaning and impact of each on Tony's identity. This differentiation validated (a) the way that the Catholic church's position on homosexuality had influenced his identity and (b) his exploration of the existence of a nonjudgmental and accepting God or Higher Power from whom he could draw support.

Near the end of the intake session Sonia knew that she needed to make a recommendation. She reflected on the extent to which she and Tony could accomplish some goals in eight sessions of short-term psychotherapy in the counseling center. She wondered if she had made a connection with Tony and if he felt understood and accepted by her. Did Tony need to be seen by a Chicana/o therapist, a gay or lesbian therapist, or a gay or lesbian Chicana/o therapist? Although not lesbian, to what extent did Sonia's knowledge of and experience with the clinical issues of the intersection of race and ethnicity, gender, and sexual orientation benefit, or hinder, the work that Tony needed to do at this point? What resources did she possess and what community resources best matched Tony's needs? The critical issue at this point was that there was no one right answer. The recommendation was based on client needs, the intake counselor's knowledge and training, and knowledge of community resources.

> Sonia: We're coming to the end of our time today and I told you I'd make a recommendation. Before I give that, what else do I need to know about you? How has this been for you?
> Tony: Feels good. . . . I'm kind of surprised, but it feels good.

Tony acknowledged that his time spent with Sonia produced positive feelings. He felt validated and understood by Sonia as a Chicano, as gay, and as a gay Chicano man. Further exploration of his issues could focus on relationship development—what role models does he have for the development and maintenance of gay relationships? They could choose to explore the pros and cons and cultural considerations in coming out to family. They could explore issues of racism in the gay and lesbian community, homophobia or heterosexism in the Chicana/o community, and the expectation for someone with multiple aspects of identity to check one box only.

Several possibilities exist to help Tony deal with his issues once the therapist demonstrates acknowledgment, understanding, and acceptance of what it means to be Chicano, what it means to be gay, and the interaction effect of race and ethnicity, gender, and sexual orientation on a person's identity. Moreover, Tony most likely recognized the commonality between himself and Sonia as members of an oppressed community. These factors may also affect clinical issues, including the expressions of anxiety, depression, interpersonal problems, and self-esteem.

SUMMARY

This chapter reviewed critical issues in psychotherapy that need to be considered when working with gay Chicano men. Knowledge of identity development issues is crucial, including familia as the basis for socialization, racial or ethnic identity development patterns, the role of machismo in a Chicano's sense of self, and the role of religion or spirituality in self-concept. Understanding the multiple aspects of identity and the multiple sources of oppression that gay Chicano men face is critical for working effectively with this population. The language and terminology that clients and therapists use have a significant impact on a client's sense of feeling heard, understood, and unconditionally validated. Finally, as noted by Liu and Chan (1996) in reference to East Asian gays and lesbians, acknowledging the multiple cultural lenses through which gay Chicano men view the world can turn a perception of hardship into a perception of assets, strengths, and integrity.

We have much to learn from *nuestras hermanas* (our sisters), Chicana lesbians. In their struggles in dealing with the intersection of racism, sexism, classism, and homophobia, listening to what they have learned and how they survive can provide extremely valuable lessons for gay Chicano men. In Navarro (1991), Castillo cited the following as her message to Chicanas and Latinas:

> If you can get up, generation after generation, after hundreds of years of humiliation and repression, and you can still get up in the morning, and you can still hold your head up, and you can still look in the mirror and say: this is an attractive woman, or this is someone whose face I would show in public; who has enough inside of her to still care, to still love, to raise up loving human beings, to know that the minute she's out in the world she's subject to every kind of atrocity that society can put upon a human being, and still she has the ability to love, and to see beauty, and to offer that up, we are tremendously powerful beings, and that's very real. All those horrible things that they say about us are society's creation about us, but who we are essentially, and the essence of our being, to me, is that of a tremendous individual. (p. 131)

The redefinition of *familia* must be validated in examining the development and management of a positive gay Chicano identity. In her essay, "La Frontera," Diane Alcalá (1991) concluded:

> Being a Chicana lesbian, I carry on, holding on to what I have learned from my *familia*. My father spoke to me of the importance of family, not only my blood family, but also *mi gente*. I think of other Chicana lesbians as family. We relate, connect, and know our strength. The strength we have because of living as who we are. (p. 197)

Healthy gay Chicano men can be single, married, divorced, partnered, widowed, joto, queer, political, apolitical, English speaking, Spanish speaking, bilingual,

Spanglish speaking, *güero* (fair skinned), *moreno* (dark-skinned), macho, femme, working class, professional, and community workers. Above all else, the critical point to underscore with clients is: *Somos familia* (we are family).

ACKNOWLEDGMENT

I greatly appreciate feedback on earlier drafts of this chapter from Carla Trujillo and Robert-Jay Green.

REFERENCES

Alcalá, D. (1991). La frontera. In C. Trujillo (Ed.), *Chicana lesbians: The girls our mothers warned us about* (pp. 196–197). Berkeley, CA: Third Woman Press.

Alquijay, M. A. (1997). The relationship among self-esteem, acculturation, and lesbian identity formation in Latina lesbians. In B. Greene (Ed.), *Ethnic and cultural diversity among lesbians and gay men* (pp. 249–265). Thousand Oaks, CA: Sage.

Arias, R. (1998). *The identity development, psychosocial stressors, and coping strategies of Latino gay/bisexual youth: A qualitative analysis.* Unpublished doctoral dissertation, California School of Professional Psychology, Alameda.

Carballo-Diéguez, A. (1989). Hispanic culture, gay male culture, and AIDS: Counseling implications. *Journal of Counseling and Development, 68*, 26–30.

Carballo-Diéguez, A. (1995). The sexual identity and behavior of Puerto Rican men who have sex with men. In G. M. Herek & B. Greene (Eds.), *AIDS, identity, and community: The HIV epidemic and lesbians and gay men: Psychological perspectives on lesbian and gay issues* (pp. 105–114). Newbury Park, CA: Sage.

Carballo-Diéguez, A., & Dolezal, C. (1995). Association between history of childhood sexual abuse and adult HIV-risk sexual behavior in Puerto Rican men who have sex with men. *Child Abuse and Neglect, 19*, 595–605.

Carrier, J. M. (1985). Mexican male bisexuality. *Journal of Homosexuality, 11*, 75–85.

Carrier, J. M., & Magaña, J. R. (1991). Use of ethnosexual data on men of Mexican origin for HIV/AIDS prevention programs. *The Journal of Sex Research, 28*, 189–202.

Cass, V. (1979). Homosexual identity formation: A theoretical model. *Journal of Homosexuality, 4*, 219–235.

Cass, V. (1996). Sexual orientation identity formation: A western phenomenon. In R. P. Cabaj & T. S. Stein (Eds.), *Textbook of homosexuality and mental health* (pp. 227–251). Washington, DC: American Psychiatric Press.

Chan, C. S. (1997). Don't ask, don't tell, don't know: The formation of a homosexual identity and sexual expression among Asian American lesbians. In B. Greene (Ed.), *Ethnic and cultural diversity among lesbians and gay men* (pp. 240–248). Thousand Oaks, CA: Sage.

Coleman, E. (1982). Developmental stages of the coming out process. *Journal of Homosexuality, 7*, 31–43.

Coronado, R. (2001). Joto caucus report. *Noticias de NACCS, 28*, 6–7.

Díaz, R. M. (1998). *Latino gay men and HIV: Culture, sexuality, and risk behavior.* New York: Routledge.

Díaz, R. M., Morales, E. S., Bein, E., Dilán, E., & Rodriguez, R. A. (1999). Predictors of sexual risk in Latino gay/bisexual men: The role of demographic, developmental, social, cognitive and behavioral variables. *Hispanic Journal of Behavioral Sciences, 21*, 480–501.

Dilán, E. (1999). *The relationship of gay Latinos to their fathers: A comparison to Euro-Caucasian gays.* Unpublished doctoral dissertation, California School of Professional Psychology, Alameda.

Division 44/Committee on Lesbian, Gay, and Bisexual Concerns Joint Task Force. (2000). Guidelines for psychotherapy with lesbian, gay, and bisexual clients. *American Psychologist, 55*, 1440–1451.

Espín, O. M. (1997). Crossing borders and boundaries: The life narratives of immigrant lesbians. In B. Greene (Ed.), *Ethnic and cultural diversity among lesbians and gay men* (pp. 191–215). Thousand Oaks, CA: Sage.

Faryna, E. L., & Morales, E. (2000). Self-efficacy and HIV-related risk behaviors among multiethnic adolescents. *Cultural Diversity and Ethnic Minority Psychology, 6*, 42–56.

González, F. J., & Espín, O. M. (1996). Latino men, Latina women, and homosexuality. In R. J. Cabaj & T. S. Stein (Eds.), *Textbook of homosexuality and mental health* (pp. 583–601). Washington, DC: American Psychiatric Press.

Greene, B. (1994). Ethnic minority lesbians and gay men: Mental health and treatment issues. *Journal of Consulting and Clinical Psychology, 62,* 243–251.

Greene, B. (Ed.). (1997). *Ethnic and cultural diversity among lesbians and gay men.* Thousand Oaks, CA: Sage.

Jones, B. E., & Hill, M. J. (1996). African American lesbians, gay men, and bisexuals. In R. J. Cabaj & T. S. Stein (Eds.), *Textbook of homosexuality and mental health* (pp. 549–561). Washington, DC: American Psychiatric Press.

Kanuha, V. (1999). The social process of "passing" as a stigma management strategy: Acts of internalized oppression or acts of resistance? *Journal of Sociology and Social Welfare, 26,* 27–46.

Keefe, S. E., & Padilla, A. M. (1987). *Chicano ethnicity.* Albuquerque: University of New Mexico Press.

Laird, J., & Green, R. J. (1996). *Lesbians and gays in couples and families: A handbook for therapists.* San Francisco: Jossey-Bass.

Liu, P., & Chan, C. S. (1996). Lesbian, gay, and bisexual Asian Americans and their families. In J. Laird & R. J. Green (Eds.), *Lesbians and gays in couples and families: A handbook for therapists* (pp. 137–152). San Francisco: Jossey-Bass.

Loiacano, D. K. (1989). Gay identity issues among Black Americans: Racism, homophobia, and the need for validation. *Journal of Counseling and Development, 68,* 21–25.

López, N. (1991). Trying to be dyke and Chicana. In C. Trujillo (Ed.), *Chicana lesbians: The girls our mothers warned us about* (p. 84). Berkeley, CA: Third Woman Press.

Marín, A. (1989). AIDS prevention among Hispanics: Needs, risk behaviors, and cultural values. *Public Health Report, 104,* 411–415.

Morales, E. S. (1990). Ethnic minority families and minority gays and lesbians. In F. W. Bozett & M. B. Sussman (Eds.), *Homosexuality and family relations* (pp. 217–239). New York: Haworth Press.

Morales, E. S. (1996). Gender roles among Latino gay and bisexual men: Implications for family and couple relationships. In J. Laird & R. J. Green (Eds.) *Lesbians and gays in couples and families: A handbook for therapists* (pp. 272–297). San Francisco: Jossey-Bass.

Muñoz, C. (1989). *Youth, identity, power: The Chicano movement.* New York: Verso.

Navarro, M. A. (1991). Interview with Ana Castillo. In C. Trujillo (Ed.), *Chicana lesbians: The girls our mothers warned us about* (pp. 113–132). Berkeley, CA: Third Woman Press.

Parés-Avila, J. A., & Montano-López, R. M. (1994). Issues in the psychosocial care of Latino gay men with HIV infection. In S. A. Cadwell, R. A. Burham, & M. Forstein (Eds.), *Therapists on the front line: Psychotherapy with gay men in the age of AIDS* (pp. 339–362). Washington, DC: American Psychiatric Press.

Rocha-Singh, I. (1995). *Chicana/Chicano identity: A true story.* Unpublished manuscript.

Rodriguez, R. A. (1989). *Significant events in gay identity development: Gay men in Utah.* Unpublished master's thesis, University of Utah, Salt Lake City.

Rodriguez, R. A. (1991). *A qualitative study of identity development in gay Chicano men.* Unpublished doctoral dissertation, University of Utah, Salt Lake City.

Rodriguez, R. A. (1996). Clinical issues in identity development in gay Latino men. In C. Alexander (Ed.), *Gay and lesbian mental health: A sourcebook for practitioners* (pp. 127–157). New York: Harrington Park Press.

Rodriguez, R. A. (1998). Clinical and practical considerations in private practice with lesbians and gay men of color. In C. Alexander (Ed.), *Working with gay men and lesbians in private psychotherapy practice* (pp. 59–75). New York: Haworth Press.

Sue, D. W., & Sue, D. (1999). *Counseling the culturally different: Theory and practice* (3rd ed.). New York: Wiley and Sons.

Tafoya, T. N. (1996). Native two-spirit people. In R. P. Cabaj & T. S. Stein (Eds.), *Textbook of homosexuality and mental health* (pp. 603–617). Washington, DC: American Psychiatric Press.

Tremble, B., Schneider, M., & Appathurai, C. (1989). Growing up gay or lesbian in a multicultural context. In G. Herdt (Ed.), *Gay and lesbian youth* (pp. 253–267). New York: Haworth Press.

Trujillo, C. (Ed.). (1991). *Chicana lesbians: The girls our mothers warned us about.* Berkeley, CA: Third Woman Press.

Trujillo, C. (1997). Sexual identity and the discontents of difference. In B. Greene (Ed.), *Ethnic and cultural diversity among lesbians and gay men* (pp. 266–278). Thousand Oaks, CA: Sage.

Appendix

INTERNET RESOURCES FOR ORGANIZATIONS AND MENTAL HEALTH RESOURCES

Alternative Family Institute. Counseling agency for lesbian, gay, bisexual, and transgender couples and families (www.altfamily.org).

Dignity. National organization for lesbian, gay, bisexual, and transgender Catholics (www.dignityusa.org) En español: Dignidad (www.dignityusa.org/spanish/index.html).

LLEGO: National Latina/o Lesbian, Gay, Bisexual, & Transgender Organization (www.llego.org).

NACCS: National Association for Chicana and Chicano Studies (www.naccs.org).

PFLAG: Parents, Families and Friends of Lesbians and Gays (www.pflag.org).

Society for the Psychological Study of Lesbian, Gay, and Bisexual Issues: Division 44 of the American Psychological Association (www.apa.org/divisions/div44/).

Multiracial Feminism for Chicana/o Psychology

Leticia M. Arellano
University of La Verne

Christina Ayala-Alcantar
California State University, Northridge

> *Numerous persons and events influenced my identity as a feminist. For example, my older sister significantly influenced my identity during my late adolescence. As a college student she often encouraged my family and me to boycott grapes. She also exposed me to Chicana feminism. My family interactions influenced my identity as a feminist as well. As the youngest child with older brothers, I often protested against the double standards within my family. My brothers were often granted special privileges that my sisters and I were denied. My participation in various Chicana/o and Latina/o organizations played a role in shaping my feminist identity. I often found myself at odds with sexist and homophobic counterparts. Challenging gender oppression and homophobia within these organizations often resulted in an array of negative responses and heated debates and internal conflict frequently ensued. Ironically, these encounters galvanized my public acknowledgement as a feminist.*
> —Leticia Arellano

> *My graduate career began at California State University, Los Angeles, where I took my first class with a Chicana psychologist, Dr. Gloria Romero. Gloria is a Chicana feminist and was one of the first people to expose me to the world of feminism. Interestingly, most of what I learned from her occurred outside of the classroom. For example, during the Clarence Thomas-Anita Hill hearings, Gloria wrote several editorials for the L. A. Times discussing the struggle women of color experience between nationalism and feminism. She asked if, in settings where men of color are in positions of power and engage in sexist behaviors, women of color should remain silent to support national solidarity or speak out against sexist men and support a feminist perspective. Although Gloria challenged my thinking regarding gender and I became more progressive with respect to women's issues, I did not identify as a feminist. Although Gloria was a feminist, I still felt that feminism was a "White thing."*
> —Christina Ayala-Alcantar

Although many Chicanas do not consider or publicly acknowledge themselves to be feminists, we find that their research, clinical practice, teaching, activism, and attitudes indicate the contrary. It appears that the "F" word remains taboo, even today. In light of the history of elitism and racism by White feminists and the retaliation from Chicana/o communities during the Chicana/o movement, we concede that feminism remains controversial and, in many instances, unappealing. This begs the question: Does feminism have any utility for the field of Chicana/o psychology?

As Chicana psychologists, we recognize the need for a conceptual framework within which a vast array of issues confronted by Chicanas can be analyzed. We argue that feminism has great utility, not simply for Chicanas, but for our community as well. This idea was heightened for both of us as doctoral students enrolled in a course taught by Chicana sociologist Dr. Maxine Baca Zinn at Michigan State University, entitled "Gender and Power." We were exposed to an array of contemporary feminisms (e.g., gender reform, gender resistance, and gender rebellion) and learned about an inclusive form of feminism known as multiracial feminism (Baca Zinn & Dill, 1996).

As an analytical framework, multiracial feminism is inclusive, as it acknowledges the experiences of both women and men, unlike other forms of second-wave feminism. This framework recognizes that gender is experienced not in a vacuum, but, rather, concurrently with numerous factors such as race, ethnicity, class, and sexual orientation. More importantly, it acknowledges that different social locations (e.g., gender, race, class) and settings interact, resulting in a differential experience of power, that is, a Chicana/o can feel powerful and powerless depending on the setting and situation.

It is our contention that multiracial feminism provides Chicana/o psychology with a framework for research, theory, and practice that extends beyond focusing solely on the examination of intrapsychic factors, a practice in which the impact and power of social structures remain obscure and in which it is hard to identify areas of strength and resilience. In this chapter we seek to relocate our gendered experiences in Chicana/o psychology within the framework of multiracial feminism.

FEMINIST THEORY AND PRACTICE

Eurocentric notions mistakenly assume that White women were the foremothers of activism in the United States (Comas-Díaz, 1991; Cotera, 1973; Mirandé & Enriquez, 1979). As Cotera argued, "the Mexicana has a long and wonderful history of Mexicano feminism which is not Anglo inspired, imposed or oriented" (p. 30). Despite this legacy, many Chicanas in psychology do not identify as feminists and tend to view feminism as a pursuit of "White women" (Espín, 1995).

Two significant factors contribute to this antifeminist perspective in the Chicana/o community. One is cultural nationalism. Chicanismo, embedded in cultural nationalism, advocated for "cultural survival within an Anglo-dominated society" (García, 1997b, p. 125). As an ideology, Chicanismo also emphasized cultural pride as a source of unity and strength within the political landscape. Accordingly, the fight for personal and political empowerment for Chicana/os was paramount. However, women who advocated for gender equality encountered internal conflict. Chicanas who challenged the sexism and gender oppression within the Chicana/o movement were often subjected to an array of negative responses (García, 1997a; Hurtado, 1998; Moraga, 1993; Nieto-Gomez, 1974). Moraga lamented that "the Chicana feminist attempting to critique the sexism in the Chicano community is certainly between a personal rock and a political hard place" (p. 207). Among various epithets, Chicana feminists were viewed as "anti-family, anti-cultural, anti-man, and anti-Chicano movement" (Nieto-Gomez, p. 35). They were also regarded with suspicion or perceived as selfish for placing their own needs above the needs of the greater community (Cotera; García, 1997a; Nieto-Gomez).

Accusations of lesbianism by homophobic Chicana/os were an attempt to further intimidate and ostracize Chicana feminists (Hurtado, 1998). Regrettably, women who openly claimed their lesbianism or sexual liberation also encountered harsh treatment from Chicana/o communities (Hurtado; Moraga, 1993; Trujillo, 1991). Sexual and emotional bonding among women was often regarded as cultural genocide, as it challenged the fabric of *la familia* (the family). Sexual liberation was also deemed deviant (Trujillo). Moraga asserted that a woman who defies her subservient roles and assumes control of her sexuality is ostracized by being regarded as a lesbian, and even if she is not.

Ironically, Chicana lesbians have profound voices within contemporary Chicana/o scholarship. Literature such as *Borderlands/La Frontera: The New Mestiza* (Anzaldúa, 1987), *This Bridge Called My Back: Writings by Radical Women of Color* (Moraga & Anzaldúa, 1983), *Making Face, Making Soul/Haciendo Caras: Creative and Critical Perspectives by Feminists of Color* (Anzaldúa, 1990), *Massacre of the Dreamers: Essays on Xicanisma* (Castillo, 1995), and other works challenge the intellectual canons of Chicana/o studies.

Another factor preventing Chicanas from identifying with the feminist movement are the exclusionary practices of White feminists (Comas-Díaz, 1991; Espín, 1995; Flores-Ortiz, 1998; García, 1997b). Feminist theory and practice were largely developed by White middle-class women (Brown, 1994; Espín, 1995; Espín & Gawelek, 1992); it does not reflect the concerns of women of color (Baca Zinn & Dill, 1996; Bing & Reid, 1996; Brown; Espín, 1994, 1995) or Chicanas (Flores-Ortiz; Gloria, 2001; Hurtado, 1998). Regrettably, criticisms of feminism include insensitivity, racism, and elitism (Bing & Reid; Espín, 1994, 1995) and such criticisms challenge the utility of feminist theory and practice for Chicanas (Gloria).

Feminist theory assumes a universal identity among women, based on the tenet that women share the same experiences, including economic oppression, commercial exploitation, and legal discrimination (Bing & Reid, 1996). Although women do experience gender oppression, their experience is influenced by individual, historical, social, economic, ecological, and psychological realities (Greene et al., 1997). Therefore, the primacy of gender ignores the inseparability of gender, ethnicity, class, sexuality, and other identities in the lives of women of color (Comas-Díaz, 1991). In addition, the realities of older, ethnic, working-class, disabled, and non-North American women are excluded from feminist theory and practice (Brown, 1994). Only a few White feminist scholars openly acknowledge exclusionary practices within feminist psychology. Brown also argued that White middle-class lesbians have been the only marginalized group consistently represented in the feminist therapy literature.

Bing and Reid (1996) noted that, although feminist ideology opposes patriarchy and social oppression, its philosophical underpinnings do not include opposition to racist or classist perspectives. Moreover, affluent and White feminist women hold a position of power afforded by their race and social class that is seldom acknowledged (Espín & Gawelek, 1992). Given these positions of privilege, White feminists frequently fail to recognize that women of color simultaneously experience race, class, sexuality, and gender subordination (Bing & Reid; Espín & Gawelek). Clearly, this exclusionary perspective marginalizes the experiences of Chicanas and asks that they leave their cultural identity, along with other identities, at the door.

Feminist Therapy

Women of color continue to challenge feminist theories that, primarily constructed around the lives of White middle-class women, exclude or misrepresent their experiences (Baca Zinn & Dill, 1996). For instance, Espín (1995) noted that "women of color, feminist or not, are seldom idealized, respected, valued, or presented as role models in whose footsteps other women would want to follow" (p. 127). She futher pointed out that, as theoreticians and feminist foremothers, women of color are rendered invisible. With respect to feminist epistemology, Espín argued, "For the most part, women of color continue to be mentioned in small asides, footnotes, or digressions from the main topic and almost always as the *object* of theorizing, rather than as the *subject* who theorizes and whose theories are part of the common knowledge" (p. 131). Nevertheless, Chicana and Latina psychologists continue to make important contributions to feminist understandings of psychotherapy and provide insight into the existence of both gender and racial biases in the treatment of women and in psychological theories (Comas-Díaz, 1987; Espín, 1993, 1995; Greene, 1986; Root, 1992). They also demonstrate how an awareness of oppressive factors and sociopolitical forces allows for culturally sensitive therapy with Latinas (Comas-Díaz; Espín, 1993, 1995; Vasquez, 1994).

Specifically focusing on feminist therapy with mainland Puerto Rican women, Comas-Díaz (1987) asserted that feminist therapy and its tenet of empowerment allow Puerto Rican women to: (a) acknowledge the deleterious effects of racism and sexism, (b) address feelings of anger and self-degradation imposed by their status as ethnic minorities, (c) perceive themselves as causal agents in achieving solutions to their problems, (d) understand the interplay between the external environment and their inner reality, and (e) perceive opportunities to change responses from the wider society. Similarly, Flores-Ortiz (1995) illustrated the applicability of feminist therapy with Chicanas at midlife by integrating feminist theory into a cultural context. She argued that a feminist psychological approach within a therapeutic setting allows for a critical analysis of the confluence of class, racial, economic, sexual, and gender oppression of Chicanas. Most importantly, this approach enables Chicanas to reclaim their voices and find balance within their lives.

MULTIRACIAL FEMINIST FRAMEWORK

Given the exclusionary practices of many White feminists, multiracial feminism was developed to build a coalition among feminists of color (Baca Zinn, personal communication, November 13, 2001). The primary goal of the coalition was to bring to the forefront the idea of race as a power system that interacts with other oppressive social structures in the construction of gender. This idea is the cornerstone of multiracial feminism and differentiates this paradigm of thinking from those developed by White feminists who do not recognize race as a critical factor of power. By grounding the experience of gender in race, one begins to understand the "social construction of various group memberships and their varying degrees of advantage and power" (Baca Zinn & Dill, 2000, p. 25).

Multiracial feminism also differs from most forms of feminism, as certain guiding principles do not focus solely on women, but include both men and women. As Chicana feminists, we acknowledge the potential controversy in advocating for an analytical framework that includes men, particularly in light of the history of sexism, violence, exclusion, and oppression by Chicanos. However, the endorsement of a universal perspective on men mimics the White feminists' failure to acknowledge the role of culture in our lives (Espín, 1995). Moreover, we recognize that power relations and social structures disenfranchise Chicanos, in particular, young boys and older, poor, disabled, immigrant, undocumented, and gay or bisexual men. We believe that it is critical to include Chicanos as subjects of study and as partners in the development of a new theory in Chicana/o psychology.

Multiracial feminism also illuminates oppressive power structures that affect the psychological well-being of Chicanas. In addition, it provides a venue for identifying areas of strength, resilience, and other psychological resources among Chicanas, which are often overlooked in the psychological literature. Building upon various intellectual perspectives, multiracial feminism, developed by Baca Zinn and Dill (1996), integrates several emergent views articulated by women of color. As an "evolving body of theory and practice," multiracial feminism is informed by six basic tenets (Baca Zinn & Dill, p. 26).

Interlocking Inequalities

The first tenet of multiracial feminism is that gender is not a binary, categorical variable. Gender is not a descriptive characteristic nor is it a variable that independently explains differences across groups. Gender is a social structure. Furthermore, gender is experienced simultaneously with other social structures such as race, class, and sexuality. The experience of being a man or woman is interlocked with the experience of other social locations (e.g., being Chicana/o, working class), leading to multiple ways that individuals experience themselves as gendered beings (Baca Zinn & Dill, 2000, p. 26).

This tenet also maintains that the range of gendered experiences created by these interlocking social locations results in inequalities, stemming from differences in a person's social location in the structures of race, class, gender, and sexuality. Certain locations are more oppressive than others, as they are at the intersection of two or more systems of domination. For example, by virtue of gender, ethnicity, and social class systems of domination, Chicanas are frequently regarded as a "triple minority" (Flores-Ortiz, 1998; Gloria, 2001; Mirandé & Enriquez, 1979; Vasquez, 1984). For bisexual and lesbian Chicanas, sexual orientation produces "quadruple oppression" (Gloria; Yep, 1995).

The experience of multiple forms of oppression and disenfranchisement poses challenges to Chicanas' mental health (Comas-Díaz, 1987; Vasquez, 1984). For example, Chicanas find themselves in organizational environments where subtle forms of discriminatory practices deplete their energy. As major socializing agents, institutions erect barriers that Chicanas must confront. Zambrana (1988) suggested that Latina/os experience "cultural assault" due to injury to their identity and self-esteem. The continuous experience of assault leads to stress and marginalization. Exposure to stressful events also increases vulnerability to psychophysiological conditions such as cardiovascular disease, diabetes, gastrointestinal problems, and borderline hypertension (Argueta-Bernal, 1991).

Interlocking social locations were further illustrated by Bernal (1994) in a discussion of her experience as a Chicana psychologist in academia. Despite her status as a prominent Chicana scholar, she was not immune to acts of oppression. She cogently articulated her professional experience with multiple forms of oppression and their inseparability:

> As a member of an ethnic minority and a woman, I have experienced the combined effects of racism and sexism in academic life. Separation of the source of these effects is impossible, however. In any given situation, I cannot tell whether my gender or my ethnicity elicits prejudice and discrimination, although I feel their dual effects. Other women also can be racist and sexist, and I have experienced comparable oppression from female and male colleagues. So while I believe that the process of sexism is oppressive and destructive to minority women in academia, and that it exacerbates the effects of the other processes about which I will write, I will not treat it separately. (Bernal, p. 406)

Intersectional Nature of Hierarchies

The second tenet of multiracial feminism is that all hierarchies of social life are intersectional. Social structures are interactive and social locations are rooted in different hierarchies. Social locations lead to differential forms of power and subjugation. The intersectional nature of gender, class, race, and age means that older Chicanas are embedded in different positions created by the hierarchies of social life. It is often suggested that Chicanas gain status as they age because they are held in high esteem due to their role as *abuelitas* (an endearing term for grandmothers; Facio, 1996). In addition, they are frequently at the pinnacle of the social hierarchy in extended family networks among Chicana/os because of their age status: Mothers and grandmothers are regarded as "powerful forces" within Chicana/o families and culture (Arredondo, 2002). However, even though they possess power in their families, they simultaneously experience powerlessness in other contexts.

Chicano families are experiencing structural and ideological changes in their familial relationships. Facio (1996) suggested that familial networks no longer reflect the "romanticized" extended families frequently described in previous literature on the Chicano elderly (p. 88). For instance, her ethnographic study of older Chicanas challenged prior research by examining their social locations. Interestingly, her findings revealed that women placed importance on independence. Despite their limited finances, of the 30 Chicanas interviewed only 4 did not live alone. Independent living enabled them to protect themselves from childcare responsibilities and potential exploitation by their families. Although they valued family obligations and assistance, older Chicanas did not regard themselves solely as caregivers, and sought to determine their lives independently from cultural expectations associated with grandmotherhood. Therefore, they defined their relationships with their families on equal or reciprocal terms, such as cultural teachers. By defining themselves in this way, they reinforced cultural values of symbolic respect. As cultural teachers, older Chicanas socialize their grandchildren and great-grandchildren with cultural values and traditions, especially respect toward older adults.

Facio's (1996) findings also demonstrated how the cultural prescription of grand-motherhood contributed to a status of powerlessness. Powerlessness was demonstrated in the potential exploitation of older Chicanas as caregivers or convenient babysitters. Power struggles were also exposed as older Chicanas strived to redefine their womanhood. They challenged cultural expectations at the risk of being disrespected. For example, although the family simultaneously provided support, care, and respect, it also stressed conformity and control. Older Chicanas were expected to remain single and refrain from seeking male companionship to respect the memory of their deceased spouse or partner, to avoid being judged as "a bad woman" by their families and communities. Strong objections from their children also resulted in the withholding of financial support, discontinued regular visits and phone calls, or attempts to impose guilt.

As this example demonstrates, older Chicanas may find themselves both power-less and powerful in their roles as grandmothers. Given that family members are embedded in the same social location of race, Chicana grandmothers' social location as elders provides them access to power, but the intersection of race, class, and gender means they may struggle for control over their sexuality and finances.

Relational Nature of Dominance and Subordination

The third tenet of multiracial feminism challenges the notion of a universal experience of womanhood. Baca Zinn and Dill (1996) proposed that dominance and subordination occur between women, that is, that race is a decisive social structure that creates differences among women and assists in the subjugation of women of color by White women.

Hurtado (1989) suggested that the experience of subordination for different groups of women is determined by social positions of power. More specifically, "each oppressed group in the United States is positioned in a particular and distinct relationship to white men, and each form of subordination is shaped by this relational position" (Hurtado, p. 833). Hurtado further argued that White women's oppression by White men takes the form of seduction through psychological and material rewards, whereas the oppression of women of color takes the form of rejection. Therefore, women of color have less access to positions of power and privilege than their White counterparts because White men do not regard them as providers of racially pure offspring. Relationships with affluent White men also provide White women with a social position of power. Yet, White women seldom acknowledge these positions of power and privilege.

Also examining social locations, Romero (1997) demonstrated how class-based social order is maintained between immigrant Mexican maids and their White middle-class employers. Using standpoint epistemology, she exposed how White female employers use their race and class privilege to shift the burden of sexism onto

Mexican maids.[1] White female employers also relied on the labor of their maids to assist in the reproduction of their gendered class status. As an illustration, the household labor of Mexican maids was expanded to accommodate the males and to preserve their privilege. Their physical labor also enabled White female employers to increase their leisure time.

White women oppress women of color in many different arenas and the ivory tower is no exception. In the following example, Romero (1991) discussed the work of a White female psychologist who uses Guatemalan women to advance her research career:

> Her well-received book surveyed the research literature on the mother-infant bonding practices following birth. The bulk of the studies reviewed had employed a methodology in which an infant was removed from its mother immediately following delivery and placed in a nursery as opposed to allowing the infant to remain with its mother. Who were the *"subjects"* of the research (please note the archaic yet standard aristocratic language of psychological research)? Women from Guatemala. . . . Guatemalan women were used as guinea pigs so that, in the application of her work, North American women can enjoy more humane conditions of childbirth. Not one word was even written about the use of Third World women to advance the standard of living for North American women. Not one word questioned the ethics of such research. (pp. 143–144)

Resilience and Strengths of Chicanas

The fourth tenet of multiracial feminism is that women possess strength and resilience. Although many women of color encounter barriers due to social structures such as race and class, they fight and "create viable lives for themselves, their families, and communities" (Baca Zinn & Dill, 2000, p. 27). Chicanas are no exception.

Chicanas resist and defy powerful forces that control them. This is clearly seen in our history. For instance, Mexican women actively participated in the 1810 War for Independence and subsequent wars for reform (Cotera, 1973; Salas 1990). Their participation as women warriors resulted in names such as *coronelas, soldaderas,* and *Adelitas* (Salas). Mexican women also founded radical publications, formed feminist organizations, and participated in numerous protests for liberation for the oppressed, including the poor, indigenous persons, workers, and women (Cotera, 1977; Mirandé & Enriquez, 1979). Consequently, they were harassed by the government and sometimes imprisoned or exiled. The Mexican revolution of 1910 provided Chicanas with numerous female role models, a rich feminist legacy, and an impetus to Chicana feminism (Cotera, 1973, 1977; Mirandé & Enriquez). For example, in their activities as clerks, secretaries, smugglers, telegraphers, journalists, financiers, and soldiers, Mexican women developed their potential on a large scale. Traditional gender roles were altered when women worked alongside their male counterparts (Cotera, 1973). However, their activism did not end with the Mexican revolution. Historical writings chronicle how Mexican and Mexican American women worked together, as they

---

[1] Female employers used their race and class privilege over their Mexican, often immigrant, female maids to shift the burden of responsibility of devalued work—housework and child care. In so doing, they increased their leisure time and maintained the male privilege of their husbands or sons. Simply put, they exploited their maids and maintained a class-based, racist social order in the daily tasks of domestic service, which includes physical, mental, and emotional labor.

were oppressed on both sides of the border (Cotera, 1973; Mirandé & Enriquez). In the following decades, Chicanas distinguished themselves in many areas, but Chicana feminists lament that these contributions are largely unrecognized.

More recently, Chicanas' resilience and dedication are evidenced in the Chicano movement. Although it is beyond the scope of this chapter to provide an extensive historical account of early Chicana feminism, a brief review is presented. For further historical accounts, *Chicana Feminist Thought: The Basic Historical Writings* (García, 1997a) and *The Chicana Feminist* (Cotera, 1977) can be consulted. Historical writings suggest that, alongside their Chicano counterparts, Chicana activists sought to eradicate various forms of oppression and strived for social, political, and economic self-determination (García).

Like their Mexican and Chicana foremothers (Mirandé & Enriquez, 1979), Chicanas in the Movimiento unequivocally supported empowerment for women, families, and communities. Activists included academics, students, labor organizers, agricultural workers, musicians, poets, and actors (Hurtado, 1998). In their activism and scholarship, they advocated for adequate jobs, decent wages, adequate working conditions, public safety, welfare rights, bilingual child care, legal rights, and control over their own reproductive capacities (García, 1997a; Hurtado; Moraga, 1993).

Chicanas also recognize the need for political action and strategies of resistance. Pardo's (1990) research on the Mothers of East Los Angeles (MELA) illustrated the ways in which working-class Mexican American women transformed traditional familial and cultural networks, politically mobilizing themselves to prevent the building of a prison and toxic waste dump in their neighborhood. The inclusion of their spouses and family members demonstrated their political astuteness and their creative strategies of resistance. For example, although they elected men as presidents of their organization, women held complete authority and control of the day-to-day activities. Their subversion was demonstrated when a male president attempted to exert his power by insisting they hold their fundraiser on Mother's Day. Pardo reported that, on the day of the fundraiser, only the president and his wife appeared. After this incident, the president no longer attempted to impose his will.

Inclusion of Diverse Methodologies and Theoretical Approaches

The fifth tenet of multiracial feminism is that an array of methodological and theoretical tools assist in understanding the experience of gender. Unfortunately, the epistemology of conventional psychology and research methodology tends to "embody male Anglo-American values and worldviews" (Comas-Díaz, 1991, p. 602) and limits the scope of inquiry by restricting what research questions are asked, how data are collected and interpreted, and how graduate students are trained to conduct research (Rabinowitz & Martin, 2001). Although Chicana/os and other marginalized groups challenge the exclusionary research practices of psychology, much work is still needed in this arena.

Standpoint theory is one tool that can assist with this process. Standpoint theory recognizes the critical position Chicanas and other women of color have in observing and understanding phenomena that are not apparent to White men and women because of their race- and class-privileged vantage point. Espín (1995) expanded upon this idea when she compared privilege to a glass pane that is not seen by individuals in positions of power. She stated:

> Those who do not partake of that privilege, however, know very well the existence of that pane of glass; they know it is impossible for them to go through this barrier—the more effective precisely because it is unseen. In fact, the non-privileged can be better "knowers" and more knowledgeable. Their vision tends to be clearer; they see themselves, they see the glass pane, and they know who is on the other side of that glass. That is why women and other oppressed people have a clearer vision of reality than white males and other oppressors. (p. 129)

Given this vantage point, it is imperative that Chicana feminists continue to challenge theoretical models that essentialize the experience of gender and ignore the influential role of social structures in the construction of gender. Lived experience is an alternative way to understand the social world and the experience of various women. Moreover, marginalized locations are appropriate for understanding social relations that remain concealed from privileged vantage points. Chicanas challenge dominant conceptions of truth by using their own voices and experiences.

Qualitative research also allows for the examination of the lived experiences of Chicanas while addressing psychological issues. For example, Torres (1996) examined the process by which Chicana psychologists attained their doctorates and found that they encountered cultural and institutional barriers. While in graduate school, they experienced conflict with their families of origin due to lack of family understanding and gender role conflicts. Institutional barriers also created feelings of isolation, estrangement, prejudice, and anger. However, despite these conflicts and dilemmas, Chicanas demonstrated personal strengths, vision, and a sense of responsibility during their graduate work and professional development. Their success in completing their doctorates was also attributed to a clear sense of purpose sustained by the development of interdependence with a community and a sense of social responsibility.

Chicana Image and Identity

The final tenet of multiracial feminism is that women's experiences are diverse and continuously changing. Chicanas are no exception. Although they share rich cultural legacies, Chicanas represent a group of heterogeneous women (Flores-Ortiz, 1998; Gloria, 2001; Vasquez, 1984; Zavella, 1997) and each selects her own self-referent based on political, social, historical, and economic realities. As an illustration, Zavella noted, "We are Chicanas, Mexicans, Mexican Americans, Spanish Americans, Tejanas, Hispanas, Mestizas, Indias, or Latinas, and the terms of identification vary according to the context" (p. 187). Similarly, their identities are created and influenced by numerous social categories, such as gender, age, sexual orientation, class, physical capacities, ethnic identity, language, religious affiliation, mental and physical characteristics, educational level, occupational status, generational status, geographical location, and political outlook (Gloria; Zavella).

Unfortunately, portrayals of Chicanas are often inaccurate or based on stereotypes. Literature on Chicanas also inaccurately suggests that their main identity is derived from motherhood or notions of *marianismo* (marianism), and often addresses exclusively their gender roles. Although gender roles are indeed important, they change and vary based on numerous factors. To assume that their identities are primarily centered around their families or males also negates their multifaceted identities, particularly with respect to less traditional Chicanas.

Chicanas are currently integrating multiple roles and realities (Anzaldúa, 1987; Gloria, 2001) as they create their own identities. The use of Spanish also establishes their distinctiveness from White mainstream culture (Hurtado, 1998) and enables them to resist cultural and linguistic domination (Montoya, 1997). Chicana feminist narratives become "outlaw genres" in documenting political and personal struggles of Chicanas (Elenes, 2000, p. 105). Similarly, the use of narratives and code switching enables Chicanas to explore cultural borders in the shaping of a new unadulterated identity (Anzaldúa). According to Montoya, "as we reinvent ourselves we import words and concepts into English and into academic discourse from formerly prohibited languages and taboo knowledge" (p. 42).

FUTURE DIRECTIONS

Despite the gains made, considerable effort is needed to advance theory, clinical practice, and research. We believe that a multiracial feminist framework will facilitate a better understanding of the Chicana/o experience. As psychologists, we can no longer maintain a narrow focus on intrapsychic and psychological variables. The need to describe the psychological realities of Chicanas, as well as their individual, historical, social, economic, and ecological realities remains. However, radical departures from our traditional training are required if it is to be met.

THEORY

Chicana feminists will continue to question theoretical models that essentialize the experience of gender and ignore the influential role of social structures in the construction of gender. Lived experience is an alternative way to understand the social world and the experience of various Chicanas. Chicana discourse often focuses on the multiplicity of experiences and the confluence of race, gender, social class, and sexual orientation. Chicana feminist theory also provides a political backdrop of various Chicana voices and experiences that challenge dominant conceptions of truth. Because these voices are not static, various forms of Chicana feminisms exist and diverse methods and approaches are used to inform their perspectives.

Given the diversity of Chicana feminisms, each is evolutionary as well as revolutionary. Chicana feminist theory will continue to evolve because of the new and fresh perspectives of Chicanas. As noted by Hurtado (1998), younger Chicanas will have more varied social, ethnic, and class experiences than current writers. Consequently, conceptions of Chicana identity and nationalistic affinity will also evolve. Undoubtedly, Chicana feminist theory will continue to document resistance and advocacy for political mobilization and social justice. Despite the educational, economical, and political gains within the last decades, Chicana/os are not at parity. Unfortunately, high dropout rates, poverty, limited political representation, governmental neglect, and other plights continue to plague our communities.

Therefore, the need to address various forms of oppression and subordination remain. Centuries of colonization, capitalism, and sociopolitical forces have certainly affected the Chicano family, often creating subordination and oppression. While the exposure of oppression within the Chicana/o community is especially delicate, the need to address violence and oppression within our families and communities is critical. Feminist theory provides us with the opportunity to identify and analyze sources of oppression that continuously shape the lives of Chicanas. Similarly, Chicana feminist theory illuminates the multiple sources of inequality encountered by Chicanas in both public and private spheres (García, 1997a).

Various disciplines, such as Chicana/o studies and sociology, have developed sophisticated theories to examine the Chicana experience within public and private spheres. However, the psychology of the Chicana experience appears embryonic. As noted by Flores-Ortiz (1998), "a psychology of Chicanas that incorporates a social, gender, and class analysis does not exist" (p. 103). A merger between Chicana/o psychology and Chicana feminist theory is needed to create a psychology of the Chicana. Such a merger will allow for the understanding and valuing of differences among Chicanas and the creation of theory. As creators of knowledge and theory, we can begin to understand the multiple realities faced by Chicanas at the intersections of gender, ethnicity, class, and sexual orientation. Increased attention must be paid to issues of sexuality, age, physical ability, and other social markers that create subjugation and affect the well-being of Chicanas.

CLINICAL PRACTICE

Chicanas and their families need cultural and ethical service delivery. As Chicanas challenge traditionally trained mental health providers, cultural competency is paramount, regardless of theoretical orientation. Recognizing that gender is not the primary locus of oppression (Greene et al., 1997), many Chicanas experience multiple forms of domination. Indeed, the experience of being a Chicana often creates conflicting loyalties, particularly among Chicanas who challenge structural and ideological underpinnings within their families and communities. However, it is important to note that familial constraints are not the only area of concern for Chicanas. Certainly, the experience of being a triple or quadruple minority affects the well-being of many.

In light of the diversity of Chicanas and their lived experiences, revisions in diagnostic criteria regarding eurocentric concepts of normalcy, adaptive behaviors, and therapeutic success are needed. Caution must be taken to ensure that Chicanas are not pathologized or regarded as helpless victims during their assessment or treatment. Mental health providers must not replicate inequity or oppression within the therapeutic relationship (Vasquez, 1994). Culturally sensitive therapy includes the understanding and awareness of oppressive factors and sociopolitical forces in the lives of Chicanas.

As noted in this volume by Baca and Hernandez (chap. 13) and Arredondo (chap. 12), clinical interventions with Chicanas require a safe therapeutic environment for them to move *entre fronteras*, or within the borders, of their bicultural worlds, an experience that must be affirmed for Chicanas. The inconsistencies that emerge from living in two different worlds must also be validated in order to reduce their acculturative stress. Moreover, such a journey may require the use of nontraditional helpers and nontraditional therapeutic approaches.

Clinical interventions require integrative and comprehensive approaches to the multiple contexts in which Chicanas reside. Feminist therapy provides an avenue toward understand their lived experience through therapeutic dialogue (Flores-Ortiz, 1995, 1998). Similarly, in combination with other theoretical orientations, feminist therapy enables Chicanas to address complex issues. However, additional empirical support is needed to document the efficacy of these theoretical approaches with Chicanas.

RESEARCH

We believe the framework of multiracial feminism has much to offer psychological research on Chicana/os. More specifically, divergent theoretical and methodological models will assist in improving the research-practitioner model. We understand that embracing such a framework will prove challenging at times, but we believe that, in the long run, it will benefit the well-being of our *communidad* (community). We propose some changes in research that will assist in this process.

First, we must move away from research that is focused only at the individual or intrapsychic level of analysis (Dalton, Elias, & Wandersman, 2000; Heller, Price, Reinharz, Riger, & Wandersman, 1984). By including other levels of analysis, we begin to take into account the complexity of our lives and the influence of contextual and structural factors that create power differentials. We also must challenge psychological paradigms that limit the understanding of gender, that is, we can no longer endorse a conceptual framework that treats gender, culture, and other demographic characteristics (e.g., sexual orientation, socioeconomic status) as nominal variables (Comas-Díaz, 1991).

Second, methodology should support a strengths-based approach. Research that pathologizes or utilizes a deficiency model when studying our communidad should not be endorsed. The recognition of the resilience of our *gente* (people) and empirical documentation of this resilience are long overdue.

Third, we must unlearn certain aspects of our psychological training. For instance, we must release the fallacy that nontraditional research approaches lack vigor. A substantial number of studies employing alternative research methods and theoretical underpinnings have clearly expanded our understanding of an array of phenomena and assisted in implementing an action-research model. For example, Kahan (2001) found that the use of focus groups was instrumental in the policy-making arena. We must also unlearn the idea of universal truths (Reid, 1993), which may be fewer in number than originally thought.

Fourth, Chicana feminists must hold tight to their experiential knowledge. As Gonzales (1995) eloquently stated, "It is not true that we do not know who we are. If anything, we should suffer the accusation we know too much who we are" (p. 43). Our knowledge base of experience can play a decisive role in creating and promoting a transformative framework of research on the Chicana/o experience. Research methods such as standpoint theory can assist in tapping into this underutilized knowledge.

Last, we must translate our research into social action (Dalton et al., 2000; Heller et al., 1984). We cannot be creators of knowledge that simply remains on the shelf. A key feature of the Chicana/o movement is the idea of giving back to the community. Therefore, it is important to continue this tradition in our research. As we move forward in the construction of this new framework for theory, research, and practice, it is helpful to look back on the evolution of Chicana/o psychology—an evolution in which an understanding of gender and the ideas of Chicana psychologists played very little part until recently.

ACKNOWLEDGMENTS

The authors extend their deepest appreciation to Dr. Maxine Baca Zinn for her invaluable comments and support. The first author received a Summer Research Grant from the University of La Verne's College of Arts & Sciences to support the writing of this chapter.

REFERENCES

Anzaldúa, G. (1987). *Borderlands/La frontera: The new mestiza*. San Francisco: Aunt Lute.

Anzaldúa, G. (1990). La conciencia de la mestiza: Towards a new consciousness. In G. Anzaldúa (Ed.), *Making face, making soul/Haciendo caras: Creative and critical perspectives by feminists of color* (pp. 377–389). San Francisco: Aunt Lute.

Argueta-Bernal, G. A. (1991). Stress and stress-related disorders in Hispanics: Biobehavioral approaches to treatment. In F. C. Serafica, A. I. Schwebel, R. K. Russell, P. D. Isaac, & L. B. Myers (Eds.), *Mental health of ethnic minorities* (pp. 202–221). New York: Praeger.

Baca Zinn, M., & Dill, B. T. (1996). Theorizing difference from multiracial feminism. *Feminist Studies, 22*, 321–331.

Baca Zinn, M., & Dill, B. T. (2000). Theorizing difference from multiracial feminism. In M. Baca Zinn, P. Hondagneu-Sotelo, & M. A. Messner (Eds.), *Gender through the prism of difference* (pp. 23–29). Boston: Allyn and Bacon.

Bernal, M. E. (1994). Integration of ethnic minorities into academic psychology: How it has been and what it could be. In E. J. Trickett, R. J. Watts, & D. Birman (Eds.), *Human diversity: Perspectives on people in context* (pp. 404–423). San Francisco, CA: Jossey-Bass.

Bing, V. M., & Reid, P. T. (1996). Unknown women and unknowing research: Consequences of color and class in feminist psychology. In N. R. Goldberger, J. M. Tarule, B. M. Clinchy, & M. F. Belenky (Eds.), *Knowlege, difference, and power: Essays inspired by women's ways of knowing* (pp. 175–202). New York: Basic Books.

Brown, L. S. (1994). *Subversive dialogues: Theory in feminist therapy*. New York: Basic Books.

Castillo, A. (1995). *Massacre of the dreamers: Essays on Xicanisma*. New York: Plume.

Comas-Díaz, L. (1987). Feminist therapy with mainland Puerto Rican women. *Psychology of Women Quarterly, 11*, 461–474.

Comas-Díaz, L. (1991). Feminism and diversity in psychology: The case of women of color. *Psychology of Women Quarterly, 15*, 597–609.

Cotera, M. (1973). Mexican feminism. *Magazín, 4*, 30–32.

Cotera, M. (Ed.) (1977). *The Chicana feminist*. Austin, TX: Information Systems Development.

Dalton, J., Elias, M., & Wandersman, A. (2000). *Community psychology: Linking individuals and communities*. New York: Wadsworth.

Elenes, C. A. (2000). Chicana feminist narratives and the politics of the self. *Frontiers, 21*, 105–123.

Espín, O. M. (1993). Feminist therapy: Not for or by White women only. *The Counseling Psychologist, 21*, 103–108.

Espín, O. M. (1994). Feminist approaches. In L. Comas-Díaz & B. Greene (Eds.), *Women of color: Integrating ethnic and gender identities in psychotherapy* (pp. 265–286). New York: Guilford Press.

Espín, O. M. (1995). On knowing you are the unknown: Women of color constructing psychology. In J. Adleman & G. M. Enguidanos (Eds.), *Racism in the lives of women: Testimony, theory, and guides to antiracist practice* (pp. 251–259). Binghamton, NY: Harrington Park Press.

Espín, O. M., & Gawelek, M. A. (1992). Women's diversity: Ethnicity, race, class, and gender in theories of feminist psychology. In L. S. Brown & M. Ballou (Eds.), *Personality and psychopathology: Feminist reappraisals* (pp. 88–107). New York: Guilford Press.

Facio, E. (1996). Understanding older Chicanas. Thousand Oaks, CA: Sage.

Flores-Ortiz, Y. G. (1995). Psychotherapy with Chicanas at midlife: Cultural/clinical considerations. In J. Adleman & G. M. Enguidanos (Eds.), *Racism in the lives of women: Testimony, theory, and guides to antiracist practice* (pp. 251–259). Binghamton, NY: Harrington Park Press.

Flores-Ortiz, Y. G. (1998). Voices from the couch: The co-creation of a Chicana psychology. In C. Trujillo (Ed.), *Living Chicana theory* (pp. 102–122). Berkeley, CA: Third Woman Press.

García, A. M. (Ed.). (1997a). *Chicana feminist thought: The basic historical writings.* New York: Routledge.

García, A. M. (1997b). The development of Chicana feminist discourse. In D. J. Bixler-Marquez, C. F. Ortega, R. Solorzano Torres, & L. LaFarelle (Eds.), *Chicano studies: Survey and analysis* (pp. 123–130). Dubuque, IA: Kendall/Hunt.

Gloria, A. M. (2001). The cultural construction of Latinas: Practice implications of multiple realities and identities. In D. B. Pope-Davis & H. L. K. Coleman (Eds.), *The intersection of race, class, and gender in multicultural counseling* (pp. 3–24). Thousand Oaks, CA: Sage.

Gonzalez, D. (1995). Chicana identity matters. In A. Darder (Ed.), *Culture and difference: Critical perspectives on the bicultural experience in the United States* (pp. 41–54). New York: Bergin and Garvey.

Greene, B., Sanchez-Hucles, J., Banks, M., Civish, G., Contratto, S., Griffith, J., Hinderly, H., Jenkins, Y., & Roberson, M. K. (1997). Diversity: Advancing an inclusive feminist psychology. In J. Worell & N. G. Johnson (Eds.), *Shaping the future of feminist psychology: Education, research, and practice* (pp. 173–202). Washington, DC: American Psychological Association.

Greene, B. A. (1986). When the therapist is White and the patient is Black: Considerations for psychotherapy in the feminist heterosexual and lesbian communities. In D. Howard (Ed.), *The dynamics of feminist therapy* (pp. 41–65). New York: Haworth Press.

Heller, K., Price, R. H., Reinharz, S., Riger, S., & Wandersman, A. (1984). *Psychology and community change: Challenges of the future.* Pacific Grove, CA: Brooks/Cole.

Hurtado, A. (1989). Relating to privilege: Seduction and rejection in the subordination of White women and women of color. *Signs, 14,* 833–855.

Hurtado, A. (1998). Sitio y lengua: Chicanas theorize feminisms. *Hypatia, 13,* 134–161.

Kahan, J. P. (2001). Focus groups as a tool for policy analysis. *Analysis of Social Issues and Public Policy, 1,* 129–146.

Mirandé, A., & Enriquez, E. (1979). *La Chicana: The Mexican-American woman.* Chicago: University of Chicago Press.

Montoya, M. E. (1997). Masks and identity. In A. K. Wing (Ed.), *Critical race feminism: A reader* (pp. 37–43). New York: New York University Press.

Moraga, C. (1993). Women's subordination through the lens of sex/gender, sexuality, class, and race: Multicultural feminism. In A. M. Jaggar & P. S. Rothenberg (Eds.), *Feminist frameworks: Alternative accounts of the relations between women and men* (3rd ed., pp. 203–212). San Francisco: McGraw-Hill.

Moraga, C., & Anzaldúa, G. (Eds.). (1983). *This bridge called my back: Writings by radical women of color.* New York: Kitchen Table.

Nieto-Gomez, A. (1974). La feminista. *Encuentro Femenil, 1,* 34–37.

Pardo, M. (1990). Mexican American women grassroots community activists: Mothers of east Los Angeles. *Frontiers, 21,* 1–7.

Rabinowitz, V. C., & Martin, D. (2001). Choices and consequences: Methodological issues in the study of gender. In R. K. Unger (Ed.), *Handbook of the psychology of women and gender* (pp. 29–52). New York: Wiley and Sons.

Reid, P. (1993). Poor women in psychological research: Shut up and shut out. *Psychology of Women Quarterly, 17,* 133–150.

Romero, G. J. (1991). "No se raje, chicanita": Some thoughts on race, class, and gender in the classroom. *California Sociologist: A Journal of Sociology and Social Work, 14,* 135–148.

Romero, M. (1997). Life as the maid's daughter: An exploration of the everyday boundaries of race, class, and gender. In R. Romero, P. Hondagneu-Sotelo, & V. Ortiz (Eds.), *Challenging fronteras: Structuring Latina and Latino lives in the U.S.* (pp. 196–209). New York: Routledge.

Root, M. P. P. (1992). The impact of trauma on personality: The second reconstruction. In L. S. Brown & M. Ballou (Eds.), *Personality and psychopathology: Feminist reappraisals* (pp. 229–265). New York: Guilford Press.

Salas, E. (1990). *Soldaderas in the Mexican military: Myth and history.* Austin: University of Texas Press.

Torres, E. C. (1996). Mexican-American female psychologists: An exploratory study of the journey to the doctorate. *Dissertation Abstracts International, 57*(2-A), 0636. (University Microfilms No. 9619495)

Trujillo, C. (1991). Chicana lesbians: Fear and loathing in the Chicano community. In C. Trujillo (Ed.), *Chicana lesbians: The girls our mothers warned us about* (pp. 86–194). Berkeley, CA: Third Woman Press.

Vasquez, M. J. T. (1984). Power and status of the Chicana: A social-psychological perspective. In J. Martinez & R. H. Mendoza (Eds.), *Chicano psychology* (2nd ed., pp. 269–287). San Diego, CA: Academic Press.

Vasquez, M. J. T. (1994). Latinas. In L. Comas-Díaz & B. Greene (Eds.), *Women of color: Integrating ethnic and gender identities in psychotherapy* (pp. 114–138). New York: Guilford Press.

Yep, G. A. (1995). Communicating the HIV/AIDS risk to Hispanic populations. In A. M. Padilla (Ed.), *Hispanic psychology: Critical issues in theory and research* (pp. 196–212). Thousand Oaks, CA: Sage.

Zambrana, R. E. (1988). Toward understanding the educational trajectory and socialization of Latina women. In T. McKenna & F. A. Ortiz (Eds.), *The broken web: The educational experience of Hispanic American women* (pp. 61–77). Claremont, CA: The Tomas Rivera Center.

Zavella, P. (1997). Reflections on the diversity of Chicanas. In R. Romero, P. Hondagneu-Sotelo, & V. Ortiz (Eds.), *Challenging fronteras: Structuring Latina and Latino lives in the U.S.* (pp. 187–194). New York: Routledge.

Psychotherapy With Chicanas

Patricia Arredondo
Arizona State University

LIFE BETWEEN BORDERS

Entre Fronteras—Between Borders

"Living in a state of psychic unrest, in a borderland, is what makes poets write and artists create," according to Gloria Anzaldúa (1987, p. 73). In her classic book of poetry and prose, Anzaldúa articulated a historical landscape and images about Chicanas and Mejicanas. "Between borders" and life in the "wild zone" (Candelaria, 1980; Chávez Candelaria, 1993) are other metaphors used by writers to speak to the experiences of contemporary Mestizas. These are the unconscious and conscious backdrops for Chicanas who find their way into therapy. Though not a place where they are naturally inclined to go according to cultural socialization norms, the therapy room and session become another between-borders reality where women can explore the ambiguity and double messages about what it is to be a *santa* (saint), *princesa* (princess), and Chicana at the same time. The familial and societal expectations are of being *una mujer cumplida*—a complete and accomplished woman.

The pressures on Chicanas are many, evidenced by the confusion and burden many feel to declare their identity with particular terminology. All women of Mexican heritage, however, do not embrace the term *Chicana*, which, like *Chicano*, carries many personal and sociopolitical meanings. For many, Chicana was a southwestern term, not something for people in Ohio or on the east coast unless they were politically active and took it on. In her essay, "Art in America con Acento," Moraga (1995) asserted that "to be a Chicana is not merely to name one's racial/cultural identity, but also to name a politic that refuses assimilation into the U.S. mainstream. It acknowledges our *mestizaje*—Indian, Spanish, and *africano*" (p. 215). Of course, not all individuals of Mexican heritage like to use the term *Chicana/o* for self-reference. Other preferences include Mexican American, Mexican, Mejicana, Hispana, and Latina.

The origin of the term is debated. Some writers indicate that it is derived from Nahuatl for "Mexican" or "Aztec." For some, it is pejorative, whereas others see it as an Americanized term for "Mexicano" (Mirandé & Enríquez, 1979). Regardless, there are particular attributes that give meaning to the Chicana identity and experience, including a shared history as colonized women of Mestizo or Mexican heritage, living in the United States, and bicultural beings, influenced by both U.S. and Mexican cultures along a continuum. In this chapter, the terms *Chicana* and *Mexican American* are used interchangeably.

The Landscape

There are many possible starting points for a discussion on psychotherapy with Chicanas. During the past 20 to 25 years, there have been literary contributions by Chicanas narrating through prose and poetry the multiple lenses, experiences, roles, and attenuating conflicts of being a *mujer Mejicana* or Chicana (Anzaldúa, 1987; Chavez, 1994, 2001; Cisneros, 1989; Hinojosa, 1999; Mora, 1986; Moraga, 1995). These narratives are essential because they help to place women in the multiple contexts—historical, sociopolitical, and cultural or ethnic—that have surrounded the Chicana since the arrival of Hernán Cortes in 1519.

Scholarly publications have increased in number. Special issues on counseling with Chicana/os and Mexican Americans further support classics such as Mirandé & Enríquez' *La Chicana* (1979). (Velesquez, 1997, and McNeill et al., 2001 are two examples.) Of course, *The Hispanic Journal of Behavioral Sciences* has consistently reported findings on a range of topics and issues relevant to Latina/o ethnic groups, including Chicanas. These publications have been broad based, with sprinklings of studies in reference to Chicanas across different contexts and developmental perspectives, who are facing innumerable challenges, and who seem to offer us a glimpse into the strengths and struggles of other Latinas not studied or written about.

It is anticipated that this chapter will add to the literature through an integrated, Chicana-focused presentation. Moreover, although the topic is psychotherapy, there is a much broader landscape to be introduced into the discussion. To accomplish this, I draw upon several personal motivators, including a long-standing fascination with *mujeres* (women) Mejicanas and Chicanas who transcended the odds stacked against them, clinical work with Chicanas from varying backgrounds for nearly 20 years, delivery of workshops and other presentations to Chicanas and other Latinas on the topic of mujeres Latinas, developing and teaching a graduate course, "Counseling Latina/os," and reading and creating new publications about Chicanas and Latinas.

Why another chapter? To date, we do not have a sufficiently broad body of research exploring the strengths of Chicanas. To understand the Chicana from a strength versus deficit perspective, multiple contexts must be examined. There are the contexts of *la familia y la comunidad* (the family and the community) and the norms transmitted there about female values and morals. In society, a Chicana must move across different settings alongside similar and different others. Classrooms, work places, churches and temples, recreational settings, and *la casa* (the home) are all domains and spaces with multiple requirements and expectations for Chicanas. Even if it appears as though there is a script that la mujer can or should follow, the emotional, physical, and spiritual stress will not allow for easy answers.

Overview of the Chapter

The objective of this chapter is to illustrate the between-borders experiences of Chicanas who participated in therapy. From these examples, numerous themes emerge about beliefs and value orientations, various dimensions of identity, developmental tasks, and cultural landscapes. These various streams in the landscape further relate to cultural reframing for the purposes of culturally informed and ethical assessment, diagnosis, and intervention planning. It is hoped that the recommendations made will allow for a juxtaposition to the Eurocentric medical model templates regarding psychological well-being and offer new ways of framing the varying persona(s) of Chicanas.

Though the therapy examples are not numerous, they illustrate the tensions and delicacy of being a bicultural woman in a society that does not believe that culture counts. Furthermore, the cases invite exploration of issues and concepts from a culture-centered perspective.

There has been limited research conducted about the experiences of Chicana/os in psychotherapy and, where there is data, the samples are limited because there were different issues being studied (Barón & Constantine, 1997; Facio, 1996; Flores-Ortiz, 1995; Hurtado, 2000; Zuniga, 1988). Nevertheless, there is a convergence in these reports and studies about factors that affect the Chicana across the age span. Findings on both men and women of Mexican heritage corroborate what is found for women alone (Barriga, 2001; Gonzales, Castillo-Canez, Tarke, & Soriano, 1997; Flores Niemann, 2001). In this respect, the culture-gender nexus is unmistakable.

In keeping with the culture-centered focus, there is a discussion of key cultural terms that give meaning to experiences. The Mexican American Dimensions of Personal Identity Model (Arredondo & Arciniega, 2001), models of Mexican identity (Ruiz, 1990), messages based on the 10 commandments of *marianismo* (marianism; Gil & Vazquez, 1996) and other relevant models are introduced to provide a fuller profile of la mujer in terms of her evolving personal and societal status. To support this discussion, references are made to writings about Latinas in general, as they share many of the same concerns and challenges. The closing discussion offers culture-specific guidelines for working with Chicanas in therapy, including psycho-educational approaches, and for mainstreaming Chicana issues and concepts into traditional counseling and psychotherapy.

CHICANAS' VENTURE INTO THERAPY

These vignettes come from my clinical practice. Additional examples are drawn from conversations with Chicanas from all walks of life.

Sonia

Sonia was a first-year medical student from an Ivy League institution in an eastern city. She came to therapy willingly, upon the recommendation of a friend. If it were not for her name, Sonia Garcia, one might assume, based on her blonde curly hair, blue eyes, and very white phenotype, that she was an Anglo American. In her initial visit, Sonia disclosed that she was embarrassed about having to seek help because of her confusion. Her expressed belief was that she should just try to figure things out alone.

The oldest of five children, Sonia had made a physical separation from her family in Tucson when she accepted a 4-year scholarship to an eastern women's college. Though this accomplishment was a source of pride for her family, it also created stress in her relationship with her mother. As the oldest child, Sonia had been a great support to her mother, as a caretaker of the younger children and source of stability within the tightly knit family. Sonia's father was a regional salesman for a supermarket chain in the Southwest and, although his travels never took him very far, he was gone frequently. Thus, at the time of moving East, she experienced a dilemma in choosing whether to go to the state university or accept the scholarship in a new world. Though her parents and siblings openly supported her, she knew that her mother really wanted her to remain in Tucson. She reported that ambivalence about her decision had nagged at her the entire 4 years. She always felt her mother's mixed voice of happiness *para mi hija* (for my daughter) and wishes that she were not *tan lejos* (so far).

Accepting admission to the highly regarded medical school also brought mixed emotions. Although her parents expressed pride in her accomplishment, they also made clear their wish that she could attend the state university medical school instead. Sonia admitted that it was with great reluctance and a sense of guilt that she accepted the "full ride" from the Ivy League. The decision, however, had tormented her throughout the summer and after she left home to resume her studies, she frequently worried about not seeing her younger siblings grow up and not being there for her mother. Her continued emotional turmoil was affecting her ability to concentrate on her studies and, for a first-year medical student, she knew that this was too risky. She said that she did not want to fail and disappoint her family, but she also felt the strain of trying to belong in a world that was very foreign to her Mexican American upbringing. "I'm the only Chicana again. Not only do I have to deal with the academic pressures, but hearing racist comments drives me crazy. They don't know I'm Chicana unless I tell them, and then you know the next line? 'You don't look Mexican!'"

Self-awareness and honesty were two strengths that served Sonia well in therapy and in life in general. Although she had never been in therapy before, she took to it very readily, seemingly relieved to dump her distress elsewhere. As she told her story, it became clear that Sonia was experiencing major identity confusion about her future role as a physician and her ethnic identity. More specifically, she was worried about living up to societal and family expectations about being una mujer Chicana.

Esperanza

Esperanza was working as an executive secretary in a high-tech firm when she first came to therapy. Sleepless nights, trembling eyelids, and general uncertainty seemed to plague her. A well-dressed, proper woman, originally from Mexico City, she experienced many stressors associated with what she described as workplace racism and her ongoing attempts to adjust to an unfriendly and cold setting. She explained that her supervisor spoke to her in harsh, disrespectful ways, never making eye contact, never acknowledging her morning greetings, and avoiding any exchange unless it was to give her an assignment. When she tried to get feedback about her performance, Esperanza reported that the supervisor summarily dismissed her; "She always acts as though *le estoy molestando* (that I'm bothering her]. Now I'm afraid I'm going to lose my job."

Professionally well dressed at all times, Esperanza always came prepared with a notepad so that she could report on live issues at work. She spoke English with a noticeable accent, was petite and phenotypically more brown with Mestiza features. In our sessions, she manifested mannerisms of deference and anxiousness. She called me *doctora* and spoke in a manner that seemed intended to elicit my approval. Her distress was obvious and she was seeking a sympathetic ear. The opportunity to participate in bilingual therapy was very important to her because she felt she could more fully express herself and be understood. "Quiero tener confianza con alguien" (I want to be able to trust someone).

Esperanza had started her employment in the United States as a babysitter and then worked her way up to being a Spanish tutor before securing employment as an administrative assistant in the well-known international high-tech company. In Mexico, she had graduated from the national university (UNAM) and worked as an accountant. She met her American-born, non-Spanish-speaking, Jewish husband when he was visiting mutual friends on a vacation to Mexico. With his help, she came to the United States. He was self-employed in a family business and worked long hours, making his availability to her very limited.

Esperanza was the youngest of six children. Her parents had divorced when she was a child due to the father's alcoholism and physical abuse of the mother and older children. Though she reported that her father had not harmed her, as therapy progressed, she described vividly what she had witnessed and the fear it had engendered. The work situation seemed to be stirring up latent fears about safety, inadequacy, and competence.

Graciela

Graciela found herself at a large eastern university with a 4-year scholarship. Originally from a Mexico-Texas border town, she struggled with the decision between completing her 4 years or moving with her boyfriend to California, where he was about to begin graduate school. Graciela was majoring in justice studies and her boyfriend Javier studied political science. They met at a migrant farm-worker rally. They were both Chicana/os away from home and fired up about the rights of farm workers.

Graciela struggled with the idea of following Javier to California before completing her own degree. Contributing to her turmoil was her desire not to disappoint her parents. There had been a struggle when she originally left her Rio Grande town to accept the scholarship at the big eastern university. Her grandmother, a retired baker, had offered to supplement her financial needs, noting that it was important that Graciela get away from home and find a new world outside of Tejas (Texas). This was controversial in the family, but, because *la abuela* (the grandmother) was well respected, even Graciela's parents deferred. Their admonitions to Graciela about doing well and not coming back *con desgracia* (disgraceful) like other Chicanas who had tried college away from *la frontera* (the border) plagued her. Even though she had full intentions of applying to a university in California to complete her studies, she knew that, more than anyone, it was her abuelita that she must not disappoint. "No quiero quedar mal" (I don't want to do something wrong or look bad).

The Struggles

These cases, among others, point to different sets of struggles faced by contemporary women, struggles that are influenced by forces of socialization from *la cultura* (ethnic background), *la familia* (family), gender, the local and mainstream communities, and peers. Embedded in these forces are issues of value orientations, acculturation, ethnic and gender identity, developmental tasks, and experiences of bias and discrimination in a society that does not value *gente Mejicana* or *Chicana* (Mexican and Chicana/o people). Although self-efficacy and a sense of personal empowerment with respect to the presenting dilemmas seemed logical, all of the women talked about their issues in relation to others. Thus, the struggles carried by these clients were really about the family as well and their role conflicts in a dominant White, male, and xenophobic society.

CULTURAL AND CLINICAL CONSIDERATIONS

Assessment and Diagnosis

Before each woman is discussed, a number of practices and concepts are reviewed. Conceptualization of clinical issues typically occurs during the treatment planning process. It could be fairly easy to view these four women from a deficit perspective. Without culture and gender-specific education and supervision, clinicians are likely to base their assessments, treatment planning, and projected outcomes on traditional male-defined norms regarding psychological maturity. Additionally, working from limited information presented in single classes on multicultural counseling and based on the philosophy of the particular instructor, students and practitioners may leave with reinforced stereotyped thinking about Chicanas, if they are discussed at all, and a less than holistic way of understanding the Chicana client in context. A few examples of misdiagnosis are described in the following discussion.

Cultural Misdiagnosis

A culturally uninformed therapist may see the presenting issues of these women strictly through an individualistic world-view lens and according to male models that promote individuation and autonomy. Sonia, the medical student, might be viewed as having a dependent or fused personality because she talked so much about her relationship with her mother. Another possibility is that her potential departure from a prestigious medical school might be termed self-sabotage and a manifestation of ethnic and gender self-hatred. A clinician without appreciation for the family decision-making process involved in Sonia's career plans may not understand the cultural conflict it presents. Moreover, the failure to consider the role of cultural world views, respect for parents' counsel, loyalty to family, the good of the entire *familia,* and the value of *familismo* may prejudice a clinician's assessment. Using descriptions from the *Diagnostic and Statistical Manual of Mental Disorders* (American Psychological Association, 2000) without consideration of cultural and gender-based value orientations leads to misdiagnosis and inappropriate treatment planning. Through cultural reframing, Sonia's allegiances may be seen as strengths rather than developmental deficits.

Esperanza, the worker under stress, might be labeled histrionic with a dependent personality as well, for complaining about her supervisor and not standing up for herself. Chicanas are the targets of both sexism and racism. If they are lesbians, homophobic oppression is also likely to occur. If the clinician is untrained in the issues of adult children of alcoholics or in posttraumatic stress symptoms, Esperanza's reactions to the supervisor might be minimized to issues of low self-esteem. A culturally unskilled clinician operating with stereotyped thinking about Latinas might believe that Esperanza should be grateful for having her job, that she was only whining, and that, with attitude change, she would get along better with her coworkers and supervisor.

Another factor contributing to cultural misreading is a lack of knowledge about the sociopolitical climate with respect to negative views of affirmative action, which could cause the clinician to see only Esperanza, the individual, not Esperanza in a sociopolitical context that is not affirming of Latina/o or Mexican immigrants. Immigrant women experience loss and acculturative stress at many levels. If the therapist views this as only job-related stress, rather than one of many stressors in the acculturation process, other factors compounding the work situation would be ignored.

Finally, Graciela's indecision about leaving school to join her boyfriend in California might indicate that she is a woman with a dependent personality following her man because that is what the culture dictates. This is where a little information can be dangerous. The therapist may be aware of the concept of marianismo and assume that the client is buying in to its 10 commandments, such as "Do not be single, self-supporting, or independent-minded" or "Do not put your own needs first" (Gil & Vazquez, 1996, p. 8). Given this perspective, a therapist may misunderstand the cultural conflict that is occurring for Graciela: She has an abuela who fosters emancipation, parents who foster more traditional socialization where roles for girls and women are clearly defined, and her own desires as an evolving, intelligent, and politically active Chicana.

Graciela's quandary also might be labeled an anxiety disorder rather than a normal response to a stressful situation. Studies indicate that Latina/os are more likely to be given a more severe diagnosis than Whites (Gonzalez, 1997; Roll, Millen, & Martinez, 1980).

CULTURE-SPECIFIC REFRAMING

The preceding discussion of the possible assessments and misdiagnoses of three Chicanas is not impossible to believe. According to Gonzales et al. (1997), Chicana/os are often pathologized and face considerable difficulty in getting beyond that label. If one becomes part of a managed care system, the diagnosis is likely to follow and, apart from this, misdiagnosis affects a Chicana's self-efficacy, self-esteem, personal empowerment, and future options.

To begin a discussion of cultural reframing, the topics that most often converge in the treatment of Chicana/os are briefly reviewed, including Latina and Chicana value orientations and cultural norms, family relations and responsibilities, gender socialization and religious prescriptions, ethnic and gender identity development, role conflicts, and acculturation. This is the multidimensional tapestry that influences the reality of contemporary Chicanas, contributing to our perpetual entre fronteras existence.

Historical Heterogeneity: From Traditional to Contemporary

It is the 21st century and Latina/os, according to the census, now number 38.8 million, or 12.8% of the U.S. population (Armas, 2001; Cohn, 2003; U.S. Bureau of the Census, 2000) and are projected to be 50 million by the year 2020. Persons of Mexican descent were 67% of the Latina/o population in 1998 and this dominant representation among the subgroups is expected to continue in the new century.

References to U.S.-Mexican history are reminders that the southwestern United States were formerly Mexican territory and that the growth of this part of the country has been and continues to be accomplished through the labor of people of Mexican descent. Individuals and families in California, Texas, New Mexico, and Arizona proudly claim their multigenerational residence on this land while new Mexican immigrants and second- and third-generation families contribute to the expanding heterogeneity of the population. Mestizos, or bicultural and biracial persons, are a direct outcome of this ancestry and interethnic marriages.

In many discussions, the Mexican culture is described as traditional, often suggesting that it is an old-fashioned approach to 21st-century life. However, the term *traditional* has to be contextualized. Certainly, the Mexican culture is steeped in rich culture and traditional values that have been transmitted across the generations through different practices. The extent to which these traditional values remain the same is open to critical analysis, which requires consideration of the values in existence in 1521 when Hernán Cortes defeated Montezuma, in 1810 when Mexico gained its independence from Spain, in 1848 when the United States annexed the Southwest, in the 1900s during the raids of Pancho Villa, and during the Hispanic civil rights era of the late 1960s and 1970s. Do contemporary Chicana/os still believe in the importance of la familia, kinship systems, *respeto* (respect), the Spanish language, spiritual support, and other mestizo principles? According to a study of multigenerational Latino families, la familia still remains the primary value for immigrants and third-generation Latina/os (Santiago-Rivera, Arredondo, & Gallardo-Cooper, 2002; *The Washington Post*, 2000). Many intervening situations and forces continue to create Mexican-centered culture change, affecting individual Chicana/os and families alike.

Deconstructing the Concepts of Traditional and Contemporary

In the literature, the terms *traditional* and *contemporary* are typically polarized, creating almost a forced choice for the Chicana, who is viewed in a very linear way as being

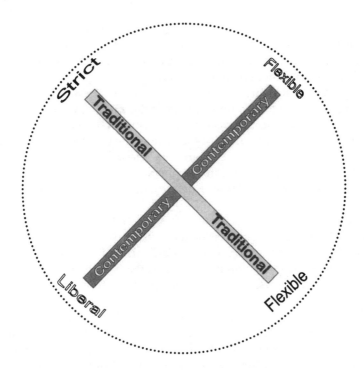

FIG. 12.1.   The traditional-contemporary nexus for Chicanas (Arredondo, 2003).

more or less one or the other. However, as we know, from one of the examples in this chapter, Sonia is a high-achieving Chicana in medical school, yet still feels loyal to her familia, particularly her mother. How would she be placed on this bipolar continuum? Studies of ethnic identity (Bernal & Knight, 1993; Ruiz, 1990) have used particular Chicana/o-specific behaviors as indicators, including "speaks Spanish, listens to Chicano/Mexican music, and has same ethnic friends." To place Chicanas at a particular ethnic identity stage based on the terms *traditional* and *contemporary* obscures the complexity and fluidity of ethnic identity. Ruiz suggested that there is a culture-specific explanation for the identity of Chicana/os and other Latina/os and families as it relates to marginal status, forced assimilation, and other ethnic-stripping experiences.

It is apparent that today's Chicana does exist psychologically, emotionally, spiritually, and physically entre fronteras, because she lives in a bicultural inner and outer world. If there is an insistence on using the concepts of traditional and contemporary, another interacting paradigm is suggested. Fig. 12.1 is a diagram of two intersecting lines labeled "traditional" and "contemporary," suggesting that Chicanas move across both dimensions. We are more or less contemporary and traditional simultaneously because modern life introduces more conflicts, choices, and opportunities. Intervening societal and political forces continue to influence the world view and behavior of immigrant Mejicanas and fifth-generation Chicanas on a daily basis. For the client Graciela, the decision to go to California with Javier or to stay on the East coast to complete her studies seemed like a force choice. However, through informed cultural analysis, the therapist could point out the conscious and unconscious dynamics that made this a major life decision. She could normalize the conflicts based on the contradictions between traditional thinking about family loyalty, and a contemporary, feminist, and more flexible lifestyle.

Contributing to this identity confusion and role conflict are the dominant White majority norms that seem to require assimilation for women who can never be White because of phenotype or other expectations of American beauty. From the Mexican culture, traditional norms about purity and marianismo clash with contemporary celebrity models from Jennifer Lopez to the late Selena. Images of Chicanas are not of physicians, teachers, or even successful mothers. Movie and television scripts, other than those by directors such as James Edward Olmos, have not portrayed Chicanas in a positive way.

So what does *traditional* really mean? How do 21st-century Chicanas bridge the multiplicity of double messages in a society where some still think of feminists as bra burners, Chicanas are forming women's organizations to support their entrepreneurial goals, and low-income immigrant Mejicanas are developing computer skills only to be told by their spouses or partners that they are forbidden to work outside of the home?

By most metrics in U.S. society, Chicanas carry multiple minority status: They are women and Chicanas to begin with, with other, less desirable, attributes such as immigrant, low income, undocumented, college student, teenage mother, and so forth. Rarely is the woman, regardless of her role, visibly acknowledged or celebrated. Therefore, to view girls and women on this traditional benchmark as a way of defining their issues is to ignore the sociopolitical context and ongoing process of border walking (Anzaldúa, 1987) that also imposes on self-efficacy.

Interfacing with legislative processes that become barriers to earning power, education, and personal growth are ever-present stereotyping practices (Flores Niemann, 2001). Chicana/os are still viewed predominantly in negative terms as individuals and as a cultural group and it is this very perception that may become a barrier between a client who seeks help and a therapist lacking in cultural competence (Arredondo, 1991; Flores Niemann; Santiago-Rivera et al., 2002; Zuniga, 1988). Traditionalism need not be viewed for its disabling value orientation, but for what it means in a family-centered culture. Conversely "mainstream" desirable behavior need not be seen as a woman forgetting her roots, but rather as a woman evolving according to personal goals and other multiple influences and supports.

Conceptos Culturales—Key Cultural Terms

For the benefit of readers who are non-Latina/os and monolingual English speakers, a few cultural concepts are introduced, followed by a discussion of value orientations that sometimes emerge as key terms.

Raza is a self- or group-referent term often used by politically aware individuals and refers to *la gente* (the people). Although it translates "race," it has a far deeper historical meaning. In discussions about being *Mestiza/o*, Ramirez (1998) used the expression *la raza cósmica* or the cosmic race. In effect, all Chicanas are Mestizas, reflecting the lineage introduced through the intermarriage of Spaniards and Aztec Indians.

Two other terms that seem to naturally follow are *orgullo* (pride) and *dignidad* (dignity). *Hay que tener orgullo* (One must have pride) is a frequently heard expression about being Mejicana/o or Chicana/o. *Ser digno* (be dignified) or, more simply stated, "behave yourself," particularly in public, is another motivating phrase that gets imbedded in the Chicana psyche. The antithesis is found in words such as *verguenza* (shame), *sin verguenza* (without pride or conscience), and *desgracia* (disgrace). *Qué desgracia* (what a disgrace) is the expression often heard.

In the context of being ambitious and goal oriented, *tener ganas* (to have desire or determination) is often invoked. In the film "Stand and Deliver" (1987), the math teacher Mr. Escalante tried to motivate his Chicana/o students by telling them, "*Hay que tener ganas*" (you must have desire or determination).

Spirituality and formal religion are a cornerstone for the Mexican culture, with the Virgen de Guadalupe as the supreme being for women and men alike who are Catholic. Chicanas vary on their religious orientation and practices and, depending on their degree of acculturation, they may be more or less familiar with certain invocations such as *si díos quiere* (if it's God's will) or *sea por díos*. Expressions such as these have caused culturally insensitive social scientists to suggest that Latina/os are fatalistic, failing to appreciate the use of language in a cultural context or the central role that spirituality plays in the lives of many Latinas.

World Views and Value Orientations

The discussion thus far indicates that Chicanas share many experiences based on historical and sociopolitical forces. Fundamental manifestations of the culture are further experienced and expressed through Latina/o value orientations. Although it can be argued that acculturation, age, generational status, region of residence, and ethnic identity status are variable for all Chicanas, there is still a framework of cultural concepts that serve as underpinnings. *La cultura* (culture) is transmitted through beliefs, values, and practices, consciously and unconsciously, and it is the blueprint of the mind for contemporary Chicanas.

In this family-centered, allocentric culture, the concepts of *familismo* and *personalismo* (personalism) must be appreciated. These speak to the importance of family and personal relationships that must be approached *con respeto* (with respect). *Falta de respeto* (lack of respect) is a cultural transgression (Falicov, 1998). For clinicians, this means that formality should guide initial communications until the client indicates that more informal discussion is acceptable. When working with an older, perhaps less acculturated Chicana, the clinician must address her as Mrs., *señora*, or *doña*. For younger, usually unmarried women like Sonia and Graciela, *señorita* is frequently used.

With older Chicanas, who are unfamiliar with therapy, there may be a tendency to inquire about the clinician's personal life. This should not be construed as informality, but rather *platíca* (small talk). According to researchers (Marín & Marín, 1991), *platíca* is a good way to build rapport or break the ice. For the clinician who engages in *platíca*, this is a demonstration of *personalismo*.

It has been suggested that the culture is hierarchical and paternalistic, however, this does not mean that Chicanas are passive and powerless. In fact, Chicanas and their mothers and abuelas are seen as very powerful forces in the family and the culture. Gloria Anzaldúa (1987, p. 108) wrote of her abuela:

> She never lived with us
> we had no bed for her
> but she always came to visit
> a gift for m'ijita
> two folded dollar bills secretly put in my hand.

The behavior of la abuela mirrors the practice of my own abuela, always generous with dollar bills and other *centavitos* (spare change) for the *nietas* (grandaughters) and *nietos* (grandsons). Unselfish, caring, and patient, she was the classic abuela.

Siendo Mujer—Becoming a Woman

Growing up Chicana requires more discussion than what is found in the Euro American literature on female development in terms of relationships, specifically mother-daughter relationships and self in relationships (Jordan, Kaplan, Miller, & Surrey, 1991). Chicana development has a different historical context, shaped by forces of historical colonization, marginality, or entre fronteras experiences based on Mestiza and bicultural identity, religious prescriptions, and la Chicana's own ongoing, feminist efforts toward self-empowerment (Anzaldúa, 1987; Gonzalez, 1999; Mora, 1986; Moraga, 1995).

Like women in most cultural groups, Chicanas are socialized to be in roles of secondary or marginal status in their communities and families (Arredondo, Psalti, & Cella, 1993). As *esposas* (wives), *hijas* (daughters), *hermanas* (sisters), *tías* (aunts), or *comadres* (godmothers or close family friends), the expectation to serve is there. Perhaps the two roles that receive the most *respeto* are those of the *abuelas* (grandmothers) and *madres* (mothers). In *Loving Pedro Infante* (Chavez, 2001), the protagonist Tere indicated that, when you think of Pedro's mother, you have to "place her up on the altar where all Mejicanos place their mothers, next to God" (p. 229).

This *santa* (saintly) expectation also brings with it very pronounced expectations for daughters: They are to remain virgins until marriage, become wives and mothers foremost, and be caring and compassionate women. It goes without saying that living up to the image of *La Virgen* (the Virgin Mary) is idealized, particularly among recently arrived Mexican families. Although Catholicism continues to be the dominant religion for Chicana/os, other denominations also seem to promote women's secondary status.

Earlier references to marianismo are significant to this discussion, because many of the 10 commandments of marianismo are still in force today. According to Gil and Vazquez (1996), they are:

1. Do not forget a woman's place.
2. Do not forsake tradition.
3. Do not be single, self-supporting, or independent minded.
4. Do not put your needs first.
5. Do not forget that sex is for making babies, not for pleasure.

6. Do not wish for more in life than being a housewife.
7. Do not be unhappy with your man, no matter what he does to you.
8. Do not ask for help.
9. Do not discuss personal problems outside the home.
10. Do not change.

For more contemporary Chicanas seeking to go beyond these mantras and traditional role expectations, cultural conflict will likely ensue. In recent courses specific to counseling with Latina/os, Chicana participants have offered varying perspectives on this concept. They report: (a) recognizing through family behavior, in particular, how the commandments are reinforced; (b) personal conflicts in not wanting to be complicit by supporting the commandments; (c) a sense of liberation in knowing that there is a cultural or academic term to attribute to these patterns of behavior; and (d) a strong desire to break the cycle, particularly of disabling commandments for Chicanas and Chicanos alike. Thus, the dicho *Mujer preparada vale por dos* (one prepared woman is better than two) can be heard as an empowering and validating expression.

Acculturation and Ethnic Identity

Acculturative stress is a phenomenon discussed in reference to immigrants as well as Chicanas who continuously find themselves adjusting to new contexts and norms that are not culturally validating. Stressors include insufficient finances, the lack of a support system resulting in isolation, psychological and physical losses associated with migration, inability to be understood because of language differences, and working in circumstances that are physically demanding. Sexism and racism are stressors as well.

The literature suggests that acculturation is a process experienced by immigrant women as well as Chicanas born in the United States. Our bicultural, Mestiza identity and marginal status in U.S. society suggest that there are different levels of acculturation, perhaps operating within the same family. The ways in which one participates in the mainstream, Mexican, and feminist cultures reveals more about one's Chicana identity. Most ethnic and racial identity models blur the genders, suggesting that women and men have similar experiences of oppression, racism, and marginalization based on their Mexican or Chicana/o identity. We posit that, for Chicanas, sexism is a barrier as well.

In her political essay, Moraga (1995) described her experiences as a Latina and writer in the United States as being one *con acento*. In her poem, "The Welder," she can not forsake her essence as a woman or as a Chicana. Rather, she stated, "women must continue to examine choice points for fusion or temporary adhesion by ultimately taking power into [their] own hands" (p. 219).

Ongoing work with ethnic identity models has introduced a composite profile of Mexican Personal Dimensions of Identity, as shown in Fig. 12.2 (Arredondo & Arciniega, 2000), adapted from the Dimensions of Personal Identity Model (Arredondo & Glauner, 1992). The Mexican version reflects varying dimensions of identity that intersect with ethnicity and gender. The C dimension in the model also affects these fixed and fluid dimensions and reflects historical, economic, and sociopolitical

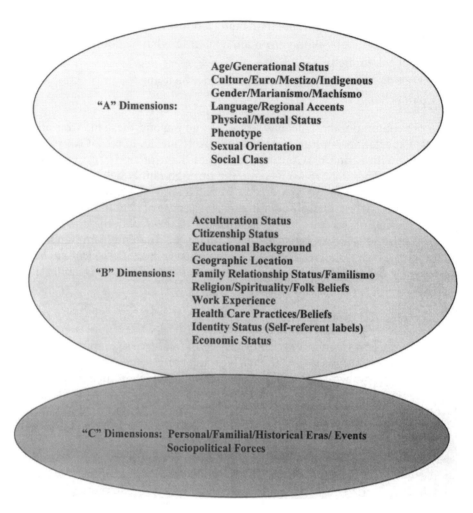

FIG. 12.2.   Mexican American dimensions of family and personal identity (Arredondo & Arciniega, 2001).

forces. It is posited that the A and C dimensions have a direct effect on opportunities and choices, whereas the B dimensions (e.g., education), do not.

For Chicana immigrants or first- and second-generation women, it is also important to examine the psychological effects of the immigration process. Not only is identity confusion a consequence of immigration, but so too is a sense of loss, grief, and posttraumatic stress reactions (Arredondo-Dowd, 1981).

RECOMMENDATIONS FOR WORKING WITH CHICANAS

Although the match between a Chicana client and therapist would seem ideal according to some literature regarding ethnic identity similarity in therapy, therapist

cultural competence is still essential. To assume similarity based on the ethnic identity would be to diminish the richness of the individuals and their life scripts. Furthermore, clinicians not in touch with their own ethnic identity struggles could easily
misread their client's confusion based on an allocentric upbringing, in conflict with
contemporary messages about being una Chicana in a White-dominated society.

As with all therapy relationships, transference and countertransference occur. With
two women sharing the same ethnic identity, caution is a necessity for a number
of reasons. First, overidentification with the client's concerns can motivate a therapist to be more solicitous and helpful, almost taking on a caretaker role. If unchecked
subjectivity or countertransference begin to occur, collaborative engagement may
become problematic. Second, unchecked biases and attitudes about one's identity—
based on ethnic, gender, or other factors—may cause a therapist to have either
higher or lower expectations of the client based on stereotyped thinking and his or
her own unresolved ethnic identity issues. Third, in the most obvious manifestations
of negative countertransference, the Chicana client may personify a female family
figure the clinician disdains. For example, if Esperanza's deference and approval-
seeking behavior remind the clinician of her mother, she might become impatient
and even critical of the client.

For the clinician who is not Chicana, there are also issues of countertransference.
Negative associations with the client may accrue through stereotyped images of half-
dressed Latinas performing on stage, abuelas praying to la Virgen de Guadalupe, or
farm workers living in poverty. Inadequate and culturally uninformed preparation
may render the clinician with feelings of incompetence that could be inadvertently
imposed on the client. Rather than owning her sense of inadequacy, the clinician dis-
places these feelings onto the unsuspecting, help-seeking Chicana client. However,
this need not be the continuing saga in the 21st century. There are guidelines for education and practice that can improve psychotherapy with Chicanas.

PROPOSED CHICANA-SPECIFIC COMPETENCIES

The Multicultural Counseling Competencies (MCC) documents (Arredondo et al.,
1996; Sue, Arredondo, & McDavis, 1992) outlined specific areas of awareness, knowledge, and skill essential for culturally competent practice. The generic nature of these
competencies allows for adaptation to working with more specific populations (e.g.,
gay, lesbian, transgendered) in particular contexts (e.g., school settings) and with
particular applications (e.g., group procedures).

It seems appropriate, therefore, to use the MCC as a reference point for the development of Chicana-specific guidelines. Keeping in mind that these statements are a
living document, it is possible to add and modify them as more outcome research on
treatment is conducted. The proposed competencies emerge from a cross-section of
literature of the past 20 to 25 years (Arredondo, 1991, 1992; Padilla, 1995; Santiago-
Rivera et al., 2002) that articulates consistent messages about contextual factors,
world views, acculturation, ethnic identity development, and other dimensions of a
Chicana's identity and roles such as age, relationship status, and religion. Adding to
this discussion is the aforementioned Mexican Dimensions of Personal Identity (see
Fig. 12.2).

The proposed competencies refer to clinicians' self-awareness and self-under-standing, their awareness and knowledge about Chicana culture and world views, and their ongoing clinical skill development. In a sense, the competencies are both personal and technical, with the technical referring to essential knowledge and skills that are respectful of the Chicana's ethnicity and gender.

Clinician Self-Awareness and Understanding

Culturally competent clinicians:

1. Recognize their cultural heritage and how it has influenced how they are in the world.
2. Understand their nuclear and extended family systems and how they have influenced their views on family relationships and dynamics.
3. Are aware of their gender socialization and the influence it has had on their perspective on women cross-culturally.
4. Understand their career development path, including enablers and barriers along the way.
5. Are aware of the cultural limitations of existing counseling theories, models of psychological development, the *DSM-IV*, research with Chicanas, and other academic- and society-sanctioned psychological statements.
6. Understand how power and privilege accrue based on one's cultural her-itage, gender, phenotype, socioeconomic status, sexual orientation, relation-ship status, citizenship, language, education, and occupation (see Fig. 12.2).
7. Recognize historical and sociopolitical institutional barriers.

**Clinician Understanding and Knowledge
of Chicana World Views**

Culturally competent counselors:

1. Are knowledgeable about the entre fronteras metaphor and how it may oper-ate for Chicanas.
2. Are knowledgeable about communication practices that may impede or enhance a trusting and positive relationship between a Chicana client and a counselor.
3. Can identify specific Chicana value orientations and interpersonal etiquette that may facilitate rapport.
4. Are knowledgeable about historical contexts and contacts that affect a Chi-cana's view of some non-Latinos, particularly Caucasians.
5. Are knowledgeable about regional sociopolitical practices, including anti-bilingual education legislation, that have adversely affected Chicanas and others of Mexican descent.
6. Understand the role of language in assessment and treatment and know when to encourage the Chicana, if Spanish is her first language, to use it in counseling sessions, particularly for the expression of emotions.

7. Are knowledgeable about ethnic and gender identity models that may be relevant for counseling with Chicanas.
8. Know about Chicana or Mejicana resources, agencies, churches, and other culturally appropriate organizations.

Culturally Competent Skill Application

Culturally competent counselors:

1. Can differentiate and describe what is culturally driven and what is idiosyncratic to the Chicana's family functioning.
2. Apply a cultural-linguistic approach in the early stages of counseling, if applicable.
3. May be bilingual and, if not, they ensure that the individual and her family are assisted by a competent clinician who speaks the family's preferred language.
4. Can interject key Spanish words, phrases, and dichos during counseling.
5. Are able to use an integration of counseling strategies and methods that take into account the multiple realities of Chicana clients.
6. Are able to adapt different kinds of family therapy models to Chicanas and their families.
7. Can develop a treatment plan that uses a multidimensional framework, incorporating aspects of the culture- and gender-centered protocols (Santiago-Rivera et al., 2002).
8. Integrate multiple frameworks for gathering initial information, developing a diagnosis, and outlining a treatment plan and interventions that will address the presenting issues in terms of the client's developmental, acculturation, and identity status, and her support network (*red de apoyo*).
9. Refer clients to other resources including indigenous healers and other spiritual guides (e.g., priests and ministers) that provide necessary support.
10. Share with Chicanas reading lists and other materials that may validate the clients' ethnic- and gender-related concerns.
11. Can discuss with clients in layperson language issues of acculturative stress, ethnic identity confusion, and gender role conflict.
12. Have broad knowledge of family systems theories as well as cultural family therapy models and are able to use them in counseling when appropriate.
13. Can identify possible barriers to family interventions with Chicano families.

RECOMMENDATIONS FOR INTERVENTION PLANNING AND TREATMENT

Throughout this chapter, the objective has been to encourage therapists and educators to think creatively and in more expansive ways about Chicanas. This requires deliberate self-assessments, as outlined with the competency statements, and intentional

educational strategies to learn more about the Latina or Chicana world view, historical and contemporary challenges, and resources for culturally competent consultation from Chicana and non-Chicana clinicians and educators. This is a preliminary
and concomitant step to creating treatment plans that are in the best interest of the
Chicana client.

Discussion has pointed to various cultural and contextual considerations that are
required for working with Chicanas. This conceptualization must occur; otherwise,
specific intervention strategies will be ungrounded. In order words, therapists must
have a multidimensional rationale for their intervention approaches; it cannot simply be only clinically based. If clinicians recognize the cultural conflicts that may be
present for clients like Sonia, Esperanza, and Graciela, they may draw upon Chicana
or Latina-specific literature to validate some of the women's experiences. In so doing,
however, they must be mindful of the Chicana's ethnic and gender identity status,
degree of difficulty of the presenting problem, available support system, and financial resources to purchase materials or to participate in activities recommended. A
few suggestions follow:

1. Have clients read excerpts from *The House on Mango Street* (Cisneros, 1989),
   Face of an Angel (Chavez, 1994), *Loving Pedro Infante* (Chavez, 2001), or *La
   Chicana* (Mirandé & Enríquez, 1979).
2. Invite clients to speak in Spanish whenever they wish, but, in particular,
   encourage this when emotions seem strong, provided the client is bilingual
   or Spanish is her first language.
3. Invite clients to prepare an autobiographical statement about growing up
   Chicana—what they remember most about family gatherings and so forth.
4. Recommend that clients see the movies "Stand and Deliver" (1998), "Mi
   Familia" (1995), "Real Women Have Curves" (2003), or "Tortilla Soup"
   (2001), all Chicana/o or Mejicana/o-centered films.
5. Ask the client to share dichos or stories that they heard from abuelas or other
   family members.
6. Have clients prepare a cultural genogram, tracing family systems back two to
   three generations.
7. Invite clients to talk about cultural artifacts that are most meaningful to them.
   These can be used as "transitional objects" in therapy, depending on the difficulty of the cultural conflict.
8. Provide clients with references to literature about La Malinche and Sor Juana
   de la Cruz, both historical Chicana icons.
9. Depending on the client's religious affiliation, inquire about the client's and
   the family's attention to La Virgen de Guadalupe, praying, and other rituals.
10. Use culture- and gender-centered intake forms. This allows for data gather-
    ing over two to three sessions about valuable cultural background informa-
    tion such as spirituality.

Chicanas in psychotherapy mirror all women. They are family members foremost,
educators, victims of domestic violence, legislators, farm workers, performers, house-

keepers, small business owners, activists, students, teenage mothers, psychotherapists, writers, artists, physicians, immigration officers, attorneys, factory workers, and any and all other roles held by other men and women in the United States. Clinicians' expectations of Chicana clients must be neither high nor low; rather, they must be suspended. Chicanas must be allowed to tell their stories and then clinicians may engage. They are the protagonists of the entre fronteras existence. It is the clinicians' privilege to play a small part in their life stories.

REFERENCES

American Psychiatric Association. (2000). *Diagnostic and statistical manual of mental disorders* (4th ed.). Washington, DC: Author.

Anzaldúa, G. (1987). *Borderlands/La Frontera.* San Francisco, CA: Spinsters/Aunt Lute.

Armas, G. (2001, May 8). Hispanic population exceeds predictions. *The Daily Gazette,* pp. 1A, 6A.

Arredondo, P. (1991). Counseling Latinas. In C. Lee & C. Richardson (Eds.), *Strategies and techniques for multicultural counseling* (pp. 143–157). Alexandria, VA: American Association of Counseling and Development Press.

Arredondo, P. (1992). Promoting the empowerment of women through counseling interventions. *Counseling and Human Development, 24,* 1–12.

Arredondo, P., & Arciniega, G. M. (2001). *Mexican American dimensions of personal identity.* Unpublished manuscript, Arizona State University.

Arredondo, P., & Glauner, T. (1992). *Personal dimensions of identity model.* Boston: Empowerment Workshops.

Arredondo, P., Psalti, A., & Cella, K. (1993). The woman factor in multicultural counseling. *Counseling and Human Development, 24,* 1–8.

Arredondo, P., Toporek, R., Brown, S. P., Jones, J., Locke, D. C., Sanchez, J., & Stadler, H. (1996). Operationalization of the multicultural counseling competencies. *Journal of Multicultural Counseling and Development, 24,* 42–78.

Arredondo-Dowd, P. M. (1981). Personal loss and grief as a result of immigration. *The Personnel and Guidance Journal, 58,* 657–661.

Barón, A., & Constantine, M. G. (1997). A conceptual framework for conducting psychotherapy with Mexican American college students. In J. G. Garcia & M. Zea (Eds.), *Psychological interventions and research with Latino populations* (pp. 108–124). Needham, MA: Allyn and Bacon.

Barriga, M. D. (2001). Verguenza and changing Chicano and Chicana narratives. *Men and Masculinities in Latin America, 3,* 278–298.

Bernal, M. E., & Knight, G. P. (Eds.). (1993). *Ethnic identity: Formation and transmission among Hispanics and other minorities.* Albany: State University of New York Press.

Candelaria, C. (1980). La Malinche, feminist prototype. *Frontiers, 5,* 1–6.

Chavez, D. (1994). *Face of an angel.* New York: Farrar, Straus, and Giroux.

Chavez, D. (2001). *Loving Pedro Infante.* New York: Farrar, Straus, and Giroux.

Chávez-Candelaria, C. (1993). The "wild zone" thesis as gloss in Chicana literary study. In R. R. Warhol & D. P. Herndl (Eds.), *About feminisms* (1997, pp. 248–256). New Brunswick, NJ: Rutgers University Press.

Cisneros, S. (1989). *The house on Mango street.* New York: Vintage Books.

Cohn, D. (2003, June 18). Hispanics are nation's largest minority. The Washington Post Company: washingtonpost.com.

Facio, E. (1996). *Understanding older Chicanas.* Thousand Oaks, CA: Sage.

Falicov, C. J. (1998). *Latino families in therapy: A guide to multicultural practice.* New York: Guilford Press.

Flores Niemann, Y. (2001). Stereotypes about Chicanas and Chicanos: Implications for counseling. *The Counseling Psychologist, 29,* 55–90.

Flores-Ortiz, Y. G. (1995). Psychotherapy with Chicanas at midlife: Cultural/clinical considerations. In J. Adelman & M. Gloria (Eds.), *Racism in the lives of women: Testimony, theory, and guides to antiracist practice.* New York: Harrington Park Press/Haworth Press.

Gil, R. M., & Vazquez, C. N. (1996). *The Maria paradox.* New York: Perigee Books.

Gonzalez, F. E. (1999). The formations of "Mexicananess": Trenzas de identidades multiples. *Dissertation Abstracts International, 60,* 1360.

Gonzalez, G. (1997). The emergence of Chicanos in the twenty-first century: Implications for counseling, research, and policy. *Journal of Multicultural Counseling and Development, 25,* 94–106.

Gonzalez, M., Castillo-Canez, I., Tarke, H., & Soriano, F. (1997). Promoting the culturally sensitive diagnosis of Mexican Americans: Some personal insights. *Journal of Multicultural Counseling and Development, 25,* 156–161.

Hinojosa, M. (1999). *Raising Raúl.* New York: Penguin Books.

Hurtado, A. (2000). "La cultura cura": Cultural spaces for generating Chicana feminist consciousness. In L. Weis & M. Fine (Eds.), *Construction sites: Excavating race, class, and gender among urban youth* (pp. 274–289). New York: Teachers College Press.

Jordan, J., Kaplan, A., Miller, J. B., & Surrey, J. (1991). *Women's growth in connection.* New York: Guilford Press.

Latinos in America: A journey in stages. (2000, January 15). *The Washington Post* [On-line]. Available: www.washingtonpost.com/wp-dyn/article/a51043–2000jan15.html

Marin, G., & Marin, B. (1991). *Research with Hispanic populations.* Newbury Park, CA: Sage.

McNeill, B. W., Prieto, L. R., Flores Niemann, Y., Pizarro, M., Vera, E. M., & Gómez, S. P. (2001). Current directions in Chicana/o psychology. *The Counseling Psychologist, 29,* 5–17.

Mirandé, A., & Enríquez, E. (1979). *La Chicana.* Chicago: University of Chicago Press.

Mora, P. (1986). *Borders.* Houston, TX: Arte Público Press.

Moraga, C. (1995). Art in America con acento. In L. Castillo-Speed (Ed.), *Women's voices from the borderland* (pp. 211–220). New York: Simon and Schuster.

Padilla, A. M. (Ed.). (1995). *Hispanic psychology.* Thousand Oaks, CA: Sage.

Ramirez, M. (1998). *Multicultural/multiracial psychology.* Northvale, NJ: Aronson.

Roll, S., Millen, L., & Martinez, R. (1980). Common errors in psychotherapy with Chicanos: Extrapolations from research and clinical experience. *Psychotherapy: Theory, Research, and Practice, 17,* 158–168.

Ruiz, A. S. (1990). Ethnic identity: Crisis and resolution. *Journal of Multicultural Counseling and Development, 18,* 29–40.

Santiago-Rivera, A., Arredondo, P., & Gallardo-Cooper, M. (2002). *Counseling Latino families: A guide for practitioners.* Thousand Oaks, CA: Sage.

Sue, D. W., Arredondo, P., & McDavis, R. (1992). Multicultural competencies and standards: A call to the profession. *Journal of Counseling and Development, 70,* 477-486.

Velázquez, R. J. (Ed.). (1997). Counseling Mexican Americans/Chicanos [Special issue]. *Journal of Multicultural Counseling and Development, 25*(2).

U.S. Bureau of the Census. (2000). *The Hispanic population in the United States: March 2000* (Report No. P20-535). Washington, DC: U.S. Government Printing Office.

Zuniga, M. E. (1988). Assessment issues with Chicanas: Practice implications. *Psychotherapy, 25,* 288–293.

13

Group Therapy With Chicanas

Louise Baca
Patricia Hernandez
Argosy University, Phoenix

This chapter illustrates group therapy work with Chicanas and other Latinas in a higher education setting. We use the term *Chicanas* while recognizing that much of what we say is relevant to all Latinas. We attempt to offer practical information for both practitioners and researchers.

The clinical work we describe represents over a decade of experience of actual implementation of group therapy programs for Chicanas. In addition, we provide information about the sociopolitical context, history, and philosophical assumptions that play a role in implementing a culturally responsive therapeutic modality for Chicanas in a higher education setting.

First, we recount the history of the development of a culturally responsive therapeutic modality for Chicanas. We then discuss the stresses and coping mechanisms experienced by Chicanas as they attempt to earn undergraduate and graduate degrees. Next, we describe the kinds of settings, contexts, and guiding philosophies that facilitate successful implementation of group therapy programs for Chicanas. We articulate the process of conducting effective groups for Chicanas with a richness of clinical detail that we hope will spur research efforts by other scholars. Additionally, we provide an illustrative case example, with changes in some details to protect client confidentiality. Finally, we discuss the implications of our work and propose recommendations for training and research in this area.

HISTORICAL BACKDROP

The historical backdrop is pertinent in that it affords an understanding of how the specific need for a culturally responsive treatment modality emerged. There was a spoken need by Chicanas to not be alone in their attempt to understand the ever-changing social landscape. Chicanas reported needing a group tailored to their unique challenges. An empathic response from a Chicana psychologist led to an attempt to tailor the group for Chicanas and to offer them an experience that was validating, growth enhancing, and meaningful. Administrative response initially requested a rationale for providing a group tailored specifically for Chicanas. The rationale included the history of the Chicana/o community within institutions of higher education.

Lessons From the 1960s and 1970s

The *Movimiento* (movement) led to ethnic identity and self-definition based on terms like *Chicana* and *Chicano*. This is the era of the first important scholarship addressing the concerns of the Chicana/o community related to mental health utilization (i.e., Barrera, 1978; Burruel & Chavez, 1974). The first Chicana/o scholars emerged to become role models and a course was set with scholarship at the forefront. From this era, it was learned that much could be accomplished with solidarity, compassion, and united voices expressing group needs and concerns. Chicana/os also learned to live with setbacks, challenges, and reality that many continue to live without education, in poverty, and with many unmet social and mental health needs (Maciel & Ortiz, 1996).

Lessons From the 1980s and 1990s

The 1980s were characterized by a conservative political backlash, but scholarship continued with classic works on Chicano ethnicity (Keefe & Padilla, 1987) and Chicana/o psychology (Martinez & Mendoza, 1984). Chicana/o studies departments were established in major universities. The importance and emphasis on education for Chicanas was correlated with increasing economic opportunity and decreasing fertility rates (Gonzalez-Baker, 1996). It became apparent that Chicanas would need additional social support to maintain gains in education and economic opportunities, especially as more of them became the heads of households following divorce (Chavez & Martinez, 1996). It was in the 1980s that the first support groups for Chicanas were established in institutions of higher education. A second generation of Chicana/o scholars and clinicians began to call for attention to the specific needs of Chicanas (Roll, Millen, & Martinez, 1980; Vasquez, 1984; Zuniga, 1988).

The 1990s were characterized by studies focusing on specific competencies needed to do psychotherapy with Chicanas (Arredondo, Psalti & Cella, 1993; Baca & Koss-Chioino, 1997; Flores-Ortiz, 1995). The need to consider historical and contextual factors of the Chicana/o experience came to the foreground in the 1990s, as did a call to create and research culturally responsive treatment modalities.

Creating a culturally responsive modality requires addressing cultural issues directly, within the group format. For example, the therapist must create cohesion between Chicanas and Mexicanas and often other Latinas. Self-labeling of personal ethnic identification can be disparate and predictive of tension between group members unless it is addressed directly by the group leader. The therapist must discuss issues related to ethnic identification such as immigration and regional history. Such discussion involves creating an understanding of the social, political, and economic factors associated with these issues. Addressing ethnic identity issues directly and in depth leads to discussion that is often complex. Chicanas identify to varying degrees with their Indian, African, and Caucasian mixtures. Furthermore, there is a need for the therapist to address a range of linguistic backgrounds within the group. Documentation of such specific skill sets, as well as the call for culturally responsive treatment, can be considered some of the major lessons from the 1990s.

In summary, all therapists who work with Chicanas need to keep the historical and cultural context in mind as they proceed with therapeutic work. It is important for therapists to attend to the sociopolitical realities of their clients and not make assumptions based on stereotypes. Remaining cognizant of the historical backdrop to the lives of a full range of Chicanas from different places and eras is critically important in tailoring the therapeutic process.

CHICANAS IN HIGHER EDUCATION

Vargas and Koss-Chioino (1992) introduced the ideas of the complex interaction of culture and the structure of group therapy for the formation of a culturally responsive therapeutic modality. Baca and Koss-Chioino (1997) further articulated the concept of a fourth life space.

To articulate the process of developing a culturally responsive therapeutic modality, an attempt was made to define a fourth life space by providing a location for personal and emotional growth that was not available in the family, school, or extracurricular areas of a Chicana's daily life. Culturally responsive group therapy becomes the vehicle for exploration beyond the narrow, imposed definitions of personhood often established in the other life spaces. Thus, culturally responsive group therapy primarily offers the freedom for self-definition that is missing in the other life spaces but that is critically important for Chicanas' success in higher education and for their general life satisfaction.

Chicanas are entering higher education at greater rates than their Chicano peers and they are matriculating toward graduation at increasing rates (Gloria, 1999), despite the association of higher relationship stress with the pursuit of increased education by Chicana and Native American women (Guerrero-Avila, 2001). Women who are confronted with strained relationships with men, families, and familiar community and religious leaders may need to look for a fourth life space to heal and gather strength (Baca & Koss-Chioino, 1998; Vasquez, 1984). Within the fourth life space of a Chicana therapy group the following needs are met:

- Need for affiliation under stress
- Need for validation
- Need for a sense of belonging and support
- Need to be understood
- Need to be in a culturally familiar environment
- Need to be seen as normal when discussing their world view, including spirituality
- Need to be given permission or a blessing to succeed in higher education
- Need for a safe place to let down their guard
- Need to foster faith, hope, and love, preparing the groundwork for further healing
- Need to learn new or recover lost coping and self-care strategies

These needs are addressed in the language and style most conducive to enhancing health and growth in Chicanas within the group format.

COPING STRATEGIES FOR CHICANAS

One of the difficult areas for Chicanas to negotiate is the tremendous amount of stress and multiple-role overload that may characterize their lives (Davalos, Chavez, & Guardiola, 1999; Vasquez, 1984). Chicanas are considered as caregivers in the roles of mother, wife or girlfriend, sister, daughter, granddaughter, friend, godmother, aunt, cousin, and neighbor. Culturally, a woman is expected to fulfill all of these roles. Even for the more acculturated Chicana, the role of a student would be in addition to all of the traditional roles. The stress of fulfilling all of these roles is overwhelming for many Chicanas. Effective coping with the stress becomes one of the variables most predictive of academic persistence (Gloria, 1999).

Acculturative stress may be evident for women who come from ethnic or racial enclaves onto a university campus that is primarily Eurocentric. Pressure to assimilate to the dominant group is often addressed in Chicana therapy groups. Such pressure may be countered using both didactic material and the opportunity to process acculturation pressures. For example, material on ethnic identity development may be presented to the group. Discussion in group therapy may focus on empowering women to self-define based on ethnic identity and other aspects of their personhood. Caring for the emerging self is a theme often supported by other group members. Thus, this work often leads to a discussion of more general coping strategies.

Effective coping for Chicanas can be defined according to the Western world view or from indigenous perspectives. For example, to treat a stomach ache, the Western medical model would endorse the use of a pill to decrease stomach pain. The indigenous perspective would rely on *la platica* (brief conversations) and *yerba buena* (spearmint tea; Harris, Renteria & White, 2002; Neff, 2001).

La platica is used diagnostically to probe for a possible mind-body discord or underlying cause of the stomach ache, such as relational discord or prolonged stress. The Western world view may not take the time to typically discern the mind-body discord and would not usually probe for disharmony within the interpersonal sphere. Instead, it often offers short-term symptom relief that may in turn create other problems such as constipation (from too many tablets for stomach distress). The key, for Chicanas, is to learn when to use the traditional remedies and when to rely on Western medicine.

Both systems of healing are of value for Chicanas. However, Chicanas need role models and a safe place to dialogue and learn the discernment critical to the maintenance of their health and well-being. Thus, groups designed for Chicanas are critically important. They do not take the place of family, but underscore the healthy negotiation between modern ways and traditional wisdom.

THERAPIST CHARACTERISTICS

As with traditional group therapy, the role modeling of a Chicana group leader is of critical importance for the group process. The leader must know some of the methods of a *curandera,* or folk healer, and also rely on sound clinical training. Many Chicanas have never known another Chicana who is a professional, a wife, and a mother. Many Chicanas are first-generation college students who want a role model to guide them as they move toward dreams for bettering themselves, their families, and their communities. Chicana therapists need not follow traditional female roles, but may need to self-disclose choices related to gender role in order to gain trust from group members.

The attributes for the Chicana group leader would ideally include the following: clear ethnic identity regardless of ethnicity, empathy regarding Chicana issues, knowledge of traditional values and customs (or the willingness to learn), and some Spanish language ability, given that many Spanish-speaking Chicanas have learned to label their emotions in Spanish allowing for fine distinctions that may not be possible in English. However, the ability to speak fluent Spanish is not always a necessity if the Chicanas in the group are fluent in English. In fact, the mixture of Spanish and English is probably the norm in any Chicana group, due to the range of acculturation levels that are often found there.

SETTING THE STAGE FOR GROUP WORK

Ideally, the reception area is welcoming and staff members are courteous, helpful, and bilingual. Decor should be attentive to the cultural nuances of colors, form configurations, textures, and faces of Chicanas. Background music is from a Spanish radio station or includes a Latin genre of music. Purposeful informality includes the use of beanbags or large pillows for sitting on the floor in a circle. Lighting is soft and music plays softly in the background as Chicanas gather for group. Food and nonalcoholic drinks are often present.

Screening clients is done carefully, when possible, to create the ideal composition of a group for Chicanas. The ideal group is diverse. Such heterogeneity may stand in direct contradiction to the screening that is normally done for forming process groups from other perspectives, such as an experiential perspective (Yalom, 1995). It is important to have a range with regard to age, urban or rural lifestyle, acculturation status, socioeconomic status, sexual orientation, language preference, level of education, major of study, and families of origin. This allows Chicanas to find the answers to often unspoken questions related to issues such as ethnic identity formation and the pressure to find acceptance from a larger cultural group. This process of valuing difference is particularly important in embracing Chicanas of mixed ethnic or racial heritage, who often wonder where and how they fit into the larger cultural picture.

Diversity within the group allows Chicanas to learn from each other in positive ways. For example, a highly acculturated woman may learn to value the traditional wisdom of another, much less acculturated, woman. The less acculturated, traditional Chicana may learn to associate pride rather than shame with traditional cultural understanding and language preference. Thus, all Chicanas are provided the opportunity to validate each other as they recognize that culture evolves and has room for personal choices within the larger group structure.

Chicanas are encouraged to ask questions before making a commitment to the group and flexibility on the part of the therapist is often helpful. For example, a young child may attend group with a family member who does not have other child-care options.

Often, it is challenging to find a time and day that works for eight Chicanas. The lunch hour (90 min) was convenient for most Chicanas once a week. Self-care is modeled and encouraged by bringing lunches and drinks and spending a few minutes in light social discourse before the official start of group. Ceremonial tools such as candles, sage, cedar, and sweetgrass are also visible (to be discussed or used upon request).

It may take time for the women to realize that group is often the treatment of choice. For some women, group does follow some individual therapy, but for many women who experience similar stresses and adjustments, therapy consists of one or more semesters of group therapy designed specifically for Chicanas in a higher education setting.

An important skill for the group leader is to actively counteract the many negative stereotypes that may deplete and diminish the Chicana woman. A recent study documented the implications of negative stereotypes for Chicanas (Niemann, 2001). Group therapy for Chicanas requires the active confrontation of internalized racism and negative stereotypes and attempts to replace these stereotypes with cultural understanding and cultural pride.

Teaching and modeling protective coping strategies from both the Western and the traditional world views becomes a critical component of group therapy. Weaving the best of Western health knowledge with an indigenous philosophy of life and healing stresses balance in all areas of life. In group, women learn the value of traditional coping strategies that incorporate herbal remedies, massage, la platica or talking out stress, meditation, and prayer as part of the spiritual coping that is often pivotal to Chicana mind-body health.

In group, Chicanas discuss curanderismo and its place in the maintenance of health (Harris et al., 2002). Often, it is important for the group to acknowledge and validate the benefits of culturally based health practices that have been in existence for literally thousands of years and are only recently becoming the subjects of inquiry by medical and social scientists (Harris, Velásquez, White, & Renteria, chap. 6, this volume; Neff, 2001).

Curanderas are often our mothers, aunties, and grandmothers, though they may not use the label of curandera (traditional healer) even if they possess many of the attributes and have at least some of the traditional knowledge of a curandera. For example, in the kitchens of most Chicanas, there is usually at least one herbal remedy used to treat family members who exhibit mild ailments ranging from stomach aches to anxiety. La platica is often part of the ritual of drinking tea together to discern the underlying cause of the symptom and *consejo* or advice is often part of the healing remedy. Helping young ones cope with the stresses of life is part of the role of mother, sister, auntie, and godmother. All Chicanas are curanderas, to some extent.

There are prevention-intervention aspects of this work attributable to the culturally prescribed skills of the curandera. The protective effects of cultural coping could be described as "wisdom ways" in English and "curanderismo" in Spanish. Traditional patterns of healing and related protective factors associated with mind-body health are likely to be the subject of scientific inquiry in the new millennium as therapists move toward more culturally responsive treatment modalities.

Some techniques of psychotherapy that deserve more scientific inquiry include the use of music, story, and imagery. As noted earlier, music often sets the stage for group. Music often leads to the discussion of memories and may invoke a feeling that can be used therapeutically. The use of music in group requires both creativity and skill as the leader weaves the discourse toward a therapeutic goal. For example, one woman commented that mariachi music was "old-fashioned" and that only her grandparents listen to "that stuff." Upon reflection, she realized that her preference for hip hop coincided with her preference for dating African American men. This realization helped her to articulate some of the gains and losses she experienced in navigating between two cultures.

In the group therapy with Chicanas, there is often an opportunity for the leader or a group member to tell a *cuento* or story to the entire group. These stories indirectly provide guidance to aid in problem solving. The cuento can be adapted to fit the circumstances of the group. For example, although the leader may have learned a story with the primarily male characters, it could be changed to revolve around women.

Imagery can be used in group for stress management and for discerning opportunities. Group members are taught to create images as they learn relaxation techniques. They can learn to imagine solutions to obstacles and can project themselves into the future with desired realistic outcomes in mind. Overall, imagery has been shown to be powerful (Shorr, Sobel, Robin, & Connella, 1980), but further empirical research is needed to support its role in the healing process.

Techniques such, music, storytelling, and imagery that are practiced today have their beginnings in traditional wisdom. These techniques have been passed down orally from the cultural roots of Africans, Moors, Mexican Indian and Native American tribes, and Spanish cultural and spiritual traditions of both Jewish and Catholic influence.

WISDOM WAYS

There are ancient philosophies of life and healing that have been transmitted via oral tradition in many indigenous cultures. Latina/o cultures often incorporate such learning in ways that seem second nature, ways that are often deeply ingrained but not always attributed to indigenous ancestors. Chicana/o people have a link to their indigenous ancestors that they are often only partially aware of.

The role of culturally responsive therapy is to point toward the awareness and knowledge of the sacred that resides in the mystery of the Chicana/o people, who are all survivors of a history filled with pain and oppression. Yet, in the concealed depths of the soul is an inborn ability to grow, heal, and find meaning (Duran & Duran, 1995). In group therapy for Chicanas, one goal is to embrace the wisdom ways of Chicana/o ancestors. Teaching the traditional wisdom ways promotes healing not only for Chicana/os but also for the Earth. The survival of both lies in acknowledging that the solutions lie not only in technology and science, but also in a spiritual revolution that sets different priorities in how energy is expended.

In the group setting, the leader is both a teacher and a healer who helps Chicanas refocus toward the spiritual wealth that is part of their ancestral heritage. Their vision of health must include the assessment of the spiritual dimensions of existence. If it is supposed that indeed *susto* (soul loss), *envidia* (envy), and *bilis* (rage) are part of the spiritual ills in need of healing, then the bodily manifestations of these ills must be assessed. These ills are sometimes literally tattooed upon the bodies of tough Chicanas, who often benefit from learning the literal definition of the word *tattoo*, which is the beat of a drum and horn calling home the warrior at night (Merriam-Webster's Collegiate Dictionary, 1993). Thus, in the ills lie the answers. The spirit must return home at night to greet the dawn and reenact the mystery of the death and rebirth cycle that metaphorically is still present, as it was with our ancestors. The acceptance of the symbolism of the reenactment promotes healing and has implications for the treatment of addiction, gang violence, and domestic unrest that plague the families and communities of many Chicanas. Holistic assessment goes far beyond standardized tests, raw scores, and treatment implications that ignore the spiritual realities of Chicanas attending group therapy. Even the type of tattoo adorning a Chicana's body can be used as an assessment device.

In group therapy, discussion often focuses on the participants' ills in families and communities. It is important to offer hope and coping skills in order to keep the group relevant via an intentional focus on the cultural context of each problem.

Those who embrace their indigenous roots are aware of the history of oppression that has led to transgenerational distress. Centuries of oppression fuels grief (*la tristeza*), rage (*el bilis*), and subsequent trauma. The collective soul wound or soul loss is at the core of the suffering, along with la envidia, the disharmony that grows with the gap between the haves and have nots in the American economy. The virus of materialism perpetuates the denial of spiritual truths as people try to buy health and happiness under the guise of consumerism. Spiritual awareness may be lost during the acculturative process. Mainstream values replace spiritual values with those of materialism and logical positivistic approaches that deny meaning in suffering. The core of Chicanas' cultural awareness is the place where the soul wound occurs: the place where mythology, dreams, and culture emerge (Duran & Duran, 1995). It is imperative that group members discuss the ravages of American imperialism and materialism on the souls of *nuestra raza*, our people. The discussion needs to include what is lost when traditional values are exchanged for mainstream American values and what gains may be incurred in the acculturative process.

TRADITIONAL VALUES AS PROTECTIVE FACTORS

Chicana therapy groups often include members with different levels of acculturation, resulting in the need to discuss the tension between the dominant culture and Chicana cultural reality. Some traditional cultural values may be protective factors for Chicanas offering hope for mental and physical health, and should therefore be articulated to call attention to their health-promoting effects. Identification of the protective factors provides not only a rationale for the maintenance of some traditional values for Chicanas within the United States, but also avenues for research with treatment implications for American culture at large.

For example, *Dia de Los Muertos*, or Day of the Dead, is a pre-Columbian and Mexican holiday, with traditions that include protective factors for at least two major conditions: depression related to loss or bereavement and eating disorders. The deceased ancestors are honored at this time and the pre-Columbian tradition focuses attention on spirituality. The belief that the spirit goes on after death is embraced emphatically by less acculturated Chicanas. Although the honoring of the deceased varies regionally, the underlying values remain remarkably intact. First, thanks are given to the Creator for all those who have come before and all who touched one's life with their birth and death. During this time, it is expected that the spirit of these individual family members will return to rejoice about life on Earth and beyond. Each family ritually enacts the building of an altar with *cajas,* or boxes, that include representations of the beloved deceased. In the cajas are *ofrendas,* or offerings, that are placed to please the spirit of the loved one. Favorite foods surround the caja and joyous decorations are made to welcome the return of the spirits of the loved ones. Flowers lead the spirits to their families and incense ensures that no evil spirits follow along. Ritual and ceremony occur within the family in communal processions and in celebrations at the cemetery. Mass is offered for the souls of the deceased in many regions, bringing together Spanish Catholicism and the indigenous reverence for the deceased. Music, prayers, dance, and food are central to the celebration.

In some regions, there are actually three days of celebration. On October 31, there is preparation for the *angelitos,* or little angels, the children in the family who have died. The food is simple and delicious, reflecting the preferences of the children. On November 1, the recently deceased are welcomed home and on November 2 the ancestors are honored. In the United States, modifications have occurred but the traditions continue. There are also some protective factors that can be identified for those who hold on to the traditional values regardless of the fluidity of the actual customs. Annually, all members of the family and community prepare for Dia de Los Muertos by remembering those who have died. Every member makes a decoration that is unique and beautiful and all types of physical beauty are often discussed, particularly the beauty of the old. The opportunity to work on grief and loss issues is expected to go on for a lifetime, a belief that stands in sharp contrast to the views of the dominant American culture with respect to death. Athough Dia de Los Muertos may seem morbid to some, it is important to think about the stories, love, tears, joy that are shared in a way that makes death normal, real, and close at hand versus something to fear and shun. Dia de Los Muertos offers an opportunity to heal wounds, repair relationships, and bond with intimacy and affection following the loss of a loved one. The embracing of the spiritual proclaims that love is stronger than death and the soul lives on.

Related to the role of food in the Dia de Los Muertos celebration is the concept that one can bring on illness by putting pressure on family members to eat, resulting in *empacho,* a stomach ache. No good mother ever wishes empacho on a child and great care is given to acknowledge the food preferences of the individual. Much attention is given to the matter of food in such a collectivistic culture that refuses to embrace individualism as a core value. Why is there so much attention and care around food? To keep the focus on the nurturing aspect of the food, great care is exercised in keeping the family table sacred. Many dichos prohibit tension and discord around food in order to keep people from getting ill. These are protective factors for the culture-bound syndrome of eating disorders, which have reached epidemic proportions in the United States. Eating disorders have not been reported in Chicanas until this past century, when the acculturation process moved at warp speed, driven by the mass media and a single, idealized standard of beauty. Pointing out the value of internal beauty and the many different types of physical beauty that have traditionally been valued is reported to be very validating for Chicanas in the group.

A CASE EXAMPLE

The following case example is representative of the strengths and challenges inherent in the formation and conduction of group therapy for Chicanas. The identifying information has been changed for protection of the confidentiality of the actual group members.

Eight Chicana women ranging in age, acculturation level, socioeconomic status, and educational level gathered weekly for support and for their personal and collective growth and development. With the help of their Chicana leader, they recognized that the bulk of their time in group therapy that particular semester had been spent coping with loss. More specifically, the Chicanas had focused on recent deaths within families and the termination of romantic relationships. The Chicanas felt that a ceremony was needed to fully grieve in a culturally responsive manner. They decided to create a ritual that included Mexican music, candles, photos, and incense and asked to hold the ceremony outside, even after the leader brought up the possible breech of confidentiality and implications for therapeutic alliances. These Chicanas made it clear that they would meet, if necessary, without the leader in order to accomplish their therapeutic goal. The leader had taught the women to advocate for their needs and own unique ways of healing. It became clear that an adjustment to the usual group routine was necessary. The Chicana leader went to her Asian American supervisor to secure permission to possibly breech confidentiality by taking the group outside. In this case, the supervisor and the leader decided that the gains outweighed the therapeutic costs given that precautions were taken to protect client confidentiality.

The women met in a semiprivate location outside and proceeded to talk about their losses with great emotion. Music, candles, photos, and incense were appropriately incorporated. Interestingly, the Chicanas chose to meet under a lilac tree that rained purple petals on the women as they spoke and sang. The outcome of the session was a culmination of a semester's worth of work on grief and loss issues that were particularly salient for these Chicanas. Indeed, they reported that the ceremony was the most beneficial aspect of the therapeutic work.

Empowering themselves to decide how to achieve closure in a culturally responsive manner was most likely the greatest therapeutic gain for the entire group. However, this accomplishment was difficult to achieve for the leader because of traditional contextual requirements that were set forth during her training in group therapy. Clearly, consultations with an ethnic minority supervisor were invaluable in order to optimally exercise judgment and provide a truly culturally responsive adjustment to the therapeutic context.

There are two main lessons to be gleaned from this case example. First, clients often know what they need in order to truly heal. Second, it is important for the leader to advocate on behalf of the clients in order to demonstrate cultural competency.

THE ROLE OF PSYCHOLOGY

The question now is: What role will psychology have in the new millenium? Will psychology be the arm of social control and maintainer of the status quo or will it be a vessel of change, integrity, diversity, and healing? Will our students be taught to blindly adopt a medical model, devoid of emotion and spirituality? Will others be inspired to adopt the best of the wisdom ways, partnering with traditional folk healers and clergy who are not limited by an archaic separation between mind and the body? Will the American paradox of at once creating great health care providers and health care technology but not providing a method for most Chicana/os to access humane care be addressed? What role will psychology play in enhancing and empowering those with traditional cultures? Will psychology collude with the dominant culture to strip away these lifelines, only to replace them with cultural values that are actually vulnerability factors such as exclusive media portrayals of young, thin, blonde, blue-eyed models of "ideal" beauty?

There are some general changes that need to be endorsed by psychology as a profession in order to create culturally responsive modalities for healing:

- The active role of the psychologist as healer
- The incorporation of ceremony and ritual in healing
- The cooperation of psychologists with folk healers or clergy
- The identification of cultural factors that are vulnerability factors related to sickness in mind and body
- The recognition of cultural strengthsas protective factors
- The creation of prevention-focused events that celebrate cultural protective factors

TRAINING ISSUES AND IMPLICATIONS FOR FUTURE RESEARCH

It is important to research and study the effectiveness of traditional wisdom ways that may hold promise for wellness and vitality in Chicana/o families and communities. Equally important is the identification of cultural variables (from all cultures) that may be vulnerability factors related to illness.

The foremost values held by most Chicanas are those of interdependence and collectivism. Chicanas generally believe all humans are children of the Earth, dependent on a Creator and intricately connected to all living and nonliving entities. This spiritual perspective is often ridiculed, but needs empirical study to ascertain the protective and vulnerability factors associated with such cultural beliefs. Spirituality may be the cornerstone for the health and well-being of our Chicana/o communities and is time for psychology to acknowledge this reality and respond in a way that validates it. As practitioners and scholars in the field of psychology, we must dedicate ourselves to learning and sharing the knowledge that comes from practice and empirical efforts in order to better serve our communities and our profession. Groups of Chicanas need to continue to meet, share knowledge, and support their culturally responsive approaches to mind-body health.

It is imperative that concepts and facts no longer be taught outside of their social context, independent of their social and ethical implications (Estrin & Nelson-Barber, 1995). In order to avoid this mistake, all courses in psychology need to emphasize social context, as well as attend to behaviors and symptomatology. Furthermore, it should be a goal within the classroom to promote discussion of diversity issues and to encourage harmony. It is possible to recognize the belief systems of all people and to allow different world views into the classroom. Harmony and balance can be modeled in the classroom, even when there are large value differences that emerge. For example, Chicanas vary in their degree of adherence to values of individualism or collectivism based on level of acculturation, socioeconomic status, and level of education attained in U.S. school systems: More education and higher socioeconomic status are generally associated with greater individualism, which indicates a better fit for treatment modalities that are based on individualistic values and beliefs. Poor immigrants from rural sectors are likely to value collectivism and will thus have the greatest difficulty with treatment modalities that are not culturally responsive.

The beginning of a new century marks the beginning of a reexamination of values and priorities for psychology. Chicana/o psychologists are in a unique position to offer psychology a new vision that embraces the old as well as the modern. What has endured and remained despite colonization, disease, and war is an indigenous philosophy of life and healing. It is time to embrace these indigenous views and bring social science back to the art of healing. It is time to create new culturally responsive treatment modalities, utilize them in therapy, and conduct research to determine their efficacy.

REFERENCES

Arredondo, P. (1992). Promoting the empowerment of women through counseling interventions. *Counseling and Human Development, 24,* 1–8.

Arredondo, P., Psalti, A., & Cella, K. (1993). The woman factor in multicultural counseling. *Counseling and Human Development, 24,* 42–78.

Baca, L., & Koss-Chioino, J. (1997). Development of a culturally responsive group counseling model for Mexican American adolescents. *Journal of Multicultural Counseling and Development, 25,* 130–141.

Barrera, M. (1978). Mexican American mental health service utilization. *Community Mental Health Journal, 14,* 35–45.

Benibo, B., Meyer, P., & Villarreal (1999). Anglo and Mexican American attitudes towards Selena's memorialization. *Hispanic Journal of Behavioral Sciences, 21,* 78–88.

Burruel, G., & Chavez, N. (1974). *Mental health outpatient centers relevant or irrelevant to Mexican Americans: Beyond clinic walls.* Montgomery: University of Alabama Press.

Chavez, L. R., & Martinez, R. G. (1996). Mexican immigration in the 1980's and beyond: Implications for Chicanas/os. In D. R. Maciel & I. D. Ortiz (Eds.), *Chicanas/Chicanos at the crossroads: Social, economic, and political change* (pp. 25–52). Tucson: University of Arizona Press.

Davalos, D., Chavez, E., & Guardiola, R. (1999). The effects of extracurricular activity, ethnic identification, and perception of school on student dropout rates. *Hispanic Journal of Behavior Sciences, 21,* 61–77.

Duran, E., & Duran, B. (1995). *Native American postcolonial psychology.* Albany: State University of New York Press.

Estrin, E. T., & Nelson-Barber, S. (1995). *Issues in cross-cultural assessment: American Indian and Alaskan Native students.* San Francisco: Far West Laboratory.

Federal State Press (Eds.). (1993). *Merriam-Webster's collegiate dictionary* (10th ed.). Springfield MA: Merriam-Webster.

Flores-Ortiz, Y. G. (1995). Psychotherapy with Chicanas at midlife: Cultural/clinical considerations. In J. Adelman & A. Gloria (Eds.), *Racism in the lives of women: Testimony, theory and guides to antiracist practice*. New York: Harrington Park Press/Haworth Press.

Gloria, A. (1998, April). *Comunidad: Promoting the educational persistence and success of Chicana/o college students*. Paper presented at the Julian Zamora Research Institute Conference Innovations in Chicano Psychology: Looking Towards the 21st Century, Kalamazoo, MI.

Gnaulati, E., & Heine, B. (2001). Separation-individuation in late adolescence: An investigation of gender and ethnic differences. *The Journal of Psychology, 135*, 59–70.

Gonzalez-Baker, S. (1996). Demographic trends in the Chicano population: Policy implication for the twenty-first century. In D. R. Maciel & I. D. Ortiz (Eds.), *Chicanas/Chicanos at the crossroads: Social, economic, and political change* (pp. 5–24). Tucson: University of Arizona Press.

Guerrero-Avila, J. (2001). *Hispanic experience in higher education*. Lanham, MD: University Press of America.

Keefe, S. E., & Padilla, A. M. (1987). *Chicano ethnicity*. Albuquerque: University of New Mexico Press.

Maciel, D. R., & Ortiz, I. D. (Eds.). (1996). *Chicanas/Chicanos at the crossroads: Social, economic, and political change*. Tucson: University of Arizona Press.

Markides, K., Roberts-Jolly, J., Ray, L., Hoppe, S., & Rudkin, L. (1999). Changes in marital satisfaction in three generations of Mexican Americans. *Research on Aging, 21*, 36–45.

Martinez, J. L., & Mendoza, R. H. (1984). *Chicano psychology*. Orlando, FL. Academic Press.

Neff, N. (2001, May 24). *Module VII: Folk medicine in Hispanics in the southwestern United States* [On-line]. Available: http://riceinfo.rice.edu/projects/HispanicHealth/Courses/mod7/mod7.html

Niemann, Y. (2001). Stereotypes about Chicanas and Chicanos: Implications for counseling. *The Counseling Psychologist, 29*, 55–90.

Niemann, Y., Romero, A., Arredondo, J., & Rodriguez, V. (1999). What does it mean to be "Mexican"? Social construction of an ethnic identity. *Hispanic Journal of Behavioral Sciences, 21*, 47–60.

Rehm, R. (1999). Religiousness in Mexican-American families dealing with chronic childhood illness. *Image: Journal of Nursing Scholarship, 31*, 33–38.

Roll, S., Millen, L., & Martinez, R. (1980). Common errors in psychotherapy with Chicanos: Extrapolations from research and clinical experience. *Psychotherapy: Theory, Research, and Practice, 17*, 158–168.

Ross, K. (1999). Can diversity and community coexist in higher education? *American Behavioral Scientist, 42*, 1024–1040.

Shorr, J. E., Sobel, P. R., & Connella, J. A. (Eds.). (1980). *Imagery: Its many dimensions and applications*. New York: Plenum Press.

Yalom, I. (1995). *The theory and practice of group psychotherapy*. New York: Basic Books.

Zuniga, M. E. (1988). Assessment issues with Chicanas: Practice implications. *Psychotherapy, 25*, 288–293.

IV

Conceptualizing Effective Intervention:
La Familia

Domestic Violence in Chicana/o Families

Yvette G. Flores-Ortiz
University of California, Davis

> *La violencia empieza desde el primer momento en que se te falta el respeto.*
> —Ana, 35 años

> *En mi matrimonio solo he conocido golpes, insultos y pena. Eso no es ser familia.*
> —Sofia, 40 años

Domestic or intimate violence rates in the United States have reached epidemic proportions. Between 1993 and 1998, women ages 16 to 24 experienced the highest per capita rates of intimate violence (19.6 per 1,000 women). During the same time period, only about half the intimate partner violence against women was reported to the police; Black women were more likely than other women to report such violence (U.S. Department of Justice, 1999).

Intimate violence, however, is not just a crime against women: Nearly half of the female victims of intimate partner violence lived in households with children under age 12, which represent 27% of U.S. households. Thus, although women may be the primary victims in cases of intimate violence, children are also significantly affected (Flores-Ortiz, 2000b).

Although intimate violence is not generally lethal, serious injury can occur, particularly in situations of long-term abuse. Between 1993 and 1998, half of female victims of intimate partner violence reported a physical injury, but only about 4 in 10 of these victims sought professional medical treatment. Detection of the abuse increased when medical personnel were trained to investigate injuries and to assess for the possibility of domestic violence (Rodriguez, Bauer, & Flores-Ortiz, 2001; Rodriguez, Bauer, Flores-Ortiz, & Skupinski-Quiroga, 1998).

Straus et al. (1989) operationalized violent behaviors as efforts by individuals and couples to resolve conflict. These efforts may be productive, as in the case of negotiation, or abusive, resulting in psychological aggression, physical aggression, sexual coercion, and injuries. These five dimensions of conflict resolution can be measured in terms of frequency and severity utilizing the Conflict Tactics Scale (Flores-Ortiz, Valdez Curiel & Andrade Palos, in press; Straus et al., 1998).

It is not clear how socioeconomic status, race, and ethnicity contribute to the incidence of domestic violence. Intimate violence occurs in all social classes. However,
detection and reporting of these crimes is more likely among the poor and working
class, thus creating the false impression that domestic violence is more prevalent
among the economically disadvantaged. Overall, in terms of reported cases of
domestic violence between 1993 and 1998, African Americans were victimized by
intimate partners at significantly higher rates than persons of any other race. Black
females experienced intimate partner violence at a rate 35% higher than that of White
females, and about 22 times the rate of women of other races. Black males experienced intimate partner violence at a rate about 62% higher than that of White males
and about 22 times the rate of men of other races. No difference in intimate partner
victimization rates between Hispanics and non-Hispanics emerged, regardless of
gender. Specific figures concerning the rates of domestic violence among Chicana/os
are not available, as the government does not disaggregate data in terms of national
origin or ethnic identification among Hispanics. Straus et al. (1989) found high rates
of domestic violence, particularly serious physical abuse, in a sample of Hispanics
who participated in his national study. However, the national origin of these respondents is unknown. Clinical and anecdotal data do suggest a serious violence problem
within Chicana/o families (Flores-Ortiz, Esteban, & Carrillo, 1994; Flores-Ortiz,
Valdez Curiel, & Andrade Palos, in press; Rodriguez et al., 2001).

The manner in which Chicana/os understand and define violence may have a
bearing on rates of reporting and tolerance of the problem within Chicana/o families,
thus it is crucial to examine the context within which intimate violence occurs in
these families. This chapter offers an empirically based model of understanding and
treating domestic violence among Chicana/os in the United States.

THE CONTEXT OF DOMESTIC VIOLENCE

Definitions

From a legal standpoint, domestic violence includes the physical, emotional, psychological, and sexual abuse of an intimate partner (Straus et al., 1989). At the core
of intimate violence is the abuse of power inherent in the relational contract made
by two people (Almeida et al., 1996). Walker (1979) described domestic violence as
a cyclical process that begins with a buildup of stress in which one partner is unable
to release in more appropriate ways. The pent-up stress may generate a number of
psychological sequelae: anxiety, fear of loss, fear of intimacy, and so on, depending
on the psychological makeup of the individual and the patterns of interaction
developed by the couple. When the stress becomes intolerable, the individual may
express this internal affective state through an act of aggression, causing physical
injury or psychological and emotional harm to the other. If the aggrieved partner
does not leave the relationship, set clear limits of what is acceptable, or views such
aggression as normal (because of childhood exposure to domestic violence, for
example), the violence is likely to recur. In the early stages of domestic violence, the
aggression of one partner may be followed by a period of remorse, acts of repen-

tance, and a honeymoon phase in which the aggressor promises never to hurt the partner again. When stress and tension build up again, the cycle may be repeated. Over time, the honeymoon phase is replaced with fear on the part of the aggrieved, a state of hypervigilance, and, at times, violent responses from the partner who has been victimized. Ultimately, the cycle may run quickly from tension buildup to violent release. In some couples, the violence is frequent, resulting in a certain degree of predictability; in others, it is intermittent and unpredictable. In both instances, over time intimate violence becomes normalized. One or both partners take the position that "this is just how things are," which can lead in turn to feelings of hopelessness and disempowerment (Flores-Ortiz, Esteban, & Carrillo, 1994; Walker).

From a clinical standpoint, domestic violence also includes the use of anger and intimidation, threats and humiliation, isolation and restriction of freedom, abuse of male privilege, use of children to control the actions of women, and sexual, economic, emotional, and moral exploitation (Roberts, 1984; Walker, 1979). For individuals who did not grow up believing that intimate violence was normal, disrespect is often viewed as the first act of aggression.

In many couples, violence becomes a way of life, and it may no longer be clear who initiated the aggression. In heterosexual couples where the males utilize physical aggression and psychological control of the women, women may respond with verbal abuse and emotional withholding. In gay and lesbian couples, similar patterns of interaction may occur, or both partners may use physical violence to exert control in situations of perceived loss of control. Thus, from a prevention and treatment standpoint, domestic violence must be viewed and understood systemically as a complex set of multidetermined and maintained interactions.

ETIOLOGICAL EXPLANATIONS

Theoretical Formulations

The interpersonal dynamics of violent couples and the psychological characteristics of perpetrators and victims have been explained from a number of theoretical perspectives, including psychoanalysis, social learning, family systems, and feminist theory (Flores-Ortiz, 1993a). Although these theories differ in their explanations of the causes of intimate violence, they concur on the description of the victim and the perpetrator. Victims of intimate violence are described as individuals who lack self-esteem, experience difficulty expressing their own needs, often demonstrate a long-suffering, martyr-like endurance of frustration, and manifest depressive or hysterical symptoms, stress disorders, and psychosomatic complaints. From a psychodynamic perspective, these individuals, particularly when they are women, are described as masochistic. Such theories clearly disregard the larger social context of violence against women and ultimately blame women for their own victimization (Luepnitz, 1998; Yllo, 1984).

Male perpetrators of intimate violence are described as lacking self-esteem and appropriate avenues for expressing anger and rage. Their lack of impulse control is viewed as as a function of unsatisfied ego needs, often the result of childhood deprivation and poor mothering. Consequently, their interpersonal relationships are characterized by mistrust, insecurity, and jealousy. The batterer may himself have been an abused child or a witness of domestic violence. His childhood victimization is believed to culminate in an insatiable need to control others, particularly women, through force, intimidation, and violence. These behaviors may be used in the name of love, protection of the woman, and preservation of the family.

Whereas psychodynamic theories explicate intimate violence in terms of intrapsychic processes and personality characteristics, social learning theories argue that intimate violence is learned. Men who batter have learned to be violent because they have observed the behavior of other men and because their aggression has been normalized and reinforced. Moreover, they have not learned more effective and appropriate ways of problem solving. Women, on the other hand, have been socialized to accept and even reinforce the behaviors of men, whether appropriate or not. Gender role socialization, in fact, encourages male aggression and female passivity; thus, societies and cultures that emphasize rigid sex role differentiation are believed to produce a familial context ripe for spousal and child abuse (Almeida et al., 1996; Flores-Ortiz, 1993a).

Though helping to explain psychological factors and socialization influences, psychoanalytic and social learning theories do not provide an analysis of the larger context in which violence occurs. Family systems theories begin to offer a more comprehensive analysis of the context of intimate violence by viewing it as a family problem, grounded in dysfunctional patterns learned generationally or over time, specifically, imbalances of power (Madanes, 1994), rigid boundaries (Minuchin, 1974), rigid sex roles, and rigid efforts to maintain family cohesion (Flores-Ortiz 1993a, 2000b; Flores-Ortiz et al., 1994).

Feminist theorists (Almeida, Woods, Messineo, & Font, 1996; Luepnitz, 1998), however, critique both individual and systemic theories for their disregard of the gender issues inherent in the problem of violence against women. They argue that domestic violence is rooted in patriarchal systems and values that privilege men over women and adults over children, objectify women, and dehumanize men (Yllo, 1984). Thus, solutions to the problem of family violence hinge on the empowerment of women and on radical change within social institutions, including marriage and parenthood. It was certainly the advocacy of feminist groups that resulted in legislation criminalizing domestic violence late in the 20th century.

Feminist theories, however, only partially explain the increase in female aggression toward intimate partners (U.S. Department of Justice, 2000). It may be that women respond violently in situations of intimate violence due to their psychological characteristics, frustration, or fear, or as a way to gain control in situations of chronic disempowerment (Morales, 2001).

Existing etiological explanations continue to lack a class and race analysis, thus ignoring the impact of migration, colonization, and neocolonization on the psychological and familial development of women and men, particularly those whose nations and cultures have been conquered, colonized, or occupied. The absence of such an analysis tends to create etiological explanations and theoretical formulations that blame the culture or the individual while obscuring the impact of state violence on people's lives.

SOCIOCULTURAL CORRELATES
OF DOMESTIC VIOLENCE

Elsewhere, I described a model for analyzing and treating domestic violence among Chicana/os (Flores-Ortiz, 2000b). At the core of this model is the proposition that the roots of interpersonal injustice within the family and society are located in a historical legacy of oppression and colonization. In addition, the stratified caste system based on race, ethnicity, religion, sexuality, and ability became instituted when the first world collided with the American continent. Injustice was historically institutionalized through limited access to education, employment, and sources of power, resulting in a pyramid of oppression in which those in power predicated belonging and dispossession on degree of acceptance. In the Americas, from the time of the conquest, Europeans (and those who looked European) were privileged over Mestiza/os and men were privileged over women (Almeida et al., 1996).

Thus, the patriarchal legacies in the Americas were racialized. All men and women were not considered equal. Rigid sex role socialization mandated a different code of behaviors for men and women; moreover, women who were considered European and from higher social classes had more access to power and privilege than indigenous or Mestiza women. In the colonial era in the Americas, European men could possess anything not considered holy; thus, indigenous women could be raped, enslaved, or made concubines. From a psychodynamic perspective, such massive domination affected men and women differentially. According to Diaz-Guerrero (1954, 1994), the conquest and colonization of Mexico created a complex in Mexican men who felt historically dispossessed, *el ser chingado*, literally, to be existentially raped, and has led many Mexican men to overcompensate feelings of powerlessness and dispossession with exaggerated bravado and machismo. Women, in turn, were made to feel inferior to men, subject to their rage, and responsible for their psychological and emotional well-being (Baker Miller, 1976). This led to a culture of abnegation and quiet suffering where men are taught to aggress and women to tolerate (Flores-Ortiz, 1998). In fact, such gender roles have been reified and reinforced through the use of religious symbolism. Women are taught to emulate the abnegation and silent strength of the Virgin Mary. Cultural values of self-sacrifice, submission, and passivity for women and stoicism and endurance for men become the cultural templates for the socialization of children and the negotiation of intimate relationships.

In summary, injustice results in a hierarchy of oppression in which those with more power use it over those perceived as having less. At an interpersonal and intrafamilial level, power over relationships lead to a culture of terror and disrespect where violence can easily occur. Moreover, the influence of structural factors on intrafamily abuse has not been examined empirically. Clinical data do suggest that men who feel oppressed in their work and larger social context and who hold rigid sex role views are more likely to be violent toward those they love (Flores-Ortiz, 1993a, 1998, 1999; Flores-Ortiz et al., 1994).

In order to examine empirically the relationship between spousal interaction and marital satisfaction among Mexicans, Diaz-Loving and Andrade Palos (1996) investigated a couple's desire for interaction, desire to know each other, frustration or dissatisfaction, and fear distancing. Their findings suggested that, when women experience frustration with or fear of their partner, their desire to know and interact with him decreases. For men, however, only fear was related to a reduction in desire to interact with the partner. Flores-Ortiz, Valdez Curiel, and Andrade Palos (2004) examined these same variables and their relationship to conflict resolution among 500 Mexican individuals in long-term couple relationships in the state of Mexico and 500 couples in the state of Jalisco. Their findings indicated that physically violent couples experienced fear of the partner and a reduction in desire to know and interact with the other. Moreover, violent couples (both men and women) espoused a greater belief in male superiority and female passivity, as measured by the machismo scale of Diaz-Guerrero (1994). These data suggest that men and women who use violent tactics with their partners also experience fear of interaction and a distancing from their partners. Likewise, the data support the theoretical proposition that traditional and rigid gender roles that support male superiority and female abnegation and submission contribute to intimate violence. To what extent these patterns are present in Chicana/os is unknown, as no large-scale empirical studies have been conducted with this population.

MIGRATION AND TRANSCULTURATION

Falicov (1998) and Sluzki (1979) identified the disruptive influence of migration on family functioning. Particularly affected are gender roles, the relationship between parents and children, and role expectations among family members, as the process of migration challenges the cultural, economic, and psychological resources of individuals and families. The greater the difference between the country of origin and the host country, the more likely postmigration difficulties are. Furthermore, the challenges of transculturation may take generations to resolve. Likewise, the disruptive influence of migration may not be initially apparent, but becomes visible at critical developmental points in the life of a family, when children enter school and begin to learn a new language, when women enter the paid work force for the first time, when men are unable to find work, or when children leave home. Language differences, economic disparities between the immigrant and the receiving countries, and racial differences exacerbate the normative adjustments of migration. In the case of Chicana/os, the United States migrated to those Mexicana/os already living in the Southwest, creating a colonial and neocolonial context where Mexicans became incorporated into a nation that occupied them with concomitant losses of language, status, and material possessions. Thus, Mexicana/os in what is now the Southwest experienced what their ancestors had endured centuries earlier when the Europeans first arrived on the American continent. It could be argued that the same psychological sequelae of marginality and dispossession described by Diaz-Guerrero (1994) affecting Mexicana/os have also affected Chicana/os, increasing their risk for psychological distress and intimate violence.

According to the 2000 census, 39.1% of the U.S. Latina/o population were foreign born. Of these 12.8 million people, the majority are Mexican. Historically, Mexicana/os have migrated for economic reasons. Generally the men migrated first and eventually emigrated their wives and children. In recent years, Mexican women have migrated alone or with their partners, because it is often easier for women to find employment as domestics than it is for men to find work (Falicov, 1998). A number of studies (De la Torre & Pesquera, 1993; Flores-Ortiz, 2000a; Pesquera, 2000) outlined the impact of migration on the traditional gender roles of Mexicana/os. One significant sequela of migration is the creation of power imbalances in the couple relationship as women enter the labor force and begin to experience greater economic freedom. If their male partners can exhibit flexibility and less rigid attitudes toward sex roles, the couple may cope with the stress of role transition and find harmony. Some men, however, experience a loss of self-esteem, develop psychiatric symptomatology, and potentially behave violently, creating further stress and difficulties for the couple. Over time, these couples may experience frustration, distancing, fear, and a reduction in positive attitudes and feelings toward each other (Flores-Ortiz, 1993a, 1998).

Transgenerational Violence and Sequelae of Intimate Violence

The impact of long-term exposure to state or family violence has not been studied empirically with Chicana/os. Clinical data do suggest that individuals suffering from posttraumatic stress disorder as a result of exposure to war, childhood victimization, domestic violence, or traumatic migrations may be more prone to intimate relationships where violence occurs (Bauer et al., 2000; Flores-Ortiz 1997a, 1999, 2000b; Rodriguez et al., 2001). Furthermore, imprisoned women and men were typically victimized as children. Alcohol and other drug abuse often correlates with childhood victimization, which in turn leads to other problems, including delinquency, adult criminality, and intimate violence (Flores-Ortiz, 1999; Morales, 2001).

In summary, Chicano families must deal with a complex interaction of experiences that can contribute to domestic violence (Bernal & Flores-Ortiz, 1982; Falicov, 1982; Flores-Ortiz, 1982), including migration, acculturation, underemployment, undereducation, and economic stress. The long-term impact of colonization in the country of origin and neocolonization in the U.S. context can create a "victim system" (Pinderhughes, 1982) characterized as an expectation of suffering and exploitation, an expectation often reinforced by patriarchal and religious influences. The identification and treatment of intimate violence thus requires a comprehensive assessment of historical, ecological, systemic, and individual factors.

GUIDELINES FOR EVALUATING AND TREATING DOMESTIC VIOLENCE

The goal of treatment for Chicana/os is to seek in the culture of the family and the individuals within the family the resources and solutions to end the violence, exploitation, and pain. The key to treating the problem of domestic violence in a culturally integrated way is to offer services for the entire family, irrespective of which family member first seeks them (Flores-Ortiz, 1993a). Regardless of the specific interventions offered, the agency or professional must be committed to addressing the needs of the entire family through direct intervention or appropriate referral (Carrillo & Goubaud-Reyna, 1998; Flores-Ortiz et al., 1994).

Assessment

The first step in the treatment of domestic violence is the assessment of lethality (i.e., the likelihood that a homicide will occur) and of the safety of all family members. Lethality is generally determined on the basis of the degree of physical violence resulting in injuries, the frequency of all types of abuse, and the duration of the violence. For example, long-term abuse that is frequent and results in physical harm may culminate in serious injury or a fatality. In such cases, it is in everyone's best interests for the family to separate. The aggressor may need to be incarcerated temporarily and should be mandated to treatment (Almeida et al., 1996) until the danger is acknowledged and accountability is established (Flores-Ortiz, 1998, 1999). Presented as efforts to save the family and protect everyone, such recommendations, even when enforced legally, are more likely to be accepted and followed through by the family. It must be noted that, when women are socialized and expected to protect men and be loyal to the family, they may be less likely to report abuse. Therefore, it is essential for health and mental health personnel to routinely inquire about intimate violence, whether or not it is a presenting problem (Bauer et al., 2000; Rodriguez et al., 2001).

Following an assessment of lethality and appropriate follow-up, the evaluation needs to focus on the historical and ecological context of the family or individual, including the woman's economic viability, familial and cultural resources in the event of a prolonged separation, level of acculturation, cultural connection, and familial (including extended family) resources. Part of an integrated case management includes the identification of social and cultural needs. Psychological evaluations of the children and adults can be helpful in determining need for individual psychotherapy as well as in assessing child abuse or neglect. Subsequently, in order to determine the most appropriate type of treatment, the following areas of assessment are recommended:

- History of migration: stages, reasons, traumas, postmigration experiences, and stressors.
- History of exposure to violence (including state, social, intrafamilial and intimate) in the country of origin and the United States; for U.S.-born Chicana/os, examination of their knowledge of the family's history of intimate violence over time.
- History of coping strategies (pre- and postmigration).
- Degree of daily indignities and feelings of marginality, discrimination, and oppression experienced by each family member.
- Level of biculturality, cultural connection and disconnection, and ethnic identity.
- Level of bilingualism, comfort with use of each language, context of language use (e.g., English at work, Spanish with spouse, with children, and in the social milieu).
- Socioeconomic and cultural resources (including material, familial, and spiritual support).
- Cultural meaning of alcohol use.
- Use of alcohol and other drugs.

- Intergenerational and cultural conflicts.
- Patterns of communication.
- Family organization and structure.
- Role expectations.
- Patterns of cultural freezing.
- Parentification of children.

On the basis of this detailed history, determinations are made on the most appropriate treatment method. If the perpetrator is a man who is living with his family, the involvement of the family in some type of treatment is essential. It facilitates the continuing evaluation of lethality and the protection of the woman and children. If the perpetrator is a woman, methods of de-escalating the violence must be implemented and the safety of the children must be ensured. In summary, an assessment of the family or individual's ecological context provides the clinician with a more comprehensive view of the factors that may have contributed to the onset of violence or that help maintain unfair ways of relating. Furthermore, the evaluation helps to identify specific family dynamics that are associated with domestic violence (Flores-Ortiz, 1993a).

Family Dynamics Associated With Intimate Violence

Dysfunctional Chicano families demonstrate a number of characteristics that contribute to the development of family violence (Flores-Ortiz & Bernal, 1990; Flores-Ortiz et al., 1994). Among these are frozen cultural patterns, parentification of children, indirect or intrusive patterns of communication, and intergenerational problems.

Cultural Freezing

Cultural freezing refers to the development of rigid, stereotyped values and behaviors as a result of a difficult migration process (Sluzki, 1979) in which cut-offs (an extreme form of disengagement) from family and culture of origin occur. The immigrant family or individual attempts to recreate, in the new context, an ideal of how a Mexican family should be. This ideal may be based on distorted or rigid notions of Latino culture. In addition, to maintain family unity and to protect the family from external threat, rigid boundaries may be formed around the family, minimizing contact with Anglos and even other Mexicans. The development of this pattern of isolation is facilitated by structural factors such as racism and discrimination, which separate individuals and families from the Anglo world and restrict their full participation in Anglo society. The excessive protection of the family eventually may result in social isolation, lack of trust in the new culture, and fears for the safety of women and children. In situations where the family has limited economic or cultural resources, frustration and despair may grow, potentially leading to violent behavior as individuals find themselves unable to cope with the challenges of a new ecological context (Falicov, 1998).

In families where cultural freezing has occurred, a pattern of rigid sex role expectations typically develops. The man perceives his primary role as provider and negotiator with the outside world; he expects the woman to create for him a safe haven to which he can retreat. Stereotypical cultural patterns of machismo (male superiority and privilege and female submission) prevail, where the man may feel entitled to all freedoms and the woman to none. If his perceived supremacy is threatened by unemployment, the forced entry of the woman into the labor force, or outside threats to his role, the man may experience unbearable stress and engage in violent behaviors in order to regain control.

At an individual psychological level, cultural freezing can result in the internalization of negative cultural stereotypes of machismo. For example, men tend to have little trust in women (with the possible exception of their mothers). They view women as treacherous, and therefore in need of being controlled, protected, and guided. The experience of colonization and neocolonization also affects the self-esteem of Chicano men. Men who batter often describe themselves as *burros,* beasts of burden, or surplus people. The psychological effect of such self-perception is typically overwhelming anger and hostility that cannot be expressed directly toward the aggressor (who may be a boss or structural factors that are faceless and nameless). The rage, however, can be expressed within the safe haven of the home, toward those perceived as weaker, responsible for the stress, or expected to *aguantar* (tolerate and hold) the pain of men (i.e., women and children).

Men who exhibit excessive machismo tend to mask their vulnerability with a veneer of stoicism; they attempt to control their emotions and not appear weak. Therefore, they may narcotize their pain through substance use, which in turn allows them to feel the pain and contributes to violence. However, if the man acts violently while under the influence, he tends to blame the substance and not himself for the actions. Moreover, a frozen cultural view that all Mexicanos and Chicanos drink supports inappropriate drinking patterns that can exacerbate the problem of violence.

Cultural freezing, the colonial legacy, and the racism of the new context also have an impact on Mexicana/os and Chicana/os. Women in battering relationships are affected by cultural variables that contribute to the cycle of violence, key among these the myth of martyrdom (Bernal & Alvarez, 1983). Through religious and cultural symbols (the Virgin, Malinche, Mary Magdalene, etc.), ideal women are depicted as self-sacrificing, self-effacing, long-suffering martyrs or as treacherous harlots. These cultural stereotypes have been reified by social scientists on both sides of the border (Diaz-Guerrero, 1954) and can be internalized not as stereotypes, but as cultural mandates and ideals that, when frozen, translate into how a Chicana should be. Influenced by these mandates, Chicanas may feel that it is their lot in life to suffer. As women, they are to be defined by their family roles; their primary obligation is to preserve the family at all costs, under any circumstances. Thus, a bad marriage, even a violent one, is a cross that a woman must bear.

The socialization process in families with frozen cultural values tends to make women feel primarily responsible for the emotional well-being of men. It is their responsibility to make the home into a safe haven, reduce family-related stress, and, if necessary, become the primary parent so that the men will not have to deal with the stress of parenting. Eventually, the women come to see the man as a *pobrecito,* a vulnerable person who is incapable of holding and managing his own emotions, facing the stress of everyday life, and nurturing his children or partner. Over time, the woman's efforts to protect the man further imbalance the family relationships; she becomes overburdened and perhaps symptomatic (depression, somatization) and he may eventually resent and blame her for the emotional distance between himself and his children. If he beats her, she is made to feel responsible for her own victimization. From a cultural perspective, machismo without control and excessive martyrdom create a perfect context for family violence. Thus, in a context of cultural freezing, particularly when economic and social victimization also occur, violence may begin as a result of external stress and eventually be maintained for generations.

Parentification of Children

The psychological make-up of people who grow up in violent families differs. Not all children of batterers grow up to be violent men or victimized women. Family theorists explain these differences on the basis of the concepts of parentification (Bernal, 1980; Minuchin, 1974) and family loyalty (Boszormenyi-Nagy & Spark, 1984). Certain children in violent families are consciously or unconsciously picked by their parents to fulfill the role of surrogate parents and to become responsible for satisfying the unmet psychological needs of the adults. The parents are unable to provide the child with the basic love, nurturance, and security all human beings need in order to develop psychological integrity and emotional security. Instead, the child is expected to provide these for the adults. Because the child will fail, the parent may become excessively punitive as he or she continues to believe the world fails him or her. Thus, the child and parent become bound in an exploitative relationship wherein the child must sacrifice him or herself for the parent. This child may develop into a disentitled adult who expects to suffer, or a destructively entitled adult who feels the world owes him or her and collects this existential debt from future partners and children.

In violent Chicano families, parentification is exemplified by overreliance on one child, usually the eldest, to help raise the other children, become mother's confidant or protector or father's ally, or mediate family disputes. Parentified children usually do not feel entitled to ask for any emotional, spiritual, or physical support from their parents. Rather, they feel they must take care of everyone else at the expense of their own independence, well-being, and emotional health. Women tend to suppress their feelings of outrage at the injustices in their lives, as they can only express their rage in indirect ways. Men, however, have the social and cultural sanction to express their anger in violent ways, although typically they do not see the relationship between their actions and their childhood victimization.

In families where substance abuse is also present, children can be further victimized through physical neglect, abuse, and incest. As children are fundamentally loyal to and depend on their parents for their very existence (Boszormenyi-Nagy & Spark, 1984), efforts to change learned patterns of abuse in adulthood may invoke feelings of disloyalty. Thus, parentified and exploited children may be more likely to enter dysfunctional relationships where continuing victimization may occur, in this way perpetuating family violence across generations.

Family Communication

Family communication refers to the overt and covert rules according to which a family operates, including the expectations of sex role behavior, child-rearing patterns, and conflict resolution strategies learned in families of origin. Violent families are characterized by indirect communication, mind reading, difficulty expressing feelings, emotional withdrawal, fear, and explosive displays of anger. Emotional, verbal, psychological, and moral abuse are ways in which family members communicate distress, anxiety, fear, and powerlessness. Although these forms of abuse leave no visible scars or bruises, they are destructive to the emotional well-being of all family members. Emotional withholding, expressions of excessive jealousy, and verbal expressions of rage assault individuals' own sense of self and integrity (Walker, 1979).

Chicana/os who are violent often are unable to express any feelings other than anger; they order, command, yell, and offend verbally. Their partners may be afraid of their moods, particularly if they also drink. This fear can translate into violent behavior for the women as well. These patterns of interaction reinforce the frozen roles already existing in the family, particularly when the family is isolated or lacks outside resources.

Moreover, because many Chicana/os are guarded and demonstrate a reluctance to discuss family problems with outsiders, it is critical to differentiate between culturally appropriate manifestations of stoicism and strong boundaries, and dysfunctional patterns that may be associated with abuse.

Intergenerational and Cultural Value Conflicts

In immigrant families, one of the major postmigration crises is the acculturation of the children and the subsequent value change away from parental expectations, as these changes may pose a threat to desired family unity. In families where cultural freezing is occurring and where the conditions for family violence exist, conflicts between the parents and the children may escalate into violence. Invariably, the mother is blamed for any deviation from expected child behavior because she is responsible for raising the children properly. The man may feel the need to exercise greater control to prevent further acculturation. When this inevitably fails, he may feel more frustrated, powerless, and disrespected by the family, and respond with physical violence.

A variant of this crisis occurs when the female partner acculturates due to entry into the labor force and begins to desire greater role equity. Likewise, when a traditional immigrant man partners with a more acculturated or U.S.-born Chicana or a Latina from a higher class background. The value differences may be profound, particularly in terms of the role of women. If the man believes the woman should be controlled and she resists, he may respond with violence, to "get her in line."

In summary, Chicano families with a problem of violence are characterized by cultural freezing and a concomitant rigidity and isolation, cultural value differences, dysfunctional communication, and a repetition of learned patterns of communication, problem solving, and child rearing that maintains the problem of violence. As with most other cultural groups (Bauer et al., 2000), Chicanas who are battered are typically blamed for their own victimization by the batterer, the larger cultural system, and the social institutions that exist to help her. If she is the violent partner, or if she responds to abuse with violence, she is further ostracized and often considered to be mentally ill.

Chicanas who are battered tend not to leave their partners or husbands for very long. They may temporarily use shelters, social service resources, or family support, but eventually they return home. An understanding of why this happens requires an analysis of socioeconomic, cultural, and psychological factors. The battered woman may lack financial resources and may respond to the abuse with depression and learned helplessness (Walker, 1979), unable to see alternatives. If she was victimized as a child, she may see further victimization as her lot in life. Furthermore, the woman's relatives may pressure her to return in order to preserve the family. The social construction of men as *pobrecitos* encourages women to repeatedly forgive abusers and give them another chance. Even if she has financial, legal, and familial resources to seek safety and protect herself, a battered Chicana may still need to contend with feelings of cultural and familial disloyalty that will come as a result of her leaving, particularly if she was raised and socialized to put herself and her needs last. Often, social service workers become frustrated at the seeming inability of battered Chicanas to leave abusive situations. Unwittingly, the woman or her culture is blamed for the abuse and the woman's inability to stop it.

To end the violence, Chicana/os must confront and understand the historical roots of their oppression and seek cultural solutions to the problem of abuse. Clinicians also must understand the historical, ecological, and cultural context of domestic violence among Chicana/os in order to provide culturally attuned and effective treatments.

Considerations for Family Therapists

Elsewhere, I outlined group therapies for batterers (Flores-Ortiz, 1993a) and specific family interventions for immigrant Latina/os (Flores-Ortiz, 1997b, 1998). The focus here is on family-centered interventions with U.S.-born Chicana/os. With the use of a case example, systemic-intergenerational and justice-based treatment approaches are demonstrated.

Justice-Based Approaches

The treatment of domestic violence from a justice-based perspective rests on several assumptions. Social injustice, or any form of oppression, leads to unfairness in intimate relationships. If oppression occurs, it can lead to isolation, family breakup, development of dysfunctional patterns of relating, loss of identity, and even destruction of culturally healthy patterns of relating (Aboriginal Health Council of South Australia, 1995). Relationships may suffer, leading to inauthentic connections as individuals isolate, disconnect from feelings, and develop a veneer of stoicism and invulnerability. If unchallenged, such patterns of relating may be generationally transmitted as legacies of disempowerment, hopelessness, and despair, thus creating a reservoir of pain on multiple levels. Not only is the individual and his or her family affected, but neighborhoods, communities, and larger systems may suffer as well (Flores-Ortiz, 2000a).

The pain of injustice may turn into explosive anger or rage. Intimate violence, social violence, self-abuse, and the maltreatment of children are some of the expressions of injustice and despair. However, in a more optimistic light, the pain of injustice may also be transformed into creativity, *entereza* (wholeness), and resilience (Flores-Ortiz, 1998).

The Gutierrez Family

Rolando and Yolanda sought marital therapy due to "relationship conflicts." Both were very attractive, successful attorneys in their mid-30s. Married for 8 years, the couple was faced with a developmental challenge: Rolando wanted to have a child, but Yolanda felt that a pregnancy would jeopardize her chances of making partner at a very competitive and high-profile firm. Although Rolando had always supported Yolanda's education (they met while in college) and aspirations, he now felt that she should take time out to have a child, as he could easily support them both. Yolanda argued that they should wait until she made partner. During a particularly difficult argument, Rolando accused Yolanda of being disloyal and not Chicana enough, and struck her. Yolanda hit him back. The police were called by the neighbors and interrupted the fight. At the time of the first session, both felt ashamed of the arrest and frightened that violence might recur, as they had become increasingly disconnected from each other and verbally abusive.

This was a couple in a relational impasse; each felt equally justified in his or her respective position and was unwilling to negotiate. The assessment obtained significant information, which helped clarify how a previously harmonious relationship had suddenly turned violent.

Psychosocial and Cultural Considerations. Both partners were first-generation professionals. They had struggled with economic hardship and major structural barriers to obtain their degrees. They both came from large farm worker families and had helped their siblings through college as well. Although they both espoused highly familistic views, Rolando held more traditional gender role attitudes. Rolando wanted a large family; Yolanda did not. He felt women should prioritize family over career and had become increasingly concerned that Yolanda was "stalling" on the family enterprise. Yolanda accused him of being *machista* and insensitive. This argument became recursive until it erupted into violence. A few days prior to the fight, Rolando had been turned down as partner. His future with the firm felt uncertain and he admitted to feeling jealous of his wife's apparent greater professional success.

Although this couple did not have financial concerns, they were not immune from work-related stress. Yolanda felt that her husband's firm was ethnically discriminating against him. Even though he did not agree with her, he did acknowledge feeling excluded from many important decisions. His stress had been building for some time. He felt invisible, unappreciated, and disrespected. In his words, Yolanda's refusal to have a child was the last straw and he "lost it." Intellectually, Rolando understood the unfairness of blaming her for his difficulties and of venting his rage on her. Emotionally, however, he did not know what else to do. He felt his masculinity and role functioning were being challenged.

Through a reconstructive dialogue (Boszormenyi-Nagy & Spark, 1984; Flores-Ortiz, 1998), the couple explored alternative solutions to their impasse. Rolando began to look for a different job, which increased his firm's interest in him. The couple agreed to postpone having children for 2 years; at that time they would begin to try to have a child whether or not Yolanda had made partner. The couple reinstated their daily 5-minute *pláticas* (brief talks), which had been forgotten as they became engrossed in their careers. Since courtship, they had developed a habit of spending a few minutes "connecting" and checking in with each other authentically. This was a sacred time for them, when each could hear and be present for the other. Sometimes the time spent together was indeed only 5 minutes, but often it continued as they took care of household chores or shared sexual intimacy. Both partners agreed that, if either ever felt drawn to violence again, they would take time out or meditate until they felt in greater control.

Given the psychological and material resources of this couple, interrupting the cycle of violence was not difficult. Both partners could discuss and come to understand how their sex role expectations had influenced, albeit invisibly, how each approached marriage and parenthood. They also understood how, as professionals from marginalized communities, the stakes were greater and success and failure had meaning beyond themselves. They were role models for their family and community. Once they could voice these invisible pressures, they felt capable of supporting each other, rather than engaging in intimate warfare over structural issues. For couples that face more serious challenges, the interventions may need to be multimodal and long term.

The Lopez Family

A couple in their late 30s, Jose worked as a janitor and his wife as a secretary for a large corporation. Jose did not finish high school but Jane enrolled in night school to earn her GED. Jose had struggled with alcoholism since young adulthood. The couple had two children, boys ages 7 and 9, and the couple was referred to treatment after Jose was arrested for domestic violence.

The couple met and married while still in high school. Since then, they had struggled with financial problems and Jose's drinking. He saw his drinking as a "cultural thing" that helped him cope. Jane saw it as a drain on the family's finances and mental health. The couple had had a fairly stable relationship early on, but as his drinking increased Jose began to beat Jane. Jane was too ashamed to tell the family and tried to hide the bruises, even from her children. She felt she needed to support her husband and explained his behavior as loss of control while intoxicated. However, it was harder for her to understand his violence when sober. On two occasions, Jane had hit Jose back. This escalated the violence until a neighbor called the police and the arrest occurred. Jose entered court-mandated treatment for domestic violence and, at Jane's request, entered family therapy.

Psychosocial and Cultural Factors. Both partners held very traditional views of marriage and family life. Jane saw herself primarily as a nurturer and caregiver who was principally responsible for parenting the boys. She expected Jose to be the provider, but worked because both incomes were needed. Jose did not want Jane to work and resented and was suspicious of her going to school. He had become very jealous and controlling, forbidding her to go. Because she "disobeyed," he had struck her to make her "fall in line." He felt badly that he did not earn enough money to support his family. Both felt unappreciated by the other. Jose and Jane loved their children and wanted to treat each other better for their sake. Jose worried that his "temper" was going to hurt the children.

In the men's group, Jose learned how his violence was triggered by feelings of powerlessness; in couple's therapy he learned to share his distress with his wife in more just ways. Neither had grown up with mothers who worked outside the home, so they needed to approach Jane's work and her desire for education as something that would be of benefit to the family. The metaphor of *compañerismo* was used. The couple explored how a traditional family arrangement was not possible, and perhaps not even desirable, so they could negotiate how to live as a young couple with children, without alcohol and violence, but with respect and authenticity. Because each saw their life as a struggle, the idea of being comrades in the struggle, *compañeros* or companions, was amenable to them.

Jane was willing to forgive Jose the pain that his violence had caused her, as long as he continued to learn ways to manage stress more effectively. Jose began to volunteer at a domestic violence hotline as a way to make restitution for his abuse. He also joined a Chicano men's group where issues of identity, masculinity, and solidarity were explored. He became more involved in parenting his children.

The couple stayed in treatment for 6 months and subsequently attended sessions once a month for 1 year. They remained violence free and committed to finding nonviolent solutions to the challenges in their lives.

Intimate violence can have multiple causes. However, understanding the particularities of the Chicana/o experience and the myriad stressors that Chicana/os face is critical for prevention and treatment. Oversimplified analyses that blame the culture or cultural patterns (machismo, marianismo, etc.) can be experienced as further oppression. The treatment of couples and families affected by violence requires respect, sensitivity, and authenticity on the part of the clinician. The mental health provider can respectfully challenge unjust ways of relating while encouraging the individual or couple to find culturally congruent alternatives to injustice.

An exploration of how couples resolve conflict and experience disrespect and injustice would provide a strong base for further investigations of the impact of social stratification and discrimination and their psychological sequelae on intimate relations. Likewise, a better understanding of how couples negotiate differences nonviolently would instruct those who have not learned adaptive and fair ways of coping with life's dilemmas. Finally, a more thorough investigation of the role of gender attitudes, socioeconomics, and frozen cultural values on domestic violence would assist the development of more effective prevention and treatment strategies. Clearly, research and practice that examine both the resources couples possess and the challenges they face will help decrease the incidence and prevalence of domestic violence.

REFERENCES

Aboriginal Health Council of South Australia. (1995). Reclaiming our stories, reclaiming our lives. *Dulwich Centre Newsletter, 1*, 1–23.

Almeida, R., Woods, R. M., Messineo, T., & Font, R. (1996). The cultural context model. In M. McGodrick, J. Giordano, & J. K. Pearce (Eds.), *Ethnic identity and family therapy* (2nd ed., pp. 120–130). New York: Guilford Press.

Baker-Miller, J. (1976). *Toward a new psychology of women.* Boston: Beacon Press.

Bauer, H., Rodriguez, M., Skupinski-Quiroga, S., & Flores-Ortiz, Y. (2000). Barriers to health care for abused Latina and Asian immigrant women. *Journal of Health Care for the Poor and the Underserved, 11*(1), 33–44.

Bernal, G. (1980). Parentification and de-parentification in family therapy. In A. S. Gurman (Ed.), *Questions and answers in family therapy* (pp. 125–142). New York: Brunner Mazel.

Bernal, G., & Alvarez, A. I. (1983). Culture and class in the study of families. In C. Falicov (Ed.), *Cultural perspectives in family therapy* (pp. 33–50). Rockville, MD: Aspen.

Bernal, G., & Flores-Ortiz, Y. (1982). Latino families in therapy: Engagement and evaluation. *Journal of Marital and Family Therapy, 8,* 357–365.

Boszormenyi-Nagy, I., & Spark, G. M. (1984) *Invisible loyalties.* New York: Brunner Mazel.

Carrillo, R., & Goubaud-Reyna, R. (1998). Clinical treatment of Latino domestic violence offenders. In R. Carrillo & J. Tello (Eds.), *Family violence and men of color: Healing the wounded male spirit* (pp. 53–73). New York: Springer.

De la Torre, A., & Pesquera, B. (Eds.). (1993). *Building with our hands: New directions in Chicana studies.* Berkeley: University of California Press.

Diaz-Guerrero, R. (1954). Neurosis and the Mexican family structure. *American Journal of Psychiatry, 112,* 411–417.

Diaz-Guerrero, R. (1994). *Psicologia del Mexicano.* Mexico, D.F., Mexico: Trillas.

Diaz-Loving, R., & Andrade Palos, P. (1996). Desarrollo y validacion del inventario de reacciones ante la pareja (IRIP). *Revista de Psicologica Contemporanea, 3*(3), 90–96.

Falicov, C. (1998). *Latino families in therapy: A guide to multicultural practice.* New York: Guilford Press.

Flores-Ortiz, Y. (1993a). La mujer y la violencia: A culturally based model for the understanding and treatment of domestic violence in Chicana/Latina communities. In N. Alarcon, R. Castro, E. Perez, B. Pesquera, A. Sosa Riddell, & P. Zavella (Eds.), *Chicana critical issues* (pp. 169–182). Berkeley, CA: Third Woman Press.

Flores-Ortiz, Y. (1993b). Level of acculturation, marital satisfaction, and depression among Chicana workers: A psychological perspective. *Aztlan: Journal of Chicana/o Studies, 20,* 51–175.

Flores-Ortiz, Y. (1997a). The broken covenant: Incest in Latino families. *In Voces: A Journal of Chicana/Latina Studies, 1,* 48–70.

Flores-Ortiz, Y. (1997b). Voices from the couch: The co-construction of a Chicana psychology. In C. Trujillo (Ed.), *Living Chicana theory* (pp. 102–122). Berkeley, CA: Third Woman Press.

Flores-Ortiz, Y. (1998). Fostering accountability: A reconstructive dialogue with a couple with a history of violence. In T. Nelson & T. Trepper (Eds.), *101 more interventions in family therapy* (pp. 389–396). New York: Haworth Press.

Flores-Ortiz, Y. (1999). Migracion, identidad y violencia/Migration, identity and violence. In M. Mock, L. Hill, & D. Tucker (Eds.), *Breaking barriers: Diversity in clinical practice* (pp. 29–33). Sacramento: California State Psychological Association.

Flores-Ortiz, Y. (2000a). From margin to center: Family therapy with Latinas. In M. Flores & G. Carey (Eds.), *Family therapy with Hispanics* (pp. 59–76). Boston: Allyn and Bacon.

Flores-Ortiz, Y. (2000b). Injustice in the family. In M. Flores & G. Carey (Eds.), *Family therapy with Hispanics* (pp. 251–263). Boston: Allyn and Bacon.

Flores-Ortiz, Y., & Bernal, G. (1990). Contextual family therapy of addiction with Latinos. In G. W. Saba, B. M. Karrer, & K. V. Hardy (Eds.), *Minorities and family therapy* (pp. 123–142). New York: Haworth Press.

Flores-Ortiz, Y., Esteban, M., & Carrillo, R. (1994). La violencia en la familia: Un modelo. Contextual de terapia intergeneracional. *Revista Interamericana de Psicologia, 28,* 235–250.

Flores-Ortiz, Y., Valdez Curiel, E., & Andrade Palos, P. (2004). Intimate partner violence and couple interaction among women from Mexico City and Jalisco, Mexico. *Journal of Border Health, 35*(5).

Luepnitz, D. A. (1989). *The family interpreted: Feminist theory in clinical practice.* New York: Basic Books.

Madanes, C. (1994). *Sex, love, and violence.* New York: Guilford Press.

Minuchin, S. (1974). *Families and family therapy.* Cambridge, MA: Harvard University Press.

Morales, A. (2001, September). *Why women in death row killed their children.* Workshop presentation, Latino Behavioral Health Institute, Los Angeles, CA.

Pesquera, B. (2000). Work gave me a lot of confianza: Chicanas' work commitment and work identity. *Aztlan: A Journal of Chicana/o Studies, 1,* 161–180.

Pinderhughes, E. (1982). Afro-American families and the victim system. In M. McGoldrick, J. K. Pearce, & J. Giordano (Eds.), *Ethnicity and family therapy* (pp. 108–122). New York: Guilford Press.

Roberts, A. R. (Ed.). (1984). *Battered women and their families: Intervention strategies and treatment programs.* New York: Springer.

Rodriguez, M., Bauer, H., & Flores-Ortiz, Y. (2001). Domestic violence in the Latino population. In A. G. Lopez & E. Carrillo (Eds.), *The Latino psychiatric patient: Assessment and treatment* (pp. 163–179). Washington, DC: American Psychiatric.

Rodriguez, M., Bauer, H., Flores-Ortiz, Y., & Skipinski-Quiroga, S. (1998). Factors affecting patient-physician communication for abused Latina and Asian immigrant women. *Journal of Family Practice, 47,* 309–311.

Sluzki, C. E. (1979). Migration and family conflict. *Family Process, 18,* 379–390.

Straus, M. A., & Gelles, R. J. (1998). *Physical violence in American families: Risk factors and adaptations to violence in 8,145 families.* New Brunswick, NJ: Transaction.

U.S. Department of the Census. (2000). *Population reports: Hispanics in the U.S.* Washington, DC: U.S. Government Printing Office.

U.S. Department of Justice. (1999). *Crime in the United States.* Washington, DC: U.S. Government Printing Office.

Walker, L. (1979). *Battered women.* New York: Springer.

Yllo, K. A. (1984). Patriarchy and violence against wives: The impact of structural and normative factors. *Journal of International and Comparative Social Welfare, 1,* 16–29.

Family Therapy With Chicana/os

Joseph M. Cervantes
California State University, Fullerton

Lisa I. Sweatt
California Polytechnic State University

> From the Chicano movement we discovered, affirmed, confirmed and reaffirmed our
> "Indianness." . . . So today the struggle within our Mejicanidad es una lucha antigua
> entre lo Indio y lo Europeo—and from there the struggle/joda vacillates entre Chicano/
> Hispano, Mejicano/Indio y hasta Latino eres tu, bruto! . . . So the lines are drawn and it's
> not an Apache or even an imperious Aztec or Tewa or two against some Moor in Spain
> from Africa or Visigoth from up North. It is about those of us who are neither from Mayan
> splendor nor Iberian Gypsy—We who didn't make it whole but almost, casi—were not ni
> Moros ni Negros, ni Blancos, somos mas, Casi!
>
> —Montoya (1992, p. 232)

Chicana/os, or Americana/os of Mexican descent, have become a significant part of
the acknowledged United States landscape for decades (Comas-Díaz, 2001; Griswold
Del Castillo, 1984; U.S. Bureau of the Census, 1993). As noted by Olmos, Ybarra, and
Monterrey (1999), these Latina/os are not strangers to this country, due to its integral
role in the nation's construction, its participation in society, and its intricate weaving
of social-community fibers to become a dynamic presence. The uniqueness of this
population is further underscored by its ethnic and cultural roots, including the
indigenous native, Spanish or European, African, and Asian. In brief, multiracial
groupings of people are emphasized in the heart, spirit, and physical presentation of
the Chicana/o.

As implied and addressed by several authors (i.e., Cervantes & Ramirez, 1992; Falicov, 1998a; Montoya, 1992; Morones & Mikawa, 1992; Ramirez, 1983), most Mexican
Americans are Mestiza/os, of mixed Spanish and Indian roots. Thus, this fusion of
cultures, belief systems, language, and spirituality has resulted in a unique philosophical outlook, which is further delineated by the contextual issues (Falicov, 1998a)
that have become additional, defining factors in the Mexican American culture: resi-
dency in the United States, immigrant status, acculturative stress, and varying levels
of integration of ethnic identity. The label "Chicana/o," which historically defined
the radical college student movement of the late 1960s and early 1970s, has become
an accepted identifying label for the broader Mexican American population in the

Southwest. We use the term to refer globally to this population of Mexican Americans. (For a more detailed discussion of the various other cultural labels employed to define the Mexican American population as a group, see Lampe, 1984; Comas-Díaz, 2001; McNeill et al., 2001.)

Family has historically been the overriding cultural theme among Chicana/os (Alvarez, 1987; Falicov, 1998a; Griswold Del Castillo, 1984; Hoobler & Hoobler, 1994; Martinez, 1988; Murillo, 1971) and is a central part of the discussion in this chapter. This chapter is intended to provide a conceptual, research, and clinical practice overview to Chicana/o practitioners, and an innovative perspective on family therapy in the new millennia. Family intervention is defined in the context of family therapy. The advantages of an increased literature base, professional experience with Chicano families, and the challenges of the variety of Chicano family structure (i.e., acculturation, language, socioeconomic, and regional differences) necessitate a fresh and creative approach to the psychological understanding of this population.

Our discussion includes conceptual, structural, and cultural aspects of the Chicano family. We develop a family psychology with Chicano families and provide a review of family intervention studies with Chicano families and assessment and treatment issues. We then outline a conceptual model for family therapy of Chicana/os and present recommendations for professional training and education, professional practice, and research.

CONCEPTUAL, STRUCTURAL, AND CULTURAL ASPECTS OF THE CHICANO FAMILY

> This is an altar of women,
> a woman's altar,
> constructed for the goddess inside the heart
> of each woman and man.
> Come to us, Diosa, and work through us,
> Diosa,
> to heal the wounds of flesh and dreams,
> to plant the seeds of strength.
> This is an altar of women,
> a woman's altar,
> and here no woman will be sacrificed. (Quiñonez, 1998, p. 21)[1]

An understanding of the Chicano family has been defined and expressed from diverse viewpoints, influenced primary by ethnic and cultural belief systems and sociohistorical backgrounds. Family among Latina/os has historically been identified with the woman or mother as the figurehead (Alvarez, 1987; Falicov, 1998a; Griswold Del Castillo, 1984; Hoobler & Hoobler, 1994). The poet and writer Anzaldúa (1987) commented that *la familia* is rooted in indigenous attributes, images, symbols, magic, and myth that houses and celebrates the feminine archetype. The Chicano family has been defined historically as both matriarchal and patriarchal, depending on the existing familial structure and the historical backdrop (Alvarez; Griswold Del Castillo). One of the earliest characterizations of the Mexican (and, by association,

---

[1]Naomi Helena Quiñonez, "La Diosa in Every Woman" (excerpt) from *The Smoking Mirror*. Copyright © 1998 by Namoi Helena Quiñonez. Reprinted with the permission of West End Press, Albuquerque, New Mexico.

the Mexican American family) was described by Diaz-Guerrero (1955, 1984), who utilized a psychoanalytic framework to comment on the development of the Mexican personality as well as the Mexican family. As a result, his view of sociocultural premises supported the existence of rigid family structures and stereotyped roles that both males and females demonstrate throughout their lives. Beliefs about how the Chicano family was characterized in early writings also negatively affected cultural beliefs and values because they were described as antiquated abstractions that were typically pejorative and nonfunctional (Diaz-Guerrero, 1955, 1984). The Mexican American family was cast into stereotyped male and female roles that were dysfunctional and thus inconsistent with the values espoused by the majority culture.

A shift in thinking about the Chicano family became evident in the work of Romano (1968, 1970) and Murillo (1971), who strongly criticized prior stereotypes of Chicana/os described by Diaz-Guerrero (1955, 1984) and reaffirmed the family as a stable and nurturing structure that provides its members a loving, supportive, and growth-enhancing environment. Mirandé (1985) argued that Diaz-Guerrero's influence in the literature also supported the transfer of those views onto Chicana/o families, characterizing them as pathological. Thus, concepts of being macho, mother as self-sacrificing, and men as unfaithful in the marriage, for example, were ascribed values that were inherited from Mexico. Nevertheless, the old stereotypes such as the family lacking motivation to advance itself or to support social or academic achievement for its members continued to be advanced by later writers who promoted similar views (i.e., Heller, 1966; Madsen, 1964).

A more evolved discussion about Chicano families was provided by Ramirez and Arce (1981). In their empirically based review, they provided a salient foundation for a more modern understanding of Chicana/os. Their conceptual reformulations of family structure, gender roles, and conjugal decision-making processes, based on current research at the time, assisted in making an effective transition from stereotypes to novel and fresh perspectives on Chicano families. According to Ramirez and Arce, their, "findings portray a distinctive institution that has been and continues to be dynamic, creative, and supportive" (p. 24).

Mirandé (1985) supported the discussion by Ramirez and Arce (1981) in his description of Chicano families as multivaried and highly stratified with several distinct structures influenced by both internal forces (i.e., age, single parent vs. intact family) and external forces (i.e., region, migration period, acculturative level, education, social class). Thus, the Chicano family was viewed as a dynamic and evolving system, not an antiquated imitation of the Mexican from Mexico.

These changes in stereotypes about the Chicano family have continued to evolve over the last 25 years, with new interpretations, images, and discussions of family process (Cervantes & Ramirez, 1992; Falicov, 1982, 1998b; Ho, 1987; Martinez, 1988; Paniagua, 1998; Ponterotto, 1987; Ramirez, 1991; Ramirez & Castañeda, 1974). The prominent themes and values noted by these authors include the following:

- Members display pre-eminent commitment and loyalty to the family.
- Family tends to maintain a patriarchal exterior but has a mother-centered base.
- Family extends its influence through the *compadrazco* system of godparentage.
- Ritual, religion, and spirituality are salient dimensions that underscore the family's commitment to its individual members, the extended family, and its respective broader community.

- Reliance and integration of extended family into the core nuclear group is common, expected, and respected.
- Development of empathetic personal relationships between, within, and among families and their community is perceived as a strong value of those who are *bien educada/o.*
- Family is multifaceted and diverse, influenced by various factors: migration, history, acculturation, ethnic or cultural integration, and experience with oppression and racism.

We acknowledge the strong reliance on the stability, engagement, support, and expectation of the role of family for Chicana/os. These observations and family themes are a major conceptual shift from the early writings of Diaz-Guerrero (1955, 1984), who had influenced social science literature and, subsequently, social and community behavior for decades.

The development of a family psychology is a reflection of the belief system of a particular ethnic or cultural group. Chicano families have a strong identification with family loyalty, respectful relationships, a maternal base, and diverse familial structures. An understanding of this family psychology is now addressed.

FAMILY PSYCHOLOGY AND CHICANO FAMILIES

A circle begins in a meadow by a snowmelt creek
where hands weave a house of thin green saplings
it is a way of song
a way of breathing
a pine womb to center oneself through sweat
a way of blessing and being blessed
a circle of humanity, prayer, and asking
and there are no clocks to measure time
but the beating of our singing hearts. (Littlebird, 1982, p. 10)

Family psychology as a conceptual and professional subdiscipline has only recently been given status as a division of the American Psychological Association (1987). Early in its development, Kaye (1985) offered a tentative definition of family psychology as the study of the larger social system to include those living within the unit. A shift to the psychological study of the family system moved beyond a family therapy perspective to that of understanding behavior, process, interaction, and incorporation of the larger community system (L'Abate, 1983, 1985; Liddle, 1987; Miller & Sableman, 1985). An adjoining paradigm was addressed by Carter and McGoldrick (1989) in their edited volume on the incorporation of the life span developmental approach to working with families in therapy. This perspective further assisted in the building of a foundation to understanding family development. Thus, the family came to be viewed as a growth model, in that the developmental expectations and demands of families change from birth through old age, with each state marked by psychosocial transitions.

The transition from the conceptualization of an individual psychology to that of a systemic psychology in understanding families was a difficult one (Miller & Sabelman, 1985). The understanding of Chicano families, in contrast, had historically been viewed more systematically, as noted in early psychological definitions of the family reported by Murillo (1971), Padilla, Carlos, and Keefe (1976), and Peñalosa (1968), who underscored the importance of the family system for Mexican Americans. They described the Chicano family as paternalistically hierarchical, gender bound (with males given higher status and freedom), emphasizing family unity, respect, and loyalty as significant cultural expectations, and relying on extended family for added social and emotional support. Thus, familism was viewed as a significant and consistent characteristic central to the Chicano family (Goodman & Beman, 1971; Mirandé, 1985). In addition, Mirandé (1985) observed that the Chicano family has its own unique characteristics, but there is significant variation in family type. He argued, as did many others (i.e., Alvarez, 1987; Griswold Del Castillo, 1984; Hoobler & Hoobler, 1994) that: "The Chicano family is not a transplanted, traditional patriarchal Mexican family, but a dynamic and evolving unit. The family has changed and adapted to external conditions and structural forces in the United States, but such change has not simply resulted from acculturation to American life" (Mirandé, p. 104). This discussion thus further outlines a family psychology with Chicana/os as composed of varying acculturative patterns, is highly adaptive, and allows for increased freedom to chart a more variable cultural life course.

A family psychology for the Chicana/o is also defined in its uniqueness by social and political circumstances that have influenced its identity, namely, migration and acculturation. Sanchez (1941), later described by Murillo (1984), initiated this understanding of the roles of environment, educational equality, and acculturation in his writing on Mexican American children. He was one of the first to put forth the idea that social and cultural experiences significantly affect family functioning while being minimally related to intelligence. Sanchez referred specifically to ethnic discrimination experiences as a salient factor in shaping family process and adaptation. Other authors commented on this understanding as well (Alvarez, 1987; Griswold Del Castillo, 1984).

Later, Keefe and Padilla (1987), in their qualitative work on ethnicity, presented case studies showing how ethnic identity is constructed among individuals. For example, cultural knowledge, ethnic identification, and acculturation were primary factors in defining Chicana/os. They also found that Chicano families are complex and vary structurally. Their work indicated that ethnic labeling as Chicana/o has various subjective interpretations and internal definitions, depending on the course of life experience and ethnic or cultural exposure.

Although their work does not specifically address Chicano families, Szapocznik and Kurtines' (1993) research on Cuban American adolescents and their families is relevant to our discussion. Their work further developed the concept of contextualism, or the view that behavior cannot be understood outside of the context in which it occurs. They described the individual as embedded within the larger context of family, community, and society, and emphasized the continuous interplay between the person and the environment. Their work seemed to anticipate the growing awareness that Latino families vary with respect to dynamic, structural, and ethnic or cultural permutations that had direct relevance for Chicano families. Thus, as already noted by Mirandé (1985) and Murillo (1971): "The reality is that there is no Mexican American family 'type' . . . there are significant regional, historical, political, socioeconomic, acculturation, and assimilation factors which result in a multitude of family patterns of living and coping with each other and with their Anglo environments" (p. 97).

The experience of racism and oppression has been important in developing a family psychology for the Chicana/o. As noted in Jones (1997), the sociopolitical environment for people of color has generally been affected by poor professional service, ill-equipped professionals, and biased theories and counseling approaches (Sue & Sue, 1999). With Chicano families, oppression and prejudicial assessments in the school (Sanchez, 1934), discrimination in mental health delivery systems (Morales, 1976), and biased attitudes have affected perceptions and compromised equal participation on many levels (Falicov, 1998; Olson, 2000). Thus, ethnic identity, family stability, and the opportunity to integrate bicultural or multicultural perspectives have not been supported or appreciated by the larger majority culture.

Falicov's (1995, 1998) guide to multicultural practice with Latino families was one of the most instructive works on psychological intervention with this population. Her work addressed the role of family psychology without directly using this concept as a defined paradigm. Her detailed discussion of context, especially for Chicano families, incorporated the uniqueness of each family system according to a number of factors: generation, acculturation, bi-ethnicity, Spanish or English language, migration status, socioeconomic level, and religious preference.

The model of family psychology that has emerged from the literature indicates that the dimensions of acculturation, familial or community context, integration of ethnic identity, and oppression and racism are important constructs. We highlight here the relevant parameters for a family psychology of Chicano families that have been indicated in research (Carter & McGoldrick, 1989; Falicov, 1998a, 1998b; Jones, 1997; Keefe & Padilla, 1987; Mirandé, 1985; Murillo, 1971; Sanchez, 1941; Sue & Sue, 1999; Szapocznik & Kurtines, 1993):

1. Chicana/os are multiethnic and enter into partnerships characterized by within-ethnic similarity to Latino-ethnic dissimilarity to majority culture intermarriage.
2. Familial structure and interactional patterns are varied, influenced by generational, regional, and ethnic or cultural background.
3. Identification with, reliance on, and loyalty to family as a primary base of operation continue to be significant and enduring.
4. Extended family, both blood relationships and those acquired through religious ceremony (compadrazco), is a relevant and meaningful support system that maintains legitimacy.
5. Social and familial roles and expectations are complex and diverse.
6. Language communication in Chicano households continues to vary, from Spanish in less acculturated families to bilingual or monolingual English in more acculturated families.
7. Ethnic or racial oppression and discrimination continue to be salient factors in identity formation and family process.
8. Additional issues of acculturation, immigration status, and migration history are relevant contextual parameters that affect and influence family development.

FAMILY INTERVENTION STUDIES
WITH CHICANO FAMILIES

> You bring out the Mexican in me . . . the Dolores del Rio in me.
> The Mexican spit fire in me. The raw Navajas, glint and passion in me.
> The Raise Caine and dance with the rooster-footed devil in me.
> The Spangled sequin in me. The eagle and serpent in me.
> The Aztec love of war in me.
> The fierce obsidian of the tongue in me.
> The berrinchuda, bien—cabrona in me.
> The Pandora's curiosity in me.
> The pre-Columbian death and destruction in me.
> The Rainforest disaster, nuclear threat in me . . .
> Yes, you do. Yes, you do. (Cisneros, 1994, pp. 4–5)

Family intervention is defined in the context of family therapy. In support of the arguments made by Soto-Fulp and Del Campo (1994), Ho (1987), Paniagua (1998), Garcia-Preto (1996), Martinez (1988), and Falicov (1998a), family therapy is the preferred, psychotherapeutic medium for working with Latina/o populations, including Mexican American families. One of the earliest examples of family research and treatment was provided by Minuchin, Montalvo, Guerney, Rosman, and Schumer (1967). Although the study did not include Chicano families, it was one of the first, documented family therapy programs to describe relevant concepts and sociocultural issues of people of color. The population studied and treated included low income, Puerto Rican and African American youth and their families living in tenement housing on the east coast. Work with these populations initiated the development of structural family concepts that were more clearly presented in later writing (Minuchin, 1974). Thus, the concepts of boundaries, power hierarchies, and enmeshment, for example, formed an understanding of families that assisted in the definition of goals and treatment success. The research by Minuchin et al. highlighted the interaction of low-income status, culture and ethnicity, and disorganized familial structure with these two distinct types of families.

The counseling literature has recently developed a strong base in writing about multicultural counseling and various psychotherapeutic approaches with people of color. Some earlier work was more generic (Acosta, Yamamoto, & Evans, 1982; Lee & Richardson, 1991; Marsella & Pedersen, 1981), offering a broad scope of counseling models with several distinct, culturally diverse populations. Others were more focused on treatment issues specific to each group (Atkinson, Morten, & Sue, 1993; Falicov, 1998a; Vargas & Koss-Chioino, 1992).

One of the earliest discussions of culture and family interventions was provided by McGoldrick, Pearce, and Giordano (1982) in their volume on ethnicity and family therapy (updated in McGoldrick, Pearce, & Giordano, 1996), in which they provided an overview of various ethnic or cultural families and potential themes and models of intervention. Ho (1987) followed with a conceptual volume on family-centered approaches to problem solving that included six ethnic minority family groups: Asians, Pacific Americans, American Indians, Alaskan Natives, Hispanic Americans, and Black Americans. Ho presented interventions from an ecological family systemic approach, which was defined as a framework that considered the "ethnic minority's reality, culture, and biculturalism, ethnicity status, language, and social class" (p. 11). Ho's chapter on family therapy with Hispanic Americans was based on a generic assessment of Latina/os, thus the observations made were not specific to Chicano families. Furthermore, Ho's recommendations for therapeutic interventions were frequently discussed from a Bowenian theory perspective (Bowen, 1978), which resulted in stereotypical generalizations and inaccuracy.

Cervantes and Ramirez (1992) initiated a discussion of integrating spirituality into counseling, provided a conceptual framework for this, and compared the treatment approaches of a family therapist and an indigenous healer. Their chapter included two case examples of family therapy treatment and discussed a treatment paradigm taking into consideration the clients' religious or spiritual orientation. Their study participants were families from a Mexican American population.

Family therapy intervention with Chicana/o populations has not been well described in the literature, despite numerous studies over the past decade that have addressed treatment paradigms with various Latina/o groups (Bean, Perry, & Bedell, 2001; Falicov, 1998b; Szapocznik & Kurtines, 1993). As stated earlier, most discussions have not been specific to Mexican Americans or Chicana/os, but have instead considered Latino families generally. Second, the modality of family therapy, with its variety of schools of thought and systems of intervention, has not been clearly addressed with Latina/o groups, especially with Chicana/o families.

Some of the earliest discussions of family intervention with Latina/o populations, apart from Minuchin et al.'s (1967) work, focused on Cuban American adolescents and their families. This treatment protocol by Szapocznik, Santisteban, Perez-Vidal, and Hervis (1984) was designed to assist with acculturation problems between teenagers and parents. Szapocznik, Kurtines, Foote, Perez-Vidal, and Hervis (1983, 1986) discussed the effectiveness of one-person family therapy over treatment with all or most family members present. Their focus was more behavioral and educational, highlighted Cuban American families, and emphasized specific development in family treatment that demonstrated positive results. Bean, Perry, and Bedell (2001) reported in their review that structural family therapy (Minuchin, 1974) had become the principal treatment modality consistently noted in the literature.

Structural family intervention, with Minuchin (1974) as its principal spokesperson, has been understood as a systematic orientation that addresses the roles that relationship boundaries, power hierarchy, decision making, and levels of family organization, for example, play in a given family. Minuchin, a Latino from Argentina, was consistent with his own perspective of familia as a salient cultural value. No other studies or discussions were found that systematically considered other family therapy approaches with Latino or Chicano families. However, there has been significant discussion in the literature regarding contextual factors in working with Latino families. A review of these studies follows.

Szapocznik and Kurtines (1993, 1997) developed the structural ecosystems theory for working with Latino families. The structural orientation of this approach draws from both the structural (Minuchin, 1974; Minuchin & Fishman, 1981; Minuchin, Rosman, & Baker, 1978) and strategic (Haley, 1976; Madanes, 1981) traditions in family systems theory, whereas the ecosystemic orientation was influenced by the social ecological theory of Bronfenbrenner (1977, 1979, 1986). The structural ecosystemic approach has been applied to the prevention and treatment of behavioral problems and drug abuse among Latina/o youth and families, primarily Cuban Americans.

Aponte (1994) applied an ecostructural model to the assessment and treatment of poor and ethnic minorities. The ecostructural model is an expansion of structural family therapy (Minuchin, 1974) that includes both the individual and the community. The ecostructural approach to assessment attempts to take into account the present issue, the ecosystemic context of the family, and both immediate and long-term goals. Aponte offered a systematic and dynamic "presentation outline" that guides the therapist in defining the focal issue(s) of the therapy, diagnostic hypotheses (structural conditions and reasons underlying the family dynamics), and therapeutic hypotheses (about the family and the therapist in relation to the family). Aponte emphasized that assessment and intervention with the poor (an increasing number of which are Chicana/o) "need to address a family's present urgencies, understand the past in the context of today's need, and speak to how to help *today*" (p. 32). More research needs to be done to assess this model's salience, given the diversity of Chicano families.

Boyd-Franklin's (1989) multisystems model of family therapy incorporates family therapy techniques from structural, strategic, and Bowenian schools, and applies them in a culturally sensitive manner to the treatment of individuals and families. This model requires the family therapist to move beyond the traditional nuclear family model and flexibly intervene on individual, family, extended-family, and community levels. This approach has been used with Latinas and their families (Boyd-Franklin & Garcia-Preto, 1994)

Though not derived from a family psychology perspective, Greiger and Ponterotto (1995) offered a generic framework for assessment in multicultural counseling. Drawing from the acculturation literature and their own clinical experiences, they identified four components of world view and acculturation deemed useful in the context of multicultural counseling assessment: the client's level of psychological mindedness (defined as familiarity with Western middle-class values), the family's level of psychological mindedness, the client's and family's attitude toward counseling, and the client system's level and attitudes toward acculturation. Other helpful cultural assessment tools are Ho's (1987) cultural transition map, Comas-Diaz's (1994) ethnocultural assessment, and McGill's (1992) cultural story. Though outlining important elements of assessment with diverse populations, they fall short of providing a comprehensive model of assessment and intervention with Chicano families.

The most recent conceptual model that attempted to illuminate common cultural themes within Latino families, while attending to the extreme diversity within and between Latino families and cultural groups, is the multidimensional ecosystemic comparative approach by Falicov (1998a). Although clinical observations and commentary are directed generally toward Latina/o groups, her frame of reference appears to be influenced primarily by her experience with Mexican American families. Falicov, like Minuchin (1974), is of Argentinean descent, and their respective conceptual lenses support the therapeutic emphasis on familial structure and organization and the roles that migration and acculturation play. Falicov provided a comprehensive framework of the interaction between cultural relevance and sociocultural factors in family therapy.

Falicov's (1998a) ecosystemic comparative approach (MECA) identified four dimensions—migration, ecological context, family organization, and family life cycle—that were used to describe and compare similarities and differences among Latina/o cultural groups. Her research demonstrated MECA's usefulness in the evaluation and treatment of Latino families. Furthermore, Falicov utilized this framework to examine the cultural maps of the treating therapist, who brings in his or her own sociocultural background, ethnic or cultural biases, and relevant life experiences to the consulting office (Haraway, 1991). Cultural maps are referred to as the internalized emotional and cognitive mental sets that are specific to the therapist. The Latina/o groups discussed by Falicov included Mexicans, Puerto Ricans, and Cubans; she did not focus exclusively on Chicana/o families. However, the MECA model and the themes identified by Falicov as relevant to Latino families are useful in developing a framework for understanding Chicano families as well.

In addition to Falicov (1998a), researchers have begun to address more specific family therapy treatment protocols with Chicana/os. Martinez (1994) provided a case example of a grieving family that was suffering because of several generations of suicide among its members. He emphasized the need to understand not just interfamily dynamics as supported by structural family therapy, but also intrafamilial dynamics, such as socioecological awareness (i.e., home and neighborhood living conditions), possible single-parent households, and employment status of parental caretakers. Soto-Fulp and Del Campo (1994) reported on their assessment of Mexican American families and the family rules that are part of their cultural systems. They provided three case discussions to highlight the family diversity of this cultural group, but also commented on possible structural and strategic family approaches in their recommendations. Their findings were consistent with the observation made by Baca Zinn (1999) that therapists need to appreciate the wide range of family structures within Chicano families, and not interpret a culturally normative relationship as pathological.

Bean et al. (2001), in their content analysis of available treatment literature with Latina/o groups, provided a set of guidelines supporting culturally competent therapy. Although their guidelines are intended to be generic to most Latino families, their observations and cited research are directly applicable to Chicano families as well. These guidelines include interfamilial dynamics (i.e., assessment of beliefs in folk medicine, bilingual fluency, and respect for established power hierarchy), intrafamilial dynamics (i.e., assessment of immigration experience and level of acculturation), and practical recommendations to support the therapeutic relationship (i.e., facilitate family with other community agencies as needed, provide helpful suggestions early on).

A summary of the findings from these studies reveals that Chicano families vary substantially over multiple dimensions, including ethnic identity integration (Keefe & Padilla, 1987), sociocultural belief systems, bilingual language ability, socioeconomic status, and religious or spiritual beliefs (Bach-y-Rita, 1982). Furthermore, in spite of differences across these dimensions, the psychological importance of family remains salient (Bean et al., 2001; Paniagua, 1998). Contextual factors in the assessment and treatment of Chicano families were outlined by several authors (Garcia-Preto, 1996; Falicov, 1998a, 1998b; Paniagua, 1998; Soto-Fulp & Del Camp, 1994). The role of sociopolitical forces and assessment for discriminatory factors in family functioning was also noted (Cross & Maldonado, 1971; Takaki, 1993). Still, additional family treatment studies that highlight Chicana/os are needed.

ASSESSMENT AND TREATMENT ISSUES WITH CHICANO FAMILIES

Mujer,
Branch of an Ancient tree,
Cactus Flower, tender
Niña
Reaping sugar cane wisdom
Abuelita's gifts—
Consejos, cuentos, remedies,
Bendicions—
Strength for tomorrow . . .
Mujer, Rose of varied hues,
Blossoming
Beyond old barriers
Your gente's pride
Visionary woman
Obstacle victor
Mujer, Mujer
Receive your pueblo's
Embrace. (Aparicio, 1999, p. 146)[2]

It has been asserted that assessment and treatment issues with Chicano families are most effectively understood as a relationship between the family, the social and cultural contexts of family therapy theory, and the therapist. Ecological context as a principal shaper of individual and family life has often been left out of the dialogue on therapy, assessment, and interventions. The dangers of excessive emphasis on specific, and often stereotypical, ethnic styles and traditions, without acknowledging the interaction of the Latino or Chicano family with macrosystems such as school, work, social services, and public policy, have been exemplified (Falicov, 1998a, 1998b; Montalvo & Gutiérrez, 1983, 1988, 1989). In particular, family therapy theory needs to be understood as a complex, interwoven, dynamic interaction that has significant impact on how therapists conceptualize families, in this case, the Chicano families.

A variety of traditional family therapy models, such as structural (Aponte, 1976; Haley, 1976; Minuchin, 1974; Soto-Fulp & Del Campo, 1994), Bowenian (Bowen, 1976, 1978; Guerin, 1976; McGoldrick & Gerson, 1985), and strategic (Boyd-Franklin & Garcia-Preto, 1994; Haley, 1973; Madanes, 1981; Papp, 1981), have been consistently cited as useful in the assessment and treatment of families. Some authors have specified issues and treatments with Latino families, only a few with Chicano families in particular. The blanket application of these models to Chicana/os and other people of color, without critical examination of the constructs embedded in them, has come under debate in recent years (Falicov, 1998a, 1998b; McGoldrick, 1998). For example, Falicov (1998a, 1998b) addressed how "triangles" have been essential constructs in family therapy for attributing distress and dysfunction. In particular, the

[2]From *Americanos: Latino Life in the United States,* ed. E. J. Olmos, L. Ybarra, & M. Monterrey, Published by Little, Brown and Company.

alliance between two members of different generations, such as one parent and child against the other parent, called a cross-generational coalition, has been cited as especially destructive. Falicov (1995) argued, however, that the pathologizing of triangles, specifically cross-generational coalitions, and the subsequent goal of restoring the boundary around the marital dyad, are based on specific cultural constructions that reflect and support the ideology of a particular kind of family, namely, the mainstream Anglo, middle-class, nuclear family. Thus, the meanings and implications of constructs within family therapy theories must be examined in relation to the social and cultural context in which they are embedded prior to their implementation with Chicano families.

In the creation of the therapeutic system, the family therapist defines not only what family is, but also what is problematic, what or who is responsible for the problems, and what or who is responsible for resolving them (Minuchin & Fishman, 1981). The therapist's internalized model of intervention, whether conscious or unconscious, is a salient part of this process. Furthermore, the therapist's entire world view—attitudes, values, opinions, emotions about self and others as shaped by personal and cultural upbringing and experience—is extremely influential in forming the lens through which family definition, assessment, and intervention are viewed. In working with Chicano families, it is essential that the family therapist, regardless of ethnic or cultural background, critically examine his or her social and cultural context in relation to the application of theory and practice.

A novel understanding of this contextual backdrop of both therapist and family and the resulting clinical applications lies in the development of a culturally appropriate, theoretical metaphor called "Trensas." This model involves a multiple, contextual interweaving of theory, therapist, and Chicano family and is presented in the next section of this chapter.

We take the position that assessment does not simply occur during the first or second meeting with the family, but rather throughout the family's treatment and is an element of intervention itself. Assessment and treatment should be ecologically valid in that they reflect the complexity of Chicano families and can accommodate the differences among individual family members. The contextual factors that affect this dynamic interaction between theory, the family therapist, and the client-family system include:

- Understanding the sociocultural context of therapy
- Gathering appropriate family, migration, and acculturation history
- Evaluating gender and generational hierarchies
- Language dominance and preference
- Spiritual and religious belief systems in understanding health
- Social advocacy role of the therapist

The family therapy literature offers little regarding specific assessment and treatment frameworks for Latino, let alone Chicano, families. Although there is no one "right" theoretical approach to working with Chicana/os, the aforementioned dimensions form a culturally syntonic and ecologically valid mind-set for the therapist. Each of these areas is now presented and illustrated with treatment case material on two Chicano families.

Sociocultural Context of Therapy

An extensive body of literature concerning the use of mental health services by Chicana/os has consistently shown that this population seeks mental health services less often than European Americans and tends to terminate services earlier (Casas, 1984; Echeverry, 1997; Sue, Zane, & Young, 1994). The reasons for this underuse and early termination of therapeutic services have been identified and addressed elsewhere (e.g., Prieto, McNeill, Walls, & Gómez, 2001). In particular, Chicano families must navigate multiple obstacles within the community mental health system in order to secure assistance. Some of these obstacles include: cultural insensitivity, lack of professional skill level, misdiagnosis of major psychological disorders, lack of knowledge about acculturative process and stressors, and disregard for the need for Spanish-speaking health systems. Thus, a therapeutic process that communicates an effective, culturally responsive understanding to the helping relationship is a significant determiner of continued service for Chicana/os (Paniagua, 1998; Sue & Sue, 1999).

This cultural understanding can be effectively communicated with an awareness and utilization of the concepts of *respeto, personalismo,* and *sympatia,* which provide the necessary bridge to the family's development of *confianza,* or trust, in the therapist (Falicov, 1998a; McNeill et al., 2001). Within the Mexican American culture, *respeto,* or respect, governs all family relationships, as well as interpersonal relationships outside the family, and manifests as reciprocity of perceived worth between equals and deferential behavior to perceived authority figures. *Personalismo* is a communication style that emphasizes the preference for personal, although not necessarily informal, contacts over distant and institutional ones and invites more intimate sharing of information. *Simpatia* is a cultural pattern of social interaction that emphasizes the promotion and maintenance of harmonious or smooth social and interpersonal relationships. Whereas personalismo emphasizes the importance of relationships among Mexican Americans, simpatia emphasizes the way in which relationships are enacted. The following case example helps to illustrate the integration of culturally congruent relationship and communication behaviors.

The intake sheet for Maria and her grandmother, Señora Gomez (Maria's guardian), indicated numerous brief attempts at family therapy and multiple family difficulties. This current venture into therapy occurred through a referral by child protective services because of a report of excessive use of corporal punishment with Maria. When Maria and Sra. Gomez were approached in the waiting area, Sra. Gomez's posture appeared anxious and fearful. Her reactions were fueled by the shame of social services involvement in her family and the accusation of physically abusing her granddaughter; resentment of being forced into counseling and extreme discomfort in discussing family issues with a stranger; previous, perhaps negative, experiences in therapy; and the significant age difference between the treating therapist and Sra. Gomez and the concomitant cultural implication of receiving help from someone younger than she. Although not fully literate in Spanish, Sra. Gomez (a Spanish-English bilingual) was greeted first in Spanish and was directed to have a seat in the most comfortable chair in the therapy room. Maria's beautifully knitted vest was commented on and immediately Maria reported that her grandmother had made it for her and was teaching her how to knit. The therapist told Sra. Gomez that she wished that she had paid more attention to her own grandmother's knitting instructions when she was younger so that she could make such beautiful things. The therapist commented that the closest thing to knitting that she did now was tying her shoe; Sra. Gomez smiled. The therapist noticed that she had her knitting bag with her and asked her what she was currently working on. Sra. Gomez became increasingly more animated as she described the blanket she was making for the upcoming birth of another grandchild. As the conversation of knitting and family unfolded, it was discovered that the therapist's grandmother grew up in the town neighboring that of Sra. Gomez's childhood home. The conversation continued to weave stories of the past and present family lives of Sra. Gomez, Maria, and the therapist. When the session had reached its end, Sra. Gomez seemed surprised. "So soon?" she questioned and "Don't we have to talk about why we are here?" The therapist indicated that they would have plenty of time next week and said she looked forward to seeing her and Maria and the progression of the baby blanket. Sra. Gomez appeared very satisfied and grateful at the close of this first visit.

Although there were multiple factors that played into their persistence in therapy, awareness and employment of a culturally appropriate relationship and communication style in the first session laid the foundation for a successful therapeutic experience for the Gomez family. The understanding and use of respeto, personalismo, and sympatia are relevant not only to the initial phases of the therapy process, but also throughout treatment, so that confianza develops effectively.

Gathering Appropriate Family, Migrational, and Acculturation History

By definition, Chicana/os are U.S.-born persons of Mexican decent (Comas-Díaz, 2001; McNeill et al., 2001; Padilla, 1995). Whether one is a first- or fourth-generation Chicana/o, there is a family history of migration that is salient to both acculturation and the development of ethnic identity. The when, why, and how of a family's migration and the meaning family members attribute to this history are important for understanding current realities, including present stressors and difficulties within the Chicano family (Falicov, 1998a; Mirkin, 1998). Falicov suggested that facilitating the family's migration narrative is a useful tool in helping the therapist and family to understand their current life circumstances. Embedded in these narratives are often tales of family separation and loss, both literal and symbolic, as well as experiences of discrimination, racism, and oppression that continue to the present. There are also stories of triumph and perseverance that are useful in understanding a family's strengths and their coping and problem-solving abilities and style. These stories are the essence of resilient people who have overcome adversity (Olmos et al., 1999).

Theories about migration and acculturation processes and their psychological impact have received considerable attention and undergone serious debate and revision over the past several decades (Cuéllar, Harris, & Jasso, 1980; Montalvo & Gutiérrez, 1988; Olmedo, Martinez, & Martinez, 1978; Padilla, 1980; Sluzki, 1979; Smart & Smart, 1995). In addition, ethnic identity development has been described as being influenced by several variables, including the acculturation process (Knight, Cota, & Bernal, 1993). Variations in racial and ethnic identity among family members are affected by a host of factors, including increasing numbers of interethnic and interracial relations, as well as experiences of racism and oppression. From the time of the Spaniard conquest of Latin America, to be White (or *guero*) has afforded the power and privilege of a higher social class, whereas to be dark (or *indio*) has signified being conquered, dominated, and intellectually inferior, or *tonto* (Fortes de Leff & Espejel, 1995, as cited in Falicov, 1998a). Therefore, addressing the meaning of skin-tone variations and the experiences of racism and prejudice within and outside families is essential to understanding Chicanos' experiential contexts, beliefs, and values. For example, an important issue in working with Chicana/o youth is the incorporation of ethnic or racial identity into their evolving self-concept.

Family identity issues are interwoven with the dynamic of acculturation, which impacts personal and family development at many levels. In working with Chicano families, it is important to understand that family members may be at various levels of acculturation in terms of integrating the dominant culture into their Chicana/o identity development (Keefe & Padilla, 1987). These differences within families may contribute to the emergence of intergenerational and gender-based conflicts (Cervantes & Ramirez, 1992; Falicov, 1998a). The therapist's understanding of the links between family history, acculturation, and ethnic identity development are critical to a culturally meaningful conceptualization and treatment of Chicano families. Encouraging families to tell their stories is a salient parameter of treatment.

The Hernandez family, composed of father, mother, Jorge (13 years old), and Carlos (8 years old), was referred for outpatient family therapy services by Jorge's school because of his declining school performance, social withdrawal, frequent somatic complaints (e.g., headaches, stomach aches), and ruminations about health concerns (belief that he was suffering from a brain tumor, although medical evaluations had ruled this out). Upon their first visit, it was apparent that Mr. and Mrs. Hernandez were extremely anxious and reluctant to be there. Jorge sat as far away from his parents as was possible in the small therapy room and did not look at them. A familial history, as well as individual histories, began to unfold in the first few sessions that illuminated current family functioning difficulties and laid the foundation for positive intervention. Jorge and his brother had lived their entire lives in a suburban town in southern California. Mr. and Mrs. Hernandez were born and raised in central Mexico and migrated to the United States just prior to Jorge's birth, seeking the "American dream." In Mexico, Mr. Hernandez had been a prominent member of the community and grocery business owner, whereas Mrs. Hernandez worked in the home. Since arriving in California, Mr. Hernandez had been unable to find suitable employment that met his experience and qualifications, and had thus worked intermittently as a day laborer for the past 14 years. Mrs. Hernandez had been employed as a full-time housekeeper for a wealthy family. Over the past several years, Mr. Hernandez had become increasingly despondent about his personal employment situation and his family's increasing economic difficulties and began drinking excessively. At the same time, Jorge had entered a predominantly White middle school and began to experience academic, familial, and peer difficulties. Mrs. Hernandez reported that it was at this time that Jorge began to angrily accuse his parents of being "too Mexican" and to distance himself from his family, especially his father. (It is important to note that Jorge was very dark in complexion, like his father.)

The migration and acculturation history of the Hernandez family illuminates themes common to the Chicano family experience, such as discrimination, loss of

personal and financial status, and familial conflict due to family members' differences in acculturation and struggles with ethnic identity and internalized racism.
Illustrated in the Hernandez family case is a frequent therapeutic observation found
among experienced Chicana/o mental health professionals, a syndrome known as
the overacculturation of the child and the underacculturation of the parent (Cervantes & Romero, 1983). The therapist's understanding of the interrelationship of
these familial experiences and dynamics, of the ties between the past and present, is
essential to the formulation of culturally congruent treatment interventions.

Evaluating Gender and Generational Hierarchies

Traditionally, Mexican American families have been considered patriarchal in terms
of gender roles. Fathers are expected to be authoritarian, rational, strong, independent, and brave and to fulfill a machismo identity that is often defined negatively as
involving physical dominance of women, excessive alcohol use, and sexual promiscuity regardless of marital status (Flores Niemann, 2001). Women, in contrast, are
expected to be submissive, docile, gentle, dependent, and intuitive and embody a
marianismo identity that requires them to be chaste and virginal until marriage and
completely self-sacrificing for the sake of their children and husband afterward (Falicov, 1998a; Flores Niemann, 2001).

The counseling literature has been criticized for portraying Latina/o populations
in stereotypical and pathological ways that are not reflective of their true variability
(Quinoñes, 2000). Increasingly, a wide range of structures and processes characterize
Chicano family life, from patriarchal to egalitarian and everything in between (Vega,
1990). Gender roles for Chicana/os are influenced by a number of factors, including
educational level, socioeconomic status, family constellation, and sexual orientation.
Indeed, feminist writers have discussed the need to understand the interaction of
gender, family, and ethnicity in shaping the identities of Chicanas (Anzaldúa, 1987;
Castillo, 1994; Moraga, 1983). Assessing gender roles in the family in relation to their
cultural context is an essential task of the family therapist.

Although Chicano families may organize in a variety of ways, their meaning systems and interactional patterns tend to flow from a collective rather than an individual ideology (Castañeda, 1984). *Familismo,* or family interdependence, involves the
sharing of extended family members for parenting tasks such as nurturing and disci-
plining of children, financial responsibilities, and problem solving (Falicov, 1996,
1998). In Chicano families, rules organized around age and relationship are the most
important determinants of authority, with older men and women granted the greatest leadership and influence, parents more than children. Family cohesiveness and
parental authority are expressed throughout the life span. The parent-child dyad
often takes precedence over the marital dyad, the mother-son bond being especially
significant. Sibling ties are also strong, as are the connections among cousins. The
strength of these ties continues into adulthood; even when siblings form families of
their own, loyalties to blood remain strong. Thus, pathologizing and employing
diagnostic labels for human attachment functions (i.e., dependency, enmeshment) is
conceptually and theoretically inappropriate for Chicano families (Ramirez & Arce,
1981; Rueschenberg & Buriel, 1989). The therapist needs to be aware of these culturally appropriate alliances and assess them contextually rather than regarding them

as pathological, as in the case of "triangulation" (Falicov, 1998a, 1998b). In brief, a cultural framework has evolved within a family system that establishes several distinct meanings and functions of attachment. Emotional connectedness necessitates a different continuum of dysfunction that has yet to be delineated. The interplay of gender and generational hierarchies is further illustrated in the case of the Gomez family.

While working with Maria and her grandmother, Sra. Gomez, it was learned (via Maria) that Sra. Gomez's youngest son, Hector (27 years old), lived with her intermittently and had a serious drinking problem. Hector's alcohol abuse greatly frightened Maria as he became destructive and verbally aggressive toward Sra. Gomez and Maria when he was intoxicated. Neighbors had called the police in the past about Hector's inebriated outbursts and had threatened to call the Department of Children and Family Services because of concerns regarding Maria's well-being. Hector's behavior was obviously very stressful for Sra. Gomez, who thought the situation hopeless and lamented, "What am I to do? I know this is not good for Maria or for me, but I can't kick him out, he is my son, mi niñito." Sra. Gomez expressed great concern about what the therapist was going to do with this information—was the system going to report her as others had threatened to do? The therapist expressed concern while communicating an understanding of the family's situation and her desire to help resolve it. In assessing resources in the family that could be of assistance, it was learned that Maria's godparents had been very useful in solving family disputes in the past, but that Sra. Gomez had not gone to them because of her feelings of guilt and shame over her son's behavior. It was also learned that Sra. Gomez's oldest son, Raul, had taken over the role as the "senior" of the family since the passing of his father, even though he lived 5 hours away from the rest of the family. The idea of including Hector, Maria's godparents, and, if possible, Raul in the next therapy session to assist in finding ways to approach the family dilemma was discussed. Sra. Gomez agreed to this change in treatment. A meeting was set up during a date and time when Raul was in town and the godparents were available. Although Hector did not come, the session proved successful for the family. To Sra. Gomez's relief, the godparents demonstrated understanding and a desire to help. Raul initially expressed anger and disgust over his brother's behavior, but also admitted regret and guilt about not being able to live closer to fulfill his family obligations. It was agreed that Raul would confront Hector about his behavior and attempt to direct him toward alcohol abuse treatment with the help of this therapist. The godparents suggested that they be called if Hector became intoxicated, so that they could come over and pick up Maria and Sra. Gomez and remove them from a possibly explosive situation. During the next couple of weeks, Raul traveled into town to spend time with Hector and eventually convinced him to move in with him and get treatment. Sra. Gomez called the godparents once regarding Hector's violent behavior and the godparents began to stop by the home more frequently to check in with her and Maria. Even after Hector moved out, the godparents continued to serve as an important source of strength and support for Sra. Gomez and Maria as they continued treatment together on other issues.

The therapist's ability to understand culturally based gender and generational hierarchies and to recognize the strengths of such familial roles and relationships is demonstrated in the case of the Gomez family. Pathologizing and condemning such alliances would have driven the family into further crisis. Family therapists must reconceptualize their family systems frameworks with a culturally congruent lens if they are to work effectively with Chicano families.

Language

Language use goes beyond fluency and is symbolic of memory, affect, places, family alliances, and intimate and public situations (Falicov, 1998a). Chicano family members often differ widely in language proficiency and usage and in their positive or negative regard for Spanish or English. Although often reported in the literature as a significant cultural expression that bonds Latina/os, many Chicana/os are primarily monolingual English speakers (Hayes-Bautista, Hurtado, Valdez, & Hernandez, 1992). Ability and comfort level in speaking Spanish have also been used to define those who are "more" or "less" Latina/o in their identity. Labeling who is "really" Chicana/o can often fall along language lines for Chicana/os themselves, as illustrated in the following poem:

> Her steady hand outlines inside bottom eyelid,
> thick
> darkening to deep velvet black.
> A finishing touch ends sixty-minute routine
> for this raccoon eyed beauty.
> Turning from the mirror she says:
> "You know what you are? A Chicana falsa."
> "MEChA don't mean shit,
> and that sloppy Spanish of yours
> will never get you any discount at Bob's market."
> "HOMOGENIZED HISPANIC,
> that's what you are . . ." (Serros, 1993, p. 1)[3]

For Chicana/os, language development and use are related to a multigenerational, experiential history of racism and oppression and the negation of a Mexican cultural heritage (Cross & Maldonado, 1971; Davis, 1990; Falicov, 1998a; Rodriguez, 1989, 1992; Takaki, 1993). Thus, assessment of language use and function in the family may be a salient key to a family's difficulties (Paniagua, 1998), as was the case for the Hernandez family.

Jorge's first language was Spanish, but he and his parents claimed that he had "lost his language" and was not currently fluent in Spanish. On the other hand, Jorge's parents spoke Spanish exclusively. Jorge's great difficulty in communicating effectively with his parents was a tremendous source of frustration and conflict between them. The Hernandez family was initially assigned a Spanish-English bilingual Latina social worker, but Jorge refused to respond to her questioning even when directed in both English and Spanish. A consulting therapist was asked to join the social worker as a cotherapist to see if Jorge would respond any differently. Upon meeting the Hernandez family for the first time, the therapist disclosed some background information about herself in English as the social worker translated into Spanish: As a third-generation Chicana (Mexican American mother and Caucasian

---

[3]Reprinted with permission.

father), the therapist indicated that she had grown up surrounded by the Spanish language, but not speaking it. Her Spanish comprehension skills were good, but she had difficulty producing. The therapist requested their patience because she would only be able to respond in English in session, although, with the help of the cotherapist, she would make sure everyone was understood and had a voice. Mr. and Mrs. Hernandez were agreeable to the arrangement. Jorge smiled and began to ask the therapist questions about her upbringing and her parents and to quiz her on some Spanish words that he "remembered." The complexity of the role of language in the Hernandez family unfolded in the early phases of assessment and treatment. It was learned that Jorge had begun to refrain from speaking Spanish upon entering kindergarten, where he was first exposed to English and was teased for not being able to speak or understand it. At first, his parents encouraged his exclusive use of English. In one session, Mr. Hernandez recalled the following: "You don't get any respect here if you speak Spanish, they look down on you. I have given up trying to learn English because if you speak it with an accent, they still won't accept you! I am proud that my sons know English! I wish I did. I also wish I could talk with my son." As both the social worker and the therapist helped the Hernandez family uncover and process the meanings and experiences of language for family members, Jorge's interest in relearning the Spanish language grew, as did his interest in things "Chicano" (e.g., Chicano art and low riders).

Spiritual and Religious Belief Systems and Health

Religion, particularly Catholicism, has historically played a significant role in the lives of Chicana/os (Bach-y-Rita, 1982; Cervantes & Ramirez, 1992; Falicov & Karrer, 1984; Morones & Mikawa, 1992). It is estimated that Catholicism provides religious guidance for more than 90% of Chicana/os and is thus a common denominator of beliefs and values for many families (Falicov, 1996). Despite the growing diversity of religious affiliations among Latina/os, the role of spirituality remains a unifying characteristic (Cervantes & Ramirez, 1992; Padilla & Salgado de Snyder, 1988; Ramirez, 1983). Cervantes and Ramirez defined spirituality as "a transcendent level of consciousness that allows for existential purpose and mission, the search for harmony and wholeness, and a fundamental belief in the existence of a greater, all-loving presence in the universe" (p. 104). Central to conducting therapy with Chicana/os is understanding spirituality from a Mestizo perspective (Cervantes & Ramirez, 1992; Ramirez, 1983). *Mestizo* refers to the intermingling of physical, psychological, cultural, and spiritual ties between Spanish and Indian ancestry. In brief, Mestizo spirituality emphasizes harmony, interdependence, and respect for the sacredness of one's place in the world (Cervantes & Ramirez).

In spite of the importance of religious and spiritual beliefs and practices for Chicana/os, very little has been written about the interaction of religion, spirituality, and psychotherapy for this population. A notable exception is the work by Cervantes and Ramirez (1992), in which they created a model of family therapy based on their conceptualization of a Mestizo spirituality. By expanding general tenets of family therapy, they evolved effective strategies for family therapy with Chicana/os that emphasize the Mestizo psychology perspective (Ramirez, 1983), Mestizo spirituality, and the philosophy and practice of *curanderismo* (Mexican faith healing). This approach recognizes the integrated world view held by Chicana/os and other Latina/os regarding the intricate connection between mind, body, and spirit. Thus, health and illness are viewed as interactive dynamics of harmony and disharmony, balance and unbalance between the mind, body, and spirit. Therefore, it is not unusual for Latina/os, including Chicana/os, to maintain a dual system of beliefs and practices concerning physical and mental problems that includes mainstream medical and psychotherapeutic approaches alongside traditional folk-oriented approaches. Thus, it is important that family therapists not only recognize Chicana/os' holistic understanding of health, illness, spirituality, and healing, but also actively acknowledge and incorporate these beliefs into the therapy itself. The therapy must fit the experience and world view of each Chicano family, as demonstrated in the work with the Hernandez family.

During the course of treatment of the Hernandez family, Mr. Hernandez's drinking became worse and he refused all referrals for alcohol abuse treatment. Verbal arguments increased between Mr. and Mrs. Hernandez and Mr. Hernandez moved out of the home at one point. Jorge's depression and social withdrawal increased. He reported feelings of guilt for the "bad things" that had happened to him and his family. When probed further about this, Jorge reported that God was "punishing" him for not attending church consistently, for dropping out of the church youth group, and for the "bad thoughts" he had when he did attend (meeting girls there). The Hernandez family was devoutly Catholic. In addition, Mrs. Hernandez had sought the help of a curandera on several occasions in the past for family illnesses. Mrs. Hernandez, upon consultation with the curandera, was convinced that the family had displeased God and that Jorge and Mr. Hernandez had lost their "spirit," tying them together in misery. In order for their spirit to be regained, one or the other of them would have to regain favor and connection with God with a set of prescribed prayer rituals and herbs. Although Jorge agreed that he had lost his spirit, he was skeptical that the use of curanderismo alone would cure him. Jorge was helped to understand what was needed to regain favor and connection with God again. Jorge stated that he additionally would need to confess his sins to God through the priest at his church and to do penance, but was unsure he would be accepted after such a long absence. Jorge was encouraged to approach the priest over the next week to begin his reconciliation with God as a means for regaining not only his spirit, but also that of the family. Mrs. Hernandez and Jorge were also encouraged to follow the recommendation of the curandera if they felt comfortable doing so. Over the following several weeks, Jorge and his mother reconnected with the church and practiced prayer rituals prescribed by the curandera. Jorge eventually approached the priest with his "confession" and the priest's order of penance was for Jorge to involve himself in the church youth group again. Jorge's symptoms of depression and social isolation began to decrease and a sense of hopefulness in the family began to emerge as Mr. Hernandez also began to frequent church more regularly, although he still refused treatment for alcohol abuse.

Therapist as Social Advocate

Traditional therapy and counseling have been criticized as lacking multicultural relevance and being oppressive by serving the status quo of the dominant societal group with its primary goal of prompting individuals to adjust and adapt to its overriding values (Ivey, 1995; Sue & Sue, 1999; Szasz, 1974). Multicultural psychology has gained momentum in recent years as a means not only to illuminate the sociopolitical nature of psychology and therapy, but also to offer alternative, contextualized frameworks for theory, research, and practice. This growing movement to expand the traditional intrapsychic focus of counseling to include the negative impact of extrapsychic forces on the health and well-being of clients has been commonly referred to as "advocacy counseling," "social action," and "social justice" perspectives to counseling and psychotherapy (Kieselica & Robinson, 2001). Thus, it is becoming more evident that competent multiculturalism must include not only an awareness of and respect for diverse people, meanings, and values, but also a social justice perspective.

Working with Chicano families, members of an oppressed ethnic minority group within the United States, demands that therapists take a social justice perspective (Falicov, 1998a). A social justice orientation focuses the attention of therapists and clients on life conditions and power differentials that negatively affect their health and well-being and are intertwined with the sociopolitical forces of prejudice, internalized racism, poverty, sexism, and unequal access to opportunity for those who fall outside of society's mainstream (Falicov, 1998a; Kieselica & Robinson, 2001). Freire (1970, 1973) defined *conscientizacào*, or the process of developing a critical consciousness, as "learning to perceive social, political, and economic contradictions, and to take action against the oppressive elements of reality" (p. 19), and further stated that one of the major purposes in education should be to make people aware of themselves in these social contexts. Ivey (1995) applied Friere's *conscientizacào* to a developmental counseling and therapy model that asserts that effective therapy must consider how oppressive conditions contribute to clients' present reality in order to transform that reality. Additionally, psychotherapy as liberation demands two or more people working together to examine their relationship with each other and their social context as well (Ivey, 1995). In summary, this focus on the sociopolitical aspects of a family's life difficulties should occur within a collaborative context, where the therapist's relevant beliefs and values may need to be shared with the family, and the social context of the therapeutic relationship and situation is illuminated.

Taking a social justice perspective in Chicano family therapy is not just providing psychological services, but is complemented by macrosystem forms of advocacy that influence the people and institutions that directly and indirectly affect the lives of Chicana/os (Kieselica, 1995, 1999, 2000). Psychologists' social responsibility to "apply and make public their knowledge of psychology in order to contribute to human welfare" (American Psychological Association, 1992) is explicitly stated within the profession's ethical code of conduct. Furthermore, the degree to which psychologists should be involved in social advocacy efforts outside of the therapeutic consulting office is supported by the American Psychological Association (APA) task force on the delivery of mental health services to ethnically and culturally different people (APA, 1993). It is argued that a culturally competent practice with Chicana/os, inclusive of a social justice approach, must strive to change organizations, institutions, and policies that impede the health and well-being of Chicano families. Dinsmore, Chapman, and McCollum (2000) suggested general organizational interventions for therapists' social advocacy efforts that also appear useful for specific advocacy work with Chicana/os. According to the authors, therapists should (a) facilitate client access to information provided by institutions that is critical to clients' well-being, (b) serve as a mediator between clients and institutions (e.g., social services, education, medical care), (c) negotiate with outside agencies and institutions to provide better services for clients, (d) direct complaints about inadequate services or oppressive policies to funding agencies, and (e) influence policy makers through educational lobbying efforts. Any of these social advocacy actions can and should be part of a therapist's socially just practice with Chicana/os. The therapeutic work with the Gomez family provides an example of the many forms that advocacy can take in Chicano family therapy.

It was the middle of a Chicago winter and Maria and her grandmother had missed two therapy sessions. Contact by phone was not possible because the line had been disconnected. They were sent a letter expressing concern regarding their absence, which led Sra. Gomez to call and apologize. She stated that Maria had been very ill because their heat had been shut off; they had been without heat for 2 weeks in weather that dipped below freezing at times. Because of the Gomez family's income status and Maria's medical condition (chronic kidney disorder), they qualified for a special program that paid for the cost of their gas during the winter months. Sra. Gomez had the documentation to prove their qualification, but had received no help from social services or the gas company. Their social worker and their contact at the gas company were called, the gravity of the situation was discussed, and it was requested that their gas services be immediately resumed. This family's situation took on a broader meaning when it was learned that other professionals in the hospital where Maria was receiving treatment had seen similar situations, with their patients' having difficulty obtaining basic home services for which they were qualified and deserving. This awareness prompted hospital staff to call on the gas company and social services to better remedy such situations in the future, a collaborative effort that resulted in formal communication from the hospital that would quickly verify a patient's medical and financial qualifications to receive certain services, including heat and electricity. Fewer reports for survival services were noted following this crucial intervention.

CONCEPTUAL MODEL FOR A FAMILY THERAPY OF CHICANO FAMILIES

> Tonatzin . . . Mother
> are you here with us?
> wipe up our sweat, our tears,
> Coatlicue . . . you who rule over snakes,
> Chalchiuhcueye . . . grant us our request
> Citlalcueye . . . let your stars guide us,
> Guadalupe . . . be our dawn, our hope,
> the flag and the fire of our rebellion! (Alarcón, 1992, p. 125)[4]

The assessment and treatment literature has provided numerous suggestions over the past decade to assist in the counseling process with people of color (APA, 1993;

---

[4]From *Snake Poems* © 1992 by Francisco X. Alarcón. Used with permission of Chronicle Books LLC, San Francisco. Visit ChronicleBooks.com

Sue, Arredondo, & McDavis, 1992; Sue & Sue, 1999). Some authors have paid specific attention to the family counseling of Chicana/os (Arredondo, 1996; Bernal & Flores-Ortiz, 1983; Falicov, 1998a; Soto-Fulp & Del Campo, 1994). The majority of these authors demonstrate a strong sensitivity to contextual factors in concert with multicultural guidelines for practice. In addition, Falicov incorporated a life span development approach to practice with Chicano families. Not addressed is a model of intervention that provides an increased understanding of the various dynamics that affect the treatment process. A treatment model of family therapy with Chicana/os needs to accommodate three salient dimensions: the therapist's sociocultural history and experiences, the conceptualization or theory that is being advanced in a particular treatment case, and the Chicano family's sociocultural history and experiences.

Analysis of the therapist's sociocultural experience and history would include attention to his or her own: familial experiences, racial or ethnic identity development, socioeconomic status, gender, religious, and spiritual beliefs, professional training experiences, and other salient contextual factors that make up the therapist's world view. A conceptualization of a case from a family systems perspective would ask: How is *family* defined in this theory? What is defined as *normal* versus *pathological* in evaluating family dynamics and functioning? What needs to be changed when familial problems are identified? How is change achieved and who is involved in making that change happen? What is the therapist's role? An analysis and understanding of the Chicano family's sociocultural experiences and history would consider several factors, including: generational and migrational history, acculturation level, English or Spanish bias, experiences of racism and oppression, gender and generational hierarchies, religious and spiritual beliefs, structural integrity (single vs. intact family), level of crisis, and other contextual factors pertinent to individual families (e.g., socioeconomic status). What follows is an illustrative counseling model that can integrate a wide diversity of issues with Chicano families.

We developed a culturally syntonic concept referred to as TRENSA (Treatment of the Relationship Encounter as Nested between Self-disclosure and professional Awareness) to illustrate the professional relationship that is interwoven contextually between theory, therapist, and Chicano family. From the Spanish, *trenza* refers to a braided hairstyle worn frequently by female children, adolescents, and adults. It is the visual and imagined symbol of interweaving, TRENSA, that provides the therapeutic metaphor for effective counseling with Chicano families.

The dimensions described earlier in the chapter in the building of a model of family psychology with Chicana/os are relevant in the development of an effective, multivaried approach for working with this population. The sociocultural experiences and history of the presenting Chicano family are intertwined with the sociocultural experiences and history of the treating therapist, which in turn are intertwined with the beliefs and values of the family therapy model being utilized. The result is a holistic framework for understanding the Chicano family's therapeutic needs and experiences. The intent of this model is to understand the relevant narrative themes as they affect the dialogue between therapist and the family, a dialogue that affects the professional relationship through appropriate self-disclosure and clinical interventions that are woven throughout the encounter. This is graphically illustrated in Fig. 15.1.

As shown in Fig. 15.1, the process of family therapy or systems intervention encourages the therapist to critically examine his or her own therapeutic premises as

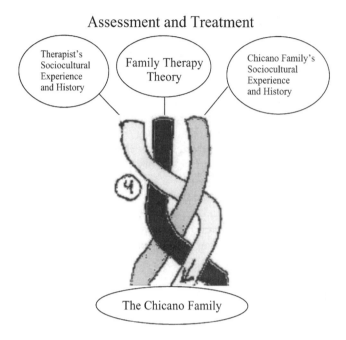

FIG. 15.1.   The TRENSA model for effective Chicano family therapy.

influenced by sociocultural history and experiences. Challenges are posed when the discrepancies listed in Table 15.1 are evident in professional interaction between the therapist and the referred family.

Similar challenges are noted with specific dynamics that are an inherent part of all families. These include, along with the contextual factors noted in Table 15.1, several unique and specific family disorders: history and presence of severe mental illness, abuse and molestation, substance abuse, developmental disorders such as mental retardation and childhood autism, blended families where step-parent is from a different ethnic or cultural background, and imminent deportation of family members.

TABLE 15.1
Discrepancies Between Therapist and Family

Therapist Variables	Family Variables
High acculturation level	Moderate to low acculturation level
Minimal to moderate Spanish-speaking ability	Bilingual children with monolingual Spanish-speaking parents
Unresolved ethnic identification	Stable Mexican or Chicana/o ethnic identification
Family background devoid of apparent experiences of oppression	History of oppression and racism in present or generational history
Specific Latina/o cultural background	Biracial background of family
Middle income, upwardly mobile	Low income, unmotivated family
U.S. citizen or resident	Undocumented status

Although this is not a comprehensive list, it does provide a wide spectrum of life problems and conditions that characterize Chicano families.

Theory is interwoven with related therapist factors to address the dynamics of the family needing intervention and the contextual dimensions evident. Relevant questions to pursue in the clinical assessment are given in Table 15.2.

How are theory and the appropriate treatment approach systemically bridged given the multilayered assessment between therapist and the family system? As noted by Lewin (1936) and Kuhn (1970) several decades ago, theory is only as good as it is useful in understanding the problem. Thus, treatment approaches to working with the broad spectrum of Chicano families require an eclectic orientation and a theoretical grounding in a variety of family therapy models (i.e., structural, Bowenian, strategic, narrative). This orientation must be rooted in a conceptual awareness of the factors that affect the professional relationship with Chicana/os (Falicov, 1998a). Table 15.3 illustrates the usefulness of this paradigm in the interaction between acculturation, family contextual factors, ethnic identity, and awareness of oppression and racism.

We now present two case studies that demonstrate the interweaving of therapist and family contextual factors with the developing treatment approach.

The first case is that of an 8-year-old Mexican American boy who was seen along with his parents and sisters. The referral question involved oppositional behavior on the part of the boy and the ensuing struggle that the parents had in managing his behavior and their own acculturation challenges.

Mario had two older sisters and a younger sister and brother. The parents were formally uneducated immigrants who had only been in the country for approximately

TABLE 15.2
Clinical Assessment Questions

Family Psychology Factors	Relevant Treatment Questions
Acculturation	Are acculturation and related stress factors in the presenting problems and the identified client? Are the potential differences in acculturation a bias that could affect the development of the therapeutic relationship?
Family community and contextual factors	Are the family background and related dynamics of the therapist and the client system so dissimilar as to warrant some extended self-disclosure in order to assess motivation and treatment progress?
Ethnic identification	Are there struggles with ethnic identity that may be important to the treatment process for the family, the therapist, or both? Is identity part of a bi- or multiracial issue that needs to be addressed?
Experience of oppression and racism	Is discrimination toward the family by a school system or other institution a relevant factor that should be addressed? How does the therapist reconcile his or her involvement outside of the consulting office in confronting institutional oppression and racism?

TABLE 15.3
Potential Strategies With Chicano Families

Family Psychology Dimensions	Potential Theory Strategies
Acculturation	Low acculturation increases risk of alcohol abuse and domestic violence in some families. Coping with acculturative stress should be evaluated and treatment may include a social learning approach, depending on family dynamics. Moderate level of acculturation may signal a transition state of values and beliefs. Structural family work may be needed if roles and parental expectations are confused or unbalanced.
Family community or contextual factors	Issues related to unresolved trauma of migration experiences and generational and language differences may require crisis management or supportive counseling, and some treatment may need to be conducted in Spanish. Severe relationship pathology like mental illness or domestic violence may require more traditional interventions.
Ethnic identification	Confusion over ethnic identity or loyalty is often part of the acculturation process. Cognitive-behavioral and psychodynamic interventions may be helpful. Multiethnic identity from interracial families may necessitate a dialogue on values clarification in order to understand related psychological symptoms.
Experience of oppression and racism	Anger and frustration caused by past discriminatory experiences based on ethnicity or race may require some cathartic work followed by role-playing techniques to teach empowerment. Institutional racism may require professional interaction, particularly as it affects the stability of the family system.

10 years prior to the intake interview. The problems that brought Mario and his family to family therapy were Mario's increasing oppositional behavior and the parents' inability to provide the necessary guidance and parental discipline. As Mario was trying to navigate the third grade in a mainstream classroom, the parents found themselves immediately handicapped by both the language system in English and their own limited experience in the educational system, each having only completed the first grade in their native country of Mexico. The family was seen at different points in Mario's life over the next 10 years, during which various educational and family crises required intervention. As Mario and his sisters grew older, the discrepancy of acculturation status became more evident in the parents' retreat to a "Mexican" discipline that emphasized unquestioned respect and adherence to family obligations. The children themselves had to wrestle with the integration of their parents' cultural values and expectations with mainstream values that emphasized more independence and reliance on peer relationships. They also had to handle, on their own, direct and indirect racism and discrimination in their respective school environments, which prevented Mario from fitting in with any of his peer group and led him to feel more accepted by those involved in gangs. Mario's discriminatory experiences became more evident in his self-defeating behavior, his poor self-esteem,

and his feeling that his Mexican-Chicano background was the reason he was unable to succeed in life. After several kinds of interventions over the 10 years of counseling with Mario and his family, he was able to graduate from high school and enroll in the California Conservation Corps. This renewed start allowed him to develop a future and new life skills for himself that would inevitably assist him in defining his career goals.

This case illustrates the conflict that often ensues for families with low levels of acculturation who become subsequently threatened by the mainstream values taught in public school systems. Issues often become more complex for children who are trying to resolve the discrepancies between the home environment and school, where independence and a future orientation are emphasized, and primary instruction is in English. Attacks on self-esteem by way of language and value biases affected these children, especially Mario, very profoundly. The family therapy was structural (Minuchin, 1974) and interwoven with social advocacy instruction about how to effectively deal with the school system. Numerous telephone consultations were made by the treating therapist in order to help advise teachers on interpreting Mario's behavior. Crisis intervention work helped to stabilize his home environment when he became involved with a gang peer group. Ethnic identification became conflictual for Mario during his early adolescent years, an issue that was addressed in treatment (Quintana & Vera, 1999). Therapy approaches were influenced by the family's low acculturative level and their continuous state of crisis. During the early phases of treatment, this caused the therapist to overidentify with the family because of her own past experiences of acculturative stress and discrimination in school. The therapist's awareness of these treatment bias issues permitted more cogent and directive strategies that were eventually helpful to Mario and his family.

The second case involves a 13-year-old female who was seen with her mother and older and younger brothers. The father was a wealthy Mexican businessman who had been estranged from the family and was only peripherally involved in his children's lives. This second case illustrates the challenge for the 13-year-old daughter to integrate Mexican and Chicana/o cultures while understanding the sense of family unity and loyalty in the face of the multiple affairs that her father was having.

Maria was the daughter of a young immigrant from Mexico whose desire was to become a wealthy businessman and a Chicana from the Southwest. Maria had one older sister and two younger sisters who were close to both parents. Maria began therapy because of the parents' separation after a 15-year marriage. Crucial in this therapeutic relationship was the observation by the mother that she had dedicated her life to helping her husband become successful from the humble roots they both shared as children of Mexican immigrants who worked in assembly line factory jobs in the 1940s and 1950s. During the first half of the marriage, the husband became extremely successful as a result of strategic involvement in the real estate market as a young man, and earning millions of dollars in a short time. This newly found wealth caused significant dissention between the parents because of the privileged status they were beginning to earn and because of the father's multiple affairs with various business partners. The father flew to Mexico on a weekly basis, where he purchased properties, developed real estate markets, and enhanced his wealth through other business transactions. Alternatively, his wife had given up her position as an elementary school teacher in order to manage her husband's business transactions. Caught in the middle of these various marital and financial changes were all the daughters, particularly Maria, who was most sensitive to these changes. The inevitable separation of the parents and their ensuing divorce caused Maria significant emotional turmoil, prompting antisocial activity, poor school performance, and abuse of drugs. The family was seen intermittently during a 3-year period in which Maria learned to handle her feelings toward her father more adaptively and to not blame her mother for the divorce. Furthermore, Maria became increasingly more secure about her ability to reconcile the strong sense of entitlement that she had learned from her father with humility for those who were economically less fortunate than her. Toward the end of the treatment, Maria chose to live with her father, who by that point had set up his home environment in Mexico. Maria's decision caused significant grief for her mother, who felt that this change would not be beneficial for her daughter. Treatment ended with Maria being more functional in school, less angry at her parents, and more prepared to handle the difficulties brought on by the rupture of her parents' relationship and the inevitable changes that would occur living with her father in Mexico.

This second case demonstrates a dramatic shift in acculturation as a result of rapidly accumulated financial wealth. The parental system became further compromised because of increasingly distant behavioral patterns brought on by the dramatic changes in economic status and the father's increased business involvement in Mexico and extramarital affairs. Maria's reactions were not unusual for a pre-adolescent female already struggling with the transition to the teen years. Maria had historically had a strong allegiance to her father, however, the shift in values and his disloyalty to the family prompted further impairment in the familial security she had come to know. Self-destructive behavior followed, with significant demonstrations of anger towards her parents. The mother and daughters were seen for family treatment, with intermittent visits on a regular schedule for Maria. Single-parent work with this family involved a rebalance of parental authority in combination with a renewed learning of beliefs and values still taught by both maternal and paternal grandparents. Thus, extended family played an important role in the treatment process, assisting in the stabilization of Maria and her sisters. This demonstration of support from grandparents was crucial in Maria's decrease in self-hate dialogue and subsequent improvement in social behavior. Maria's decision to move to Mexico with her father came about as a result of her desire to maintain contact with him and to restore a once fragile father-daughter relationship with some degree of health and integrity.

RECOMMENDATIONS FOR TRAINING, PROFESSIONAL EDUCATION, AND RESEARCH

> ... carnalas y carnales, chicaspatas
> por vida y bien entacuchaus, adding style and class
> to being half-breeds who took their Indianess
> and His panishness and became Chicanos—
> los Nuevos Mexicanos! Que Curada!
> ... ultimamente, we are still here, —no nos echen
> la bendicion yet—Octavio, Peace, brother,
> didn't get us in his labyrinth, and yet,
> was made the nobler for it!

> ... como jodidos que no nos vamos a curar?
> Orale! La Curada!
> ... heal yes, simón que sí! (Montoya, 1992, pp. 235–236)

A principal theme stated throughout this chapter is that Chicano families are a dominant force in this country, with a unique blend of ethnic and cultural history and a salient diversity in familial structure, language, and migration and acculturation experience. This uniqueness requires innovative professional tools for effective and culturally appropriate mental health practice with this population. We now present a number of critical areas of professional development that must be addressed.

Professional Training and Education

Recent surveys demonstrate that graduate education still does not include coursework relevant to working effectively with culturally diverse populations (Bernal & Castro, 1994). The increased presence of Chicano families across communities in the country (Garcia & Marotta, 1997; U.S. Bureau of the Census, 1993) indicates that the demand for appropriately defined mental health delivery services is increasing. This increased population will need more sophisticated expertise (Casas, Pavelski, Furlong, & Zanglis, in press) and comprehensive and coordinated treatment approaches (Boles & Curtin-Boles, 1996) than are currently available. Professional training must not only address the lack of appropriately conceptualized service, but also make it relevant to a family psychology for Chicana/os, incorporating meaningful and effective treatment parameters.

Though they share similar values and cultural expectations, each Chicana/o community has unique and specific family psychology issues (Alvarez, 1987; Griswold Del Castillo, 1984; Hoobler & Hoobler, 1994). We recommend that Chicana/o faculty and professionals in every community (i.e., Fresno, Orange County, Tucson, Albuquerque) develop a training model, unique to their region, that addresses the specific mental health issues of Chicano families. This could lead to the development of a data bank to which effective delivery systems of psychological care for this population can be more consistently directed. In the meantime, meaningful in-service training about specific community concerns should be provided to professionals.

The uniqueness of the Chicana/o experience has likely been a salient factor in the creation of a unique training program for mental health professionals wanting to work with Spanish-speaking individuals and families. Our Lady of the Lake University in San Antonio, Texas, developed a summer institute for bilingual (Spanish-English) psychologists, providing intensive training for professionals (www.ollusa.edu). We recommend that Latina/o faculty across the country seize the opportunity to learn about this training model for professionals, and develop related coursework, workshops, and continuing education programs that refine skills in working with respective Chicana/os.

Professional Practice

This chapter has outlined factors that contribute to an understanding of a family psychology for Chicana/os: acculturation, familial and community context, integration of ethnic identity, and experiences of oppression and racism. As pointed out by Sue and Sue (1999), appropriate psychological intervention with people of color must integrate life themes and experiences that are descriptive and meaningful to the population treated. Failure to understand the acculturation level of individuals leads to improper treatment expectations (Paniagua, 1998); disregarding contextual factors for individuals leads to biased assessment (Falicov, 1998a, 1998b); making inaccurate assumptions of ethnic identification leads to stereotyping and poor development of therapeutic goals (Flores Niemann, 2001); not recognizing the impact of oppression and racism, when applicable, on individuals and families leads to discriminatory practice and unethical practice behavior (APA, 1993). It is incumbent on practitioners and faculty who teach in graduate programs in psychology and counseling to underscore those factors that are crucial to the appropriate assessment and treatment of people of color, in this case, Chicano families.

It is a difficult professional agenda to integrate the TRENSA model into real-world practice. It also demands an awareness of one's sociocultural biases and acculturation expectations, and the goodness of fit with the specific client family dynamics and the developing theoretical approach. However, it is this stage of professional development that should be the goal of those practicing with Chicana/o populations. Along with having a content base that is guided by a family psychology orientation (Kaslow, 2001), practitioners must have more sophisticated experience with acculturation, associated language dynamics (Spanish-English), and various Chicano family structural systems. This requires a commitment to continued professional learning, even for the advanced practitioner, and a consistent willingness to learn from clients. Treating families who have learned to manage difficult life challenges (i.e., migratory experience, oppression, and racism) can educate even the seasoned clinician.

The professional development of therapists, specifically the ability to navigate both generational and acculturative terrain with individuals and families, requires advanced skills, namely, awareness and management of their ethnic stereotypes (Flores Niemann, 2001) and language facility in both Spanish and English (Falicov, 1998a; Paniagua, 1998). Stereotypes in the counseling process can have a significant negative effect on the therapeutic relationship. Furthermore, facility in both languages, including relevant professional jargon in Spanish, is necessary to effectively assist those Chicano families in which acculturation is low or the need to accommodate non-English speakers is important to treatment success. We recommend that practitioners self-assess those parameters that affect their professional abilities to be helpful with respect to conscious and unconscious attitudes toward less acculturated families and ability to communicate effectively in Spanish.

The arena of practice with Chicano families is still new and the need to examine therapeutic processes and helpful conceptualizations is becoming increasingly more relevant (Casas, 2001). Hall (1997) challenged professional psychology and counseling to become more meaningful to people of color, including a systematic compilation and understanding of what works in treatment and what does not. Thus, the development of a "best practices" portfolio for Chicano families is a necessary agenda in the new millennia. This could be accomplished through published case studies and workshops given at large national conferences (i.e., APA) where increased competency is learned at the interface of the therapist's abilities, the family's sociocultural history and dynamics, and the emerging conceptualization of treatment. It is this commitment to providing the most effective care available that marks the boundary between mediocrity and underutilized services on the one hand, and advanced competency in delivering effective mental health services to the Chicana/o community on the other.

There has been increased awareness of the need to understand the role of religion and spirituality across multiple client populations (Dossey, 1999; Fukuyama & Sevig, 1999; Miller, 1999; Shafranske, 1996; Walsh, 1999). The recent success of the first National Multicultural Conference sponsored by the APA (Sue, Bingham, Porché-Burke, & Vasques, 1999) emphasized the need to implement cultural competence in all psychological endeavors. One emphasis in this call to professional and political action is the recognition of spirituality as a salient dimension of the health and mental health care of Chicano families (Bach-y-Rita, 1982; Cervantes & Ramirez, 1992; Morones & Mikawa, 1992; Ramirez, 1983). Familiarity with this area as it pertains to the healing process has become more relevant (Falicov, 1999). Practicing therapists need to incorporate the fundamentals of religious or spiritual issues into the healing process and the building of meaningful and effective professional relationships with Chicano families. This additional level of competency requires awareness of both the religious or spiritual traditions of the family and the religious or spiritual belief system of the therapist.

Research

Over the past two decades, family therapy research has increased and evolved. Some of the most promising studies in the area of family therapy have been conducted by Szapocznik and his associates at the Spanish Family Guidance Center in Miami (Letich, 1993). This clinical-based research has focused on Hispanic and Latin American families, but has significant implications for family therapy in general. Although this program of research has made notable contributions toward the understanding of effective family therapy with some Latina/o populations (mostly Cuban) as well as family therapy in general, research specific to Chicana/os is seriously lacking. We present a number recommendations to resolve this problem.

Focusing Specifically on Chicano Families. There is considerable need for Latino family research that focuses on intragroup variability and uniqueness. Specifying and including Chicano families in research is essential for a clearer understanding of the mental health needs, processes, and difficulties of Chicana/os and of culturally appropriate interventions. Going beyond ethnic identification and attending to the complexities of race, gender, acculturation, socioeconomic status, education, and region is important in illuminating the within-group and between-group differences and similarities of the Chicano family experience. In order to begin accumulating such a knowledge base, it is recommended that collaborative, multisite clinical research programs be developed and implemented with attention to a contextual, systemic family framework.

Different Treatment Approaches. It is essential to conduct research on the effectiveness of various treatment models with Chicano families. This research should attend to the complex interplay of contextual variables in discussing under what conditions certain treatment approaches are effective. This examination of conditions would include family variables (e.g., socioeconomic status, acculturation, education), issue variables (e.g., what brought the family to treatment, how the family defines the problem), and therapist variables (e.g., ethnic or racial identification, experience, theoretical orientation). There is no one-size-fits-all therapeutic approach to working with Chicano families; clinical research must delineate what works, as well as what does not work, and under what conditions.

What Is Family Therapy for Chicano Families?   The underuse of mental health services by Chicana/os, as well as some of the systemic barriers to increased utilization (e.g., lack of Spanish-speaking therapists, transportation difficulties, childcare issues, financial constraints), have been clearly documented (Casas, 1984; Echeverry, 1997; Sue et al., 1994). It has also been suggested that cultural norms (such as shame in seeking mental health services), seeking help primarily from family and friends, and the use of religious or alternative folk healing methods may affect Chicana/os' use of mental health resources (Prieto et al., 2001). However, the profession understands very little about what Chicana/os believe about family therapy and its utility in assisting them in resolving the difficulties in their lives. What are their expectations about the therapist and the therapy process? Under what conditions would they seek out family therapy services? Ideally, where would these services be provided and what services would be deemed helpful? Perhaps another reason for the underutilization of mental health services by Chicana/os is that their conceptualization of what would be helpful is different from the traditional therapeutic approaches that have been offered to them. In summary, greater input is needed from the target population, namely, Chicana/os, in order to increase the viability of family therapy and mental health services as a whole.

Empowerment Research.   Finally, there is a need for greater utilization of qualitative methods in family research with Chicana/os in order to address the various complexities and research questions outlined earlier. Instead of trying to fit the experience of Chicano families into predetermined researcher categories, practitioners should engage in the development of grounded theory through extensive interviews, oral histories, and participant observation with Chicana/os in order to legitimately understand their experiences and meaning-making processes (Pizarro & Vera, 2001). Specifically, utilizing research methods that are both participatory and transformative is essential to a social justice approach to research with disempowered communities (Pizarro, 1998). Pizarro asserted that Chicana/os do not produce and pass on knowledge in ways that other communities do. Therefore, researchers need to acknowledge the uniqueness and validity of Chicana/o epistemology if they are to construct authentic frameworks of understanding the complexities of the Chicana/o experience. This empowerment approach, then, would include and be guided by Chicano families in all phases of the research process to ensure that their voices are accurately heard and documented. Furthermore, the process and product of such research should be explicitly beneficial to participating Chicano families and their communities and generate broader implications for the theory and practice of family therapy.

REFERENCES

Acosta, F. X., Yamamoto, J., & Evans, L. A. (1982). *Effective psychotherapy for low-income and minority patients.* New York: Plenum Press.

Alarcón, F. X. (1992). *Snake poems: An Aztec invocation.* San Francisco: Chronicle Books.

Alvarez, R. R. (1987). *Familia: Migration and adaptation in Baja and Alta California, 1800–1975.* Berkeley: University of California Press.

American Psychological Association. (1992). *Ethical principles of psychologists and code of conduct.* Washington, DC: Author.

American Psychological Association. (1993). Guidelines for provider of psychological services to ethnic, linguistic, and culturally diverse populations. *American Psychologist, 48,* 45–48.

Anzaldúa, G. (1987). *Borderlands/la frontera: The new Mestiza.* San Francisco: Spinsters/Aunt Lute.

Aparicio, I. L. (1999). Mujer, mujer. In E. J. Olmos, L. Ybarra, & M. Monterrey (Eds.), *Americanos: Latino life in the United States* (p. 146). Boston: Little, Brown.

Aponte, H. J. (1976). Underorganization in the poor family. In P. J. Guerin (Ed.), *Family therapy: Theory and practice* (pp. 432–448). New York: Gardner Press.

Aponte, H. J. (1994). *Bread and spirit: Therapy with the new poor.* New York: Norton.

Arredondo, P. (1996). MCT Theory and Latina/o-American populations. In D. W. Sue, A. E. Ivey, & P. P. Pedersen (Eds.), *A theory of multicultural counseling and therapy* (pp. 217–235). Pacific Grove, CA: Brooks/Cole.

Atkinson, D. R., Morten, G., & Sue, D. W. (Eds.) (1993). *Counseling American minorities: A cross-cultural perspective.* Madison, WI: Brown and Benchmark.

Baca Zinn, M. (1999). Social science theorizing for Latino families in the age of diversity. In S. Coontz, M. Parson, & G. Ralez (Eds.), *American families: A multicultural reader* (pp. 230–241). New York: Routledge.

Bach-y-Rita, G. (1982). The Mexican American: Religious and cultural influences. In R. M. Becerra, M. Karno, & J. I. Escobar (Eds.), *Mental health and Hispanic Americans: Clinical perspectives* (pp. 29–40). New York: Grune and Stratton.

Bean, R. A., Perry, B. J., & Bedell, T. M. (2001). Developing culturally competent marriage and family therapists: Guidelines for working with Hispanic families. *Journal of Marital and Family Therapy, 27,* 43–54.

Bernal, G., & Flores-Ortiz, Y. (1983). Latino families in therapy: Engagement and evolution. *Journal of Marital and Family Therapy, 8,* 357–365.

Bernal, M., & Castro, F. (1994). Are clinical psychologists prepared for service and research with ethnic minorities? Report of a decade of progress. *American Psychologist, 49,* 797–805.

Boles, A. J., III, & Curtin-Boles, H. A. (1996). Culturally competent health and human services for emotionally troubled children and youth: Only through intensive case management. In P. Manoleas (Ed.), *The cross-cultural practice of clinical case management in mental health* (pp. 211–232). New York: Haworth Press.

Bowen, M. (1976). Theory in the practice of psychotherapy. In P. J. Guerin (Ed.), *Family therapy: Theory and practice* (pp. 245–270). New York: Gardner Press.

Bowen, M. (1978). *Family therapy in clinical practice.* New York: Aronson.

Boyd-Franklin, N. (1989). *Black families in therapy: A multisystems approach.* New York: Guilford Press.

Boyd-Franklin, N., & Garcia-Preto, N. (1994). Family therapy: The cases of African American and Hispanic Women. In L. Comas-Díaz & B. Greene (Eds.), *Women of color: Integrating ethnic and gender identities in psychotherapy* (pp. 239–264). New York: Guilford Press.

Bronfenbrenner, U. (1977). Toward an experimental ecology of human development. *American Psychologist, 32,* 513–531.

Bronfenbrenner, U. (1979). *The ecology of human development.* Cambridge, MA: Harvard University Press.

Bronfenbrenner, U. (1986). Ecology of the family as a context for human development: Research perspectives. *Developmental Psychology, 22,* 723–742.

Carter, B., & McGoldrick, M. (Eds.). (1989). *The changing of family life cycle: A framework for family therapy.* Boston: Allyn and Bacon.

Casas, J. M. (2001). Directions and redirections in Chicano psychology. *The Counseling Psychologist, 29,* 128–138.

Casas, J. M., Pavelski, R., Furlong, M. J., & Zanglis, I. (in press). Addressing the mental health needs of Latino youth with emotional and behavioral disorders: Practical perspectives and policy implications. *The Harvard Journal of Hispanic Policy.*

Casas, M. (1984). Policy, training, and research in counseling psychology: The racial/ethnic minority perspective. In S. Brown & R. Lent (Eds.), *Handbook of counseling psychology* (pp. 785–831). New York: Wiley.

Castañeda, A. (1984). Traditionalism, modernism, and ethnicity. In J. L. Martinez & R. H. Mendoza (Eds.), *Chicano psychology* (pp. 35–40). San Diego, CA: Academic Press.

Castillo, A. (1994). *Massacre of the dreamers: Essays on Xicanisma.* Albuquerque: University of New Mexico Press.

Cervantes, J. M., & Ramirez, O. (1992). Spirituality and family dynamics in psychotherapy with Latino children. In L. Vargas & J. Koss-Chioino (Eds.), *Working with culture: Psychotherapeutic interventions with ethnic minority children and adolescents* (pp. 103–128). San Francisco: Jossey-Bass.

Cervantes, J. M., & Romero, J. D. (1983). *Hispanic mental health professionals: Emerging issues and clinical models.* Paper presented at the 91st Annual Convention of the American Psychological Association, Anaheim, CA.

Cisneros, S. (1994). *Loose woman.* New York: Knopf.

Comas-Díaz, L. (1994). An integrative approach. In L. Comaz-Díaz & B. Greene (Eds.), *Women of color: Integrating ethnic and gender identities in psychotherapy* (pp. 238–261). New York: Guilford Press.

Comas-Díaz, L. (2001). Hispanics, Latinos, or Americanos: The evolution of identity. *Cultural Diversity and Ethnic Minority Psychology, 7,* 115–120.

Cross, W. C., & Maldonado, B. (1971). The counselor and the Mexican American stereotype. *Elementary School Guidance and Counseling, 6,* 27–31.

Cuéllar, I., Harris, L. C., & Jasso, R. (1980). An acculturation scale for Mexican American normal and clinical populations. *Hispanic Journal of the Behavioral Sciences, 2,* 199–217.

Davis, M. P. (1990). *Mexican voices, American dreams: An oral history of Mexican immigration to the United States.* New York: Holt.

Diaz-Guerrero, R. (1955). Neurosis and the Mexican family structure. *American Journal of Psychiatry, 112,* 411–417.

Diaz-Guerrero, R. (1984). *The psychological study of the Mexican.* In J. Martinez, Jr. & R. H. Mendoza (Eds.), *Chicano psychology* (pp. 251–268). San Diego, CA: Academic Press.

Dinsmore, J. A., Chapman, A., & McCollum, V. J. C. (2000, March). *Client advocacy and social justice: Strategies for developing trainee competence.* Paper presented at the Annual Conference of the American Counseling Association, Washington, DC.

Dossey, L. (1999). *Reinventing medicine: Beyond mind-body to a new era of healing.* San Francisco: Harper.

Echeverry, J. J. (1997). Treatment barriers to accessing and accepting professional help. In J. G. Garcia & M. C. Zea (Eds.), *Psychological interventions and research with Latina/o populations* (pp. 94–107). Boston: Allyn and Bacon.

Falicov, C. J. (1982). Mexican families. In M. McGoldrick, J. K. Pearce, & J. Giordano (Eds.), *Ethnicity and family therapy* (pp. 169–182). New York: Guilford Press.

Falicov, C. J. (1995). Training to think culturally: A multidimensional comparative framework. *Family Process, 34,* 373–388.

Falicov, C. J. (1996). Mexican families. In M. McGoldrick, J. Giordano, & J. K. Pierce (Eds.), *Ethnicity and family therapy* (pp. 169–182). New York: Guilford Press.

Falicov, C. J. (1998a). *Latino families in therapy: A guide to multicultural practice.* New York: Guilford Press.

Falicov, C. J. (1998b). The cultural meaning of family triangles. In M. McGoldrick (Ed.), *Re-visioning family therapy: Race, culture, and gender in clinical practice* (pp. 37–47). New York: Guilford Press.

Falicov, C. J. (1999). Religion and spiritual folk traditions in immigrant families: Therapeutic resources with Latinos. In F. Walsh (Ed.), *Spiritual resources in family therapy* (pp. 104–120). New York: Guilford Press.

Falicov, C. J., & Karrer, B. (1984). Therapeutic strategies for Mexican American families. *International Journal of Family Therapy, 6,* 16–30.

Flores Niemann, Y. (2001). Stereotypes about Chicanas and Chicanos: Implications for counseling. *The Counseling Psychologist, 29,* 55–90.

Freire, P. (1970). *Pedagogy of the oppressed.* New York: Herder and Herder.

Freire, P. (1973). *Education for critical consciousness.* New York: Seabury Press.

Fukuyama, M. A., & Sevig, T. D. (1999). *Integrating spirituality into multicultural counseling.* Thousand Oaks, CA: Sage.

Garcia, J. G., & Marotta, S. (1997). Characterization of the Latino population. In J. G. Garcia & M. C. Zea (Eds.), *Psychological intervention and research with Latino populations* (pp. 1–14). Boston: Allyn and Bacon.

Garcia-Preto, N. (1996). Latino families: An overview. In M. McGoldrick, J. Giordano, & J. K. Pearce (Eds.), *Ethnicity and family therapy* (pp. 141–224). New York: Guilford Press.

Goodman, M. E. & Beman, A. (1971). Child's eye view of life in an urban barrio. In N. N. Wagner & M. J. Hauge (Eds.), *Chicanos: Social and psychological perspectives* (pp. 109–122). St. Louis, MO: Mosby.

Greiger, I., & Ponterotto, J. (1995). A framework for assessment in multicultural counseling. In J. G. Ponterotto, J. M. Casas, L. A. Suzuki, & C. M. Alexander (Eds.), *Handbook of multicultural counseling* (pp. 357–374). Thousand Oaks, CA: Sage.

Griswold Del Castillo, R. (1984). *La familia: Chicano families in the urban Southwest, 1848 to the present.* South Bend, IN: University of Notre Dame Press.

Guerin, P. (1976). *Family therapy: Theory and practice.* New York: Gardner Press.

Haley, J. (1973). *Uncommon therapy: The psychiatric techniques of Milton H. Erikson.* New York: Norton.

Haley, J. (1976). *Problem-solving therapy.* San Francisco: Jossey-Bass.

Hall, C. (1997). Cultural malpractice: The growing obsolescence of psychology with the changing U.S. population. *American Psychologist, 52*, 642–651.

Haraway, D. (1991). *Simians, cyborgs, and women: The reinvention of nature.* New York: Routledge.

Hayes-Bautista, D., Hurtado, A., Valdez, R., & Hernandez, A. C. R. (1992). *No longer a minority: Latinos and social policy in California.* Los Angeles: Chicano Studies Research Center, University of California.

Heller, C. S. (1968). *Mexican American youth: Forgotten youth at the crossroads.* New York: Random House.

Ho, M. K. (1987). *Family therapy with ethnic minorities.* Newbury Park, CA: Sage.

Hoobler, D., & Hoobler, T. (1994). *The Mexican American family album.* New York: Oxford University Press.

Ivey, A. E. (1995). Psychotherapy as liberation: Toward specific skills and strategies in multicultural counseling and therapy. In J. G. Ponterotto, J. M. Casas, L. A. Suzuki, & C. M. Alexander (Eds.), *Handbook of multicultural counseling* (pp. 53–72). Thousand Oaks, CA: Sage.

Jones, J. M. (1997). *Prejudice and racism* (2nd ed.). New York: McGraw-Hill.

Kaslow, F. W. (2001). Families and family psychology at the millennium: Intersecting crossroads. *American Psychologist, 56*, 37–46.

Kaye, K. (1985). Toward a developmental psychology of the family. In L. L'Abate (Ed.), *The handbook of family psychology and therapy* (Vol. 1, pp. 38–72). Homewood, IL: Dorsey Press.

Keefe, S. E., & Padilla, A. M. (1987). *Chicano ethnicity.* Albuquerque: University of New Mexico Press.

Kieselica, M. S. (1995). *Multicultural counseling with teenage fathers: A practical guide.* Thousand Oaks, CA: Sage.

Kieselica, M. S. (1999). Culturally sensitive interventions with African American teenage fathers. In L. E. Davis (Ed.), *Working with African American males* (pp. 205–218). Thousand Oaks, CA: Sage.

Kieselica, M. S. (2000, April). *The mental health professional as advocate: Matters of the heart, matters of the mind.* Paper presented at the Great Lakes Regional Conference of Division 17 of the American Psychological Association, Muncie, IN.

Kieselica, M. S., & Robinson, M. (2001). Bringing advocacy counseling in life: The history, issues, and human dramas of social justice work in counseling. *Journal of Counseling and Development, 79*, 387–397.

Knight, G., Cota, M., & Bernal, M. (1993). The socialization of cooperative, competitive, and individualistic preferences among Mexican American children: The mediating role of ethnic identity. *Hispanic Journal of Behavioral Sciences, 15*, 291–309.

Kuhn, T. S. (1970). *The structure of scientific revolutions.* Chicago: University of Chicago Press.

L'Abate, L. (Ed.). (1983). *Family psychology: Theory, therapy and training.* Washington, DC: University Press of America.

L'Abate, L. (Ed.). (1985). *The handbook of family psychology and therapy* (Vols. 1–2). Homewood, IL: Dorsey Press.

Lampe, P. E. (1984). Mexican Americans: Labeling and mislabeling. *Hispanic Journal of Behavioral Sciences, 6*, 77–85.

Lee, C. C., & Richardson, B. L. (Eds.). (1991). *Multicultural issues in counseling: New approaches to diversity.* Alexandria, VA: American Counseling Association.

Lewin, K. (1936). *Principles of topological psychology.* New York: McGraw-Hill.

Liddle, H. A. (1987). Family psychology: The journal, the field. *Journal of Family Psychology, 1*, 5–22.

Littlebird, H. (1982). *One mountain's breath.* Santa Fe, NM: Tooth of Time Books.

Madanes, C. (1981). *Strategic family therapy.* San Francisco: Jossey-Bass.

Madsen, W. (1964). *The Mexican Americans of South Texas.* New York: Holt, Rinehart, and Winston.

Marsella, A. J., & Pedersen, P. B. (Eds.). (1981). *Cross-cultural counseling and psychotherapy.* New York: Pergamon Press.

Martinez, C. (1988). Clinical practice with special groups: Mexican Americans. In L. Comas-Diaz and E. Griffin (Eds.), *Clinical guidelines in cross-cultural mental health* (pp. 182–203). New York: Wiley and Sons.

Martinez, K. (1994). Cultural sensitivity in family therapy gone awry. *Hispanic Journal of Behavioral Sciences, 16,* 75–89.

McGill, D. (1992). The cultural story in multicultural family therapy. *Families in Society, 73,* 339–349.

McGoldrick, M. (1998). *Re-visioning family therapy: Race, culture, and gender in clinical practice.* New York: Guilford Press.

McGoldrick, M., & Gerson, R. (1985). *Genograms in family assessment.* New York: Norton.

McGoldrick, M., Pearce, J. K., & Giordano, J. (Eds.). (1982). *Ethnicity and family therapy.* New York: Guilford Press.

McNeill, B. W. (1999). Development of a course in Chicano/Latino psychology: An academic odyssey. *JSRI Occasional Paper #49.* East Lansing, MI: The Julian Samora Research Institute, Michigan State University.

McNeill, B. W., Prieto, L. R., Flores Niemann, Y., Pizarro, M., Vera, E. M., & Gómez, S. P. (2001). Current directions in Chicana/o psychology. *The Counseling Psychologist, 29,* 5–17.

Miller, D. R., & Sabelman, G. (1985). Models of the family: A critical review of alternatives. In L. L'Abate (Ed.), *The handbook of family psychology and therapy* (Vols. 1–2, pp. 3–37). Homewood, IL: Dorsey Press.

Miller, W. (Ed.). (1999). *Integrating spirituality into treatment.* Washington, DC: American Psychological Association.

Minuchin, S. (1974). *Families and family therapy.* Cambridge, MA: Harvard University Press.

Minuchin, S., & Fishman, H. C. (1981). *Family therapy techniques.* Cambridge, MA: Harvard University Press.

Minuchin, S., Montalvo, B., Guerney, B. G., Rosman, B. L., & Schumer, F. (1967). *Families of the slums: An exploration of their structure and treatment.* New York: Basic Books.

Minuchin, S., Rosman, B. L., & Baker, L. (1978). *Psychosomatic families: Anorexia nervosa in context.* Cambridge, MA: Harvard University Press.

Mirandé, A. (1985). *The Chicano experience: An alternative perspective.* South Bend, IN: University of Notre Dame Press.

Mirkin, M. P. (1998). The impact of multiple contexts on recent immigrant families. In M. McGoldrick (Ed.), *Re-visioning family therapy: Race, culture, and gender in clinical practice* (pp. 370–383). New York: Guilford Press.

Montalvo, B., & Gutiérrez, M. (1983). A perspective for the use of the cultural dimension in family therapy. In C. J. Falicov (Ed.), *Cultural perspectives in family therapy* (pp. 15–30). Rockville, MD: Aspen.

Montalvo, B., & Gutiérrez, M. (1988). The emphasis on cultural identity: A developmental-ecological constraint. In C. J. Falicov (Ed.), *Family transitions: Continuity and change over the life cycle* (pp. 181–210). New York: Guilford Press.

Montalvo, B., & Gutiérrez, M. (1989). Nine assumptions for work with ethnic minority families. *Journal of Psychotherapy and the Family, 6,* 35–52.

Montoya, J. (1992). *Information: Twenty years of Joda.* San Francisco: Chusma House.

Moraga, C. (1983). *Loving in the war years: Lo que nunca paso por sus labios.* Boston: South End Press.

Morales, A. (1976). The impact of class discrimination and white racism on the mental health of Mexican-Americans. In C. A. Hernandez, M. J. Haug, & N. N. Wagner (Eds.), *Chicanos: Social and psychological perspectives* (pp. 211–216). St. Louis, MO: Mosby.

Morones, P. A., & Mikawa, J. K. (1992). The traditional Mestizo view: Implications for modern psychotherapeutic interventions. *Psychotherapy, 29,* 458–466.

Murillo, N. (1971). The Mexican American family. In N. N. Wagner & M. J. Haug (Eds.), *Chicanos: Social and psychological perspectives* (pp. 97–108). Saint Louis, MO: Mosby.

Murillo, N. (1984). The works of George I. Sanchez: An appreciation. In J. L. Martinez & R. H. Mendoza (Eds.), *Chicano psychology* (2nd ed., pp. 23–33). Orlando, FL: Academic Press.

Olmedo, E. L., Martinez, J. L., & Martinez, S. R. (1978). Measure of acculturation for Chicano adolescents. *Psychological Reports, 42,* 159–170.

Olmos, E. J., Ybarra, L., & Monterrey, M. (1999). *Americanos: Latino life in the United States.* Boston: Little, Brown.

Olson, D. H. (2000). *Marriage and the family: Diversity and strengths* (3rd ed.). Mountain View, CA: Mayfield.

Padilla, A. M. (1980). The role of cultural awareness and ethnic loyalty in acculturation. In A. M. Padilla (Ed.), *Acculturation: Theories, models, and some new findings* (pp. 47–84). Boulder, CO: Westview Press.

Padilla, A. M. (1995). *Hispanic psychology.* Thousand Oaks, CA: Sage.

Padilla, A. M., Carlos, M. L., & Keefe, S. E. (1976). Mental health services utilization by Mexican Americans. In M. R. Miranda (Ed.), *Psychotherapy with the Spanish speaking: Issues in research and service delivery* (pp. 9–20). Los Angeles: Spanish Speaking Mental Health Research Center, University of California.

Padilla, A., & Salgado de Snyder, V. N. (1988). Psychology in pre-Columbian Mexico. *Hispanic Journal of Behavioral Sciences, 10,* 55–66.

Paniagua, F. A. (1998). *Assessing and treating culturally diverse clients.* Thousand Oaks, CA: Sage.

Papp, P. (1981). Paradoxes. In S. Minuchin & C. Fishman (Eds.), *Family therapy techniques* (pp. 244–261). Cambridge, MA: Harvard University Press.

Peñalosa, F. (1968). Mexican family roles. *Journal of Marriage and Family, 30,* 680–689.

Pizarro, M. (1998). "Chicana/o power!": Epistemology and methodology for social justice and empowerment in Chicana/o communities. *International Journal of Qualitative Studies in Education, 11,* 57–80.

Pizarro, M., & Vera, E. (2001). Chicana/o ethnic identity research: Lessons for researchers and counselors. *The Counseling Psychologist, 29,* 91–117.

Ponterotto, J. G. (1987). Counseling Mexican-Americans: A multimodal approach. *Journal of Counseling and Development, 65,* 308–312.

Prieto, L., McNeill, B. W., Walls, R. G., & Gómez, S. P. (2001). An overview of utilization, counselor preference, and assessment issues. *The Counseling Psychologist, 29,* 18–54.

Quinoñes, M. (2000). Beyond stereotypes: Exploring the complexities of Latino identity. *Family Therapy Networker, 24,* 63–66.

Quiñonez, N. H. (1998). *The smoking mirror.* Albuquerque, NM: West End Press.

Quintana, S., & Vera, E. (1999). Mexican American children's ethnic identity, understanding of ethnic prejudice, and parental ethnic socialization. *Hispanic Journal of Behavioral Sciences, 21,* 387–404.

Ramirez, M. (1983). *Psychology of the Americas.* Elmsford, NY: Pergamon Press.

Ramirez, M. (1991). *Psychology and counseling with minorities: A cognitive approach to individual and cultural differences.* New York: Pergamon Press.

Ramirez, M., & Castañeda, A. (1974). *Cultural democracy, bicognitive development and education.* New York: Academic Press.

Ramirez, O., & Arce, C. H. (1981). The contemporary Chicano family: An empirically based review. In A. Barón, Jr. (Ed.), *Explorations in Chicano psychology* (pp. 3–28). New York: Praeger.

Rodriguez, R. (1989). *Hunger of memory: The education of Richard Rodriguez.* New York: Bantam.

Rodriguez, R. (1992). *Days of obligation: An argument with my Mexican father.* New York: Viking.

Romano, O. L. V. (1968). The anthropology of sociology of the Mexican Americans: The distortion of Mexican-American history. *El Grito: A Journal of Contemporary Mexican-American Thought, 2,* 13–26.

Romano, O. L. V. (1970). Social science, objectivity, and the Chicanos. *El Grito: A Journal of Contemporary Mexican-American Thought, 2,* 4–16.

Rueschenberg, E., & Buriel, R. (1989). Mexican American family functioning and acculturation: A family systems perspective. *Hispanic Journal of Behavioral Sciences, 11,* 232–244.

Sanchez, G. I. (1934). Bilingualism and mental measures: A word of caution. *Journal of Applied Psychology, 18,* 765–772.

Sanchez, G. I. (1941). New Mexicans and acculturation. *New Mexico Quarterly Review, 11,* 61–68.

Sandoval, M. C., & De La Roza, M. C. (1986). A cultural perspective for serving the Hispanic client. In H. P. Lefley & P. B. Pedersen (Eds.), *Cross-cultural training for mental health professionals* (pp. 151–181). Springfield, IL: Charles C. Thomas.

Serros, M. (1993). *Chicana falsa and other stories of death, identity, and Oxnard.* New York: Riverhead Books.

Shafranske, E. P. (Ed.). (1996). *Religion and the clinical practice of psychology.* Washington, DC: American Psychological Association.

Sluzki, C. (1979). Migration and family conflict. *Family Process, 18,* 379–389.

Smart, J. F., & Smart, D. W. (1995). Acculturative stress: The experience of the Hispanic immigrant. *The Counseling Psychologist, 23,* 25–42.

Soto-Fulp, S., & Del Campo, R. L. (1994). Structural family therapy with Mexican-American family systems. *Contemporary Family Therapy: An International Journal, 16,* 349–362.

Sue, D. W., Arredondo, P., & McDavis, R. J. (1992). Multicultural counseling competencies and standards: A call to the profession. *Journal of Counseling and Development, 70,* 477–486.

Sue, D. W., Bingham, R. P., Porché-Burke, L., & Vasquez, M. (1999). The diversification of psychology: A multicultural revolution. *American Psychologist, 54,* 1061–1069.

Sue, D. W., & Sue, D. (1999). *Counseling the culturally different: Theory and practice* (3rd ed.). New York: Wiley and Sons.

Sue, S., Zane, N., & Young, K. (1994). Research on psychotherapy with culturally diverse populations. In A. Bergin & S. Garfield (Eds.), *Handbook of psychotherapy and behavior change* (4th ed., pp. 783–817). New York: Wiley.

Szapocznik, J., & Kurtines, W. M. (1993). Family psychology and cultural diversity: Opportunities for theory, research, and application. *American Psychologist, 48,* 400–407.

Szapocznik, J., Kurtines, W. M., Foote, F. H., Perez-Vidal, A., & Hervis, O. (1983). Conjoint versus one-person family therapy: Some evidence for the effectiveness of conducting family therapy through one person. *Journal of Consulting and Clinical Psychology, 51,* 889–899.

Szapocznik, J., Kurtines, W. M., Foote, F. H., Perez-Vidal, A., & Hervis, O. (1986). Conjoint versus one-person family therapy: Further evidence for the effectiveness of conducting family therapy through one person with drug abusing adolescents. *Journal of Consulting and Clinical Psychology, 54,* 395–397.

Szasz, T. (1974). The myth of psychotherapy. *American Journal of Psychotherapy, 28,* 517–526.

Takaki, R. (1993). *A different minor: A history of multicultural America.* Boston: Little, Brown.

U.S. Bureau of the Census. (1993). *Latino Americans today.* Washington, DC: U.S. Government Printing Office.

Vargas, L. A., & Koss-Chioino, J. D. (Eds.). (1992). *Working with culture: Psychotherapeutic interventions with ethnic minority children and adolescents.* San Francisco: Jossey-Bass.

Vega, W. A. (1990). Hispanic families in the 1980's: A decade of research. *Journal of Marriage and Family, 52,* 1015–1024.

Walsh, F. (Ed.). (1999). *Spiritual resources in family therapy.* New York: Guilford Press.

V

Risks and Prevention

Substance Abuse Among Chicanos and Other Mexican Groups

Richard C. Cervantes
Behavioral Assessment, Inc., and
California State University, Long Beach

María Félix-Ortiz
Florida International University, Miami

Chicana/os[1] are among the fastest growing groups in the United States with a growth rate six times that of non-Hispanic Whites (Giachello, 2001), one that has doubled over the last two decades. Latina/os now represent 11.7%, or around 31.7 million, of this country's total population. By 2032, Latina/os are projected to represent approximately 20% of the general population. Two thirds of Latinos are persons of Mexican descent, or Chicana/os, and are concentrated in the states of California, Arizona, New Mexico, and Texas, although their numbers are increasing in other states, including Illinois, Florida, and New York. At the same time, more and more Chicana/os are visible in a variety of institutions, including the health care, correctional, and mental health care systems. As a result, the social policy implications of social and health problems among the general Latina/o population, and Chicana/os specifically, are receiving more attention.

In this chapter, we present key information based on current research and practice regarding the problem of alcohol and other substance abuse in the Chicana/o community. The chapter is divided into four interrelated sections on prevalence data, risk and protective factors associated with substance use, treatment and prevention programs and issues, and directions for future research. It is important to note that a comprehensive search of the research literature was conducted in both the behavioral sciences, using PsycINFO and ERIC, and the medical literature, using Medline and that our review is limited to the most recent studies available for the period of

---

[1]We use this label to refer to all individuals of Mexican descent, including those who are politically identified as Chicana/o. *Latino* is used to refer to all ethnic groups who are of Latin American descent or from a Spanish-speaking country. The use of these conventions is not to say that these groups are homogeneous, but, rather, for the sake of convenience. Finally, in reviewing studies, we use the convention selected by the authors to refer to their sample.

1995 to 2002. A few studies from before 1995 are discussed when historical context relevant.

DRUG USE PREVALENCE AMONG CHICANA/OS AND OTHER LATINA/O GROUPS: AN OVERVIEW

Epidemiology of Substance Abuse Among Chicana/os and Latina/os

Despite the relative paucity of research and information on substance abuse treatment and prevention programs available for the Latina/o and the Chicana/o communities, researchers have documented the prevalence of behavioral problems and alcohol and drug use among Latina/o youth and adults in various national survey studies. One such study is the National Household Survey on Drug Abuse (NHSDA), conducted annually by the U.S. Department of Health and Human Services and the Substance Abuse and Mental Health Services Administration, Center for Substance Abuse Prevention (SAMHSA, 2001). The survey collects information from a representative sample of persons ages 12 and over who are residents and who are "non-institutionalized." It employs a multistage area probability sample design that includes oversampling of African American and Latina/o youth ages 12 to 17 years. Although the survey collects information on ethnic identification within the Latina/o sample, no recent information has been reported on specific ethnic or racial breakdowns, an issue that continues to limit findings in many epidemiologic surveys of Mexican Americans.

In a review of data from the NHSDA for the years 1985 through 2001, illicit drug use among Latina/os ages 12 to 17 years fluctuated, but with what appeared to be a steady increase in use (SAMHSA, 2001). In 1985, 8% of Latina/o youth surveyed reported illicit drug use in the past month and in 1990, the rate was 5%, but use has progressively increased from 9.4% in 1995 to 10.1% in 2001, with a high of 11.4% in 1999.

As illustrated in Table 16.1, similar increases in drug abuse were seen for adolescents the general population. For example, past-month illicit drug use in non-Latino White youth for 2001 rose to 11.3% from 10.1% in the previous year. Increases in substance use were also found among Latina/o young adults ages 18 to 25: 10.5% in 1997, 11.1% in 1998, and a dramatically higher 14.2% in 1999. In 2000, illicit drug use dropped to 10.8%, but in 2001 the rate jumped dramatically again to 13.2%. For this same age group, non-Latina/o White young adults had the highest rates of current illicit drug use (20.8% in 2001).

As seen in Table 16.1, alcohol use in the past month declined from 18.9% in 1998 to 15.1% in 2001 among Latina/o youth. The prevalence rate of binge alcohol use among Latina/o youth ages 12 to 17 years changed from 4.8 percent in 1994 to 7.4 percent in 1995. The rates of both binge (five or more drinks at least once in past month) and heavy alcohol use (five or more drinks on five or more occasions in the past month) remained quite high for Latina/o youth in 2001. For 2001, NHSDA data reflected steady increases to 9.8% (binge drinking) and 2.1% (heavy drinking). Most troubling is the rapid and steady increase in binge drinking among Latina/o youth

Table 16.1
Percentages Reporting Past-Month Use

	Age Group									
	12 to 17					18 to 25				
Demographic Characteristic	1997	1998	1999	2000	2001	1997	1998	1999	2000	2001
Any Illicit Drug										
White, non-Hispanic	11.8	10.3	10.9	10.1	11.3	15.1	17.6	18.3	17.6	20.8
Hispanic	10.5	9.9	11.4	9.5	10.1	10.5	11.1	14.2	10.8	13.2
Black	11.0	9.9	10.7	8.4	9.1	15.5	17.1	16.2	14.5	17.1
Marijuana										
White, non-Hispanic	9.8	8.7	—	—	—	13.4	14.9	—	—	—
Hispanic	8.4	7.6	—	—	—	7.8	9.0	—	—	—
Black	9.1	8.3	—	—	—	14.1	15.2	—	—	—
Cocaine										
White, non-Hispanic	1.1	0.9	—	—	—	1.2	2.2	—	—	—
Hispanic	1.0	1.4	—	—	—	1.5	2.7	—	—	—
Black	0.1	—	—	—	—	0.9	0.6	—	—	—
Alcohol										
White, non-Hispanic	22.0	20.9	19.9	18.4	19.5	63.5	65.0	63.8	63.3	64.4
Hispanic	18.8	18.9	19.8	16.8	15.1	48.5	50.8	48.6	44.7	48.7
Black	16.3	13.1	13.3	8.8	10.6	46.6	50.3	44.3	43.9	46.5
Cigarettes										
White, non-Hispanic	21.8	20.5	17.1	16.0	15.0	45.2	46.9	45.3	43.9	44.3
Hispanic	16.0	15.1	12.1	10.2	15.8	30.9	31.5	30.9	22.3	22.6
Black	14.9	13.7	8.6	6.1	6.5	30.2	30.7	25.3	25.9	25.2

Note. Information from SAMHSA, Office of Applied Studies, National Household Survey on Drug Abuse 1998–2001.

since the early 1990s. For the young adult Latina/o population (ages 18 to 25), about 48.7% reported some alcohol use in the past month, a much lower rate than that of non-Latina/o Whites (64.4%).

A second, and very important, national survey entitled Monitoring the Future (MTF), published by the National Institute on Drug Abuse (NIDA, 2000), gathers information on high school substance use rates. Whereas the NHSDA collects data through telephone interviews, the NIDA uses self-reported, paper-and-pencil surveys, which may explain why substance use rates for high school age youth from NIDA studies are typically much higher than those documented by the NHSDA study (see Table 16.2). Among eighth-grade students in the MTF study (NIDA), Latina/os had the highest prevalence of marijuana, hallucinogen, LSD, cocaine, and tranquilizer use. It appeared that, in the early 1990s Latina/o youth initiated drug use earlier than other ethnic groups.

Latina/o youth also displayed higher rates of use of dangerous drugs, such as heroin, crack, and cocaine, in the MTF survey. Concerning alcohol use, Latina/os showed a rate similar to non-Latina/o Whites, which was higher than that of Black youth (Johnston et al., 1996). More recent data for the combined period of 1999 and 2000, as seen in Table 16.2, shows Latina/o twelfth graders to have high rates of current use of any illicit drug (27.4%), and high rates for marijuana (24.6%) and for cocaine (3.6%), all of which are higher than rates reported for either non-Latina/o White or Black students. Self-reported current alcohol use rates are also quite high for Latina/o (51.2%) and non-Latina/o White (55.1%) youth. As with the NHSDA data, older youth show much higher rates of current use of any illicit drug or alcohol when compared with their younger counterparts. Finally, current cigarette smoking was found to be very high among twelfth graders, especially among non-Latina/o White students (37.9%).

Data from the 2001 NHSDA also provides an opportunity to examine alcohol and substance use rates that would be considered by medical and mental health practitioners as drug or alcohol "dependency" using specific criteria from the *Diagnostic and Statistical Manual of Mental Disorders* (American Psychiatric Association, 1994). Additional information from the 2001 NHSDA on treatment utilization for either drugs or alcohol among various ethnic and racial groups was provided. Based on the 2001 data aggregated for all age groups 12 and older, Latina/os, as shown in Table 16.3, appeared to have slightly higher rates of dependence for illicit drugs and similar rates for alcohol when compared with non-Latina/o Whites. Hipanics tend to

TABLE 16.2
Percentages of All Youth in Grades 8, 10, and 12
Reporting Past 30-Day Use

	1999 to 2000		
Demographic Characteristic	8th Grade	10th Grade	12th Grade
Any illicit drug			
White, non-Hispanic	11.2	23.0	25.9
Hispanic	15.2	23.7	27.4
Black	10.8	17.0	20.3
Marijuana			
White, non-Hispanic	8.4	20.2	22.7
Hispanic	12.7	20.5	24.6
Black	9.3	15.8	19.0
Cocaine			
White, non-Hispanic	1.1	1.8	2.5
Hispanic	2.7	3.0	3.6
Black	0.4	0.3	0.8
Alcohol			
White, non-Hispanic	24.7	43.9	55.1
Hispanic	26.7	40.5	51.2
Black	16.0	24.7	30.0
Cigarettes			
White, non-Hispanic	17.7	28.2	37.9
Hispanic	16.6	19.6	27.7
Black	9.6	11.1	14.3
Sample sizes			
White	18,900	18,200	17,700
Hispanic	4,000	3,100	2,200
Black	4,800	3,100	3,300

Note. Source: Monitoring the Future Study, University of Michigan.

TABLE 16.3
Percentages of Past-Year Dependency and Treatment
for All Youth Ages 12 or Older

Demographic Characteristic	Dependence	Treatment
Any illicit drug		
White, non-Hispanic	2.4	0.7
Hispanic	3.1	0.8
Black	2.7	1.4
Alcohol		
White, non-Hispanic	6.2	0.9
Hispanic	6.2	1.0
Black	4.7	1.3

Note. Dependence is based on the definition
found in the *Diagnostic and Statistical Manual of Mental Disorders,* American Psychological Associatio, 1994.
The sample sizes are based on the combination 1997
and 1998.

have similar rates of treatment utilization as compared to other ethnicities. As seen in Table 16.3, Blacks have slightly higher rates of treatment utilization when compared with either Latina/o or non-Latina/o Whites.

Emergency room (ER) and coroner data also indicate the dangerous trends in drug abuse.[2] Latina/os represented only 11% of ER cases, fewer than White or Black cases, and the Latina/o cases were younger (ages 18 to 25) than the Black (ages 35 to 44). Moreover, half of the young Latino male ER cases were for substance dependence, compared to only one third of the White and Black cases. An even bleaker picture emerged for young Latinas, half of whom were admitted for suicide attempts. Unfortunately, cocaine, alcohol in combination with other drugs (usually cocaine), and heroin or morphine were the drugs most frequently mentioned for Latina/o ER cases.

Many Latina/os and Chicana/os do not leave the ER. The increase in Latina/o deaths was highest, rising 28% from 1998 to 1999 (relative to around 13% for the other racial and ethnic groups). The largest increase in substance abuse deaths from 1998 to 1999, at 149%, was recorded for San Antonio, Texas. Most of these were cocaine related (46%), representing a 150% increase in cocaine-related deaths for San Antonio. However, most Latina/o deaths are heroin related (47%). This was also reflected in the San Antonio statistics: There was a 157% increase in heroin-related deaths. The case of San Antonio is important because its population is 60% Chicana/o (James Codd, personal communication, August 9, 2001). Other cities containing large numbers of Chicana/os were also experiencing huge increases in drug-related deaths, for example, Los Angeles saw a 67% increase, Phoenix, a 44% increase, and Denver, a 38% increase. Deaths were usually the result of overdoses involving multiple drugs, usually including alcohol.

---

[2]Drug Abuse Warning Network (DAWN) data are collected annually from a representative sample of 24-hour emergency departments (ED) and a nonrepresentative sample of medical examiners (ME) in the coterminus United States.

Alcohol and Drug Use in the Chicana/o-Mexican American Community

Much of what is known specifically about Chicana/o substance use comes from smaller regional or local community studies, the largest of which are the Mexican American Prevalence and Services Survey (MAPSS; Vega, Alderete, Kolody, & Aguilar-Gaxiola, 1998) and the U.S.-Mexico Border Study of Adolescents (BSA; Pumariega, Swanson, Holzer, Linskey, & Quintero-Salinas, 1992). The MAPSS was a study of Fresno County, California in which face-to-face interviews using the World Health Organization's Composite International Diagnostic Interview (CIDI) were conducted to collect drug use and other mental health data from 3,012 Chicana/os (ages 18 to 59) in 1996 and featured sampling from town and rural as well as urban areas. BSA data were collected from 4,000 South Texas Mexican American and Mexican immigrant students ages 11 to 18 via a self-administered questionnaire completed in the classroom. Other substance use data on Chicana/os is often collected by state agencies that monitor drug use in schools or in treatment facilities through admissions data.

In a recent study by Nielsen (2000), the ubiquitous use of alcohol in the Chicana/o community resulted in more Chicana/os who use alcohol having alcohol-related problems than was the case for Puerto Ricans, Cubans, or other Latina/os who use alcohol. It was also found that nearly 20% of participant men had experienced four or more alcohol-related problems such as cirrhosis, with most problems being attributed to those 18 to 29 years old. In another study, Chicana/os were more likely to use inhalants, which are often associated with brain damage and death, as compared to other Latina/o ethnic groups (Vega, Alderete, Kolody, & Aguilar-Gaxiola, 1998). In yet another study, Chicana/os who injected drugs were more likely than Whites, Puerto Ricans, or Blacks to share injection equipment and less likely to clean it prior to or after use (Estrada, 1998).

In a few studies, substance use among special populations within the Chicana/o community has been examined, including residents of rural areas, migrant farm workers, arrestees, older adults, dropouts, and the learning disabled. Urban place of residence seems to be associated with higher drug use among Chicana/os. Although, by itself, urban versus rural residence was not associated with drug use (no main effect), acculturated urban individuals were more likely to have used illicit drugs and inhalants than were acculturated rural individuals and urban U.S.-born women were 30 times more likely to have used illicit drug or inhalants in their lifetime than were rural foreign-born women (Vega et al., 1998).

Drug Use Trends in Mexico

There is a general tendency to believe that inherent in cultural change is an increased risk for substance abuse. Important cross-cultural comparisons of substance use in Mexico with that of Mexican Americans provide a better understanding of how drug use may be influenced by the interaction of Mexican and American cultures. Data from a number of studies are reviewed here.

Based on information gathered from the SAMHSA (2001) "Summary of Findings from the 1998 National Household Survey on Drug Abuse" and the Mexican Secretary of Health report "Observatorio Epidemiologico en Drogas: El Fenomeno de las Adicciones en Mexico 2001" (Consejo Nacional Contra las Adicciones, 2001), persons in the United States (13.8%) were more likely to have used marijuana in the past month than those surveyed in Mexico (3.8%). Conversely, individuals in Mexico were more likely to have used cocaine (3.6% vs. 2%), heroin (2.6% vs. 0.2%), sedatives (3.5% vs. 0.2%), tranquilizers (4.3% vs. 1%), inhalants (3.1% vs. 1.1%), and hallucinogens (3.4% to 2.7%) in the past month than U.S. survey participants. However, when the United States population was examined based on demographic characteristics, participants of Hispanic origin tended to have higher rates of any illicit drug use for the lifetime or past-month time periods. When compared to their Mexican counterparts, persons of Hispanic origin in the United States reported a 43.2% lifetime and a 13.4% past-month rate, as opposed to 19.3% lifetime and 7.8% past-month percentages in Mexico.

Comorbidity with Mental Health Disorders, Illness, and HIV and AIDS

Substance use, abuse, and dependence commonly co-occur with mental health problems, especially the need to relieve stress or to self-medicate for disorders. In one study using the NCS, Chicana/os were more likely than Puerto Ricans, "other" Hispanics, and Blacks to have both a psychiatric disorder and substance abuse or dependence (Ortega, Rosenheck, Alegria, & Desai, 2000). Distress, depressive symptoms, and suicidal ideation and attempts correlated with substance abuse (Amaro, Messinger, & Cervantes, 1996; Félix-Ortiz, Muñoz, & Newcomb, 1994; Swanson, Linskey, Quintero-Salinas, Pumariega, & Holzer, 1992). Adolescents with significant emotional and behavioral problems were much more likely to use substances than those with less serious problems, and those with severe problems were more likely to report serious substance involvement and dependence (SAMHSA, 1999, Office of Applied Studies). Among some Mexican and Central American immigrants, adjustment disorder and posttraumatic stress disorder were often accompanied by diagnoses of depression, substance abuse or dependence (usually alcohol use), and somatic complaints (Cervantes, Salgado de Snyder, & Padilla, 1989). Immigration usually involves extraordinary hardship and stress, and sometimes the tragedies of robbery, sexual assault, torture, and worse. When these immigration-related experiences are compounded by a civil war experience, as is the case for many Latin Americans, the co-occurrence of substance abuse or dependence is highly likely (Cervantes et al.).

Substance abuse or dependence also causes a variety of health problems, including infections of major organs like the heart, abscesses, stroke, and brain damage, and these patients' active substance abuse makes treatment of their primary medical problems very challenging. Substance abuse may even negatively affect the health of family members. For example, nearly half of Chicana/o youth with asthma were exposed to cigarette smoke in the home (Amaro et al., 1996). Alcohol abuse among pregnant women can result in Fetal Alcohol Syndrome and developmental delays in their children. Finally, intravenous and other drug use is associated with HIV and AIDS. When one considers that HIV infection and AIDS are in the top ten causes of death among Latina/o youth (Amaro et al.), controlling the abuse of substances, especially those that are injected or associated with the sex trade and the sex-for-drugs trade (which occurs in crack houses), is an important goal. Among Chicana/os, HIV is spread primarily through heterosexual sex that may occur because of a large number of sexual partners and the use of prostitutes, especially those who are injection drug users and use part or most of their income to support their drug use. More Latino boys were sexually active and fewer used contraception than non-Latino Whites (Amaro et al.).

Substance Abuse Risk and Protective Factors in Chicana/os and Latina/os

This section is guided by an ecological risk-resiliency framework for the prevention and treatment of alcohol, tobacco, and drug use and delinquency. This theoretical framework offers a way of classifying factors related to substance use along different levels, from individual (proximal) factors to environmental factors (distal). Figure 16.1 depicts these various levels of the ecological framework as they reflect risk-resiliency domains.

This framework has been the basis for much of the recent state-of-the-art research on substance abuse, and was adopted by SAMHSA in 1996. It suggests that there are a number of individual, peer, family, community, and societal factors that increase the risk for adolescent substance abuse (e.g., Hawkins, Catalano, & Miller, 1992; Jessor & Jessor, 1997). Consequently, intervention strategies must focus on decreasing risk and increasing resiliency in these various ecological domains.

Personal Risk Domain.   Research on drug use has historically been dominated by investigations of individual-level (proximal) factors. At this level, in general population studies, the following have been associated with drug use: low conventionality (Cloninger, Sigvardsson, & Bohman, 1988; Jessor, Donovan, & Costa, 1991; Johnston, O'Malley, & Bachman, 1986; Newcomb, Maddahian, & Bentler, 1986), low educational achievement and aspirations (Friedman & Humphrey, 1985; Gottfredson, 1988; Johnston, O'Malley, & Bachman, 1989), emotional distress (Kandel, 1978; Newcomb & Harlow, 1986; Newcomb, Maddahian, Skager, & Bentler, 1987; Shedler & Block, 1990), childhood sexual abuse (Harrison, Hoffman, & Edwall, 1989; Singer & Petchers, 1989), stressful life events (Barrera, Li, & Chassin, 1993), low self-esteem or self-derogation (Dielman, Campanelli, Shope, & Butchart, 1987; Kaplan, 1980), and health beliefs and coping style (Chassin & Barrera, 1993; Johnston et al., 1989; Kandel & Yamaguchi, 1985).

Individual Risk Domain.   The association between emotional distress and drug use among Latina/os further supports the coping hypothesis. Emotional distress was found to be associated with drug use among Latina/o youth (Félix-Ortiz et al., 1994; Zapata & Katims, 1994). For example, Félix-Ortiz et al. found that symptoms of anxiety, depression, and hostility, along with a positive history of suicide attempt, were associated with most types of substance use among predominantly Chicana/o high school youth. Swanson et al. (1992) found that a greater proportion of youth living in Mexico were free from drugs and distress than those living in the border communities of Texas, but that, in both countries, adolescents who used drugs were much more likely to be distressed than those who did not. Fraser, Piacentini, Van Rossem, Hien, & Rotheram-Borus (1998) also found that psychopathology (i.e., affective, anxiety, and conduct disorders and suicidality) was significantly related to increased drug use. Childhood abuse (both sexual and physical) in Chicanas (Gutierres & Todd, 1997) and high threat appraisal and avoidant coping in Latinas (Nyamathi, Stein, & Brecht, 1995) were associated with drug use.

If some Latina/os use substances as part of a coping response, then many may be at risk for drug use because of a recent immigration experience. Salgado de Snyder, Cervantes, and Padilla (1990) found some evidence that recent arrivals experienced more distress than those who had lived in the U.S. for more than 5 years. Indeed, both distal and more proximal "upsetting life events" were associated with more depressive symptoms and poor health in their sample of immigrant Mexican women. These investigators also found that young adult female immigrants exhibited more depressive symptoms than their male counterparts and that these symptoms were associated with cultural or family conflict. Hondagneu-Sotelo (1994) noted that Latina immigrants tend to experience unique and intense stresses because they are expected to be the *dama de la casa,* or lady of the house, a role that makes them the high authority in home matters. However, economic necessity and reality dictate that they work outside of the home and, because of the work that Latinas typically do, they often earn more than their male partners, a situation that usually causes more tension in the household. This research indicates that female immigrants may be among the most at risk for substance abuse, although epidemiologic studies have yet to bear this out.

Nontraditional living and economic conditions among Latina/os have also been associated with substance use. Being single or a full-time homemaker, a student, or an individual unable to work was associated with higher risk for drug use (Parker, Weaver, & Calhoun, 1995). Younger Latina/os were found to be more at risk for drug use than older Latina/os (Parker et al.). Regarding gender, some have found that, although girls initiate drug use later, they appear to catch up to boys, as there is no difference between boys' and girls' drug use by the ninth grade (Khoury, Warheit, Zimmerman, Vega, & Gil, 1996). Rotheram-Borus, Rosario, Van Rossem, Reid, & Gillis (1995) found that personal resources (self-esteem) were associated with lower rates of alcohol use among gay and bisexual Latina/o youth.

Various beliefs, such as expectations regarding the consequences of drug use, have also been associated with Latina/o drug use. For example, Latina/os expected more emotional and behavioral impairment and social extroversion than non-Latina/o Whites (Marín, Posner, & Kinyon, 1993). Gilbert (1993) found that Mexican American men had more positive expectations about alcohol use than women, which may account for the gender disparity described earlier.

Health beliefs were also found to be related to drug use in Latina/os (Farabee, Wallisch, & Maxwell, 1995; Rodriguez, 1995). For example, Farabee et al. reported that Latina/os as well as non-Latina/o Whites cited concern for their health as the most important reason for abstinence. Beliefs about having control are also associated with drug use: In a sample of predominantly Chicana/o middle school students in southern Texas, Zapata and Katims (1994) found that external locus of control was associated with most types of substance use among boys, but not girls.

Indicators of conventionality are also associated with drug use among Latina/os. Drug use can be part of a problem behavior syndrome (Jessor & Jessor, 1997) or, at a minimum, indicative of a culture of unconventionality among youth who are seeking to develop an identity separate from that of their family and community. Sensation seeking (Simon, Stacy, Sussman, & Dent, 1994) and deviant behavior (Vega et al., 1998; Zapata & Katims, 1994), were further predictors of drug use among Latina/os. Simon et al. (1994) found that, among Latina/os, high sensation-seeking levels were significantly related to most substance use as well as the number of drugs used, but no such association was found for the non-Latina/o White students. They hypothesized that the physiological effects of a drug may be labeled differently depending on cultural norms regarding drug effect expectancies or that, among high sensation-seeking White students, drug use was not sufficiently stimulating. It may also be that drug use plays a special role for some Chicana/o or Latina/o subcultures (e.g., gangs). *La vida loca* (the crazy life), for example, is characterized by sensation-seeking, deviant behaviors and drug use.

Vega et al. (1998) conducted an extensive analysis of longitudinal data collected from middle school children in Miami and found that early illicit drug use and early heavy alcohol use were associated with later minor and major deviance among Latina/o (predominantly Cuban American) and White students. They also found that early heavy alcohol use was associated with current and later disposition to deviance (attitudes suggesting that deviant behaviors are acceptable), a relationship that was most evident among foreign-born Latina/o students (23%) and least evident among White students (5%).

This relationship was evident among Latinas as well as Latinos. For example, Latinas who used alcohol regularly also had more sex partners (fortunately, they also used condoms more often) and more highly acculturated Latinas tended to use alcohol before sex (Marin & Flores, 1994). Other investigators reported that Latinos frequently engaged in sexual activity while under the influence of drugs or alcohol or both (Diaz, Stall, Hoff, Daigle, & Coates, 1996). A study by Brindis, Wolfe, McCarter, Ball, & Starbuck-Morales (1995) found that Latina/o students engaged in a variety of risk behaviors, including frequent sexual activity, alcohol use, cigarette and marijuana use, illicit drug use, self-inflicted violence, unintended pregnancy, carrying a weapon, or being involved in a fight. Although this substantial body of evidence indicates that deviance was a predictor or causal factor for drug use, some have found that drug use could predict or cause deviance. For example, Taylor, Biafora, Warheit, and Gil (1997) found that the best predictors of theft and vandalism were low family pride and substance abuse for Hispanics.

On the other hand, frequent church attendance, strong religious affiliation, and educational achievement and aspirations appear to buffer Latina/os against drug use (Chavez, Oetting, & Swaim, 1994; Zapata & Katims, 1994). Church attendance and religious affiliation may be forms of social support that provide a basis for meaning, identity development, and belonging that, when weak or absent, may be replaced by intimate social relationships involving drug use (e.g., sharing joints or the close and confidential relationship with a dealer; Brownfield & Sorenson, 1991). Bonding to traditional institutions such as church and school may replace weak or absent social supports.

School Risk Domain. The lack of school bonding, poor attendance, academic failure, and high dropout rates are also strongly associated with substance use and other problematic behaviors among Hispanics. Hispanic educational attainment remains significantly low, making this group the least educated major population in the United States, with very high rates of student dropout. Studies have also found that Hispanics who have not completed an elementary or high school education have higher incidences of illicit drug use than those who are high school graduates (De la Rosa, Khalsa, & Rouse, 1990). However, the blame for the shortfalls in education cannot be placed solely on the Hispanic culture, since U.S. schools suffer many shortcomings. As a risk factor, many schools have ambiguous, lax, or inconsistent policies, rules or sanctions regarding foreign (English as a Second Language) students, alcohol, tobacco, and other drug (ATOD) use, and student conduct, making it difficult to consistently address problems if identified. Unfortunately, many Latina/o immigrant students who migrate to this country and attend public schools are not provided with the necessary assistance to make a smooth transition to a new language or culture. As a result, many of these students drop out or simply do not enroll in the educational system. In addition, favorable staff and student attitudes toward ATOD use, poor student management practices, and the availability of ATOD on school premises are all major risk factors. Latina/o students entering the school system are often overwhelmed with learning a new language or have difficulties of acculturation and fall susceptible to ATOD use. Paulson et al. (1990) found that nonusers reported higher grades, fewer absences and cut classes, higher academic aspirations, more interest in school work, and stronger feelings of its importance; more Latina/o students reported lower grades, less homework, more absences, and lower personal and parental educational goals than non-Latina/o Whites.

Alternatively, a positive instructional climate, school responsiveness to student needs, and strong school policies against substance use foster improved teacher-student relationships, educational practices, and lowered drug use (SAMHSA, 2001). This can effectively address the lower education level attained by the Latina/o community as compared to other ethnic groups (Chapa & Valencia, 1993). These changes can also help to reverse the cycle of lower career aspirations, lower social status, lower self-esteem, and an increased likelihood of experimentation with ATOD.

Parental and Family Risk Domain. The process of cultural change, or acculturation, appears to challenge traditional family values and consequent healthy family functioning among some Mexican Americans. In a review of substance abuse and family issues, Kail (1993) suggested that family and drug use may be characterized by three themes: the absence of both mother and father or an extended family, family conflict conducive to drug use, which is a result of differential rates of acculturation, and family involvement in drug use or other antisocial behavior. These factors can work together to result in behavioral problems, which are in turn related to ATOD use among youth (Cervantes, 1993; Santisteban & Szapocznik, 1982). Family stress and cultural conflict tend to be the strongest predictors of depression, anxiety, and somatic problems in U.S.-born and immigrant Latina/os (Salgado de Snyder et al., 1990), with many of these factors being associated with substance use in the general population. Among the most important family-related resiliency factors is adequate family functioning, characterized by successful parental leadership and parent-child communication that is clear and direct (Szapocznik, Kurtines, Santisteban, & Rio, 1990). Moore (1990), based on her study of a female barrio gang, described what she termed a *cholo* family, characterized by long-standing gang involvement by several members, illegal income, usually from drug dealing, and imprisonment. This exposure did not kindle an early personal interest in heroin among these girls but was actually off-putting.

In a sample of 413 Mexican American early adolescents, various risk and protective factors were found to be related to drug use (Brooks, Stuewig, & LeCroy, 1998). A major finding from the study was that separate models for predicting substance use emerged for male versus female participants. For males, family substance abuse or positive attitudes toward their use was a major influence. For females, however, the family factor indirectly influenced substance use through the relationship to family and school or peer attachment. The differences between the two models were attributed to the traditional male and female roles in the Latina/o culture, where females are traditionally raised to take on the part of the family caretaker and males are usually socialized to be dominant in the family relationship. As a result, Mexican American males were more likely to resort to substance use if a disruption in the family unit was experienced and the traditional family support or structure was no longer present.

Chicana/o child-rearing norms and having children in the household are not always protective factors. In one study, those with children had an increased risk of lifetime use of illicit drugs or inhalants compared to those without (Vega et al., 1998). Chicanas do not always refrain from drug use when pregnant (Vega, Kolody, Noble, & Porter, 1997) and their partners may be smoke or use around pregnant women and the children after they are born.

Peer Risk Domain. The SAMHSA Principles of Substance Abuse Prevention Guide (2001) reported that expectations about substance use within the peer group and ties to deviant peers or gang involvement are precursors to multiple problem behaviors in adolescent youth. During the middle school years they are exposed to considerably more external negative influential risk factors than before, at a time when adult and parent supervision is less prominent. At this time, youth seeking the approval or acceptance of their peers are more likely to give in to negative peer pressures than they previously would have.

The peer bonds to individuals with norms that contradict those held by the general population may encourage ATOD use as an accepted behavior in society. According to a study by Ellickson, Collins, and Bell (1999), the prodrug environment that this may create can encourage adolescent youth to experiment with gateway drugs such as alcohol and marijuana, which can be precursors to hard core substances (amphetamines, inhalants, cocaine, and LSD) later on in life.

In one study comparing 1,636 Mexican American middle school students to non-Hispanic Whites and Blacks in the Phoenix area (Moon, Hecht, & Jackson, 2000), negative peer influences were also found within the family environment, as Chicana/o youth were more likely to be offered drugs by peer family members (brother, sister, cousin). The problem that this prodrug attitude of peer family members presents is heightened by the finding that the family environment is one of the strongest influential factors in the Chicana/o population (Markides et al., 1986; Mindel, 1980).

In addition, Mexican American youth who affiliated with delinquent peers were more likely to engage in illicit drug use, whereas those with more conventional peers showed a lower tendency to engage in ATOD use (Oetting & Beauvais, 1987).

Community Risk Domain. Higher level community and societal factors also influence drug use among Chicana/os (SAMHSA/CSAP, 2001). At the community level, protective factors include: opportunities for youth and high expectations for their success, controlling the environment around schools and other areas where youth gather, clear company policies against drug use, active community coalitions to build programs, and support for a large number of prevention activities. Risk factors include: community disorganization and deterioration, lack of community bonding, lack of cultural pride and competence in majority culture, tolerance of drug use, availability of drugs, and inadequate youth services and opportunities for prosocial involvement. Physical characteristics of the neighborhood may also influence drug use in the community. Higher level risk factors include prodrug messages in media and economic factors like low alcohol prices, impoverishment, unemployment, and discrimination. Protective factors include different kinds of legislation aimed at reducing driving under the influence, reducing the number and location of establishments serving or selling alcohol, increasing the minimum purchasing age for tobacco and alcohol, increasing excise taxes, and restricting tobacco use in public places and indoors. Training beverage servers and increasing their liability are other successful strategies to reduce driving under the influence.

ACCULTURATION, ACCULTURATIVE STRESS, AND OTHER CULTURAL PHENOMENA AS A SPECIAL RISK FACTOR

Psychological acculturation is one of the most frequently studied correlates of Latina/o drug use, but the most poorly understood. Acculturation is the process of becoming familiar with and being able to negotiate, adopt, and value the mainstream or dominant culture (Félix-Ortiz, Newcomb, & Myers, 1994). However, the recent consensus has been that acculturation is both a group and individual phenomenon and that it usually occurs for both groups (Segall, Dasen, Berry, & Poortinga, 1999). New acculturation theory includes various acculturation strategies (e.g., marginalization, separation, integration, and assimilation) and psychological outcomes (e.g., behavioral shifts, cultural learning, social skills acquisition, and cultural shedding) that ultimately result in the individual's adaptation (Segall et al.). New multidimensional acculturation and cultural identity measures that include measures of familiarity with or adaptation to both Latina/o and American culture (e.g., ARSMA-II, Cuéllar et al., 1995; CISA, Félix-Ortiz et al., 1994) provide a partial assessment of acculturation as it is described in the anthropological literature.

Historically, two hypotheses about how acculturation is related to drug use among Chicana/os have been postulated. According to the first hypothesis, individuals who are acculturated are protected from the risk for drug use. For example, in a national study of drug use using a unidimensional acculturation measure, less acculturated Chicano men drank more heavily and were more likely to engage in risky sexual behavior than those who were more acculturated (Hines & Caetano, 1998). The second hypothesis, that acculturation is risk inducing, has been supported by more studies, particularly recent studies that used birthplace or language proficiency or both (e.g., Spanish, English, and Indian languages from Mexico and other Latin American countries) as proxies for acculturation. For example, although Hines and Caetano found heavy drinking among less acculturated Chicano men, they also found heavy drinking among acculturated Chicana women. In another study, those who were more acculturated (unidimensional measure) and U.S. born were more likely to have used illicit drugs, inhalants, cocaine, or marijuana (Vega et al., 1998). Marín and Posner (1995) found that there was a lower proportion of abstainers among Chicana/os who were more acculturated, compared to those who were less acculturated. In Farabee et al. (1995), Mexican-born participants had the lowest rate of substance use and related problems, whereas those that were highly acculturated actually had higher rates of past-year alcohol and illicit drug use or alcohol or drug problems than non-Latino Whites. Having one parent born in the U.S. also increased the likelihood of having a *Diagnostic and Statistical Manual of Mental Disorders*, 3rd edition revised (*DSM-III-R;* American Psychiatric Association, 1987) substance abuse or dependence disorder (Ortega et al., 2000).

Acculturation, as measured by both scales and proxies, is associated with more substance abuse in pregnant Chicanas. In one study, more acculturated pregnant Chicanas reported more substance use than their less acculturated counterparts (Zambrana, Scrimshaw, Collins, & Dunkel-Schetter, 1997). Urine toxicology screening used in another study revealed that pregnant Chicanas born in the U.S. were eight times more likely to have used illicit drugs than immigrant Chicana women (Vega et al., 1997). Moreover, drug abuse at an early age is likely to negatively affect Chicana/o infant health and mortality because Chicana women tend to have children earlier (Giachello, 2001).

English-language usage has also been associated with drug use among Chicana/os, who were more likely to have smoked crack (Wagner-Echeagaray, Schutz, Chilcoat, & Anthony, 1994) and to have three or more *DSM-III-R* substance abuse or dependence disorders (Ortega et al., 2000). In a study that examined the differences in substance use between immigrant Indians from Mexico (e.g., Mixtecos, Zapotecos, Tarahumaras, respondents who had a parent who spoke an Indian language) and non-Indian Mexican immigrants, the substance abuse and dependence rate for Indians was 30%, or two times higher than that of non-Indians (16%). Although this difference in risk remained despite more time in the U.S., English-language usage was associated with higher rates of psychiatric and drug dependence diagnoses (Alderete, Vega, Kolody, & Aguilar-Gaxiola, 2000). This study is an important one because it was the first to deal with the especially controversial construct of race as a within-group difference that might contribute to drug use among Chicana/os. Although these results suggest that acculturation is associated with drug abuse or dependence among Chicana/os, the proxies are not actual full measures of acculturation and must be considered carefully.

As first-generation unidimensional acculturation measures are discarded for second-generation multidimensional instrumentation, two additional hypotheses are being explored. Bicultural identity can be protective or risk inducing. Fraser et al. (1998) found that highly bicultural girls were just as likely to use drugs as less bicultural girls and attributed this to strong proscriptions in traditional Mexican culture regarding female drug use, which operated even in those endorsing a mainstream identification. However, in another study, Mexican American adolescent boys and girls who were strongly Latina/o-identified and those who were strongly American-identified used alcohol most infrequently and in the smallest amounts, whereas those who were not strongly identified with either Latina/o or American culture (marginal identity) used alcohol most frequently and in the highest amounts; biculturals fell in the middle (Félix-Ortiz & Newcomb, 1995).

Confusion about the relationship between drug use and acculturation among Latina/os may exist for several reasons. First, acculturation measures and their proxies continue to be relatively atheoretical, that is, no commonly used psychological acculturation measures are based on Berry's (1990) well-developed anthropological theory of acculturation (Segall et al., 1999). As such, most acculturation measures bear more resemblance to identity measures (e.g., Phinney, 1992) than to measures of adaptation to culture. Second, the measurement of acculturation continues to be unidimensionally conceived and measured in some studies, despite the existence of second-generation measures that are multidimensional in nature (i.e., include a measure of American identity as well as Latina/o identity). As such, those who are highly bicultural are not distinguished from those who do not identify strongly with either culture. More precise assessments of acculturation and identity that are multidimensional, and that assess several domains have been demonstrated to capture many different relationships in drug use among Chicana/os. For example, Félix-Ortiz and Newcomb (1995) found that drug use among Chicano boys was significantly influenced by three components of cultural identity: greater English proficiency (Spanish proficiency did not matter), less familiarity with Latina/o culture (familiarity with American culture did not matter), and more defensive Latino activism.

Third, acculturation has usually been measured via a single domain, specifically, language spoken. Other domains in which acculturation can occur, such as behavior, knowledge, and values, are not usually assessed, precluding the identification of specific cultural influences associated with drug use among Chicana/os (Félix-Ortiz et al., 1994). Spanish-language use may also be associated with more social desirability or a reluctance to report drug use (Wagner-Echeagaray et al., 1994), but this is not usually tested when using Spanish language as a proxy. Finally, acculturation is often confounded with acculturative stress (Félix-Ortiz, 1999).

ACCULTURATIVE STRESS AND OTHER CULTURAL PHENOMENA POSSIBLY RELATED TO DRUG USE

Psychological acculturation, acculturative stress, minority stress, assimilation, enculturation, cultural identity, racial socialization, racial identity development, and privilege are examples of cultural background variables that can be considered in an emic approach to Chicana/o drug use research. Acculturation refers to a psychosocial process, the extent of an immigrant's adaptation to the host culture (characterized by their ability to negotiate and participate in the host culture). Acculturative stress, on the other hand, is the unique stress associated with learning and participating in the host culture, and has been implicated in drug abuse and other problems (Gil, Vega, &

Dimas, 1994; Vega, Gil, and associates, 1998). Acculturative stressors might be experienced because there is no mature community enclave for those who immigrate to the U.S. (Alderete et al., 2000) and compounded by racism and discrimination due to more easily identifiable differences in appearance, dress, and language accent.

Another type of acculturative and minority stress occurs when there is a difference between the child's cultural identity and the family's cultural orientation. For example, intergenerational discrepancy (ID) in cultural orientation was associated with more child problem behavior (Szapocznik, Scopetta, Aranalde, & Kurtines, 1978). However, ID produced youth problem behavior only in the pre-existing context of family stress and conflict (Vega, Gil, et al., 1993). It also appears that only certain kinds of ID are associated with problem behaviors. ID is only associated with drug use among Latina/o youth when the child is more American identified relative to the family, but not when the child is more Latina/o identified than the family (Félix-Ortiz, Fernandez, & Newcomb, 1998). There are many different acculturative and minority stressors, but they are not experienced by all Latina/os, nor are they experienced in the same way or with the intensity. When acculturation is used as an indicator or proxy for acculturative stress, the relationship to drug use is not likely to be adequately assessed.

A GENDER GAP IN LATINA/O AND CHICANA/O DRUG USE

A dramatic gender difference in alcohol and drug use prevalence rates also distinguishes Chicana/o drug use: Women tend to abstain, but men tend to be heavy users. Fifteen times as many Mexican American immigrant women abstain from drinking, compared to Mexican American immigrant men (Canino, Burnam, & Caetano, 1992). This same dramatic male-female ratio was found for cases of misuse and dependence: for Mexican immigrants, 25:0 and for Mexican Americans, 4:1 (Canino et al.). In the NHSDA, Chicanas were more likely to abstain from drinking than Chicanos and these men reported higher rates of frequent high-quantity drinking (Nielsen, 2000). Marin and Posner (1995) also found that gender was an important determinant of frequency, number, and volume of alcoholic drinks for Chicanos, and there was a lower proportion of men who reported being abstainers than women.

The MAPSS study offered data on gender difference in illicit drug use (Vega, Alderete, Kolody, & Aguilar-Gaxiola, 1998). Lifetime prevalence of any illicit drug use among Chicana/os was 46% for men, but only 23% for women, and this gap held for different types of drug use and across urban and rural areas. Drug use in the last year indicates the possibility of active drug use, drug abuse, or dependency, and 6.4% of Chicana/o men and 1.4% of women had used cocaine in the last year, that is, Chicano men in Fresno, California were over nine times more likely to have used cocaine in the last year than their female counterparts.

Age and gender seem to interact to influence drug use among Chicana/os and Mexican nationals. Black and Markides (1994) examined gender differences in drinking across four age groups (25 to 34, 35 to 44, 45 to 54, 55 to 74) in the Hispanic Health and Nutrition Examination Survey (HHANES). They found that the number of abstainers among Mexican American women was greatest for the oldest group,

Unique to Immigrants

Psychological Acculturation
The extent of immigrants' adaptation to the host culture (Berry, 1990) characterized by their ability to negotiate and partici-pate in the host culture (Félix-Ortiz, 1999). Although enculturation and racial or ethnic socialization are the first cultural influences on individuals, acculturation is the second set of cultural influences and are from the sociopolitical context out-side of their own culture (Segall et al., 1999).

Acculturative Stress
The stress associated with learning and participating in the host culture (Vega, Gil, and associates, 1998).

Experienced by U.S.-born Minority Group Members or Highly Acculturated Immigrants

Minority Stress
The stress associated with living in the host culture as an unwelcome minority (DiPlacido, 1998; Rodriguez, Myers, Morris, & Cardoza, 2000); minority stress is usually experienced by those not accepted by the host culture (e.g. people of color, reli-gious minorities, and members of the gay, lesbian, bisexual, and transgendered community.

Assimilation
Refers specifically to the case where an individual has been able to completely adapt to the host culture and be accepted by host culture members as a bona fide member (Atkinson, Morten, & Sue, 1998). Assimilation is different from acculturation because it depends on the host culture's attitude toward the minority group member; without the host culture's receptivity, a minority person cannot assimilate. Assimilation can only occur if there is minimal or no difference in physical appearance between the individual and the host culture members, therefore, only some ethnic minority group members can assimilate. The phenomenon of "passing for White" best describes the experience of assimilation.

Universal Processes of Cultural Education

Cultural Identity
A self-initiated exploration of who one is ethnically and culturally. Theoretically, it can include nonethnic identities as well. Although cultural identity development begins in childhood, it is probably influenced by sociopolitical con-text, racial or ethnic socialization, and acculturation. Therefore, commitment to a cultural identity can change throughout adulthood.

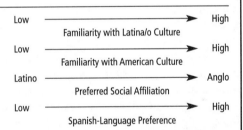

Enculturation and Racial or Ethnic Socialization
Everyone learns about race relations and ethnicity as part of childhood development (Bernal & Knight, 1997; Stevenson, 1996). Even immigrants have undergone some sort of racial or ethnic socialization in their country of origin. Racial or ethnic socialization is likely to influence racial or ethnic and cultural identity development and is a part of the enculturation pro-cess through which the nuances of a culture are absorbed through implicit or tacit learning as opposed to teaching (Lonner & Malpass, 1994; Segall et al., 1999).

Racial or Ethnic Identity
Racial or ethnic identity refers to the process of exploring race in one's identity (Cross, 1971; Phinney, 1992; Helms, 1997). Racial identity development refers to the unique experiences of someone who is considered a member of a racial minority group and probably involves racial socialization.

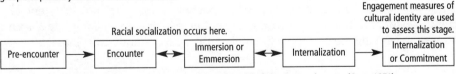

Racial Identity Stage Model: Process-Oriented Model of Identity Development (Cross, 1971)

Privilege
The advantages associated with living in the host culture as a member (Pinderhughes, 1989) can be experienced by those who are assimilated (i.e., who "pass for White"), as well as by White Americans. Everyone enjoys some sort of privilege associated with one of their identities or their socioeconomic status.

FIG. 16.1.   Cultural phenomena unique to immigrants and universal cultural education processes.

whereas the numbers of abstainers in younger groups were similar. This disappearing gender gap among young Chicana/os has been confirmed in more recent studies as well (e.g., Khoury et al., 1996; Wagner-Echeagaray et al., 1994) and is also being seen in Mexico, where generation, or age, seemed to be a more influential factor in determining drug use patterns (Gutmann, 1996).

ACCULTURATION AND THE GENDER GAP

When discussing Latina and Chicana drug use, the concept of acculturation is very relevant and appears to parsimoniously explain their use patterns. The degree to which Chicanas acculturate to the U.S. is influenced by multiple factors like age of immigration, degree of exposure to the U.S. culture, individual willingness to explore U.S. culture, and self-confidence (Mora, 1998). Canino (1994) suggested that the marked gender role differentiation typical of Latina/o culture, especially with respect to alcohol use, is protective for women. However, as recent generations are born into a less traditional Latina/o culture, the protection wanes and, as a result, acculturated women have more liberal attitudes toward drinking than do immigrant women and are more likely to use alcohol and drugs. When the effect of social disapproval of drinking by women was controlled, gender differences disappeared (Helzer & Canino, 1992). Among younger Mexican American females, acculturation is also associated with cigarette smoking and using illegal substances (Balcazar, Peterson, & Cobas, 1996; Vega et al., 1998). For example, Vega et al. found that U.S.-born Chicanas were six times more likely to have used illicit drugs or inhalants than foreign-born women, whereas U.S.-born men were only 2.4 times more likely to have used than their foreign-born compatriots.

Changes in gender role expectations may also influence drug use among Chicanas. For example, a Chicana who is employed outside the home violates traditional norms (i.e., norms that constrain the woman to the house and household duties) and is likely to experience conflict and stress due to sex role changes. Ultimately, this results in rejection or resistance from spouses, children, or other family members. These changes associated with working outside the home and being born or raised in the U.S. increased rates of heavy drinking among Chicanas (Mora, 1998). Higher education, income, and being single also increase a Chicana's likelihood of drug use (Mora). In addition to the traditional norms, which discourage alcohol and other drug use among Chicanas, there are also norms that label and severely stigmatize women who do not perfectly conform to gender role expectations and can indirectly encourage drug use (Moore, 1994). Therefore, the two extreme behaviors of complete abstention and heavy drinking are disproportionately represented among Chicanas.

TREATMENT AND PREVENTION APPROACHES
FOR SUBSTANCE ABUSE: AN OVERVIEW

Treatment Approaches

There is no question that culturally appropriate substance abuse treatment services for Chicana/os are sorely needed, yet little empirical work has been conducted to explore what constitutes a relevant service model. Substance abuse treatment service models must be able to address various risk factors, including acculturative stress and gender and socioeconomic issues. Although there are many skilled Chicana/o clinicians working to treat substance abuse problems in the community, few clinical research studies are available to document the effects of Chicana/os treating Chicana/os in a culturally competent manner.

With regard to Chicana/o and Latina/o adolescents, a specific multidimensional approach for substance abuse is needed to replace the common practice of providing treatment to adolescents using techniques developed for adults (Newcomb & Bentler, 1989). An adolescent multidimensional approach should emphasize the inadequacy of focusing exclusively on substance-related problems and include interventions that also target family functioning, psychological problems, and school and peer social functioning. Some recent studies of family-focused substance abuse prevention and early intervention programs are promising. Cervantes (1993), for example, conducted a test of the Hispanic Family Intervention Program, which was found to be an effective early intervention program for urban Latina/o youth with accompanying conduct and behavior problems, including ATOD. Similarly, Alexander et al. (1998) had success with functional family therapy in treating Latina/o juvenile offenders with multiple problems.

The Brief Strategic Family Therapy Model (BSFT; Robbins & Szapocznik, 2000) is another science-based intervention that has been tested with numerous samples of Hispanic substance-abusing adolescents. It is currently being tested for use in San Antonio, Texas, in a program targeted at substance-abusing, Mexican American, gang-affiliated adolescents. The theoretical framework of the BSFT is a dual approach (strategic and systemic), using a combination of multidimensional family therapy and multisystemic therapy, which brings the various members of the family into the therapy session to allow them to become more cohesive while solving their conflicts together.

PRIMARY PREVENTION WITH CHICANA/O ADOLESCENTS AT RISK FOR SUBSTANCE ABUSE

One of the great discoveries of the past two decades is that primary prevention for drug abuse, as an early intervention, works with youth. Many effective educational programs are available for youth regarding drugs and associated paraphernalia that increase self-esteem, change an adolescent's character, or plead to an adolescent's morality. This is after discarding ineffective programs that focused solely on content intended to scare youth or programs that were not systematic in their approach. Successful programs all rely on multiple and interrelated components: (a) interaction versus didactics, (b) community involvement in development and implementation to ensure culturally sensitive access and engagement, (c) coping and life skills building, (d) decision-making skills, (e) resistance to peer and media pressure skills, (f) parent-family and teacher involvement, (g) relationship building (to family, nonusing peers, school, and community), (h) training in a new, marketable skill or vocation, and (i) alcohol and drug education, especially regarding true rates of use (norms). All of these successful programs are focused on building caring, supportive relationships and a connection to the larger community.

The Substance Abuse and Mental Health Services Administration's Center for Substance Abuse Prevention (CSAP) has identified at least 18 effective substance abuse prevention programs for youth and, of these, six programs have been tested on, or have served a large proportion of, Chicana/o youth as well as other ethnic group youth. The programs were deemed effective only after they had been shown to be science based, to have served diverse ethnic populations, to have reduced substance abuse and other youth risk behaviors, and to have focused on individual, family, school, or community domains. A brief description of each of the six programs follows (more details are available through the CSAP Model Programs website at: www.samhsa.gov/csap/modelprograms):

- The Child Development Project (CDP), directed by Eric Schaps in Oakland, California, is a school-based program for 6- to 12-year-olds to transform the school environment into a caring community. Some strategies used included classroom and school community-building projects that foster helping, cooperation, and communication among teachers, students, and families, and home activities that involve the entire family in a reinforcement of what was learned at school. CDP was tested at 12 schools across the country (53% Latina/o, predominantly of Mexican descent). This program reduced alcohol, cigarette, and marijuana use, increased positive feelings about school and motivation to learn, and increased conflict-resolution skills and social competence.

- Life Skills Training, developed by Gilbert Botvin and colleagues at the Cornell University Medical College, targets middle and junior high school students and emphasizes the development of important personal and social skills, some general, others specifically related to the problem of drug use. This is achieved through drug education, training in decision-making skills, coping skills, social skills, and assertiveness, and a self-improvement project. Although initial tests of the program involved mostly Puerto Ricans, the program is being used in southern California and Texas with significant success. Results included decreased rates of cigarette, alcohol, and marijuana use, increased ability to refuse offers, and increased ability to find different ways to cope with stress. The effects are evident even 6 years after the intervention.

- Project ALERT, developed by Phyllis Ellickson and colleagues at the RAND Corporation in Santa Monica, California, targets middle school students, attempting to help them establish new norms against drug use, develop reasons to abstain, and resist pressures to use drugs. This is achieved through participatory activities and videos, peer interaction, intensive role playing, and parent-involved homework. The program was tested in California and Oregon and is currently used in southern California and South Texas, both of which are densely populated by Chicana/os. Results indicated reduced cigarette and marijuana use and reduced prodrug attitudes and beliefs.

- The SMART Moves Program, exclusively offered by the Boys and Girls Club of America, comprises three different age-appropriate programs and an additional program for participants' families called the Family Advocacy Network, or FAN. Structured experiential and discussion sessions, peer leadership activities, and youth activities and outings are used to develop youth leadership, resistance, interpersonal, decision-making, and coping or life skills, and to educate. FAN offers basic support for participants' families, as well as educational, socialal, and parental leadership activities. Results indicated decreased drug use, decreased perceived benefits of alcohol and marijuana use, greater ability to refuse offers, and increased knowledge of the health consequences of drug use and the prevalence of drug use. SMART Moves allows for local modifications and enhancements. At the Boys and Girls Club of Greater Fort Worth, where 47% of the participants are Chicana/o, their nationally recognized SMART Moves program has been implemented in 23 schools instead of solely at the club. It also features partnerships with a mental health agency to provide on-site individual and family counseling, with a local business to provide new children's clothes and a food bank to provide families with two grocery bags of food when their child does well academically (Sharon Driggers, personal communication, September 26, 2001).

• Project Towards No Tobacco Use, developed by Steve Sussman and colleagues at USC, comprises 10 lessons plus two booster lessons 1 year later to teach 10- to 15-year-olds about misleading social information regarding tobacco use and its prevalence, information about the physical consequences of tobacco use, resistance and interpersonal skills, decision making, and attitude change. Latina/os, predominantly of Mexican descent, accounted for 27% of the study sample. The program incorporated an interesting component: social activism letter writing to address risk factors for cigarette use in the community. Results indicated reduced tobacco use, and later initiation of tobacco use, and complete cessation of weekly or more frequent smokeless tobacco use.

Some programs target adults and, based on secondary prevention, focus on preventing dependence or harm due to drug use. One example is the Programa Latino Para Dejar de Fumar, developed by Marín and his associates at the University of San Francisco, a community-wide smoking cessation program that was designed specifically for Spanish-speaking Latina/os and included glossy booklets, bus cards, television public service announcements, and even a half-hour self-help television show on a major network. Results indicated that the program successfully disseminated smoking cessation information and that smokers reduced their daily cigarette use and made more attempts to quit (Marín & Pérez-Stable, 1995; VanOss Marín, Pérez-Stable, Marín, & Hauck, 1994).

Currently, there is only a bare patchwork quilt of Latina/o drug use research that has more holes than patches. Studies tend to use small samples that are poorly defined (e.g., key sociodemographic or mediator variables are not collected) and questionable measures or ethnic-based instruments that may have limited validity and reliability with Chicana/os and the greater Latina/o population. To date, few studies have attempted to examine within-group variability among Latina/os (e.g., Chicana/o vs. Puerto Rican). Moreover, many of the available national databases on substance use and dependence (e.g., HHANES) may now be dated given the dramatic changes in the demographics of Latina/os in the 1990s. Following are several specific recommendations based on our experiences as clinicians, researchers, and program evaluators:

1. There is a need for large, programmatic research including prospective studies in all areas of drug abuse (i.e., epidemiology and etiology, prevention, and intervention) utilizing common instruments or measures that have been validated with Latina/o subgroups such as Chicana/os, in order to replicate the studies throughout the country and perhaps even in Latin America. Use of such instrumentation would increase the comparability of results across different studies (e.g., if one were to use meta-analytic techniques). For example, a measure that appears to be appropriate for use with Chicana/os, bilinguals or English and Spanish speakers, is the Composite International Diagnostic Interview (CIDI). Many recent studies have begun to use the CIDI because it is more sensitive than other structured interviews, especially when applied to Latina/os. Alderete et al. (2000) found that the CIDI has been effectively used with Mexican nationals and Chicana/os. To date, the CIDI has been used in both the MAPSS and NCS studies to facilitate the comparison of data. In addition, the measures that are used in research studies need to be adapted for use by clinicians, who can gain much by using such data in treatment and prevention settings.

2. These studies should include instruments that measure specific ethnic identity (e.g., Chicana/o, Boricua, Nuyorican) rather than more generic labels such as Hispanic. Ethnic identity does make a major difference in how a person views and reacts to the world. For example, the term *Chicano* implies a very strong sociopolitical element of a person's identity and a person who has likely experienced prejudice or racism, or acknowledges its existence in the greater society. This identity is likely to have accompanying feelings and experiences related to community, political involvement, and so forth.

3. Recent research is uncovering new issues worthy of attention, including (a) the importance of belonging to a strong and resilient family, a strong institution (e.g., school, church), and a strong community that has in its own right been resilient and supportive, (b) the importance of social and community influences like community disintegration, (c) antidrug legislation, and (d) the role of acculturative and minority stress, cultural identity, and nationalism. There is also a need to better understand drug use in invisible Chicana subgroups such as adolescent girls who are gang affiliated, gay, lesbian, bisexual, and transgendered communities, and addicts, or *tecatos* who use heroin and cocaine at the same time. Furthermore, these explorations can employ both quantitative and qualitative methods that can be blended to respond to the complexities of the Chicana/o experience with substances.

4. Finally, there is a need to conduct research in *in vivo* or front-line settings with practitioners who treat Chicana/o substance abusers in a variety of places such as community mental health centers and private practices. In recent years, managed care has pushed Chicana/os to be treated within their own communities in mental health clinics or in the offices of private practitioners. It is important for researchers to partner with practitioners to determine whether empirically devised methods or interventions for treating substance use and dependence in Chicana/os are valid and generalizable to nonexperimental real-life settings. In order for this to happen, researchers need to extend their investigations into settings that are more likely to serve this population, where concepts such as *personalismo* (personalism) and *confianza* (trust) are practiced by the providers.

In this chapter, we have attempted to give a comprehensive overview of existing information and science on Chicana/o substance abuse. The quality and specificity of recent studies have improved dramatically over the past two decades and there is promise in new theory about culture, culture change, and individual and family adaptation as it is related to risk taking and drug use behavior. Despite these advances, we continue to call for resources and more focused efforts to understand the etiology of Chicana/o substance abuse, the development of effective prevention programs for youth, and culturally competent treatment models.

REFERENCES

Alderete, E., Vega, W. A., Kolody, B., & Aguilar-Gaxiola, S. (2000). Effects of time in the United States and Indian ethnicity on DSM-III-R psychiatric disorders among Mexican Americans in California. *The Journal of Nervous and Mental Disease, 188*, 90–100.

Alexander, J., Barton, C., Gordon, D., Grotpeter, J., Hansson, K., Harrison, R., Mears, S., Mihalic, S., Parsons, B., Pugh, C., Schulman, S., Waldron, H., & Sexton, T. (1998). *Blueprints for violence prevention, book three: Functional family therapy.* Boulder, CO: Center for the Study and Prevention of Violence.

Amaro, H., Messinger, M., & Cervantes, R. C. (1996) The health of Latino youth and challenges for prevention. In M. Kagawa-Singer, P. Katz, D. Taylor, & J. Vanderryn (Eds.), *Health issues for minority adolescents* (pp. 80–115). Lincoln: University of Nebraska Press.

American Psychiatric Association. (1987). *Diagnostic and Statistical Manual of Mental Disorders* (3rd ed., rev.). Washington, DC: Author.

American Psychiatric Association. (1994). *Diagnostic and Statistical Manual of Mental Disorders* (4th ed.). Washington, DC: Author.

Atkinson, D. R., Morten, G., & Sue, D. W. (1998). *Counseling American minorities: A cross-cultural perspective* (5th ed.) New York: McGraw-Hill.

Balcazar, H., Peterson, G., & Cobas, J. A. (1996). Acculturation and health-related risk behaviors among Mexican-American pregnant youth. *American Journal of Health Behaviors, 20*, 425–433.

Barrera, M., Li, S. A., & Chassin, L. (1993). Ethnic group differences in vulnerability to parental alcoholism and life stress: A study of Hispanic and non-Hispanic Caucasian adolescents. *American Journal of Community Psychology, 21*, 15–35.

Battistich V., Schaps E., Watson M., & Solomon D. (1996). Prevention effects of the Child Development Project: Early findings from an ongoing multisite demonstration trial. *Journal of Adolescent Research, 11*, 12–35.

Bernal, M. E., & Knight, G. P. (1997). Ethnic identity of Latino children. In J. G. Garcia & M. C. Zea (Eds.), *Psychological interventions and research with Latino populations* (pp. 15–38). Needham Heights, MA: Allyn and Bacon.

Berry, J. W. (1990). Psychology of acculturation: Understanding individuals moving between cultures. In R. W. Brislin (Ed.), *Applied cross-cultural psychology* (pp. 232–253). Newbury Park, CA: Sage.

Bosworth, K., Espelage, D., & DuBay, T. (1996). Using multimedia to teach conflict-resolution skills to young adolescents. *American Journal of Preventive Medicine, 12*(5), 65–74.

Bosworth, K., Espelage, D. L., DuBay, T., Daytner, G., & Karageorge, K. (2000). A preliminary evaluation of a multimedia violence prevention program for early adolescents. *American Journal of Health Behavior, 24*(4), 268–280.

Botvin, G. J., Epstein, J. A., Baker, E., Diaz, T., Ifill-Williams, M., Miller, N., & Cardwell, J. (1997). School-based drug abuse prevention with inner-city minority youth. *Journal of Child and Adolescent Substance Abuse, 6*(1), 5–20.

Botvin, G. J., Griffin, K. W., Diaz, T., Scheier, L. M., Williams, C., & Epstein, J. A. (2000). Preventing illicit drug use in adolescents: Long-term followup data from a randomized control trial of a school population. *Addictive Behaviors, 25*, 769–774.

Botvin, G. J., Schinke, S. P., Epstein, J. A., & Diaz, T. (1994). Effectiveness of culturally-focused and generic skills training approaches to alcohol and drug abuse prevention among minority youths. *Psychology of Addictive Behaviors, 8,* 116–127.

Brindis, C., Wolfe, A. L., McCarter, V., Ball, S., & Starbuck-Morales, S. (1995). The associations between immigrant status and risk-behavior patterns in Latino adolescents. *Journal of Adolescent Health, 17,* 99–105.

Brooks, A. J., Stuewig, J., & LeCroy, C. W. (1998). A family based model of Hispanic adolescent substance abuse. *Journal of Drug Education, 28,* 65–86

Brown, S., Myers, M. G., Mott, M. A., & Vik, P. W. (1994). Correlates of success following treatment for adolescent substance abuse. *Applied and Preventive Psychology, 3,* 61–73.

Brown, B. S., & Mills, A. R. (Eds.). (1987). *Youth at high risk for substance abuse.* Rockville, MD: National Institute on Drug Abuse.

Brownfield, D., & Sorenson, A. M. (1991). Religion and drug use among adolescents: A social support conceptualization and interpretation. *Deviant Behavior, 12,* 259–276.

Canino, G. (1994). Alcohol use and misuse among Hispanic women: Selected factors, processes and studies. *The International Journal of the Addictions, 29,* 1083–1100.

Canino, G. J., Burnam, A., & Caetano, R. (1992). The prevalence of alcohol abuse and/or dependence in two Hispanic communities. In J. E. Helzer & G. J. Canino (Eds.), *Alcoholism in North America, Europe, and Asia* (pp. 131–155). New York: Oxford University Press.

Cervantes, R. C. (1993). The Hispanic Family Intervention Program: An empirical approach toward substance abuse prevention. In B. Kail, R. Mayers, & T. Watt (Eds.), *Hispanic substance abuse* (pp. 101–114). Newbury Park, CA: Sage.

Cervantes, R. C., Padilla, A. M., & Salgado de Snyder, V. N. (1991). The Hispanic Stress Inventory: A culturally relevant approach to psychological assessment. *Psychological Assessment, 3,* 438–447.

Cervantes, R. C., Salgado de Snyder, V. N., & Padilla, A. M. (1989). Posttraumatic stress in immigrants from Central America and Mexico. *Hospital and Community Psychiatry, 40,* 615–619.

Chapa, J., & Valencia, R. R. (1993). Latino population growth, demographic characteristics, and educational stagnation: An examination of recent trends. *Hispanic Journal of Behavioral Sciences, 15,* 165–187.

Chassin, L., & Barrera, M. (1993). Substance use escalation and substance use restraint among adolescent children of alcoholics. *Psychology of Addictive Behaviors, 7,* 3–20.

Chavez, E. L., Oetting, E. R., & Swaim, R. C. (1994). Dropout and delinquency: Mexican American and Caucasian non-Hispanic youth. *Journal of Clinical Child Psychology, 23,* 47–55.

Cloninger, C. R., Sigvardsson, S., & Bohman, M. (1988). Childhood personality predicts alcohol abuse in young adults. *Alcoholism: Clinical and Experimental Research, 12,* 494–505.

Consejo Nacional Contra las Adicciones. (2001). *Observatorio epidemiológico en drogas: El fenómeno de las addiciones en México.* Mexico: Author.

Cross, W. E., Jr. (1971). The Negro-to-Black conversion experience. *Black World,* 13–27.

Cuéllar, I., Arnold, B., & Maldonado, R. (1995). Acculturation Rating Scale for Mexican Americans–II: A revision of the original ARSMA Scale. *Hispanic Journal of Behavioral Sciences, 17,* 275–304.

De la Rosa, M. R., Khalsa, J. H., & Rouse, B. A. (1990). Hispanics and illicit drug use: A review of recent findings. *International Journal of Addictions, 25,* 665–691.

Dent, C. W., Sussman, S., Stacy, A. W., Craig, S., Burton, D., & Flay, B. R. (1995). Two-year behavior outcomes of project toward no tobacco use. *Journal of Consulting and Clinical Psychology, 63* (4), 676–677.

Diaz, R. M., Stall, R. D., Hoff, C., Daigle, D., & Coates, T. J. (1996). HIV risk among Latino gay men in the southwestern United States. *AIDS Education and Prevention, 8,* 415–429.

Dielman, T. E., Campanelli, P. C., Shope, J. T., & Butchart, A. T. (1987). Susceptibility to peer pressure, self-esteem, and health locus of control as correlates of adolescent substance abuse. *Health Education Quarterly, 14,* 207–221.

DiPlacido, J. (1998). Minority stress among lesbians, gay men, and bisexuals: A consequence of heterosexism, homophobia, and stigmatization. In G. M. Herek (Ed.), *Stigma and sexual orientation: Understanding prejudice against lesbians, gay men, and bisexuals: Psychological perspectives on lesbian and gay issues* (pp. 138–159). Thousand Oaks, CA: Sage.

Drug Abuse Warning Network, SAMHSA: Office of Applied Science DAWN Report 2000.

Drug Abuse Warning Network, SAMHSA: Office of Applied Science 1999 (03/2000 update).

Ellickson, P., Bell, R., & Harrison, E. (1993). Changing adolescent propensities to use drugs: Results from Project ALERT. *Health Education Quarterly, 20* (2), 227–242.

Ellickson, P., Collins, R., & Bell, R. M. (1999). Adolescent use of illicit drugs other than marijuana: How important is social bonding and for which ethnic group? *Substance Use and Misuse, 34,* 317–346.

Estrada, A. L. (1998). Drug use and HIV risks among African-American, Mexican-American, and Puerto Rican drug injectors. *Journal of Psychoactive Drugs, 30,* 247–253.

Farabee, D., Wallisch, L., & Maxwell, J. C. (1995). Substance use among Texas Hispanics and non-Hispanics: Who's using, who's not, and why. *Hispanic Journal of Behavioral Sciences, 17,* 523–536.

Félix-Ortiz, M. (1999). Acculturative stress is important in drug use, but is limited to explaining immigrant's drug use: Comments on Vega, Gil, and associates (1998). *Contemporary Psychology, 44,* 220–224.

Félix-Ortiz, M., Fernandez, A., & Newcomb, M. D. (1998). The role of intergenerational discrepancy of cultural orientation in drug use among Latina adolescents. *Substance Use and Misuse, 33,* 967–994.

Félix-Ortiz, M., Muñoz, R., & Newcomb, M. D. (1994). The role of emotional distress in drug use among Latino and Latina adolescents. *Journal of Child and Adolescent Substance Abuse, 3,* 1–22.

Félix-Ortiz, M., & Newcomb, M. D. (1995). Cultural identity and drug use among Latino and Latina adolescents. In G. J. Botvin (Ed.), *Drug abuse prevention with multi-ethnic youth* (pp. 147–165). Newbury Park, CA: Sage.

Félix-Ortiz, M., Newcomb, M. D., & Myers, H. (1994). A multidimensional scale of cultural identity for Latino and Latina adolescents. *Hispanic Journal of Behavioral Sciences, 16,* 99–115.

Fraser, D., Piacentini, J., Van Rossem, R., Hien, D., & Rotheram-Borus, M. J. (1998). Effects of acculturation and psychopathology on sexual behavior and substance use of suicidal Hispanic adolescents. *Hispanic Journal of Behavioral Sciences, 20,* 83–101.

Friedman, J., & Humphrey, J. A. (1985). Antecedents of collegiate drinking. *Journal of Youth and Adolescence, 14,* 11–21.

Giachello, A. (2001, August). *Issues and challenges in reducing health disparities among Hispanic/Latinos in the U.S.* Paper presented at the Hispanic Cluster, National Hispanic/Latino Substance Abuse Prevention Conference, San Diego, CA.

Gil, A. G., Vega, W. A., & Dimas, J. M. (1994). Acculturative stress and personal adjustment among Hispanic adolescent boys. *Journal of Community Psychology, 22,* 43–54.

Gilbert, M. J. (1993). Intracultural variation in alcohol-related cognitions among Mexican Americans. In R. S. Mayers, B. L. Kail, & T. D. Watts (Eds.), *Hispanic substance abuse* (pp. 51–64). Springfield, IL: Thomas.

Gottfredson, D. C. (1988). An evaluation of an organization development approach to reducing school disorder. *Evaluation Review, 11,* 739–763.

Gutierres, S. E., & Todd, M. (1997). The impact of childhood abuse on treatment outcomes of substance users. *Professional Psychology: Research & Practice, 28,* 348–354.

Gutmann, M. C. (1996). *The meanings of macho: Being a man in Mexico City.* Berkeley: University of California Press.

Harrison, P. A., Hoffman, N. G., & Edwall, G. E. (1989). Sexual abuse correlates: Similarities between male and female adolescents in chemical dependency treatment. *Journal of Adolescent Research, 4,* 385–399.

Hawkins, J. D., Catalano, R. F., & Miller, J. Y. (1992). Risk and protective factors for alcohol and other drug problems in adolescent and early adulthood: Implications for substance abuse prevention. *Psychological Bulletin, 112,* 64–105.

Helms, J. E. (1997). Implications of Behrens for the validity of the White Racial Identity Attitude Scale. *Journal of Counseling Psychology, 44,* 13–16.

Helzer, J., & Canino, G. (1992). Comparative analysis of alcoholism in ten cultural regions. In J. Helzer & G. Canino (Eds.), *Alcoholism in North America, Europe, and Asia* (pp. 289–308). New York: Oxford University Press.

Hines, A. M., & Caetano, R. (1998). Alcohol and AIDS-related sexual behavior among Hispanics: Acculturation and gender differences. *AIDS Education and Prevention, 10,* 533–547.

Hondagneu-Sotelo, P. (1994). *Gendered transitions: Mexican experiences of immigration.* Berkeley: University of California Press.

Jessor, R., Donovan, J. E., & Costa, F. M. (1991). *Beyond adolescence: Problem behavior and young adult development.* New York: Cambridge University Press.

Jessor, R., & Jessor, S. L. (1997). *Problem behavior and psychosocial development: A longitudinal study of youth.* New York: Academic Press.

Johnston, L. D., O'Malley, P. M., & Bachman, J. G. (1986). *Drug use among American high school students, college students, and other young adults: National trends through 1985.* Rockville, MD: National Institute on Drug Abuse.

Johnston, L. D., O'Malley, P. M., & Bachman, J. G. (1989). *Drug use, drinking, and smoking: National survey results from high school, college, and young adults populations, 1975–1988.* Rockville, MD: National Institute on Drug Abuse.

Johnston, L. D., O'Malley, P. M., & Bachman, J. G. (1996). *National survey results on drug use from the Monitoring the Future Study, 1975–1994. Volume 1: Secondary school students.* Rockville, MD: National Institute on Drug Abuse.

Johnston, L. D., O'Malley, P. M., & Bachman, J. G. (2000). *Monitoring the future national survey results on drug use, 1975–1999. Volume I: Secondary school students* (NIH Publication No. 00-4802). Bethesda, MD: National Institute on Drug Abuse.

Kail, B. L. (1993). Patterns and predictors of drug abuse within the Chicano community. In R. S. Mayers, B. L. Kail, & T. D. Watts (Eds.), *Hispanic substance abuse* (pp. 19–36). Springfield, IL: Thomas.

Kandel, D. B. (1978). Convergences in prospective longitudinal surveys of drug use in normal populations. In D. B. Kandel (Ed.), *Longitudinal research on drug use: Empirical findings and methodological issues* (pp. 3–38). Washington, DC: Hemisphere.

Kandel, D. B., & Yamaguchi, K. (1985). Developmental patterns of the use of legal, illegal, and medically prescribed psychotropic drugs from adolescence to young adulthood. In C. L. Jones & R. J. Battjes (Eds.), *Etiology of drug abuse: Implications for prevention* (pp. 193–235). Rockville, MD: National Institute on Drug Abuse.

Kaplan, H. B. (1980). Self-esteem and self-derogation: Theory of drug abuse. In D. J. Lettieri, M. Sayers, & H. W. Pearson (Eds.), *Theories on drug abuse: Selected contemporary perspectives* (pp. 128–131). Rockville, MD: National Institute on Drug Abuse.

Khoury, E. L., Warheit, G. J., Zimmerman, R. S., Vega, W. A., & Gil, A. G. (1996). Gender and ethnic differences in the prevalence of alcohol, cigarette, and illicit drug use over time in a cohort of young Hispanic adolescents in South Florida. *Women and Health, 24,* 21–40.

Lonner, W. J., & Malpass, R. S. (1994). *Psychology and culture.* Needham Heights, MA: Allyn and Bacon.

Marin, B. V., & Flores, E. (1994). Acculturation, sexual behavior, and alcohol use among Latinas. *International Journal of the Addictions, 29,* 1101–1114.

Marín, G., & Pérez-Stable, E. J. (1995). Effectiveness of disseminating culturally appropriate smoking-cessation information: Programa Latino Para Dejar de Fumar. *Journal of the National Cancer Institute Monographs, 18,* 155–163.

Marín, G., & Posner, S. F. (1995). The role of gender and acculturation on determining the consumption of alcoholic beverages among Mexican-Americans and Central Americans in the United States. *International Journal of the Addictions, 30,* 779–794.

Marín, G., Posner, S. F., & Kinyon, J. B. (1993). Alcohol expectancies among Hispanics and non-Hispanic Whites: Role of drinking status and acculturation. *Hispanic Journal of Behavioral Sciences, 15,* 373–381.

Mindel, C. H. (1980). Extended familism among urban Mexican Americans, Anglos, and Blacks. *Hispanic Journal of Behavioral Sciences, 2,* 21–34.

Moon, D. G., Jackson, K. M., & Hecht, M. L. (2000). Family risk and resiliency factors, substance use, and the drug resistance process in adolescence. *Journal of Drug Education, 30,* 373–398.

Moore, J. (1994). The *Chola* life course: Chicana heroin users and the barrio gang. *International Journal of the Addictions, 29,* 1115–1126.

Moore, J. W. (1990). Mexican-American women addicts: The influence of family background. In J. W. Moore & R. Glick (Eds.), *Drugs in Hispanic communities* (pp. 127–153). London, CT: Rutgers University Press.

Mora, J. (1998). The treatment of alcohol dependency among Latinas: A feminist, cultural and community perspective. *Alcoholism Treatment Quarterly, 16,* 163–177.

Newcomb, M. D., & Bentler, P. M. (1989). Substance use and abuse among children and teenagers: Children and their development. Knowledge base, research agenda, and social policy application. *American Psychologist, 44,* 242–248.

Newcomb, M. D., & Harlow, L. L. (1986). Life events and substance use among adolescents: Mediating effects of perceived loss of control and meaninglessness in life. *Journal of Personality and Social Psychology, 51,* 564–577.

Newcomb, M. D., Maddahian, E., & Bentler, P. M. (1986). Risk factors for drug use among adolescents: Concurrent and longitudinal analyses. *American Journal of Public Health, 76,* 525–531.

Newcomb, M. D., Maddahian, E., Skager, R., & Bentler, P. M. (1987). Substance abuse and psychosocial risk factors among teenagers: Associations with sex, age, ethnicity, and type of school. *American Journal of Drug and Alcohol Abuse, 13,* 413–433.

Nielsen, A. L. (2000). Examining drinking patterns and problems among Hispanic groups: Results from a national survey. *Journal of Studies on Alcohol, 61,* 301–310.

Nyamathi, A., Stein, J. A., & Brecht, M. L. (1995). Psychosocial predictors of AIDS risk behavior and drug use behavior in homeless and drug addicted women of color. *Health Psychology, 14,* 265–273.

Oetting, E. R., & Beauvais, F. (1987). Common elements in youth drug abuse: Peer clusters and other psychosocial factors. *Journal of Drug Issues, 17,* 133–151.

Ortega, A. N., Rosenheck, R., Alegria, M., & Desai, R. A. (2000). Acculturation and the lifetime risk of psychiatric and substance use disorders among Hispanics. *Journal of Nervous and Mental Disease, 188,* 728–735.

Paulson, M. J., Coombs, R. H., & Richardson, M. A. (1990). School performance, academic aspirations, and drug use among children and adolescents. *Journal of Drug Education, 20,* 289–303.

Parker, K. D., Weaver, G., & Calhoun, T. (1995). Predictors of alcohol and drug use: A multi-ethnic comparison. *Journal of Social Psychology, 135,* 581–590.

Phinney, J. S. (1992). The Multigroup Ethnic Identity Measure: A new scale for use with diverse groups. *Journal of Adolescent Research, 7,* 156–176.

Pinderhughes, E. (1989). *Understanding race, ethnicity, and power: The key to efficacy in clinical practice.* New York: Free Press.

Robbins, M. S., & Szapocznik, J. (2000). *Brief strategic family therapy* (NCJ No. 179285). Washington, DC: Department of Justice, Office of Justice Programs, Office of Juvenile Justice and Delinquency Prevention.

Rodriguez, N., Myers, H. F., Morris, J. K., & Cardoza, D. (2000). Latino college student adjustment: Does an increased presence offset minority-status and acculturative stresses? *Journal of Applied Social Psychology, 30,* 1523–1550.

Rodriguez, O. (1995). Causal models of substance abuse among Puerto Rican adolescents: Implications for prevention. In G. J. Botvin, S. Schinke, & M. A. Orlandi (Eds.), *Drug abuse prevention with multiethnic youth* (pp. 130–146). Thousand Oaks, CA: Sage.

Rotherum-Borus, M. J., Rosario, M., Van Rossem, R., Reid, H., & Gillis, R. (1995). Prevalence, course and predictors of multiple problem behaviors among gay and bisexual male adolescents. *Developmental Psychology, 31,* 75–85.

Salgado de Snyder, V. N., Cervantes, R. C., & Padilla, A. M. (1990). Migration and posttraumatic stress: The case of Mexicans and Central Americans in the U.S. *Acta Psiquiatrica y Psicologica de America Latina, 36,* 137–145.

Santisteban, D., & Szapocznik, J. (1982). Substance abuse disorders among Hispanics: A focus on prevention. In R. M. Becerra, M. Karno, & J. Escobar (Eds.), *Mental health and Hispanic Americans: Clinical perspectives* (pp. 83–100). New York: Grune and Stratton.

Segall, M. H., Dasen, P. R., Berry, J. W., & Poortinga, Y. H. (1999). *Human behavior in global perspective: An introduction to cross-cultural psychology* (2nd ed.). Boston: Allyn and Bacon.

Shedler, J., & Block, J. (1990). Adolescent drug use and psychological health: A longitudinal inquiry. *American Psychologist, 45,* 612–630.

Simon, T. R., Stacy, A. W., Sussman, S., & Dent, C. W. (1994). Sensation seeking and drug use among high risk Latino and Anglo adolescents. *Personal and Indiviual Differences, 17,* 665–672.

Singer, M. I., & Petchers, M. K. (1989). The relationship between sexual abuse and substance abuse among psychiatrically hospitalized adolescents. *Child Abuse and Neglect, 13,* 319–325.

Solomon, D., Battistich, V., Watson, M., Schaps, E., & Lewis, C. (2000). A six-district study of educational change: Direct and mediated effects of the Child Development Project. *Social Psychology of Education, 4,* 3–51.

Stevenson, H. C. (in press). Theoretical considerations in measuring racial identity and socialization: Extending the self further. In R. Jones (Ed.), *Theoretical advances in Black psychology.* Hampton, VA: Cobb and Henry.

Substance Abuse and Mental Health Services Administration, Center for Substance Abuse Prevention. (2001). *Principles of substance abuse prevention* (DHHS Publication No. SMA 01-3507. Rockville, MD: U.S. Department of Health and Human Services.

Substance Abuse and Mental Health Services Administration, Office of Applied Studies. (1999). *The relationship between mental health and substance abuse among adolescents* (SAMHSA National Household Survey on Drug Abuse Series A-5). Rockville, MD: U.S. Department of Health and Human Services.

Substance Abuse and Mental Health Services Administration, Office of Applied Studies. (2000). *Drug Abuse Warning Network annual medical examiner data 1999.* DAWN Series: D-16. Rockville, MD.

Substance Abuse and Mental Health Services Administration, Office of Applied Studies. (2003). *Emergency department trends from the Drug Abuse Warning Network, final estimates 1995–2002.* DAWN Series: D-24. Rockville, MD.

Sussman, S., Dent, C. W., Stacy, A. W., Hodgson, C. S.., Burton, D., & Flay, B. R. (1993). Project toward no tobacco use: Implementation, process and post-test knowledge evaluation. *Health Education Research Theory and Practice, 8*(1), 109–123.

Swanson, J. W., Linskey, A. O., Quintero-Salinas, R., Pumariega, A. J., & Holzer, C. E., III. (1992). A binational school survey of depressive symptoms, drug use, and suicidal ideation. *Journal of the American Academy of Children and Adolescent Psychiatry, 31,* 669–678.

Szapocznik, J., Kurtines, W., Santisteban, D. A., & Rio, A. T. (1990). Interplay of advances between theory, research, and application in treatment interventions aimed at behavior problem children and adolescents. *Journal of Consulting and Clinical Psychology, 58,* 696–703.

Szapocznik, J., Scopetta, M. A., Aranalde, M., & Kurtines, W. (1978). Cuban value structure: Treatment implications. *Journal of Consulting and Clinical Psychology, 46,* 961–970.

Taylor, D. L., Biafora, F. A., Warheit, G., & Gil, A. (1997). Family factors, theft, vandalism, and major deviance among a multiracial/multiethnic sample of adolescent girls. *Journal of Social Distress and the Homeless, 6,* 71–87

VanOss Marín, B., Pérez-Stable, E. J., Marín, G., & Hauck, W. W. (1994). Effects of a community-wide intervention to change smoking behavior among Hispanics. *American Journal of Preventive Medicine, 10,* 340–347.

Vega, W., Gil, A. G., et al. (1998). *Drug use and ethnicity in early adolescence.* New York: Plenum Press.

Vega, W. A., Alderete, E., Kolody, B., & Aguilar-Gaxiola, S. (1998). Illicit drug use among Mexicans and Mexican Americans in California: The effects of gender and acculturation. *Addiction, 93,* 1839–1850.

Vega, W. A., Gil, A., Warheit, G. J., Zimmerman, R., & Apospori, E. (1993). Acculturation and delinquent behavior among Cuban American adolescents: Toward an empirical model. *American Journal of Community Psychology, 21,* 113–125.

Vega, W. A., Kolody, B., Noble, A., & Porter, P. (1997). Perinatal drug abuse among immigrant and native born Latinas. *Substance Use and Misuse, 32,* 43–60.

Wagner-Echeagaray, F. A., Schutz, C. G., Chilcoat, H. D., & Anthony, J. C. (1994). Degree of acculturation and the risk of crack cocaine smoking among Hispanic Americans. *American Journal of Public Health, 84,* 1825–1827.

Zambrana, R. E., Scrimshaw, S. C., Collins, N., & Dunkel-Schetter, C. (1997). Prenatal health behaviors and psychosocial risk factors in pregnant women of Mexican origin: The role of acculturation. *American Journal of Public Health, 87,* 1022–1026.

Zapata, J. T., & Katims, D. S. (1994). Antecedents of substance use among Mexican American school-age children. *Journal of Drug Education, 24,* 233–251.

17

Culturally and Socially Competent HIV Prevention With Mexican Farm Workers

Kurt C. Organista
University of California, Berkeley

Farm workers of Mexican descent are among the poorest, most marginalized and exploited Latina/os in America. Although they are part of a century-and-a-half-old tradition of supplying essential, labor-intensive work to billion-dollar industries and corporations, they struggle and toil at the bottom of the U.S. stratification system, where they are extremely vulnerable to numerous life-compromising problems and circumstances.

Severe and neglected health problems have been documented for farm workers for years (e.g., Rust, 1990) with increasing methodological sophistication. For example, researchers at the California Institute for Rural Studies recently published landmark studies on farm-worker health, including the first ever statewide survey to include a comprehensive physical examination (Villarejo et al., 2000), as well as a binational health survey of agricultural workers in Mexico and the United States (Mines, Mullenax, & Saca, 2001). Villarejo et al. found that risk for chronic diseases, such as heart disease, stroke, asthma, and diabetes, was startlingly high for a group composed mostly of young Mexican men who would normally be in peak physical condition. It was also found that nearly 70% of the 971 participants lacked health insurance and that only 7% were covered by government-funded programs for the poor. Similar findings were reported by Mines et al., with the addition that farm workers receive few, intermittent, uncoordinated services on both sides of the border, limiting opportunities for health promotion and disease prevention.

Reviews of the literature on HIV risk in migrant laborers on general (Organista & Balls Organista, 1997), and Mexican migrants in particular (Organista, Carillo, & Ayala, 2003), add to the problematic health profile of farm workers the possibility of an AIDS epidemic due to a variety of social and cultural factors described here. The purpose of this chapter is to provide sociodemographic and HIV risk profiles for Mexican and Chicana/o farm workers followed by a discussion of culturally competent HIV and AIDS research with this unique population. In addition, recommendations for both future research and culturally and socially appropriate HIV-prevention strategies are presented. It is worth mentioning that the frequency with which Mexican migrant laborers eventually settle in the U.S. blurs the distinction between Mexican and Chicana/o farm workers.

SOCIODEMOGRAPHIC PROFILE

Estimates of the number of farm workers in the U.S. vary between two and four million, with the higher figure including an estimation of family members (U.S. Department of Labor, 1990). As seen in Table 17.1, farm workers are predominantly foreign born, Mexican, male, low in education, and living in poverty, and half are undocumented. For the purposes of this chapter, it should also be noted that about 10% of farm workers are U.S.-born Chicana/os. Inherent in this sociodemographic profile are many formidable obstacles to conducting HIV research with Mexican farm workers, and to providing them with the numerous health and human services that they need, including HIV-prevention services. Yet, it is time to begin to struggle with these obstacles in order to prevent an AIDS epidemic in this new high-risk group.

HIV Infection-Risk Profile

HIV screening with migrant laborers is currently infrequent and sporadic. However, the few screenings that have been conducted indicate an AIDS epidemic in progress for Black farm workers in the southeastern states and the beginning of such an epidemic in Mexican farm workers. For example, HIV testing in labor camps in Florida and the Carolinas revealed infection rates ranging from 3.5% to an alarming 13% in Black farm workers from both the U.S. and the Caribbean.

TABLE 17.1
Characteristics of Migrant Farmworkers
in the U.S.

Population estimates	2.7 to 4 million
Foreign born	70%
Racial or ethnic background	
Mexican	65%
Other Latina/o	13%
White	18%
African American	2%
Other	2%
Gender (male)	80%
Undocumented	52%
Education	4 to 7 years
Income (< $10,000 annually)	75%
Poverty	60%
Illiteracy estimate	10%

Note. Data from U.S. Department of Labor (1990, 1998).

Although the results of three HIV screenings of Mexican farm workers only found infection rates of less than 2% (Carrier & Magaña, 1991; Center for Disease Control and Prevention, 1988; López & Ruiz, 1995), these studies also documented the presence of significant precursors to an AIDS epidemic in this population. For example, in López and Ruiz's HIV screening of 176 Mexican farm workers in northern California, they found a 9% history of sexually transmitted diseases and two active cases of syphilis. In addition, they noted that 9% of female respondents reported having sex with a partner who injected drugs. In their screening of 2,000 migrant laborers, Carrier and Magaña noted that epidemics of syphilis and chancroid had recently occurred in migrant laborers and prostitutes in southern California.

Major HIV Exposure Categories for Farm Workers

There are at least four major HIV exposure categories that render farm workers vulnerable to infection. These categories are related to both social and cultural factors and are now reviewed and discussed.

Prostitution Use in the United States. Worldwide prostitution use is a common part of the migrant labor experience for men far away from home for extended periods of time (Hulewicz, 1994). With regard to Mexican migrants, Organista, Balls Organista, Garcia de Alba G., Castillo Moran, and Ureta Carrillo (1997a) found that 44% of 342 male respondents from Jalisco, Mexico, had had sex with prostitutes while working in the U.S. Interestingly, married men in the survey were as likely as single men to use prostitutes, but less likely to use condoms, underscoring significant risk to wives. With regard to the complex ways in which culture, migratory labor, and economics influence behavior, it was also found that 13% of the men surveyed reported participating in a male bonding ritual in which several migrant men had sex with the same prostitute in succession. After such an experience, these men referred to themselves as *hermanos de leche* (milk brothers), presumably for sharing sperm.

The *hermanos de leche* ritual was also documented by Magaña (1991), who interviewed 50 male Mexican migrants and 38 injection-drug-using female prostitutes. Magaña reported that the prostitutes actively solicited the men at labor camps, bars, and other locations where they congregated, especially on pay day. Ironically, low condom use was reported by both the migrants and the sex workers in this study because members of each group believed that suggesting condom use would insinuate that they had AIDS or another sexually transmitted disease (STD). Efforts to promote condom use with prostitutes must consider the complex nuances of this salient HIV-exposure category.

Sex Between Men. Surveys of Mexican migrants inquiring about sex between men report rates ranging from 2% to 3.5% (Lafferty, 1991; Lopez & Ruiz, 1995; Organista, Garcia de Alba G., Castillo Moran, & Ureta Carrillo, 1997). Although these survey interviews were private and conducted by male interviewers, the figures most likely underestimate this taboo behavior. For example, when the author conducted pre-survey focus groups in rural Mexico with migrant men to discuss the issue, all participants acknowledged the common practice of heterosexual macho men occasionally having sex with other men when women were unavailable. However, when asked directly if any of them had had such experiences, all said "no," given the non-private and social nature of focus groups. Private interviews are needed to learn more about the complexities of this pertinent HIV-exposure category.

Carrier (1985, 1995) wrote extensively about the construction of (homo)sexuality in Mexico versus the United States in ways that are informative to HIV-prevention research and services. Consistent with the aforementioned focus groups, Carrier noted that masculine Mexican men who occasionally play the active inserter role with passive, effeminate men may continue to identify as heterosexual and lead predominantly heterosexual lifestyles. Such culture-based sexual behaviors are bound to be influenced by the experience of migratory labor, in which sex between men is not uncommon. For example, Bronfman and Minello (1992) conducted in-depth, qualitative interviews with Mexican migrants and concluded that homosexual contact increases with migration due to extended periods of loneliness, isolation, and emotional deprivation, as well as greater sexual freedom in the U.S. Obviously, the different constructions of sex between Mexican men need to be considered for maximally effective HIV-prevention messages.

Needle Sharing.   Needle sharing is a very interesting HIV-exposure category for Mexican migrants for many economic and culture-related reasons such as the frequent practice of lay "therapeutic injections" of vitamins and antibiotics. In Mexico, it is legal and common for people to purchase and use hypodermic needles to medicate themselves and their family members. This practice continues in the United States, especially given the low access to affordable health care. For example, Lafferty (1991) found that 20% of 411 Mexican farm workers reported lay therapeutic injections, including 3.5% who reported sharing a needle with family members. In contrast, only 2.9% of the sample reported illegal injection-drug use. More recently, McVea (1997) found that 12% of 532 Mexican farm workers surveyed admitted to lay injection with antibiotics or vitamins. Thus, HIV-prevention messages aimed at needle sharing must not be confined to illegal drug use.

Though not documented in the literature, there is discussion these days in the labor camps about the practice of young migrant men sharing needles while tattooing their bodies. This would be yet another example of HIV risk related to a rather distinct form of needle sharing.

Gender and HIV Risk.   As mentioned earlier, Mexican migrant women, as well as the wives of migrant men back in Mexico, are vulnerable to HIV due to the risky behaviors of their male sex partners, including intravenous drug use (López & Ruiz, 1995), prostitution use without condoms (Organista, Balls Organista, Garcia de Alba G., Castillo Moran, & Ureta Carrillo, 1997), sex between men, and needle sharing. Unfortunately, risk for these women is exacerbated by their lack of knowledge about STDs (Schoonover Smith, 1988) and cultural prohibitions to HIV-prevention strategies such as condom use. For example, Organista et al. found that Mexican migrants from Jalisco, Mexico, and female migrants in particular, believed that women would be seen as promiscuous for carrying condoms. As a result, 75% of the 159 women surveyed reported "never" carrying condoms, as compared to 41.4% of men.

Hence, there are considerable culture- and gender-related obstacles to initiating protective behaviors in female migrants. One indirect way is to focus on the risk behaviors of migrant men that place their female partners at risk. However, female-focused strategies warrant equal attention and one place to start is by conducting focus groups with Latinas in which their beliefs about practical prevention strategies can be discussed (Amaro, 1988).

HIV/AIDS-Related Knowledge, Attitudes, Beliefs, and Behaviors

HIV Transmission. Considering the high risk status of Mexican farm workers, what do we know about HIV- and AIDS-related knowledge in this population? Survey research conducted by myself and my associates in Jalisco, Mexico, documented that, contrary to popular belief, Mexican migrant laborers have a good deal of knowledge about the major modes of HIV transmission (e.g., blood, unprotected sex, etc.; Organista, Balls Organista, Garcia de Alba G., Castillo Moran, & Ureta Carrillo, 1997). However, they simultaneously held many misconceptions about contracting HIV from casual modes such as mosquito bites, public bathrooms, kissing on the mouth, being coughed on, and giving blood. For example, a full 50% of the 501 migrant laborers surveyed by Organista et al. believed that they could contract HIV from the HIV test, a surefire deterrent to getting tested.

Condom Knowledge and Use. The safer sex strategy of carrying and using condoms is particularly relevant to migrant laborers, given the transient and geographically isolated nature of their work and lifestyles. Unfortunately, research on condom use reveals little condom knowledge and inconsistent use. For example, Organista, Balls Organista, Garcia de Alba G., Castillo Moran, and Ureta Carrillo (1997) found that between half and two thirds of their sample either answered incorrectly or reported not knowing the answers to questions such as "Is Vaseline good lubricant for condoms?" or "Should you unroll condom before putting on penis?"

When condoms are used by Mexican migrants, they are used far more often with secondary or occasional sex partners than with primary sex partners. In pre-survey focus groups, the following reasons were given for not using condoms with intimate, regular sex partners: It would suggest infidelity, female partner already using (non-barrier) birth control, and couple's desire to have children. Consequently, only 21% of sexually active migrants reported "always" using condoms with regular sex partners during the past year, compared to 71% with secondary sex partners (Organista, Balls Organista, Garcia de Alba G., Castillo Moran, & Ureta Carrillo, 1997). Culture-related condom use and sex partner patterns need to be considered in condom-promotion strategies.

Predictors of Condom Use

In view of the low and inconsistent use of condoms on the part of Mexican migrant laborers, it is important to explore predictors of condom use. Analyses of data from a small pilot survey of 87 Mexican migrant laborers in Jalisco, Mexico, revealed that condom use with both occasional and regular sex partners, as well as carrying condoms, were correlated with the perception that friends carry and use condoms or "condom social norms" (Organista, Balls Organista, Bola, Garcia de Alba G., & Castillo Moran, 1997). Pilot study findings also showed that personally knowing someone with AIDS was a significant predictor of carrying condoms and using them with occasional sex partners. Worry about contracting AIDS also predicted carrying condoms. Thus, although secondary to the social norm variable, items tapping perceived risk were noteworthy predictors.

Predictors of condom use were also analyzed in a large follow-up survey of the 501 Mexican migrant laborers surveyed in Jalisco, Mexico (Organista, Balls Organista, Bola, Garcia de Alba G., & Castillo Moran, 2000). The purpose of this larger predictor study was threefold. First, we were interested in replicating the pilot study findings on a larger and more representative sample of Mexican migrant laborers. Second, we examined the effects of additional demographic and lifestyle control variables on the replication analyses. The larger sample size gave us the opportunity to more stringently control for variables well known in the AIDS literature for their influence on condom use (e.g., age, education, number of sex partners, etc.). Finally, we explored the added effects of several additional pertinent variables on the results of the controlled analyses. For example, we examined the variable "condom efficacy," or how confident respondents felt about negotiating condom use with sex partners in a variety of challenging situations. That is, subjects were asked how capable they would be of insisting on condom use if a prospective sex partner were to, get angry, not want to use a condom, threaten to leave, and so on. Other condom efficacy items assessed condom use with a sex partner with whom the respondent was in love, who was using another form of birth control, who wanted to have a baby, and so forth. This variable was included in the larger predictor study because previous research on U.S. Latina/os had showed that it predicts condom use with occasional sex partners (Marín, Gomez, & Tschann, 1993). In fact, Marín, Tschann, Gomez, and Gregorich (1998) recently validated a full 20-item scale of condom efficacy on a large, 10-state sample of over 1,100 U.S. Latina/o men and women. This particular scale was used to assess condom efficacy in our larger predictor study.

Results revealed that, although we were able to replicate our pilot study finding that condom use with occasional and regular sex partners and carrying condoms were predicted by condom social norms, the addition of condom efficacy as a predictor factor greatly altered the final results as described below.

Condom Use With Occasional Sex Partners. In the case of condom use with occasional sex partners, the condom social norms factor was rendered nonsignificant (as well as all other predictors) when condom efficacy was added to the final regression model. This finding indicated that the omission of condom efficacy in the pilot study overestimated the influence of condom social norms on condom use with occasional sex partners. Thus, condom efficacy appears to be a central factor in understanding condom use with occasional sex partners in Mexican migrants whose work and lifestyle accentuate this major HIV-exposure category. For example, 82% of single men and 27% of married men in the survey reported multiple sex partners during the past year (Organista, Balls Organista, Garcia de Alba G., Castillo Moran, & Ureta Carrillo, 1997).

Condom Use With Regular Sex Partners.   Condom use with a regular sex partner appears to be more complex and multidetermined than condom use with occasional sex partners. The addition of condom efficacy to the final regression model again displaced condom social norms as a significant predictor factor, but carrying condoms and low negative attitudes toward condoms remained significant predictors. Thus, for migrants to increase their condom use in presumably intimate, ongoing sexual relationships, it appears that they must feel both efficacious and positive regarding condoms and must also keep condoms readily available.

Carrying Condoms.   The regression model predicting carrying condoms contained the most significant number of predictors, suggesting that promoting this behavior is a crucial first step that requires attention to a wide variety of factors. Carrying condoms was predicted by condom efficacy as well as condom social norms, perceived vulnerability about contracting AIDS, and low negative attitudes toward condoms.

Thus, promoting the carrying of condoms may need to address all four of the previous influential factors. For example, perceived vulnerability can be increased by informing Mexican migrants of their status as a new high-risk group. All three of the other predictors could be addressed by involving Mexican migrants in condom-promotion efforts (e.g., communicating positive attitudes toward condoms, normalizing and endorsing condom use, and discussing how to insist on condom use in challenging sexual situations).

Taken together, results from the predictor studies indicate three very important forms of condom use, each with its own distinct set of predictors. In summary, our results suggested that carrying condoms is an imperative, albeit infrequent, first step in preventing AIDS in Mexican migrants that can be increased by interventions that enhance condom-related social norms, attitudes, and efficacy as well as a sense of vulnerability to contracting HIV. Although condom efficacy is only one of several factors needed to increase the frequency of carrying condoms, it appears to be the central factor in condom use with occasional sex partners and must be stressed in this important context. Finally, although condom use with regular sex partners is secondary to occasional sex partners in the target population, our findings suggest that even this infrequent and interpersonally sensitive form of condom use might be enhanced by increasing condom efficacy, positive attitudes, and carrying condoms.

Notes on Conducting Culturally Competent HIV Research

Before discussing the implications of the previously discussed research for future HIV-prevention research and services for Mexican and Chicana/o farm workers, I briefly review the considerable preparation, networking, and use of culture that went into making this research project culturally and socially responsive.

Collaboration.   The idea for this research emerged from discussions with Javier Garcia de Alba G., director of the Regional Institute of Public Health at the University of Guadalajara in Mexico during the early 1990s, who was concerned about cases of

AIDS appearing in some of the remote "sending towns" of Jalisco, Mexico, with long histories of outmigration to the United States. Indeed, research has documented a strong link between AIDS cases in Mexico and migration to the United States. For example, Bronfman, Camposortega, and Medina (1989) found that, of the 165 registered AIDS cases in Mexico in 1988, 10.4% had lived in the U.S. and 33% of the cases were from states with the highest outmigration to the U.S. (e.g., of the AIDS cases in Baja California, 20% had lived in the U.S.).

From 1983 to 1995, the Universidad de Guadalajara and the School of Social Welfare at the University of California, Berkeley (UCB), cosponsored an annual *Intercambio Academico* (Academic Exchange) program in which students and faculty visited each other's institutions for a 3-week period in order to receive didactic instruction and field experience in the areas of social work and public health. This innovative program was developed by UCB's pioneering Chicana/o social work faculty member, Joe Solis, whose vision was to enrich Latino curricula and inspire collaborative research. When Organista joined the UCB faculty in 1990, his ability to speak Spanish, as well as his Chicano background, enabled him to utilize the Intercambio Academico as a vehicle for conducting collaborative, cross-cultural, international research in Mexico.

Research Approach.   The information in this chapter is based on 7 years of labor-intensive qualitative and quantitative survey research. The state of the art in social science HIV research has now shifted to blending qualitative and quantitative research methods in ways that inform each other in an illuminating bidirectional fashion. Such an approach is consistent with current critiques of the intervention literature that urge researchers to carefully tailor AIDS-prevention programs to the sociocultural and ethnic realities of specific at-risk groups (Marín, 1995; Wyatt, 1994).

However, although blending qualitative and quantitative research represents an optimal approach, few researchers possess balanced skills in both of these research methods. As as result, interdisciplinary collaboration is imperative, as is an openness to transcend one's own typically one-sided research training, not to mention the considerable biases built into such narrow training.

As with most projects, the first step was to thoroughly review the literature in order to summarize and critique the state of current knowledge. Given the paucity of research in this area and the need to develop a knowledge base, a comprehensive review of the literature was written up and published (Organista & Balls Organista, 1997). Mishra, Conner, and Magaña (1996) similarly expanded this knowledge base with their pioneering book *AIDS Crossing Borders: The Spread of HIV Among Migrant Latinos,* the first to compile research and thinking on this topic in the previous decade.

The next step was to identify or design instruments in order to conduct an HIV and AIDS knowledge, attitudes, beliefs, and behaviors, or KABB, survey with Mexican migrant laborers. The plan was to survey a prototypic sending town in the state of Jalisco, Mexico, during the Christmas season, when migrant laborers in the U.S. return home for the holidays. Mexican colleagues were crucial in providing access to the town, given their previous work with the medical school at Universidad de Guadalajara, establishing satellite health clinics, and conducting health campaigns in poor, rural, and isolated communities. The town selected had an average of two family members per household who had lived and worked in the United States.

Barbara VanOss Marin and associates at the Center for AIDS Prevention Services (CAPS) at the University of California, San Francisco, have been at the forefront of conducting large behavioral-epidemiological HIV-related surveys with Latina/os in the United States (e.g., Marín et al., 1993). I requested a copy of Marín's Hispanic Condom Questionnaire (HCQ), a fully back-translated KABB questionnaire developed for U.S. Latina/os. My research team modified the HCQ based on our literature review, consultations with experts, and pre-survey focus groups with members of the target population at the selected study site. (Note that it would have been easier, and less culturally sensitive, to simply impose the HCQ without considering local emic issues.)

I flew to Mexico and visited the study site with Marco Antonio Castillo Moran, a trusted Universidad de Guadalajara medical doctor who had previously lived and worked in the town as a medical provider for a period of 1 year during his required *servicio social* (social service). Introduced as the doctor's colleague, we first met with an important community leader or "gate keeper" who ran the local hardware store. He offered me *pitayas* (a regional small red prickly pear) to eat while I shared my family's roots in Jalisco, noting that many of my cousins currently lived in Guadalajara. When I accepted his second offering of *pitayas*, the hardware store owner smiled and exclaimed, "So, you really are Mexican!" From that moment on, I was able to request his assistance in organizing focus groups with adult migrant men and women who had lived and worked in the United States since the early 1980s (coinciding with the beginning of the AIDS epidemic in America).

The hardware store owner took out a megaphone, climbed to the roof of his store, and broadcasted to the town my arrival, title, and the requested focus groups, incidentally mentioning that fresh eggs had arrived and could be purchased at his store. I marveled as the store owner's amplified voice echoed off the rooftops and nearby cliffs and even more when the focus group participants dutifully gathered at the designated locations at mid-day.

The previous interpersonal exchange is highlighted to illustrate the necessity of understanding and using a Latino-based relationship protocol to build *confianza* or trust on the basis of salient values such as *respeto* (respect) and *personalismo*, or a personalized approach to collaboration in which the personal dimension predominates over the task dimension of the relationship. That is, to begin such an exchange by requesting assistance with a task, as in the American style of not mixing business with pleasure, generally runs counter to traditional Latino communication protocol and can be perceived as cold or rude.

During the focus groups, the author facilitated discussions about HIV and AIDS designed to reveal what the migrants knew and believed and how they behaved sexually with respect to the disease. Discussions were tape recorded and reviewed with research team members. Ultimately, the information obtained was used to tailor the HCQ for use with Mexican migrant laborers from the town. New items were back translated by our bilingual research team members.

Mexican medical students from the Universidad de Guadalajara were trained to administer the survey instrument by a Mexican HIV expert with years of experience training HIV-agency personnel how to administer such highly personal questionnaires. Only those students evaluated to be competent by the trainer were included in the interview team. It was also imperative that I participate as both interviewer and daily team convener in order to process the ongoing experience. We were successful in surveying every household in the town and in publishing a series of reports focusing on KABB results for the entire sample (Organista, Balls Organista, Garcia de Alba G., Castillo Moran, & Carrillo, 1996), results for women only in the sample (Balls Organista, Organista, & Soloff, 1998), and the aforementioned analyses of predictors of condom use (Organista, Balls Organista, Garcia de Alba G., & Castillo Moran, 1997b).

The pilot study was most informative for ascertaining how to further modify and refine the survey instrument in preparation for a planned five-site, statewide survey in Jalisco. For example, we decided to drop a measure of depression because it revealed little statistical variance and elicited a negative response bias from participants. Conversely, pilot study findings that illuminated HIV risk or protection resulted in the creation, expansion, or adoption of scales in such areas as prostitution use, condom social norms, and condom efficacy. However, these survey modifications were proceeded by yet another round of pre-survey focus groups at prospective study sites stratified by age (younger and older migrants) in addition to gender. Again, this qualitative dimension of the research demanded an extra trip to Mexico and careful study of focus group tape recordings. The result was a collection of scales with sound psychometric properties that illuminated HIV risk and protection for the target population. For instance, a 19-item condom social norms scale was created to assess the frequency with which respondents, as well as their family and friends, condoned condom use in a variety of ways. For example, respondents were asked how frequently they had told friends or family members that they use condoms. Respondents were then asked how frequently friends or family members had told them that they use condoms. Other items assessed the frequency of recommending, criticizing, giving, and asking for condoms. Items were scored on scales ranging from 1 (never) to 4 (very frequently). The scale demonstrated high internal consistency (Cronbach's alpha = .80) and had a mean score of 2.38 (SD = .45), indicating that participants "sometimes" sanctioned condom use.

The condom social norm scale was intended to assess actual condom-related interpersonal norms in Mexican migrants, as opposed to perceived condom norms assessed in previous research (e.g., Fishbein, Middlestadt, & Trafimow, 1993). Although such condom-related norms would be expected to be associated with condom use, the use of interpersonal condom norms is designed to assess the relation between what people say or do interpersonally with regard to condoms, and the behavioral act of using condoms during sex (i.e., assessing whether people practice what they preach).

Findings from the previous research have implications for the next phase of HIV-prevention research and for informing HIV-prevention strategies with the target population.

IMPLICATIONS FOR FUTURE HIV RESEARCH WITH MEXICAN FARM WORKERS

Objectives

Although prior research suggests several possible future research directions, it seems logical to first pursue the objective of increasing proper and consistent condom use with secondary sex partners by Mexican male farm workers. This particular objective addresses many of the salient interacting factors that frame the problem of HIV risk in Mexican farm workers.

Framing the Problem. Figure 17.1 serves as a working conceptual model that depicts salient characteristics of both migratory labor in the U.S. (e.g., lonely and transient work, poverty wages, social marginality) and Mexican culture (e.g., traditional gender roles, machismo) in the attempt to portray how these two major overlapping dimensions frame a wide variety of risk scenarios. Such scenarios are in turn a function of different interactions between subgroups of farm workers (e.g., age group, gender), different HIV-exposure categories (e.g., prostitution use), and situational factors (e.g., geographical isolation, heavy drinking at local bars, etc.). This model is being used to plan a pilot study to assess the feasibility of pursuing the previously described research objective, given the formidable obstacles that this complex problem area presents to conventional social science research methods.

A Proposed Pilot: Research Methods

The proposed pilot study consists of two phases: (a) gathering pertinent information from key informants to better understand the farm worker situation in order to work out prevention service delivery issues and to refine HIV-prevention program content, and (b) pilot testing the preliminary HIV-prevention service delivery program on a small scale, complete with a plan for evaluating intervention effectiveness. Both study phases will be carried out in collaboration with community-based migrant health service providers currently serving the target population.

A recent survey of 181 California agencies that provide AIDS-prevention services to Latina/os showed that community-based agencies are more effective than federal, state, and private agencies because of their greater number of bilingual staff and volunteers and their culturally sensitive approaches to service delivery (Castañeda & Collins, 1995).

Qualitative Groundwork. Qualitative research methods in the form of a series of private, individual interviews with farm workers and focus groups with health outreach workers will be used to: (a) obtain basic, descriptive information about the farm worker experience at potential study sites (e.g., number and different types of labor camps in northern California counties, labor migration seasons and patterns, migrant population estimates, etc.), (b) obtain information on HIV and AIDS, other health, and social service delivery models currently available to farm workers (e.g., sponsored by federal, state, nonprofit, or community grass-roots agencies) and (c) obtain input on perceptions of barriers and facilitators to HIV prevention with the target population.

Innovative Interventions. Qualitative data will also be used to develop a preliminary version of the HIV-prevention program and to assess the feasibility of program delivery and evaluation. This phase of the study is important for building on prior research. For example, although condom efficacy predicts condom use with occasional sex partners, what inhibits and promotes condom efficacy with different types of sex partners such as other men, local women, and sex workers? Thus,

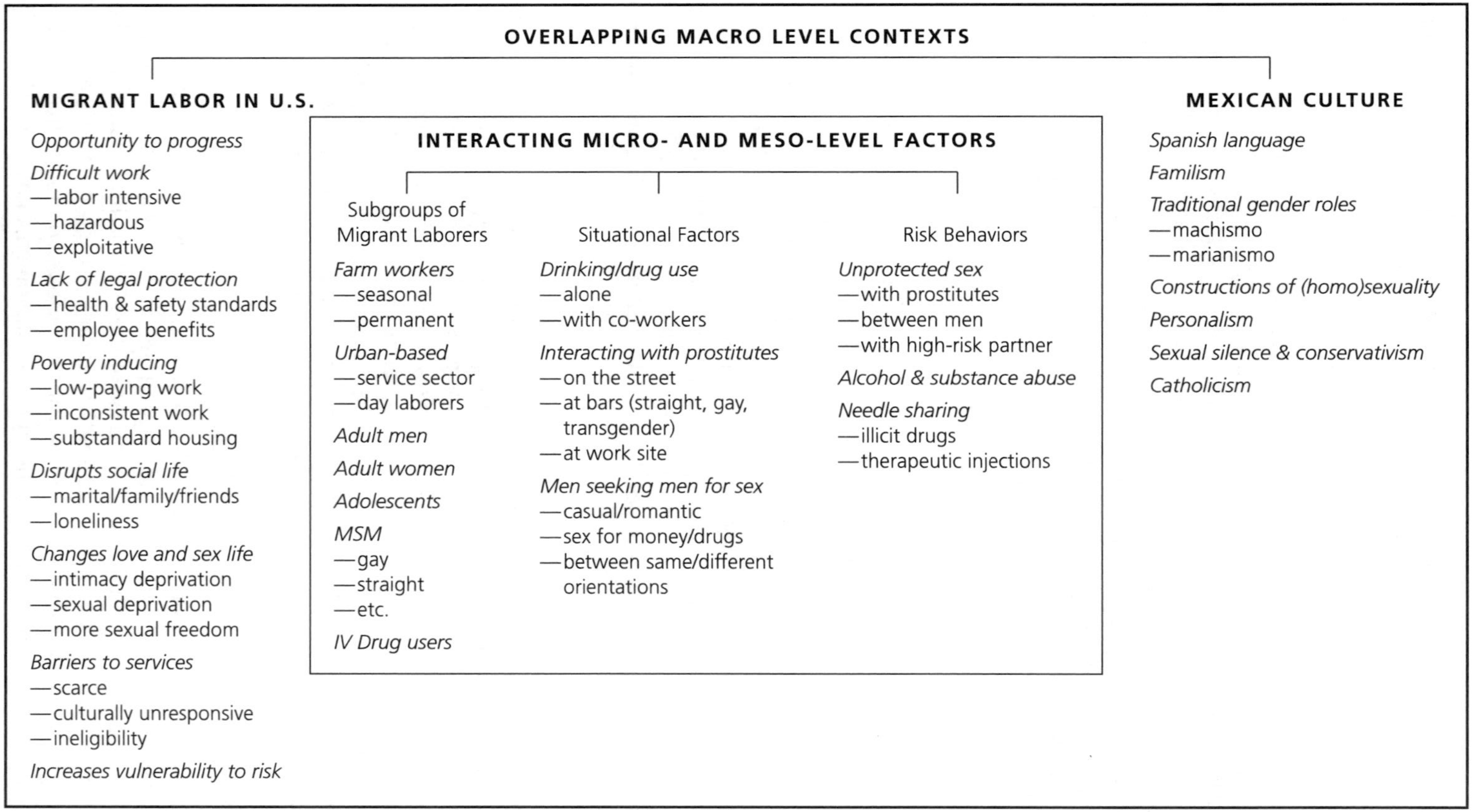

OVERLAPPING MACRO LEVEL CONTEXTS

MIGRANT LABOR IN U.S.

Opportunity to progress

Difficult work
—labor intensive
—hazardous
—exploitative

Lack of legal protection
—health & safety standards
—employee benefits

Poverty inducing
—low-paying work
—inconsistent work
—substandard housing

Disrupts social life
—marital/family/friends
—loneliness

Changes love and sex life
—intimacy deprivation
—sexual deprivation
—more sexual freedom

Barriers to services
—scarce
—culturally unresponsive
—ineligibility

Increases vulnerability to risk

MEXICAN CULTURE

Spanish language
Familism
Traditional gender roles
—machismo
—marianismo
Constructions of (homo)sexuality
Personalism
Sexual silence & conservatism
Catholicism

INTERACTING MICRO- AND MESO-LEVEL FACTORS

Subgroups of
Migrant Laborers

Farm workers
—seasonal
—permanent

Urban-based
—service sector
—day laborers

Adult men

Adult women

Adolescents

MSM
—gay
—straight
—etc.

IV Drug users

Situational Factors

Drinking/drug use
—alone
—with co-workers

Interacting with prostitutes
—on the street
—at bars (straight, gay, transgender)
—at work site

Men seeking men for sex
—casual/romantic
—sex for money/drugs
—between same/different orientations

Risk Behaviors

Unprotected sex
—with prostitutes
—between men
—with high-risk partner

Alcohol & substance abuse

Needle sharing
—illicit drugs
—therapeutic injections

FIG. 17.1.   Conceptual model of HIV risk in Mexican farm workers in the United States.

qualitative data will also be used to modify and refine variables from previous research believed to mediate condom use. For example, condom efficacy as assessed in prior research may not consider challenging sexual situations specific to farm workers at potential study sites in northern California. Qualitative data will also help in decisions about different intervention methods that can be attempted (e.g., actively involving farm workers in the HIV-prevention service vs. a more traditional didactic approach). With regard to innovative approaches, Magaña, Batista, Ferreira-Pinto, Blair, and Mata (1992) advocated *circulos de salud* (health circles) for HIV prevention with Latina/os based on the empowering and progressive work of Brazilian educator Paulo Friere. Such health circles begin by teaching participants the technical basics of HIV transmission and prevention and then involve them in an active problem-solving discussion after posing relevant hypothetical risky situations relevant to their lives. The assumption here is that participants want to prevent HIV and know much more about their reality than researchers and service providers.

Another creative intervention idea is to collaborate with the Teatro Campesino (farm worker theater) that is currently active in the area of HIV-prevention writing and delivering *actos* (brief plays) to campesinos or farm workers dealing with this topic. The Teatro Campesino is a distinctly politicized and immensely entertaining Chicano art form that has been used since the 1960s to educate and activate farm workers in issues that directly affect their lives (e.g., Cesar Chavez' United Farmworker Union). The idea of using culturally appropriate research findings to inform actos about HIV prevention is an intriguing one, given the high probability of involving participants in an enjoyable manner and delivering prevention strategies with an empirical basis.

Finally, methods of data collection for assessing intervention program effectiveness, including strategies for conducting follow-up evaluations (e.g., 2 months post-intervention) with the transient target population, will also be explored. One piece of advice on this matter, provided by a consulting health agency, is to focus on government labor camps where documented farm workers are easier to track. Obviously, the exclusion of undocumented farm workers has numerous trade-offs. On the one hand, undocumented workers are more difficult to involve in formal research; on the other hand, they constitute half of the Mexican-descent farm worker population and their exclusion would be a human disservice, as well as a strong limitation on the generalizability of study findings.

IMPLICATIONS FOR HIV-PREVENTION SERVICES FOR MEXICAN FARM WORKERS

Although research efforts are growing, people continue to become infected with HIV. Hence, it is necessary at any point in time to use state-of-the-art knowledge to inform prevention strategies as much as possible.

General Recommendations

Basic HIV and AIDS information must be communicated to Mexican farm workers in Spanish (e.g., 81% of our large survey sample spoke only or mostly Spanish). Written literature must be geared to the appropriate reading level (average years of education was 4 to 7 in survey sample). It is imperative to do HIV-prevention outreach where migrants live and work (e.g., labor camps). It is also important to develop and deliver focused, single-session interventions given the transient nature of farm work. Finally, the delivery of intervention messages may often need to be done separately for men and women given the sexual conservativism of traditional Mexican people (de la Vega, 1990).

Male-Focused Interventions (Married and Single)

Condom-promotion efforts with male Mexican farm workers must begin with providing basic instructions on proper condom use, including hands-on practice with phallic replicas. Men should be urged to carry or keep condoms handy in the spirit of being *hombres preparados* (well-educated and prepared men), a term that carries the connotation of being learned in addition to prepared. HIV transmission with different types of sex partners should be discussed. For example, the common practice of using prostitutes while in the U.S., including the occasional practice of the hermanos de leche ritual, should be addressed in detail (e.g., Can men still be hermanos de leche if condoms are used? Isn't it important for real hermanos to protect each other? Are there less risky forms of male bonding?).

The topic of sex between men (specifically unprotected anal sex) must not be restricted to "homosexual" men, but should acknowledge the occasional participation of heterosexuals or bisexuals and the need to protect their female partners by using condoms with occasional male sex partners. In a study of 190 recent Mexican immigrants, Mikawa et al. (1992) found that using condoms to "protect the woman" predicted condom use, whereas using condoms to protect one's own health did not.

Because of the apparent central role of condom efficacy in predicting condom use with secondary sex partners, sufficient discussion and role playing should be used to insist on condom use in challenging sexual situations encountered by Mexican male migrants (e.g., being solicited by prostitutes in bars while drinking with encouraging coworkers on pay day).

Female-Focused Interventions

Female migrants in our surveys were extremely low in acculturation and thus presumably high in traditional Mexican culture and adherence to conservative gender roles. Working within traditional gender roles could involve urging Mexican women to protect themselves in order to prevent the congenital transmission of HIV to children. Similarly, because Mexican women are central to their family's health and well-being, they could be reminded that their family's health is closely linked to their own. However, working outside of traditional Mexican culture is also necessary and may not be as difficult as often presumed given the changing nature of gender roles in migrant and immigrant women.

Guendelman (1987) noted that Mexican migrant and immigrant women experience "gender role expansion" as a result of their wage earnings and greater purchasing power, family decision making, sharing of household chores with husbands, and greater feelings of autonomy. Hence, empowering and proactive prevention strategies to be initiated by women need to be considered (e.g., assertively negotiating sexual matters).

Culturally and socially competent HIV-prevention research and direct services are urgently needed to prevent the high probability of an AIDS epidemic in Mexican and Chicana/o farm workers, who represent the majority of all migrant laborers in the United States. Within the large overlapping dimensions of migratory labor and Mexican culture exist a number of pertinent HIV-exposure categories and risk scenarios that need to be carefully considered and targeted. The development of culturally and socially responsive research and service approaches is imperative, despite the extra work required to adequately respond to the special needs and circumstances of Latina/os and other people of color.

The contribution of Chicana/o psychology to decreasing HIV risk in campesinos can be considerable given the emerging emphasis on interdisciplinary and binational collaboration, combining qualitative and quantitative research methods, and seeking to integrate cultural and social variables into research efforts in order to customize or tailor interventions to the lived realities of Mexican and Chicana/o farm workers. Such efforts represent a needed enhancement to the traditional behavioral science paradigm in HIV-prevention research, which has for too long overemphasized individual variables and under emphasized social, cultural, and environmental factors that can place limits on self-protection from HIV. For example, as a cost-saving device, current guest worker contracts disallow married migrant men from having their wives and children join them during seasonal work in the U.S. (Chang, 2000). However, research clearly shows that married Mexican migrant men, unaccompanied by their wives, report more lifetime sexual partners, more partners in the previous 2 years, more extramarital affairs, and more sex with prostitutes, compared to men accompanied by their wives (Viadro & Earp, 2000). Thus, environmental factors, including social policies and labor practices, also need to be targeted in our research efforts to reduce HIV risk in Mexican migrant laborers. The personal agency of Mexican migrants, in response to oppressive environmental factors, also needs to be included in future research.

REFERENCES

Amaro, H. (1988). Considerations for prevention of HIV infection among Hispanic women. *Psychology of Women Quarterly, 12*, 429–443.

Balls Organista, P., Organista, K. C., & Soloff, P. R. (1998). Exploring AIDS-related knowledge, attitudes, and behaviors of female Mexican migrant workers. *Health and Social Work, 23*, 81–160.

Bronfman, M., Camposortega, S., & Medina, H. (1989). La migración internacional y el SIDA: El caso de México y Estados Unidos. In J. Sepulveda Amor, M. Bronfman, G. Ruiz Palacios, E. Stanislawski, & J. L. Valdespino (Eds.), *SIDA, ciencia y sociedad en México* (pp. 435–456). Mexico City, Mexico: Secretaria de Salud, Instituto Nacional de Salud Publica, Fondo de Cultura Economica.

Bronfman, M., & Minello, N. (1992). *Habitos sexuales de los migrantes temporales Mexicanos a los Estados Unidos de America, practicas de riesgo para la infección por VIH.* Mexico City, Mexico: El Colegio de Mexico.

Carrier, J. (1995). *De los otros (of the others): Intimacy and homosexuality among Mexican men.* New York: Columbia University Press.

Carrier, J. M. (1985). Mexican male bisexuality. *Journal of Homosexuality, 11–12*, 75–85.

Carrier, J. M., & Magaña, J. R. (1991). Use of ethnosexual data on men of Mexican origin for HIV/AIDS prevention programs. *Journal of Sex Research, 28,* 189–202.

Castañeda, D., & Collins, B. E. (1995). The role of community agencies in HIV/AIDS education and prevention among Latinas and Latinos. *California Policy Seminar Briefs, 7*(2), 1–3.

Center for Disease Control and Prevention. (1988). HIV seroprevalence in migrant and seasonal farmworkers—North Carolina, 1987. *Morbidity and Mortality Weekly Report, 37,* 517–519.

Chang, G. (2000). *Disposable domestics: Immigrant women workers in the global economy.* Cambridge, MA: South End Press.

de la Vega, E. (1990). Considerations for reaching the Latino population with sexuality and HIV/AIDS information and education. *Siecus Report, 18,* 1–8.

Fishbein, M., Middlestadt, S. E., & Trafimow, D. (1993). Social norms for condom use with heterosexuals in the Eastern Caribbean. *Advances in Consumer Research, 20,* 292–296.

Guendelman, S. (1987). The incorporation of Mexican women in seasonal migration: A study of gender differences. *Hispanic Journal of the Behavioral Sciences, 9,* 245–264.

Hulewicz, J. M. (1994). AIDS knows no borders. *World AIDS, 35,* 6–10.

Lafferty, J. (1991). Self-injection and needle sharing among Migrant farmworkers. *American Journal of Public Health, 81,* 221.

López, R., & Ruiz, J. D. (1995). *Seroprevalence of Human Immunodeficiency Virus Type I and syphilis and assessment of risk behaviors among migrant and seasonal farmworkers in northern California.* Unpublished manuscript, Office of AIDS, California Department of Health Services, Sacramento, California.

Magaña, J. R. (1991). Sex, drugs and HIV: An ethnographic approach. *Social Science and Medicine, 33,* 5–9.

Magaña, J. R., Batista, J., Ferreira-Pinto, J. B., Blair, M., & Mata, A., Jr. (1992). Una pedagogia de concientizacion para la prevencion del VIH/SIDA. *Revista Latino Americana De Psicologia, 24,* 97–108.

Marín, B. V. (1995). *Analysis of AIDS prevention among ethnic minority populations in the United States.* Washington, DC: Office of Technology Assessment, U.S. Congress.

Marín, B. V., Gomez, C., & Tschann, J. M. (1993). Condom use among Hispanic men with multiple female partners: A nine-state study. *Public Health Reports, 25,* 742–750.

Marín, B. V., Tschann, J. M., Gomez, C. A., & Gregorich, S. (1998). Self-efficacy to use condoms in unmarried Latino adults. *American Journal of Community Psychology, 26,* 53–71.

McVea, K. L. S. P. (1997). Lay injection practices among migrant farmworkers in the age of AIDS: Evolution of a biomedical folk practice. *Social Science Medicine, 45,* 91–98.

Mikawa, J. K., Morones, P. A., Gomez, A., Case, H. L., Olsen, D., & Gonzales-Huss, M. J. (1992). Cultural practices of Hispanics: Implications for the prevention of AIDS. *Hispanic Journal of Behavioral Sciences, 14,* 421–433.

Mines, R., Mullenax, N., & Saca, L. (2001). *The binational farmworker health survey: An in-depth study of agricultral worker health in Mexico and the United States.* Davis: California Institute for Rural Studies.

Mishra, S. I., Conner, R. F., & Magaña, J. R. (Eds.). (1996). *AIDS crossing borders: The spread of HIV among migrant Latinos.* Boulder, CO: Westview Press.

Organista, K. C., & Balls Organista, P. (1997). Migrant laborers and AIDS in the United States: A review of the literature. *AIDS Education and Prevention, 9,* 83–93.

Organista, K. C., Balls Organista, P., Bola, J., Garcia de Alba G., J. E., & Castillo Moran, M. A. (2000). Predictors of condom use in Mexican migrant laborers. *American Journal of Community Psychology, 28,* 245–265.

Organista, K. C., Balls Organista, P., Garcia de Alba G., J. E., & Castillo Moran, M. A. (1997). Psychosocial predictors of condom use in Mexican migrant laborers. *Interamerican Journal of Psychology, 31,* 77–90.

Organista, K. C., Balls Organista, P., Garcia de Alba G., J. E., Castillo Moran, M. A., & Carrillo, H. (1996). AIDS and condom-related knowledge, beliefs, and behaviors in Mexican migrant laborers. *Hispanic Journal of Behavioral Sciences, 18,* 392–406.

Organista, K. C., Balls Organista, P., Garcia de Alba G., J. E., Castillo Moran, M. A., & Ureta Carrillo, L. E. (1997). Survey of condom-related beliefs, behaviors, and perceived social norms in Mexican migrant laborers. *Journal of Community Health, 22,* 185–198.

Organista, K. C., Carillo, H., & Ayala, G. (2003). *HIV prevention with Mexican migrant laborers: Review, critique, and recommendations.* Unpublished manuscript.

Rust, G. S. (1990). Health status of migrant farmworkers: A literature review and commentary. *American Journal of Public Health, 80,* 1213–1217.

Schoonover Smith, L. (1988). Ethnic differences in knowledge of sexually transmitted diseases in North American Black and Mexican American farmworkers. *Research in Nursing and Health, 11*, 51–58.

U.S. Department of Labor. (1990). *Findings from the National Agricultural Workers Survey (NAWS): A demographic and employment profile of perishable crop farmworkers.* Washington, DC: Author.

U.S. Department of Labor. (1998). *Findings from the National Agricultural Workers Survey (NAWS): A demographic and employment profile of United States farmworkers.* Washington, DC: Author.

Viadro, C. I., & Earp, J. L. (2000). The sexual behavior of married Mexican immigrant men in North Carolina. *Social Science and Medicine, 50*, 723–735.

Villarejo, D., Lighthall, D., Williams, D., III., Souter, A., Mines, R., Bade, B., Samuels, S., & McCurdy, S. A. (2000). *Suffering in silence: A report on the health of California's agricultural workers.* Davis: California Institute for Rural Studies.

Wyatt, G. E. (1994). The sociocultural relevance of sex research: Challenges for the 1990s and beyond. *American Psychologist, 49*, 748–754.

A Cultural Perspective on Prevention Interventions

Felipe González Castro
Arizona State University

Nilda Teresa Hernandez
Yavapai College

OVERVIEW OF PREVENTION RESEARCH: ISSUES RELEVANT TO LATINA/O COMMUNITIES

Issues and Challenges in Effective Prevention Intervention Research with Latina/o Communities

Culturally-Rich Prevention Research.　Disease prevention and health promotion are important public health strategies with Latina/os, given that, as a population, they are disproportionately represented within the lower socioeconomic strata of American society (Molina, Zambrana, & Aguirre-Molina, 1994). Furthermore, various cultural differences involving the Spanish language and Latina/o customs and traditions that differ from those of mainstream American society are associated with a limited access to health care and to valued social resources (Giachello, 1994; Ginsberg, 1991). As a consequence, certain sectors of the U.S. Latina/o population, including many Chicana/o subpopulations, experience greater risks for various diseases and disabilities, including alcohol abuse, obesity, Type-2 diabetes mellitus, cardiovascular disease, and cancer (Flack, Amaro, Jenkins, Kunitz, Levy, Mixon, & Yu, 1995). To address these needs, an important challenge in prevention research is to conduct culturally rich research that informs the design and development of culturally relevant health-promotion and disease-prevention programs for Latina/os (Castro, Cota, & Vega, 1999; Castro & Gutierres, 1997).

Classic prevention theory postulates three levels of prevention: (a) primary prevention that aims to prevent problems before they occur, (b) secondary prevention that aims to reduce the severity of a developing disease, and (c) tertiary prevention that consists of rehabilitation and aims to reduce disease-related injury and promote recovery toward normalcy (Botvin, 1995; Turnock, 2001). Quality in prevention research is generated from studies having high levels of scientific merit as rated according to three scientific criteria: significance, approach, and innovation (National Institutes of Health, 2000). *Significance* refers to the importance of the public health problem addressed and the study's advancement of scientific knowledge. *Approach* refers to the appropriateness and integration of a study's conceptual framework, methods, and analysis. *Innovation* refers to the originality of the study aims, concepts, approaches, and methods as these may challenge existing paradigms.

Contemporary disease prevention and health promotion emphasize targeting population subgroups who are at high risk for a specific disease or disability (McKenzie & Smeltzer, 2001). Such targeted approaches also aim to identify etiological factors (possible causal factors) and to clarify their role as either risk factors or protective factors. Successful prevention research can also help inform efforts in the cultural adaptation of existing model programs. Cultural adaptation aims to modify model programs so that they respond effectively to the unique needs of a targeted special population of consumers. Currently, culturally relevant prevention research is needed that will generate specific guidelines for program adaptation (Castro, Barrera, & Martinez, in press). That is, evidence-based strategies on the application of scientific methods to modify a model prevention program in order to make it culturally relevant for members of a special population, while also maintaining the program's effectiveness as originally designed and tested (Botvin, 1995).

In summary, clinical and community-based prevention research can contribute important scientific and practical knowledge that can guide prevention strategies for program planning, program implementation, program evaluation, and subsequent program improvement. Adding culturally relevant content to each of these steps aims to reduce health disparities and meet the public health needs of specific members of special populations (Botvin, 1995; McKenzie & Smeltzer, 2001; Turnock, 2001).

Classic Models of Health Behavior.   Within the field of health psychology and health promotion, several classic research models have been proposed to explain why people act in healthy or unhealthy ways (Frankish, Lovato, & Shannon, 1999). These classic models include: the Health Beliefs Model (Rosenstock, 1990), the Theory of Reasoned Action (Ajzen & Fishbein, 1980), the Theory of Planned Behavior (Ajzen, 1991; Albarracin, Johnson, Fishbein, & Muellerleile, 2001), Problem Behavior Theory (Jessor & Jessor, 1977; Jessor, Van den Bos, Venderryn, Costa, & Tubin, 1985), and Social Learning Theory (Bandura, 1986). Each of these theories and their related models present sets of antecedent variables (predictors) that purport to explain the occurrence of a specific health-related behavior. Table 18.1 presents these variables for two of the models: the Health Beliefs Model and the Theories of Reasoned Action and Planned Behavior.

These models also suggest the importance of certain intervening variables, variables described as *mediators* or *moderators,* that also contribute to specific health outcomes. For example, in the Health Beliefs Model, levels of self-efficacy may operate as a moderator that modifies the effects of the other predictor variables on health behavior. Similarly, in the Theory of Reasoned Action, behavioral intentions may operate as a mediator through which the antecedent variables act to influence health-related outcomes (see Table 18.1).

In the past, these and other existing theories and models of health behavior have given little or no attention to cultural variables, variables that serve as central aspects in the life experiences of many Chicana/os and other Latina/os. Table 18.2 presents a set of cultural variables that have been frequently described within the Latino literature and are regarded by many Latina/o investigators as core aspects of the life experiences of Chicana/os and other Latina/os (Castro & Hernandez-Alarcon, 2002). Among these variables, those that relate to cultural aspects of interpersonal relations are: familism (Sabogal, Marín, Otero-Sabogal, & Marín, 1987), *personalismo, respeto,* and *simpatia* (Marín & Marín, 1991). Other cultural variables that operate as personal traits are: acculturation, enculturation, biculturalism, and "cultural flex" (Ramirez, 1999); ethnic identity (Bernal & Knight, 1993; Phinney, 1990); ethnic pride, *machismo, marianismo,* traditionalism, and modernism (Ramirez); field sensitivity and field independence (Ramirez); and spirituality.

The omission of these cultural variables from the classic health research models when applied to Latina/os raises questions about the cultural relevance of these models for them. This limitation prompts the need for future research that explicitly includes these cultural variables within the classical models of health behavior when these models are applied to Latina/os (Meyerowitz, Richardson, Hudson, & Leedham, 1998).

Importance of Culture in Health and Prevention. Recently, the U.S. Surgeon General released a report on minority health that asserts that "culture counts" (Department of Health and Human Services, 2000). This report emphasized that cultural variables operate as significant determinants of the health behavior and health status of minority persons. This significant statement harkens the need for research

TABLE 18.1
Two Major Theories and Models Used in Health Research With Chicana/os

Model or Role of Variable	Constructs	Typical Health Outcome Variable	Representative Study
Health Beliefs Model			
Predictors	Cue to action Perceived susceptibility Perceived severity Perceived barriers	HIV-preventive behavior	Steers, Elliot, Nemiro, Ditman, and Oskamp (1996)
Mediators and Moderators	Self-efficacy		
Outcome	Health behavior		
Theories of reasoned action and planned behavior			
Predictors	Attitudes Norms Perceived control	Condom use Heart-healthy nutrition	Ford and Norris (1995) Apodaca, Woodruff, Candelaria, Elder, and Zlot (1997)
Mediators and Moderators	Behavioral intention	Smoking cessation	Marín, Marín, Perez-Stable, and Otero-Sabogal (1990)
Outcome	Health behavior		

TABLE 18.2
Major Cultural Variables for Mexicana/os and Chicana/os

Cultural Variable	Description or Resource
Interpersonal	
Familism	Strong family orientation, involvement, and loyalty (Sabogal, Marín, Otero-Sabogal, & Marín, 1989)
Personalismo	Preference for personalized attention and courtesy in interpersonal relations
Respeto	Emphasis on respect and attention to issues of social position in interpersonal relations, for example, respect towards elders
Simpatia	A deferential posture toward family members and others in efforts to maintain harmony in family and in interpersonal relationships (Marín & Marín, 1991)
Personal trait	
Acculturation	Level of belief and behavior that conforms to the mainstream U.S. American way of life
Enculturation	An orientation toward a return to ethnic core culture
Biculturalism or "flex"	Capacity to function effectively and to "shuttle" adaptively between two cultures (Ramirez, 1999)
Ethnic identification	Personal identification with one's ethnic cultural group or group of origin (Bernal & Knight, 1993; Phinney, 1990)
Ethnic pride	Positive feelings, pride in one's own ethnic group, and pride in belonging to the group
Machismo	A traditional gender role orientation that accepts male dominance as a proper form of male conduct
Marianismo	A traditional female role orientation that accepts motherly nurturance and the demure and pure identity of a virgin (Virgin Mary) as a proper form of female conduct
Traditionalism	An emphasis and value of cultural beliefs and behaviors, customs, and traditions as the correct and preferred ways to live one's life (Castro & Gutierres, 1997; Ramirez, 1999)
Modernism	An emphasis on accepting change and modern beliefs and behaviors as better and preferred ways to live one's life (Ramirez, 1999)
Field sensitivity	An others-oriented preference or style in ways of thinking and ways of relating to others (Ramirez, 1999)
Field independence	A self-oriented preference or style in ways of thinking and in ways of approaching work and tasks (Ramirez, 1999)
Spirituality	A belief in a higher source of strength and well-being and a related appreciation for natural and beneficial aspects of the world

that explicitly asks significant culture-related questions about health, questions that focus on relevant cultural variables as contributors to health behavior among people of color. Needed now are culturally relevant, and culturally rich models that present explicit hypotheses about the possible protective or risk-producing effects of these cultural variables. With these expanded classical models, the aim is to examine empirically the effects of these cultural variables on important health outcomes that affect Latina/os. For example, *machismo* could be examined as a risk factor for unhealthy behavior, such as the onset of Type-2 diabetes mellitus among middle-aged Mexican and other Latino males. Alternately, *machismo* might operate as a protective factor that prompts behavior to protect one's family from harm. Similarly, *marianismo* might operate as a risk factor for depression among middle-aged Mexicanas and other Latinas, but might also be protective against cigarette smoking. As another example, among Chicanas, the Latino value of familism may prompt nurturing and self-care behavior that produces positive outcomes in child birth. In contrast, within a dysfunctional family, a mother's overly protective behavior might operate as enabling behavior that maintains alcohol abuse in one of the family's siblings.

Such complex cultural situations prompt the need for the development of culturally rich models, even if exploratory, that introduce and test certain specific cultural hypotheses. In the past, investigators have proposed variations of the "Hispanic paradox," or alternatively, a Cultural Protectiveness Hypothesis, which postulates that certain cultural traits, within certain family situations or contexts, protect against disease or mental disorders (Alderete, Vega, Kolody, & Aguliar-Gaxiola, 2000). A family of such hypotheses would explain why certain traditional behaviors as practiced by Chicana/os and other Latina/os may indeed protect them from certain disease outcomes.

Issues in Methodology

Measurement and Instrumentation. Prevention-intervention research with Chicana/os and other Latina/os could be enhanced by conducting basic research that refines the conceptualization and measurement of these cultural variables. For example, the variable of ethnicity or ethnic identity has been conceptualized and measured as an invariant trait, such as race. By suggestion, race is an invariant trait established at birth. In contrast, ethnic identification typically operates as a developmental (time variant) variable, because Mexican American and other youth mature through certain stages of identity development, from a stage of ethnic nonawareness, to ethnic awareness and distress, to ethnic identity integration (Phinney, 1990). New basic research on the state, trait, and developmental characteristics of several cultural variables such as ethnic identity will help to advance the field of Chicana/o and Latina/o psychology.

Moreover, the recent 2000 Census analysis that allowed for the reporting of multiple racial or ethnic identifications underscored the actual complexity of this variable. Although only 2.4% of persons identified as having two or more racial or ethnic identities (U.S. Census Bureau, 2001), new findings on multiple ethnic identities indicate that, for many who have a more complex family and cultural heritage, ethnic identity that is encoded by a single choice from a restricted set of racial or ethnic identifiers produces inaccurate and misleading classifications. Amaro and Zambrana (2000) emphasized that Latina/os come in many shades of racial appearance. This diversity has prompted the use of various racial or ethnic descriptors such as Mestizo, Mulatto, and Criollo as indicators of the wide-ranging variation in racial or ethnic identity that exists within the Latino cultures.

Methodology and Research Design. In the past, comparative group designs have often been used to compare a group of Chicana/os with a group of Euro-Americans, in an effort to identify cultural differences that may exist between members of these two groups (Barrera, Castro, & Biglan, 1999). This often simplistic research approach, though highlighting basic group differences, has many limitations, including the potential to yield stereotypical conclusions, especially if the investigator overgeneralizes results from a small study sample. Today, more in-depth and culturally informed research is needed that asks more substantive cultural questions and uses more revealing designs and analyses to examine group differences. For example, such models include simultaneous comparison of several variables in a model-fitting analysis using latent variable models (Duncan, Duncan, Strycker, Li, & Alpert, 1999).

Confounding of Social Class and Ethnicity. Social class and ethnic status are two important sociocultural variables that must be examined separately or controlled for in health-related studies. Clearly, having lower social and educational status is different from being an ethnic person, although these characteristics often are highly correlated. For example, if within a given community the prevalence rate of Type-2 diabetes is higher for a group of Latina/os relative to Euro Americans, one may ask whether this elevated rate is attributable to the lower social class status of Latina/os or to their racial or ethnic origin. Attributing the rate to social class implicates the disease-inducing influences of poverty and limited access to health care. Attributing this outcome to ethnicity implicates aspects of being Latina/o that involve genetic or familial background. Clearly, both are contributing factors, although a greater clarity in the conceptualization and measurement of these constructs and their interactive effects will enhance future prevention research with Chicana/os and other Latina/os.

EPIDEMIOLOGY OF DISEASE, RISK, AND PROTECTIVE FACTORS IN PREVENTION RESEARCH WITH CHICANA/OS AND OTHER LATINA/OS

This section examines evidence from health research with Chicana/os and other Latina/os in the areas of mental disorder and substance abuse, HIV and AIDS, cardiovascular disease, cancer, and diabetes. Relevant research studies were selected through searches from the following databases: Medline, PsycINFO, and Health Star. The studies retrieved were screened for sufficient sample size of Chicana/os or Latina/os to yield stable and representative conclusions. Studies that were purely descriptive or anecdotal or that lacked a control group were excluded.

Overview of Prevention Research with Chicana/os

Latina/os and other ethnic minority persons, especially those from lower sociocultural backgrounds, are disproportionately affected by a number of diseases and thus exhibit higher prevalence rates for several of the chronic degenerative diseases when compared with nonminority Whites (Carter-Pokras, 1994). Factors such as gender and socioeconomic status typically interact with ethnicity and other cultural factors to produce higher rates of disease in communities of color (Anderson & Armstead, 1995). There is some evidence that certain minority communities (e.g., Cubans and some Asians) have fared better than others (Carter-Pokras, 1994). Nonetheless, when compared to nonminority White patients, marked inequities persist in minority access to health care, which contributes to the prevalence of several chronic degenerative diseases in Chicana/os and other Latina/os.

Today, Mexican and other Latina/o immigrants, some undocumented, serve as a source of inexpensive labor. Many are underemployed, working many hours in jobs that offer no insurance benefits. This process of immigration and migration in search of better employment is associated with family fragmentation and the erosion of traditional family values and structures, which may adversely affect mental well-being and physical health. In contrast, despite life stressors, some migrating individuals exhibit a resiliency to mental and somatic disorder. The Latino values of family, community, spirituality, and collaboration may operate as sources of resiliency and social support that would protect against stress and stress-related disorders. However, with increasing globalization and acculturation, the traditional support systems and healing practices of Latina/os may be eroding in favor of more modernistic beliefs, behaviors, and customs, some of which may influence health status in adverse ways. This issue merits further study.

Several studies have examined the cultural relevance of the use of Latina/o lay health workers, or *promotora/es* as a way to enhance outreach and access to health education and health care (Castro, Elder, Coe, Tafoya-Barraza, Moratto, Campbell, & Talavara, 1995; McAllister, Fernandez-Esquer, Ramirez, Treviño, Gallion, Villareal, Pulley, Hu, Torres, & Zhang, 1995). As an example, Por La Vida, a program funded by the National Cancer Institute, has used *promotoras* to promote lifestyle changes related to diet and physical activity (Navarro, Rock, McNicholas, Senn, & Moreno, 2000). Por la Vida uses a 12-session health education program to promote behavior change consistent with reducing the risk of cancer, including eating a healthy diet maintaining adequate weight. Such programs have been well received by Latina/os and other minorities and serve as a culturally relevant approach that is applicable to a wide variety of health problems, including cancer, cardiovascular disease, and AIDS. However, controlled treatment outcome studies are still needed to evaluate the full effectiveness of this approach.

Health-Promotion Studies With Chicana/os

Mental Disorders and Substance Abuse. A study by Escobar, Hoyos-Nervi, and Gara (2000) reviewed 48 journal articles and found that Mexican-born recent immigrants, in spite of their economic disadvantage, exhibited better mental health outcomes than did U.S.-born Mexican Americans. Similarly, Ortega, Rosenheck, Alegria, and Desai, (2000) examined 8,098 adults between the ages of 15 and 54 and found that Mexican Americans were less likely to have any psychiatric disorder when compared with other groups, although level of acculturation was related to a greater risk of mental disorder. Where mental health issues did appear, the presence of substance abuse disorders was associated with a higher level of acculturation. These findings from Ortega et al. corroborated the findings of Escobar et al. suggesting that, among Mexican Americans, there is a positive association between greater level of acculturation and a higher prevalence of certain types of mental disorders. These findings also suggest that low-acculturated Latina/os constitute a subpopulation distinct from higher acculturated Latina/os. Accordingly, future study designs and proposed statistical analyses must consider the within-group variation involving these and other distinct subpopulations of Latina/os to ensure quality in future Latina/o health research.

Various studies have examined the relationship between acculturative stress and mental disorders, although the relationship between these variables is not entirely clear (Rogler, Cortés, & Malgady, 1991). It remains uncertain whether increased contact with the dominant culture has a direct effect on poor health outcomes. Moreover, the reasons for variability in disease onset among subgroups of Mexican Americans and other Latina/os who have been exposed to the same risk factors have not been well explained and the interactions between level of acculturation and sociocultural variables such as immigration status, time residing in the United States, cultural values, gender, age, education level, and socioeconomic status are also not well understood (Rogler, 1994). As one complication, family and individual acculturation levels do not always coincide, and differences in parent-youth acculturation can cause conflict within families (Szapocznik & Kurtines, 1993).

Certain subpopulations of Chicana/os may be at higher risk of developing mental health problems. One study by Swenson, Baxter, Shatterly, Scarbro, and Hamman (2000), conducted with older Latinas, found that a lower level of acculturation was associated with a higher risk of depression. In addition, depressive symptomatology concurrent with chronic medical conditions was found to increase the risk of death among older Mexican Americans. In Black, Markides, and Miller (1998), nearly 26% of 2,823 subjects reported depressive symptomatology, possibly related to the greater level of isolation of older persons. In their study, female gender, lack of insurance, financial strain, chronic health conditions, and disability were identified as risk factors for depressive symptoms. Another study found an association between ethnicity and depressive symptoms among Mexican Americans, with adolescent girls in this group identified as the most vulnerable relative to girls from other ethnic groups (Joiner, Perez, Wagner, Berenson, & Marquina, 2001). Black et al. also found that female Mexican American immigrants were at significantly higher risk of developing depressive symptoms than were their male counterparts.

A study by Hovey (1998) illustrated certain associations between acculturation and mental disorder. This study examined a sample of 26 male and 28 female Mexican American students living in California. Youth who reported high levels of acculturative stress were at higher risk for depression and suicidal ideation, suggesting that monitoring acculturation-related stressors among high-risk Chicana/o youth constitutes an important strategy in suicide prevention. These studies suggest that female gender, older age, and acculturative stress constitute notable risk factors for depression among Mexican Americans; other factors that contribute to depression include isolation and the relative lack of choices experienced by both females and older persons. These results underscore the importance of developing prevention interventions that address the specific needs of members of these high-risk subpopulations.

Caetano and Raspberry (2000) conducted interviews with 250 Mexican Americans and 250 Whites in a northern California county and found that the prevalence of alcohol dependence was 29% for Whites and 27% for U.S.-born Mexican Americans, but was only 9% for those born in Mexico. In addition, prevalence rates for drug abuse were 23%, 24%, and 6% respectively for Whites, U.S.-born Mexican Americans, and those from Mexico, respectively. Mexican Americans born in the United States appear to be at significantly higher risk for substance abuse relative to Mexicans who remain in their country of origin. Factors such as immigration status, traditionalism, rural lifestyle, acculturation level, socioeconomic status, acculturative stress, and changing family and social roles may play an important part in elevating the risk of substance use (Castro & Gutierres, 1997; Vega, Alderette, Kolody, & Aguilar-Gaxiola, 1998).

For some Chicana/os, a higher level of acculturation may be related to a disconnection from native cultural and healing practices, as well as alienation from naturally occurring social support systems and extended family networks. Connections to community, social support, family, and spirituality are valued core cultural elements for many Latina/os, cultural elements that may buffer against stress and disease. These core elements of Latino cultures constitute fertile resources that can be incorporated into health-promotion interventions that foster personal and community empowerment (Freire, 1993).

Some of the foundational research on the role of personal characteristics in protecting against disease can be found in the literature on resilience. *Resilience* can be described as a self-righting capacity, or the strengths that individuals and social networks use to promote health and healing (Werner & Smith, 1982). Investigators have described some of the factors and coping skills that comprise resilience, including active and meaningful engagement in the world, a positive approach to life, openness to experience, confidence, a sense of mastery in a number of domains, good interpersonal skills, and a capacity for warm relationships (Block, 1971; Hart, Keller, Edelstein, & Hofman, 1998; Klohnen, 1996). Programs such as the Health Realization Model (Mills, 1995), Strengthening Families (Kumpfer, DeMarsh, & Child, 1989), the Rochester Child Resilience Project (Cowen, Wyman, & Work, 1990) and the Perry Preschool Program (Berruta-Clement, Schweinhart, Barnett, Epstein, & Weikart, 1984) have effectively taught resilience skills to parents, children, and youth of all ages. Among the positive outcomes of these resilience skills training programs are decreased delinquency, increased school attendance, decreased family dysfunction, decreased use of drugs by teenagers, decreased rates of child abuse and neglect, and decreased incidence of teen pregnancy.

In contrast to the factors that foster resilience, the risk factors for substance abuse among Chicana/o youth include peer drug use and current drug use (Katims, Zapata, & Yin, 1996; Mason & Roehe, 1997; McBride, Joe, & Simpson, 1991), school behavior problems and susceptibility to peer pressure (Katims et. al.; Mason & Roehe), parental drug use (Joe, Barrett, & Simpson, 1991), and poverty (Morales, 1984). There is also some evidence that families in which the parents either use drugs or condone youth drug use may place their children at higher risk for substance abuse and related problems (Moon, Hecht, Jackson, & Spellers, 2000; Vega et al., 1998). Training in resilience skills such as interpersonal problem solving and resistance to peer pressure appear to be effective preventive and treatment strategies for substance abuse problems in Latina/o communities (Botvin, Baker, Tortu, & Botvin, 1990). It is thus important to examine empirically based resilience skills training programs and to examine strategies for adapting these programs for use within various Mexican American and other Latina/o communities. Moreover, the prevention literature cites certain sociocultural factors as buffers against disease, so that including these factors in programs may enhance outcomes. Among these beneficial sociocultural factors are ethnic affirmation (Longshore, 1997; Romero, 1998) and positive family relationships (Raymond, Rhoads, & Raymond, 1981).

Overall, this line of research suggests that programs that promote resilience skills in youth and reduce neighborhood and family risk factors can decrease the incidence and prevalence of substance abuse. They also underscore the importance of the family and other social networks as resources that should be incorporated into prevention interventions with Chicana/os and other Latina/os. The current challenge involves designing prevention research that identifies how a general life-skills program can be adapted culturally for implementation with a specific subgroup of Latina/os who reside within a certain community (Castro, Barrera, & Martinez, in press).

HIV and AIDS.   Data from the Centers for Disease Control and Prevention (CDC) indicate that Hispanics constitute about 13% of the total U.S. population, but 19% of new AIDS cases (Centers for Disease Control and Prevention, 2002b). The AIDS incidence rate per 100,000 Hispanics is 25.6, much higher than for Whites (7.6), but lower than for African Americans (66.0). Economic inequality, certain aspects of traditional gender roles, and other cultural factors may interact to promote unsafe practices related to drug use and sexual behaviors. Traditional gender roles and gender stereotypes may serve to block communication about sexual practices between partners, so that the uninfected partner may not be informed of the need for protection. In traditional Mexican culture, women may have fewer choices about sexual behavior, thus decreasing the extent to which they can avoid contact with an infected partner. For example, Davila and Brackley (1999) found that Mexican and Mexican American females who requested condom use met with abuse from their male sexual partner. This aggressive male reaction reduces a woman's feelings of safety regarding sexual choices and may ultimately compromise her ability to protect herself from HIV infection.

Several studies have examined risk factors for HIV and AIDS among Latina/o groups (Carrillo & Uranga-McKane, 1994). Economic disadvantage and lack of health insurance often result in a decreased likelihood of obtaining medical attention for HIV infection and for the development of associated infections. Moreover, health disparities related to one health problem often impact other health issues. This applies to HIV infection, which often co-occurs with substance abuse, as they share many of the same risk factors. Further research is needed on the role of family risk and protective factors among Latina/os as these jointly affect the risk of HIV infection and of illicit drug use.

The model of Strategic Family Therapy, developed at the Miami Spanish Family Guidance Center, has been designed for Hispanic families with adolescents 12 to 17 years old who have been using drugs or who exhibit the behavioral precursors to drug use (Szapocznik & Kurtines, 1989). This intervention involves the use of process-oriented family groups that aim to modify family interactions so that negative family dynamics are replaced by positive interactions. Evaluations of this approach show that it can reduce adolescent behavior problems that are precursors to substance abuse.

The Preparing for the Drug-Free Years program (PDFY) is delivered by specially trained community lay health workers and has been used in multiethnic communities. This program is guided by the Social Development Model (Hawkins, Catalano, & Miller, 1992) and its goal is to empower parents to work with their children to reduce critical risk factors and enhance protective factors that promote substance use abstinence and long-range interpersonal success (Harachi, Hawkins, & Catalano, 1996). The PDFY program aims to increase opportunities for positive social interactions, teach peer resistance skills to parents and children, promote the use of consistent family management techniques, and teach skills to help manage family conflicts. Harachi et al. studied a youth sample that was 46% Hispanic and found that culturally relevant recruitment strategies led to at least 55% of the parents attending at least half of the program sessions. For Hispanics in this sample, the most effective recruitment mechanisms included access to personal networks such as churches, friends, and other informal support systems. A similar culturally relevant approach for Latina/os that focuses on enhancing the parent-child relationship and communication to prevent substance abuse is the Hablemos Con Confianza series that includes the Soy Unica, Soy Latina website developed by the Center for Substance Abuse Prevention, in collaboration with several Latina/o health experts nationally (Center for Substance Abuse Prevention, 2002).

The Strengthening Families Program (SFP), described by Kumpfer, DeMarsh, and Child (1989), has implemented a family-focused curriculum with high-risk multiethnic families. SFP includes parent, children, and family skills training to promote family cohesion, improve family communication, and reduce family conflict. The underlying models used by SFP are the Coping Skills Model, the Social Ecology of Adolescent Drug Use, and the Resiliency Model. SFP has demonstrated success in decreasing child behavior problems, reducing future intentions and actual use of drugs and alcohol, decreasing child aggressive behaviors, and increasing peer refusal skills.

Because intravenous drug use is a major HIV risk factor, programs that are effective in preventing substance abuse hold promise as long-term HIV-prevention strategies. In addition, a number of the substance abuse prevention programs are designed to teach coping skills, peer refusal skills, and resilience, which, if combined with culturally relevant family and community involvement, appear promising for reducing risk factors and promoting protective factors against substance abuse and HIV infection.

Cardiovascular Disease. Cardiovascular disease is the leading cause of death in the United States for Latina/os, as well as for the general American population (Centers for Disease Control and Prevention, 2001). Pandey, Labarthe, Goff, Chan, and Nichaman (2001) conducted a community-based surveillance in Nueces County, Texas, by examining death certificates of all the residents between ages 25 and 74 years who had died in that county between 1990 and 1994. Decedents included 519 Mexican Americans and 584 Whites who died from cardiovascular disease as validated via standardized methods and that included evaluator blindness to ethnicity. Among Mexican American women, coronary heart disease was observed to be 36 percent greater than among White women, and among Mexican American men, cardiovascular disease was 12 percent greater than among White men. Several prior studies had reported that Mexican Americans typically exhibit lower rates of cardiovascular disease relative to non-Hispanic Whites (Castro, Baezconde-Garbanati, & Beltran, 1985; Goff, Ramsey, Labarthe, & Nichaman, 1993; Mitchell, Stern, Haffner,

Hazuda, & Patterson, 1990). These conflicting findings may be explained by the fact that some of these earlier studies only used vital statistics, which may underestimate the number of Latina/o deaths, or aggregated all Latina/o groups without regard to sources of within-group variability such as nationality, level of acculturation, or socioeconomic status. Some of the more recent studies, using multiple research methods or separating Chicana/os according to acculturation level, found that higher acculturated Mexican Americans exhibit higher rates of cardiovascular disease mortality, demonstrating the importance of including variables such as socioeconomic status and level of acculturation when defining the study population so that main effects and interactions can be detected if they exist (Balcazar, Castro, & Krull, 1995).

Elevated insulin levels, high body mass index, low levels of HDL cholesterol, and obesity among Chicana/o adults and children have been found to increase the risk of cardiovascular disease (Reaven, Nader, Berry, & Hoyt, 1998; Winkleby, Kraemer, Ahn, & Varady, 1998). Evidence from recent studies suggests that the profile of risk factors for cardiovascular disease in Mexican Americans may differ from that of Whites. The Third National Health and Nutrition Survey (NHANES) for 1988 to 1994, which included 628 Mexican Americans, 700 African Americans, and 2,192 Whites, demonstrated that Mexican American women have a significantly higher prevalence of Type-2 diabetes than White women (Sundquist, Winkleby, & Pudaric, 2001). Type-2 diabetes is a risk factor for cardiovascular disease. This study controlled for both age and socioeconomic status, so that its results provide an unbiased estimate of diabetes prevalence in this population.

A second study that included data from the NHANES included 1,387 Mexican American women and 1,404 Mexican American men between the ages of 25 and 64. The age-adjusted 10-year mortality risk was highest for U.S.-born Spanish-speaking Mexican Americans, followed by U.S.-born English-speaking Mexican Americans, and lowest for Mexican-born men and women. Mexican Americans who were born in the United States had the highest incidence of cardiovascular disease risk factors (Sundquist & Winkleby, 1999). However, it is likely that level of acculturation as defined by fluency in speaking English operates as a proxy variable for a specific underlying mechanism that promotes cardiovascular disease, an issue that should be further studied. Moreover, additional study is needed to determine whether certain risk factors, such as obesity, are uniformly pathological across various ethnic or racial and sociocultural groups, or even across different subgroups of individuals within the same cultural group. Further investigation is needed on the ways in which various risk factors interact and how these interactions can be modified through changes in lifestyle.

Data from the Hispanic Health and Nutrition Examination Survey and the Hispanic Established Populations for Epidemiologic Studies of the Elderly conducted in the states of Arizona, California, Colorado, New Mexico, and Texas demonstrated that, between 1982 and 1994, there was a significant increase in the prevalence of obesity among persons ages 65 to 74 (Stroup-Benham, Markides, Espino, & Goodwin, 1999). A popular indicator of the presence of cardiovascular risk, the body mass index (BMI), measures adipose tissue present in relation to height, so that the BMI can be used as a rough estimate of obesity. Excessive adiposity is a known risk factor for cardiovascular disease and other chronic diseases among Mexican Americans and other populations. Similarly, a study using data from the NHANES found that insulin and glucose levels were significantly higher for Mexican American children than for White children and that cross-ethnic differences were evident by the third grade, indicating that risk factors for cardiovascular disease are present from an early age (Tortolero, Goff, Nichaman, Labarthe, Grunbaum, & Harris, 1997). Rainwater, Mitchell, Comuzzie, VandeBerg, Stern, and MacCluer (2000), using a population-based sample of 539 Mexican Americans in the San Antonio Heart Study, found that changes in weight were associated with increased risk for cardiovascular disease. Another study found that differences in adiposity between Mexican American and White girls were present by ages 6 to 9 (Winkleby, Robinson, Sundquist & Kraemer, 1999). Thus, the early elementary grades constitute a prime time to implement prevention programs aimed at reducing cardiovascular disease risk factors in order to prevent the onset of cardiovascular disease in adulthood.

In attempting to explain cross-cultural differences in health outcomes, previous studies described barriers to health care access among Mexican Americans. One such study, Morgenstern, Steffen-Batten, Smith, & Moye (2001), included 719 subjects identified via random-digit dialing in Corpus Christi, Texas. The sample was approximately half Mexican American and half White, with an overall cooperation rate of 58% for the survey. Mexican Americans were observed to have a higher prevalence of diabetes, but similar rates of hypertension, elevated cholesterol, and tobacco use. In addition, Mexican Americans in this sample were less able to recognize the warning signs of stroke and were more reticent to call 911 than their White cohorts, suggesting that education aimed at helping Mexican Americans to recognize stroke warning signs may be needed.

Today, many women may not identify cardiovascular disease as a health problem for their gender (Mosca et al., 2000). Evidence suggests that gender and sociocultural factors play an important part in the willingness of Mexican American women to do aerobic exercise and thus to address some of the risk factors for cardiovascular disease (Juarbe, 1998). A study by Nader, Sallis, Abramson, and Broyles (1992) found that risk-reduction education for cardiovascular disease was relatively more effective for Anglo Americans, whereas for Mexican Americans program-related dietary changes and physical activity increases disappeared at follow-up. This suggests that cardiovascular disease risk reduction and other health educational programs for Latinas should incorporate culturally relevant motivational activities that maintain program-related healthy behavior changes in order to produce lasting reductions in disease risk.

Cancer. Latin American countries are experiencing steady increases in cancer incidence and mortality and it is estimated that by the year 2020, nearly one million individuals in Latin America and the Caribbean will have died of cancer (Granda-Cameron, 1999). Glazer et al. (1999) examined data on California children who were younger than 15 and who were diagnosed with invasive cancers from 1988 to 1994. This study used California's population-based cancer registry and found that the overall incidence rate of cancer was 7% lower for Hispanic children than for White children. Hispanic children, however, had a substantially higher incidence of lymphoid leukemia than did White children.

Regarding breast cancer, recent studies suggest a positive correlation between female breast cancer and level of acculturation among Latinas. Similarly, two studies found that breast cancer incidence increased with affluence only among Latina women (Krieger, Quesenberry, Peng, Horn-Ross, Stewart, Brown, Swallen, Guillermo, Suh, Alvarez-Martinez, & Ward, 1999). This suggests a link between increasing levels of acculturation and a higher incidence of breast cancer among Latinas, a trend that needs further study. One plausible hypothesis is that increased affluence results in a higher consumption of certain foods that have a connection to breast cancer (Kushi & Foerster, 1998).

In contrast, Latino cultural values and beliefs may help or hinder a person's survival from cancer. Here, the Latino values of *personalismo* and *simpatía* are central features of Latina/o interpersonal relationships and involve courteous, deferential, warm, and caring responses to others (Granda-Cameron, 1999). Unfortunately, personalismo and simpatía are not well served in the existing health care system. Few health care providers truly integrate spirituality and alternative approaches to cancer treatment and many are unwilling to collaborate with indigenous healers, thus alienating some Latina/os from the health care system.

Diabetes.   Mexican Americans are disproportionately affected by diabetes, which has several adverse physical manifestations and is often accompanied by psychological symptoms such as depression. Several studies have found that, relative to non-Hispanic Whites, Mexican American children and adults exhibit a higher prevalence of diabetes or glucose intolerance (elevated fasting blood glucose levels; Luepker, 2001; Morgenstern et al, 2001; Sundquist et al., 2001; Tortolero et al., 1997; West et al., 2001). Black and Markides (1999) examined ethnic differences in rates of comorbid chronic health conditions, complications, and disabilities in a sample of 173 Mexican Americans, 201 African Americans, and 181 Whites. They found that the prevalence of self-reported diabetes was 17.6% for Mexican Americans, compared to 8.5% for Whites. Stroup-Benham, Makides, Espino, and Goodwin (1999) examined a national sample from the NHANES totaling 3,050 cases, including 216 Mexican Americans who were observed from 1982 to 1993. They found an increase in rates of obesity, the prevalence of diabetes, and elevated diastolic blood pressure.

Among Mexican Americans, compared with non-Hispanic Whites, some evidence exists for differences by racial or ethnic group, not only in the prevalence of diabetes and diabetes-related risk factors, but also for outcomes following hospitalization for diabetes-related complications. A study by Lavery, van Houton, Ashry, Armstrong, and Pugh (1999) examined medical records for incidence of lower leg amputations in a sample of Mexican Americans, Blacks, and Whites. Mexican Americans had more diabetes-related amputations than either Blacks or Whites, with rates of 85.9%, 74.7%, and 56.3%, respectively. Some of these disparities may be the result of a lower percentage of health insurance coverage and thus fewer health care choices among Mexican Americans (66%), compared with Whites (91%; Harris, 1999). These health disparities might thus be decreased with greater access to health insurance for Mexican Americans.

Religious and spiritual practices may play a protective and supportive role in the prevention and management of diabetes among Chicana/os and other Latina/os. For example, the health practices of Hispanic Seventh Day Adventists who eat a plant-based diet and abstain from smoking and alcohol use have been associated with a better blood lipid profile, lower blood pressure, and a lower risk of diabetes, compared to other Latina/os whose diets are different (Alexander, Lockwood, Harris, & Melby, 1999). These findings suggest that dietary modification is a promising means of reducing risk factors for a number of disorders that overwhelmingly affect Mexican Americans. In addition, Hunt, Pugh, and Valenzuela (1998) studied 51 Mexican Americans who had Type-2 diabetes and found that patients who exercised control over their diabetes adapted their self-management of the disease to fit the context of their daily lives. This suggests that diabetes-management programs for Mexican Americans should stress simplicity and consistency in order to promote compliance and adherence and to prevent more serious diabetes-related disabilities.

STRATEGIES TO PROMOTE CULTURALLY RELEVANT PREVENTION INTERVENTION RESEARCH WITH LATINA/O POPULATIONS

Implications for Prevention Research With Chicana/os

The preceding review of current literature points to certain research areas that must be addressed in order to develop more effective prevention interventions for Chicana/os and other Latina/os. Because acculturation tends to be associated with both increased stress and higher socioeconomic status, the interactions between these two variables as contributors to disease risk or protection among Latina/os should be examined. In addition, immigration status is an important variable to examine given that recent immigrants appear for some reason to be protected against certain disorders, thus the postulated Hispanic paradox. Along these lines, two research questions are especially important: (a) For Latina/os, how does contact with the dominant American culture affect incidence, prevalence, morbidity, and mortality of disease? and (b) what is the interaction between acculturation level, socioeconomic status, immigration status, and disease?

   Taking some of the central values of Latino culture into account—family, community, spirituality—a number of important research topics emerge. One area of exploration involves the roles of age and gender in disease and health promotion among Chicana/os. It is especially important to elucidate the specific aspects of age and gender roles that both help and hinder health promotion. More broadly, the role of social networks in the promotion of health, including the use of lay health workers and traditional healing practices, needs to be fully explored due to its potential health-promoting effects. Finally, prevention efforts should be directed at developing culturally relevant methods to effectively build resilience in the form of enhanced coping skills and stress management among Mexican Americans, with an additional focus on children and youth. Specifically sampling both at-risk youth and adults within high-risk families is a strategic prevention approach for decreasing the major risk factors that affect Chicana/os and other Latina/os.

Incorporating Cultural Factors Into Prevention Theory and Models

Conceptual and Strategic Issues. With the aforementioned aims in mind, the scope of contemporary prevention research must be expanded to include cultural

factors while its quality is increased. Culturally rich research should not be scientifically mediocre, but rather, the addition of cultural variables should produce a higher
quality of research by providing insight into the real-world conditions that adversely
affect the life experiences of Chicana/os and other Latina/os. Especially needed is
research that balances social action with scientific rigor (Flores, Castro, & Fernandez-
Esquer, 1995).

As another example, there is a need for process-related, longitudinal research on
the benefits and liabilities of acculturation as it affects various subgroups of Chi-
cana/os. For improved research analyses, within research designs the Latina/o population should be segmented into meaningful subgroups according to the three basic
types of acculturative status: low acculturation, bilingual bicultural, and high acculturation (Balcazar, Castro, & Krull, 1995).

Moreover, certain types of high-risk and high-payoff research are also needed. The
National Institutes of Health offers a review category of high-risk studies that affords
research review committees the opportunity to designate a study as "innovative"
and perhaps thus as "higher risk," but one that is also worthy of support for the
potential contributions that this study can make to the field if it can be conducted
effectively and ethically.

Such prevention research would strive for a deeper examination of cultural issues
by conducting hypotheses-driven analyses that are derived from culturally rich
research questions. What then is significant cultural research? It can be regarded as
problem-solving research that aims to answer questions that have a high social
significance for the daily lives of Chicana/os and other Latina/os. Such research
includes studies that have strong ecological validity that includes the use of combined qualitative and quantitative data-analytic methods that respond assertively to
community needs. Such dual-method studies (Creswell, 1994; Marshall & Rossman,
1995) add depth of analysis and understanding to the study of thematic content that
is important to the lives of Chicana/os who reside within a specific community.

Moderator Effects of a Cultural Variable.   Culture, as measured operationally by
one or more of the aforementioned cultural variables, is probably best seen as not
being a direct causal antecedent of health outcomes, but rather as an effect modifier
of these outcomes. In other words, the noted cultural variables (see Table 18.2) are
not likely to operate as direct-effect causal factors of health behavior, but may instead
operate as amplifiers or buffers of the direct influence of other causal variables of
health behavior (Aiken, Jackson, Castro, & Pero, 2000). Thus, several of the identified
cultural variables may be examined as moderators or as mediators of effect for certain health outcomes (see Fig. 18.1). The illustrated models of moderation and mediation serve as basic models that depict a hypothesized effect-modifier role for the
various cultural variables presented in Table 18.2. These models illustrate effects that
can be tested in greater detail when using the classic models of health behavior such
as the Health Belief Model and the Theory of Reasoned or Planned Action.

As one example, one can ask "Does greater ethnic pride attenuate the detrimental
effects imposed by progressively increasing levels of exposure to cigarette-smoking
peers (peer influence), as these may erode a youth's confidence (self-efficacy) in
avoiding tobacco?" First, a basic relationship may exist that involves a negative correlation (the unmoderated effect). Thus, a higher level of exposure to cigarette-

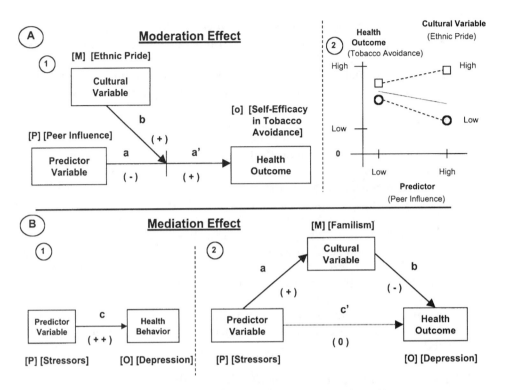

FIG. 18.1. Moderator and mediator effects of cultural variables.

smoking peers (a greater number of these as friends, peer influence) would reduce an adolescent's confidence (self-efficacy) in being able to avoid tobacco (cigarette smoking; see Fig. 18.1, panel A, frame 2). In this situation, does the cultural variable of ethnic pride operate as a moderator, that is, as a factor that, with increasing levels, modifies (either reduces or enhances) a youth's ability to avoid tobacco (the health outcome), in the presence of progressively greater levels of exposure to cigarette-smoking peers?

In this analysis, the moderator effect of ethnic pride (a cultural variable) is shown to counter the adverse effect of exposure to smoking peers as indicated by a youth's self-efficacy in avoiding tobacco (see Fig. 18.1, panel A, frames 1 and 2; Castro & Hernandez-Alarcon, 2002). In contrast, low levels of ethnic pride are shown to accentuate this detrimental effect (a steeper slope), whereas high levels of ethnic pride enhance youth capacity to avoid tobacco use. Thus, a significant Predictor-by-Moderator (P × M) interaction would indicate a significant effect of the moderator variable, ethnic pride, on the health-related outcome, self-efficacy in tobacco avoidance (Baron & Kenny, 1986). In summary, this analysis suggests that ethnic pride enhancement could operate as a protective prevention intervention to discourage tobacco use among Latina/o youth.

Mediator Effect of a Cultural Variable. A simple model of the direct effects of a predictor variable on a health outcome would postulate that increasing levels of a certain predictor, such as greater levels of life stress (frequency or intensity of stressful events), contribute to the severity of a given health outcome, such as depression (see Fig. 18.1, panel B, frame 1). In a simplified analysis, this model indicates that greater stress causes depression. However, the presence of a cultural variable that operates as a mediator, for example, increasing levels of familism (family cohesion and support) buffers (reduces) the adverse direct effects of stressors on the development of depression.

In this illustration, the strong positive correlation (+ +) between the predictor (stressors) and the health outcome (depression; Path c in Fig. 18.1, panel B, frame 1), is reduced to zero by the intervening effect of the moderator variable, familism. Here, in a temporal chain of events, an increase in stressors prompts an increase in familial support (path a in panel B, frame 2). In turn, greater familism is negatively correlated with depressive symptoms (path b). Significant path coefficients for paths a and b, and the attenuation of path c', when tested appropriately (MacKinnon, 1994; MacKinnon, Krull, & Lockwood, 2000), would indicate that the cultural variable of familism operates as a mediator and buffer against stressors. Thus, familism is shown here to reduce the effects of these stressors as antecedent conditions that cause depression. This modeled outcome suggests that strengthening families, via the enhancement of familism, could serve as a preventive intervention strategy against depression despite an exposure to life stressors. Clearly, the empirical testing of this hypothesized effect, as guided by the indicated models, would serve to confirm or refute this and related hypotheses.

Integrating Research and Community Health Practice. Culturally relevant research on Latina/os gains importance when it is integrated into community practice. One of the most important principles behind the integration of research and community practice is that research should be guided by a public health and social action perspective that aims to improve life conditions for Chicana/os and other Latina/os (Flores et al., 1995). Cultural relevance can be achieved by designing prevention research that includes community participation in research design and implementation (Minkler & Wallerstein, 2003). This research should include quantitative and qualitative methodologies and young Chicana/o researchers in leadership positions. Inclusion of those who are knowledgeable of Mexican and other Latina/o cultures and values will improve the quality of the research design, data collection, and data analysis, and will enhance program implementation.

Improving Methodology

Conceptualization and Measurement. Four major principles in the conceptualization and measurement of research and program development with Chicana/os include: (a) theories that are culturally relevant and generated by individuals from the culture, (b) measurement instruments that are culturally relevant based on their validation with samples from the culture under study, (c) consensus building with members of a targeted group regarding the cultural relevance of the proposed program and evaluation methods, and (d) input from community members from the study population at each step of the implementation and evaluation process. This participatory approach to prevention research planning and implementation is especially important in the adaptation of existing models so that cultural relevance to the targeted population is ensured (Castro, Barrera, & Martinez, in press). The proper translation and adaptation of culturally relevant intervention procedures, evaluation instruments and research methods require collaboration with knowledgeable community partners and careful attention to data collection and fidelity monitoring in protocols that purport to offer effective prevention or treatment.

Intervention Program Design.   Given the relative newness of many areas of Chicana/o psychology research, it is important to conceptualize and consider levels of research that can be conducted feasibly: exploratory, descriptive, or confirmatory. Each level introduces different types of demands and constraints. Whereas the use of well-validated measures and instruments is ideal and critical for effective confirmatory research, scientifically defensible exploratory research must also be conducted with measures of cultural variables that have been pretested, but that may not have the desired full record of standardization and validation.

Given that establishing the construct validity of a variable is the product of a long-term effort, prevention research with Chicana/os often encounters a conflict between demands for scientific rigor and the practical demands for quick outcome data that will inform programmatic decisions. Clearly, there is a need to balance scientific rigor with a responsiveness to pressing social needs. Within exploratory- and descriptive-level research, practical demands emphasize the importance of service delivery such that data collection and scientific rigor are de-emphasized in response to client needs. In contrast, where the emphasis is on scientific rigor, the focus is on accuracy in data collection with the most valid measures and service delivery issues are addressed, but secondarily in relation to fidelity in the implementation of the intervention protocol.

Accordingly, in the maturing field of Chicana/o psychology, in which there are still only a limited number of established and well-validated culturally relevant measures, there continues to be a great need to adjust research constraints involving measurement validity in direct relationship to the nature of the proposed research: exploratory, descriptive, or confirmatory. Newer acculturation measures that embody newer conceptions of acculturation and new measruement challenges include the Acculturation Rating Scale for Mexican Americans II (Cuellar, Arnold, & Maldonado, 1995), and the Bidimensional Acculturation Scale for Hispanics (Marin & Gamboa, 1996). In addressing these issues, Table 18.3 offers a prescribed balanced resolution for the implementation of effective and culturally relevant research at each of these three research levels.

Data Analysis and Interpretation.   In the analysis of qualitative text information, one basic approach to data analysis involves the extraction of thematic content via frequency or co-occurrence of word counts, in an effort to distill meaning accurately and completely (Miles & Huberman, 1994). A program such as CDC EZ-Text permits qualitative analyses of data such as narratives and can be downloaded from the CDC website (Centers for Disease Control and Prevention, 2002a). This type of software program permits the coding and analysis of transcripts from actual therapy sessions, focus groups, or other interactive encounters in order to generate a quantitative measure of interpersonal processes. Currently, more basic methodology research is needed to develop robust qualitative data-analysis protocols that establish

TABLE 18.3
Balancing Scientific and Practical Demands in Research
with Chicana/o Communities

	Scientific	*Practical*	*Balanced Resolution*
Level 1: Exploratory	High demand for validated measures	Demand for expeditious and usable results	New measures included and tested Validated measures are used as available
Level 2: Descriptive	High demands for validated measures	Demand for expeditious and usable results	New measures used as needed Validated measures are included
Level 3: Confirmatory	High demands for validated measures	Demand for expeditious and usable results	New measures used sparingly Validated measures emphasized

procedures for a truly inductive yet reliable generation of thematic categories from open-ended text narratives. Such methods, if robust, would permit the coding of thematic categories into quantitative databases that then allows for the implementation of statistical comparisons and model testing in conjunction with other quantitatively generated variables (Denne, Castro, & Harris, 2001).

Enhancing Implementation

Establishing Partnerships With Community-Based Agencies.   Community-based interventions demand an intense and sustained focus over a long period of time. To build an effective partnership with community agencies, respect, community focus, collaboration, cultural relevance, and ongoing community involvement are essential. The academic researcher who enters a community is typically an outsider and must refrain from interfering with the community's traditional values and practices. Information-exchange networks can be created with community input and by integrating advisory committees, informal support systems (e.g., church, family members, alternative and complementary medical providers), and formal health care support networks into an overall plan for community collaboration (Center for Substance Abuse Treatment, 2000; Substance Abuse and Mental Health Services Administration, 1998). Consumer and stakeholder involvement in program planning, development, and implementation can help to promote truly collaborative academic-community research partnerships (Minkler & Wallerstein, 2003).

Training and Selection of Latina/o Researchers.   The field of academic research needs to train and mentor a new generation of Latina/o researchers. It is important that Chicana/o and other Latina/o researchers attain professional competence, but they must also develop cultural competence and a commitment to serving Latina/o communities. It is crucial to provide experiential training along with didactic instruction, because many training experiences exclude the former in favor of the latter, which results in a diminished level of practical competence for the new researcher.

Training of staff should include continuing education regarding cultural competence, psychosocial stressors, and unique traumas that relate specifically to the target population (U.S. Department of Health and Human Services, Center for Mental Health Services, 2001). In addition, staff should be trained to recognize the effects of the acculturation process, as well as the interaction between sociocultural variables and health.

Cultural competence training should promote an understanding of differences in symptom expression across cultures, culture-bound syndromes, nuances of communication, cross-cultural differences in definitions of wellness and illness, differences in help-seeking behaviors across cultures, and the role of sociocultural factors in promoting health. The cultural appropriateness of assessment tools and methods should also be discussed and particular attention should be given to cross-cultural variability in response to psychotropic medications (U.S. Department of Health and Human Services, Center for Mental Health Services, 2001).

A CULTURALLY RICH APPROACH TO FUTURE PREVENTION RESEARCH WITH LATINA/OS

The Need for Culturally Rich Research with Latina/os

As noted earlier, previous prevention research studies conducted in Latina/o communities have been limited by a shallow level of cultural analysis. Culturally shallow research studies are those that, from their inception, lack substantive cultural research questions and that include a sample of Mexican Americans solely as a sample of convenience. The explicit or implicit rationale for the inclusion of Mexican Americans in such a study has been to compare them with another group, or to study them on a certain health issue because they have not been studied before. Such studies can be classified as culturally shallow, that is, they lack deep strucure, even if strong in their scientific merit (Resnikow, Soler, Braithwait, Ahluwalia, & Butler, 2000).

Such prevention research studies can be improved by taking a culturally focused approach that explicitly examines research questions according to the cultural life experiences of Latina/os, given that these life experiences usually will influence their health status. A few of the significant cultural issues involving deeper cultural context and greater cultural grounding, include the analysis of ethnic identity development, gender roles, family norms and expectations, traditional beliefs and practices, and adaptation to acculturative stressors, as these affect the health status of Latina/os.

Beyond this, examining these cultural issues using integrated cultural theory and analysis would add further depth and character to such prevention studies, thus making them culturally rich. Such studies are seen as capable of yielding more significant research outcomes and as likely to yield more meaningful research results that contribute substantive knowledge for conducting health promotion with Latina/o populations.

Some research investigators who are unresponsive to this call for cultural depth and integration may deliberately avoid the incorporation of cultural issues into their studies. They may regard cultural issues as irrelevant relative to "the real scientific question," or as content that should be avoided because it could, lower their scientific merit score. On the contrary, today in many study sections of the Center for Scientific Review (CSR) of the National Institutes of Health (NIH), avoiding the scientific analysis of cultural issues in prevention research with Latina/os is likely to detract from a higher rating of scientific merit. As one specific indicator of the growing importance of integrating cultural elements into a new generation of culturally rich research, many government-sponsored program announcements emphasize the inclusion of cultural elements, including issues of race/ethnicity, gender, and other special characteristics, as preferred or required features of proposed research projects (National Institutes of Health, 2001).

The Origins of Culturally Rich Research

A culturally rich prevention research study originates with an investigator's formal intention to conceptualize and design a study that explicitly examines cultural issues in connection with a significant research question regarding disease prevention or health promotion with Latina/os. This culturally oriented research planning constitutes an integral part of sound conceptualization and development of a research proposal. Moreover, this conceptualization and planning serves as the basis for the integration of cultural content into the research questions and hypotheses that operate as the scientific core of research conducted with Latina/os. The inclusion of Latina/o research staff and efforts to utilize a community participatory approach in the development and implementation of the proposed research project would provide additional features for a culturally rich prevention research project. Cultural issues should be afforded explicit and central significance in culturally rich prevention research for health promotion and disease prevention in Latina/o populations.

REFERENCES

Aiken, L. S., Jackson, K. M., Castro, F. G., & Pero, V. I. (2000). Mediators of the linkage from acculturation to mammography screening compliance among urban Hispanic women. *Women and Cancer, 2*, 4–16.

Ajzen, I. (1991). The theory of planned behavior. *Organizational Behavior and Human Decision Process, 50*, 179–211.

Ajzen, I., & Fishbein, M. (1980). *Understanding attitudes and predicting social behavior: Attitudes, intentions, and perceived behavioral control.* Englewood Cliffs, NJ: Prentice-Hall.

Albarracin, D., Johnson, B. T., Fishbein, M., & Muellerleile, P. A. (2001). Theories of Reasoned Action and Planned Behavior as models of condom use: A meta-analysis. *Psychological Bulletin, 127*, 142–161.

Alderete, E., Vega, W. A., Kolody, B., & Aguliar-Gaxiola, S. (2000). Lifetime prevalence of and risk factors for psychiatric disorders among Mexican migrant farmworkers in California. *American Journal of Public Health, 90*, 608–614.

Alexander, H., Lockwood, L. P., Harris, M. A., & Melby, C. L. (1999). Risk factors for cardiovascular disease and diabetes in two groups of Hispanic Americans with differing dietary habits. *Journal of the American College of Nutrition, 18*, 127–136.

Amaro, H., & Zambrana, R. E. (2000). Criollo, Mestizo, Mulato, LatiNegra, Indigena, White, or Black? The US Hispanic/Latino population and multiple responses in the 2000 Census. *American Journal of Public Health, 90*, 1724–1727.

Anderson, N. B., & Armstead, C. A. (1995). Toward understanding the association of socioeconomic status and health: A new challenge for the biopsychosocial approach. *Psychosomatic Medicine, 57*, 213–225.

Apodaca, J. X., Woodruff, S. I., Candelaria, J., Elder, J. P., & Zlot, A. (1997). Hispanic health program participant and non-participant characteristics. *American Journal of Health Behavior, 21,* 356–363.

Balcazar, H., Castro, F. G., & Krull, J. L. (1995). Cancer risk reduction in Mexican American women: The role of acculturation, education, and health risk factors. *Health Education Quarterly, 22,* 61–84.

Bandura, A. (1986). *Social foundations of thought and action: A social cognitive theory.* Englewood Cliffs, NJ: Prentice-Hall.

Baron, R. M., & Kenny, D. A. (1986). The moderator-mediator variable distinction in social psychological research: Conceptual, strategic, and statistical considerations. *Journal of Personality and Social Psychology, 51,* 1173–1182.

Barrera, M., Castro, F. G., & Biglan, A. (1999). Ethnicity, substance use, and development: Exemplars for exploring group differences and similarities. *Development and Psychopathology, 11,* 805–822.

Bernal, M. E., & Knight, G. P. (1993). *Ethnic identity: Formation and transmission among Hispanics and other minorities.* Albany: State University of New York Press.

Berruta-Clement, J., Schweinhart, L., Barnett, W., Epstein, A., & Weikart, D. (1984). *Changed lives: The effects of the Perry Preschool Program on youth age 19.* Ypsilanti, MI: High/Scope Press.

Black, S. A., & Markides, K. S. (1999). Depressive symptoms and mortality in older Mexican Americans. *Annals of Epidemiology, 9,* 45–52.

Black, S. A., Markides, K. S., & Miller, T. Q. (1998). Correlates of depressive symptomatology among older community-dwelling Mexican-Americans: The Hispanic EPESE. *Journals of Gerontology, 53,* S198–S208.

Block, J. (1971). *Lives through time.* Berkeley, CA: Bancroft Books.

Botvin, G. J. (1995). Principles of prevention. In R. H. Coombs & D. Zedonis (Eds.), *Handbook of drug abuse prevention: A comprehensive strategy to prevent the abuse of alcohol and other drugs* (pp. 19–44). Boston: Allyn and Bacon.

Botvin, G. J., Baker, E., Dusenbury, L., Tortu, S., & Botvin, E. M. (1990). Preventing adolescent drug abuse through a multimodal cognitive-behavioral approach: Results of a 3-year study. *Journal of Consulting and Clinical Psychology, 58,* 437–446.

Caetano, R., & Raspberry, K. (2000). Drinking and DSM-IV alcohol and drug dependence among White and Mexican-American DUI offenders. *Journal of Studies on Alcohol, 61,* 420–426.

Carrillo, E., & Uranga-McKane, S. (1994). HIV/AIDS. In C. W. Molina & M. Aguirre-Molina (Eds.), *Latino health in the U.S.: A growing challenge* (pp. 313–337). Washington, DC: American Public Health Association.

Carter-Pokras, O. (1994). Health profile. In C. W. Molina & M. Aguirre-Molina (Eds.), *Latino health in the U. S.: A growing challenge* (pp. 45–79). Washington, DC: American Public Health Association.

Castro, F. G., Baezconde-Garbanati, L., & Beltran, H. (1985). Risk factors for coronary heart disease in Hispanic populations: A review. *Hispanic Journal of Behavioral Sciences, 7,* 153–175.

Castro, F. G., Barrera, M., & Martinez, C. R. (in press). The cultural adaptation of prevention interventions: Resolving tensions between fidelity and fit. *Prevention Science.*

Castro, F. G., Cota, M. K., & Vega, S. C. (1999). Health promotion in Latino populations: A sociocultural model for program planning, development, and evaluation. In R. M. Huff & M. V. Kline (Eds.), *Promoting health in multicultural populations: A handbook for practitioners* (pp. 137–168). Thousand Oaks, CA: Sage.

Castro, F. G., Elder, J., Coe, K., Tafoya-Barraza, H., Moratto, S., Campbell, N., & Talavara, G. (1995). Mobilizing churches for health promotion in Latino communities: Compañeros en la Salud. *Journal of the National Cancer Institute Monographs, 18,* 127–135.

Castro, F. G., & Gutierres, S. (1997). Drug and alcohol use among rural Mexican Americans. In E. B. Robertson, Z. Sloboda, G. M. Boyd, L. Beatty, & J. Kozel (Eds.), *Rural substance abuse: State of knowledge and issues* (NIDA Research Monograph No. 168, pp. 498–533). Rockville, MD: National Institute on Drug Abuse.

Castro, F. G., & Hernandez-Alarcon, E. (2002). Integrating cultural variables into drug abuse prevention and treatment with racial/ethnic minorities. *Journal of Drug Issues, 32,* 783–810.

Center for Substance Abuse Prevention. (2002). *Soy unica, soy Latina* [On-line]. Available: http://www.samhsa.gov/centers/csap/csap.html.

Center for Substance Abuse Treatment. (2000). *Changing the conversation: Improving substance abuse treatment. The National Treatment Plan Initiative* (DHHS Publication No. SMA 00-3479). Rockville, MD: Author.

Centers for Disease Control and Prevention. (2001). *Fast stats A to Z: Minority health* [On-line]. Available: http://www.cdc/gov/nchs/faststats/minority.htm.

Centers for Disease Control and Prevention (2002a). *CDC EZ-Text* [On-line]. Available: http://www .cdc.gov/hiv/software/ex-text.htm.

Centers for Disease Control and Prevention (2002b). *HIV/AIDS among Hispanics in the United States* [On-line]. Available: http://www.cdc.gov/hiv/pubs/facts/hispanic.htm.

Cowen, E. L., Wyman, P A., & Work, W. C. (1990). The Rochester Child Resilience Project. *Developmental Psychopathology, 2,* 192–212.

Creswell, J. W. (1994). *Research design: Qualitative and quantitative approaches.* Thousand Oaks, CA: Sage.

Cuellar, I., Arnold, B., & Maldonado, R. (1995). Acculturation Rating Scale for Mexican Americans II: A revision of the original ARSMA scale. *Hispanic Journal of Behavioral Sciences, 17,* 275–304.

Davila, Y. R., & Brackley, M. H. (1999). Mexican and Mexican American women in a battered women's shelter: Barriers to condom negotiation for HIV/AIDS prevention. *Issues in Mental Health Nursing, 20,* 333–355.

Denne, R., Castro, F. G., & Harris, T. (2001, May). *Antecedents and consequences of relapse in stimulant users: Integrating qualitative and quantitative analyses.* Paper presented at the Society for Prevention Research Meeting, Washington, DC.

Department of Health and Human Services. (2000). *Culture, race and ethnicity: A supplement to mental health. A report of the Surgeon General* [On-line]. Available: http://www.mental health.org/cre/execsummary-6.asp.

Duncan, T. E., Duncan, S. C., Strycker, L. A., Li, F., & Alpert, A. (1999). *An introduction to latent growth curve modeling: Concepts, issues, and applications.* Mahwah, NJ: Lawrence Erlbaum Associates.

Escobar, J. I., Hoyos-Nervi, C., & Gara, M. A. (2000). Immigration and mental health: Mexican Americans in the United States. *Harvard Review of Psychiatry, 8,* 64–72.

Flack, J. M., Amaro, H., Jenkins, W., Kunitz, S., Levy, J., Mixom, M., & Yu, E. (1995). Panel I: Epidemiology of minority health. *Health Psychology, 14,* 592–600.

Flores, E., Castro, F. G., & Fernandez-Esquer, M. E. (1995). Social theory, social action, and intervention research: Implications for cancer prevention among Latinos. *Journal of the National Cancer Institute Monographs, 18,* 101–108.

Ford, K., & Norris, A. E. (1995). Factors related to condom use with casual partners among urban African American and Hispanic males. *AIDS Education and Prevention, 7,* 494–503.

Frankish, C. J., Lovato, C. Y., & Shannon, W. J. (1999). Models, theories, and principles of health promotion with minority populations. In R. M. Huff & M. V. Kline (Eds.), *Promoting health in multicultural populations: A handbook for practitioners* (pp. 41–72). Thousand Oaks, CA: Sage.

Freire, P. (1993). *Pedagogy of the oppressed.* New York: Continuum.

Giachello, A. L. M. (1994). Issues of access and use. In C. W. Molina & M. Aguirre-Molina (Eds.), *Latino health in the U.S.: A growing challenge* (pp. 83–111). Washington, DC: American Public Health Association.

Ginsberg, E. (1991). Access to health care for Hispanics. *Journal of the American Medical Association, 265,* 238–241.

Glazer, E. R., Perkins, C. I., Young, J. L., Schlag, R. D., Campleman, S. L., & Wright, W. E. (1999). Cancer among Hispanic children in California, 1988–1994: Comparison with non-Hispanic white children. *Cancer, 86,* 1070–1079.

Goff, D. C., Ramsey, D. J., Labarthe, D. R., & Nichaman, M. Z. (1993). Acute myocardial infarction and coronary heart disease mortality among Mexican Americans and non-Hispanic whites in Texas, 1980 through 1989. *Ethnicity and Disease, 3,* 64–69.

Granda-Cameron, C. (1999). The experience of having cancer in Latin Americans. *Cancer Nursing, 22,* 51–57.

Harachi, T. W., Hawkins, J. D., & Catalano, R. F. (1996). *Parenting for the drug-free years: Effective recruitment within ethnic minority communities.* Seattle: University of Washington Social Development Research Group.

Harris, M. I. (1999). Racial and ethnic differences in health insurance coverage for adults with diabetes. *Diabetes Care, 22,* 1679–1682.

Hart, D., Keller, M., Edelstein, W., & Hoffman, V. (1998). Childhood personality influences on social-cognitive development: A longitudinal study. *Journal of Personality and Social Psychology, 74,* 1278–1289.

Hawkins, J. D., Catalano, R. F., & Miller, J. Y. (1992). Risk and protective factors for alcohol and other drug problems in adolescence and early adulthood: Implications for substance abuse prevention. *Psychological Bulletin, 112,* 64–105.

Hovey, J. D. (1998). Acculturative stress, depression, and suicidal ideation among Mexican-American ado-lescents: Implications for the development of suicide prevention programs in schools. *Psychological Reports, 83,* 249–250.

Hunt, L. M., Pugh, J., Valenzuela, M. (1998). How patients adapt diabetes self-care recommendations in everyday life. *Journal of Family Practice, 46,* 207–215.

Jessor, R., & Jessor, S. L. (1977). *Problem behavior and psychosocial development: A longitudinal study of youth.* New York: Academic Press.

Jessor, R., Van den Bos, J., Vanderryn, J., Costa, F. M., & Tubin, M. S. (1985). Protective factors in adolescent problem behavior: Moderator effects and developmental change. *Developmental Psychology, 31,* 923–933.

Joe, G. W., Barrett, M. E., & Simpson, D. D. (1991). An integrative model for drug use severity among inhalant users. *Hispanic Journal of Behavioral Sciences, 13,* 324–340.

Joiner, T. E., Perez, M., Wagner, K. D., Berenson, A., & Marquina, G. S. (2001). On fatalism, pessimism, and depressive symptoms among Mexican-American and other adolescents attending an obstetrics-gyne-cology clinic. *Behaviour Research and Therapy, 39,* 887–896.

Juarbe, T. C. (1998). Cardiovascular disease-related diet and exercise experiences of immigrant Mexican women. *Western Journal of Nursing Research, 20,* 765–782.

Katims, D. S., Zapata, J. T., & Yin, Z. (1996). Risk factors for substance use by Mexican American youth with and without learning disabilities. *Journal of Learning Disabilities, 29,* 213–219.

Klohnen, E. C. (1996). Conceptual analysis and measurement of the construct ego-resiliency. *Journal of Personality and Social Psychology, 70,* 1067–1079.

Krieger, N., Quesenberry, C., Peng, T., Horn-Ross, P., Stewart, S., Brown, S., Swallen, K., Guillermo, T., Suh, D., Alvarez-Martinez, L., & Ward, F. (1999). Social class, race/ethnicity, and incidence of breast, cervix, colon, lung, and prostate cancer among Asian, Black, Hispanic, and White residents of the San Francisco Bay area, 1988–1992. *Cancer Causes and Control, 10,* 525–537.

Kumpfer, K. L., DeMarsh, J. P., & Child, W. (1989a). *The Strengthening Families Program: Parent Training Manual.* Salt Lake City, UT: Utah Department of Health Education, University of Utah and Alta Institute.

Kumpfer, K. L., DeMarsh, J. P., & Child, W. (1989b). *The Strengthening Families Program: Children's Training Manual.* Salt Lake City, UT: Utah Department of Health Education, University of Utah and Alta Institute.

Kumpfer, K. L., DeMarsh, J. P., & Child, W. (1989c). *The Strengthening Families Program: Family Training Manual.* Salt Lake City, UT: Utah Department of Health Education, University of Utah and Alta Institute.

Kushi, L. H., & Foerster, S. B. (1998). Diet and nutrition. In R. C. Brownson, P. L. Remington, & J. R. Davis (Eds.), *Chronic disease epidemiology and control* (2nd ed., pp. 215–259). Washington, DC: American Public Health Association.

Lavery, L. A., van Houton, W. H., Ashry, H. R., Armstrong, D. G., & Pugh, J. A. (1999). Diabetes-related lower-extremity amputations disproportionately affect Blacks and Mexican Americans. *Southern Medical Journal, 92,* 593–599.

Longshore, D. (1997). Treatment motivation among Mexican American drug-using arrestees. *Hispanic Journal of Behavioral Sciences, 19,* 214–229.

Luepker, R. V. (2001). Cardiovascular disease among Mexican Americans. *American Journal of Medicine, 110,* 147–148.

MacKinnon, D. P. (1994). Analysis of mediating variables in prevention and intervention research. In A. Cazares & L. A. Beatty (Eds.), *Scientific methods for prevention intervention research* (NIDA Research Monograph No. 139, pp. 127–153). Rockville, MD: National Institute on Drug Abuse.

MacKinnon, D. P., Krull, J. L., & Lockwood, C. M. (2000). Equivalence of the mediation, confounding and suppression effect. *Prevention Science, 1,* 173–181.

Marín, B. V., Marín, G., Perez-Stable, E., & Otero-Sabogal, R. (1990). Cultural differences in attitudes towards smoking: Developing messages using the theory of reasoned action. *Journal of Applied Social Psychology, 20,* 478–493.

Marín, G., & Gamboa, R. (1996). A new measure of acculturation for Hispanics: The Bidimensional Acculturation Scale for Hispanics (BAS). *Hispanic Journal of Behavioral Sciences, 18,* 297–316.

Marín, G., & Marín, B. V. (1991). *Research with Hispanic populations.* Newbury Park, CA: Sage.

Marshall, C., & Rossman, G. B. (1995). *Designing qualitative research* (2nd ed.). Thousand Oaks, CA: Sage.

Mason, M. J., & Roehe, C. (1997). Drug use in a Mexican American majority/border area school district. *Alcoholism Treatment Quarterly, 14,* 35–45.

McAllister, A. L., Fernandez-Esquer, M., Ramirez, A. G., Treviño, F., Gallion, K. J., Villareal, R., Pulley, L., Hu, S., Torres, I., & Zhang, Q. (1995). Community level cancer control in a Texas barrio: Part I. Base-line and preliminary outcome findings. *Journal of the National Cancer Institute Monographs, 18,* 123–126.

McBride, A. A., Joe, G. W., & Simpson, D. D. (1991). Prediction of long-term alcohol use, drug use, and criminality among inhalant users. *Hispanic Journal of Behavioral Sciences, 13,* 315–323.

McKenzie, J. F., & Smeltzer, J. L. (2001). *Planning, implementing and evaluating health promotion programs: A primer* (3rd ed.). Boston: Allyn and Bacon.

Meyerowitz, B. E., Richardson, J., Hudson, S., & Leedham, B. (1998). Ethnicity and cancer outcomes: Behavioral and psychosocial considerations. *Psychological Bulletin, 123,* 47–70.

Miles, M. B., & Huberman, A. M. (1994). *Qualitative data analysis.* Thousand Oaks, CA: Sage.

Mills, R. (1995, August). *Health realization: Thought and resiliency. Toward a comprehensive model of prevention. Building a foundation for understanding the root causes of drug abuse, alienation, and emotional disorders.* Paper presented at the American Psychological Association, New York.

Minkler, M., & Wallerstein, N. (2003). *Community-based participatory research for health.* San Francisco, CA: Jossey-Bass.

Mitchell, B. D., Stern, M. P., Haffner, S. M., Hazuda, H. P., & Patterson, J. K. (1990). Risk factors of cardiovascular mortality in Mexican Americans and non-Hispanic Whites. *American Journal of Epidemiology, 131,* 423–433.

Molina, C. W., Zambrana, R. E., & Aguirre-Molina, M. (1994). The influence of culture, class, and environment on health care. In C. W. Molina & M. Aguirre-Molina (Eds.), *Latino health in the U.S.: A growing challenge* (pp. 23–43). Washington, DC: American Public Health Association.

Moon, D. G., Hecht, M. L., Jackson, K. M., & Spellers, R. E. (2000). Family risk and resiliency factors, substance use and the drug resistance process in adolescence. *Journal of Drug Education, 30,* 373–398.

Morales, A. (1984). Substance abuse and Mexican American youth: An overview. *Journal of Drug Issues, 14,* 297–311.

Morgenstern, L. B., Steffen-Batten, L., Smith, M. A., & Moye, L. A. (2001). Barriers to acute stroke therapy and stroke prevention in Mexican Americans. *Stroke, 32,* 1360–1364.

Mosca, L., Jones, W. K., King, K. B., Ouyang, P., Redberg, R. F., & Hill, M. N. (2000). Awareness, perception, and knowledge of heart disease risk and prevention among women in the United States: American Heart Association Women's Heart Disease and Stroke Campaign Task Force. *Archives of Family Medicine, 9,* 506–515.

Nader, P. R., Sallis, J. F., Abramson, I. S., & Broyles, S. L. (1992). Family-based cardiovascular risk reduction education among Mexican- and Anglo-Americans. *Family and Community Health, 15,* 57–74.

National Institutes of Health. (2000). *Reviewer guidelines* [On-line]. Available: http://www.nih.gov/guidelines.r01.htm.

National Institutes of Health. (2001). *Social and cultural dimensions of health* [On-line]. Available: http://www.nih.gov.grants/guide/pa-files/PA-02-043.html.

Navarro, A. M., Rock, C. L., McNicholas, L. J., Senn, K. L., & Moreno, C. (2000). Community-based education in nutrition and cancer: The Por La Vida Cuidandome curriculum. *Journal of Cancer Education, 15,* 168–172.

Ortega, A. N., Rosenheck, R., Alegria, M., & Desai, R. A. (2000). Acculturation and the lifetime risk of psychiatric and substance use disorders among Hispanics. *Journal of Nervous and Mental Diseases, 188,* 736–740.

Pandey, D. K., Labarthe, D. R., Goff, D. C., Chan, W., & Nichaman, M. Z. (2001). Community-wide coronary heart disease mortality in Mexican Americans equals or exceeds that in non-Hispanic Whites: The Corpus Christi Heart Project. *American Journal of Medicine, 110,* 81–87.

Phinney, J. S. (1990). Ethnic identity in adolescents and adults: Review of research. *Psychological Bulletin, 108,* 499–514.

Rainwater, D. L., Mitchell, B. D., Comuzzie, A. G., VandeBerg, J. L., Stern, M. P., & MacCluer, J. W. (2000). Association among 5-year changes in weight, physical activity, and cardiovascular disease risk factors in Mexican Americans. *American Journal of Epidemiology, 152,* 974–982.

Ramirez, M. (1999). *Multicultural psychotherapy: An approach to individual and cultural differences* (2nd ed.). Boston: Allyn and Bacon.

Raymond, J. S., Rhoads, D. L., & Raymond, R. I. (1981). The relative impact of family and social involvement on Chicano mental health. *American Journal of Community Psychology, 8,* 557–569.

Reaven, P., Nader, P. R., Berry, C., & Hoyt, T. (1998). Cardiovascular disease insulin risk in Mexican-American and Anglo-American children and mothers. *Pediatrics, 101,* E12.

Resnikow, K., Soler, R., Braithwait, R. L., Ahluwalia, J. S., & Butler, J. (2000). Cultural sensitivity in substance abuse prevention. *Journal of Community Psychology, 28,* 271–290.

Rogler, L. H. (1994). International migrations: A framework for directing research. *American Psychologist, 49,* 701–708.

Rogler, L. H., Cortés, D. E., & Malgady, R. G. (1991). Acculturation and mental health status among Hispanics: Convergence and new directions for research. *American Psychologist, 46,* 585–597.

Romero, A. J. (1998). The impact of ethnic identity on sociopsychological stress and mental well-being in adolescents from a rural setting. *Dissertation Abstracts International, 59*(6-B), 3124.

Rosenstock, I. M. (1990). The Health Belief Model: Explaining health behavior through expectancies. In K. Glanz, F. M. Lewis, & B. K. Rimer (Eds.), *Health behavior and health education* (pp. 39–62). San Francisco: Jossey-Bass.

Sabogal, F., Marín, G., Otero-Sabogal, R., & Marín, B. (1989). Hispanic familism and acculturation: What changes and what doesn't? *Hispanic Journal of Behavioral Sciences, 9,* 397–412.

Steers, W. N., Elliot, N., Nemiro, J., Ditman, D., & Oskamp, S. (1996) Health beliefs as predictors of HIV-prevention behavior and ethnic differences in prediction. *Journal of Social Psychology, 136,* 99–110.

Stroup-Benham, C. A., Markides, K. S., Espino, D. V., & Goodwin, J. S. (1999). Changes in blood pressure and risk factors for cardiovascular disease among older Mexican-Americans from 1982–1984 to 1993–1994. *Journal of the American Geriatrics Society, 47,* 804–810.

Substance Abuse and Mental Health Services Administration. (1998). *Cultural competence performance measures for managed behavioral healthcare programs.* Rockville, MD: Center for Mental Health Services.

Sundquist, J., & Winkleby, M. A. (1999). Cardiovascular risk factors in Mexican American adults: A transcultural analysis of NHANES III, 1988–1994. *American Journal of Public Health, 89,* 723–730.

Sundquist, J., Winkleby, M. A., & Pudaric, S. (2001). Cardiovascular disease risk factors among older Black, Mexican-American, and White women and men: An analysis of NHANES III, 1988–1994. Third National Health and Nutrition Survey. *Journal of the American Geriatrics Society, 49,* 109–116.

Swenson, C. J., Baxter, J., Shatterly, S. M., Scarbro, S. L., & Hamman, R. F. (2000). Depressive symptoms in Hispanic and non-Hispanic White rural elderly: The San Luis Valley health and aging study. *American Journal of Epidemiology, 152,* 1048–1055.

Szapocznik, J., & Kurtines, W. M. (1989). *Breakthroughs in family therapy with drug abusing and problem youth.* New York: Springer.

Szapocznik, J., & Kurtines, W. M. (1993). Family psychology and cultural diversity: Opportunities for theory, research, and application. *American Psychologist, 48,* 400–407.

Tortolero, S. R., Goff, D. C., Nichaman, M. Z., Labarthe, D. R., Grunbaum, J. A., & Hanis, C. L. (1997). Cardiovascular risk factors in Mexican-American and non-Hispanic White children: The Corpus Christi Heart Study. *Circulation, 96,* 418–423.

Turnock, B. J. (2001). *Public health: What it is and how it works* (2nd ed.). Gaithersburg, MD: Aspen.

U.S. Census Bureau. (2001). *Overview of race and Hispanic origin 2000: Census 2000 brief.* Available: http://www.census.gov/population/www/cen2000/briefs.html.

U.S. Department of Health and Human Services, Center for Mental Health Services. (2001). *Cultural competence standards in managed mental health services: Four underserved/underrepresented racial/ethnic groups.* Washington, DC: Author.

Vega, W. A., Alderete, E., Kolody, B., & Aguilar-Gaxiola, S. (1998). Illicit drug use among Mexicans and Mexican Americans in California: The effects of gender and acculturation. *Addiction, 93,* 1839–1850.

Werner, E. E., & Smith, R. S. (1982). *Vulnerable but invincible: A study of resilient children.* New York: McGraw-Hill.

West, S. K., Klein, R., Rodriguez, J., Muñoz, B., Broman, A. T., Sanchez, R., & Snyder, R. (2001). Diabetes and diabetic retinopathy in a Mexican-American population: Proyecto VER. *Diabetes Care, 24,* 1204–1209.

Winkleby, M. A., Kraemer, H. C., Ahn, D. K., & Varady, A. N. (1998). Ethnic and socioeconomic differences in cardiovascular disease risk factors: Findings for women from the Third National Health and Nutrition Examination Survey, 1988–1994. *Journal of the American Medical Association, 280,* 356–362.

Winkleby, M. A., Robinson, T. N., Sundquist, J., & Kraemer, H. C. (1999). Ethnic variation in cardiovascular disease risk factors among children and young adults: Findings from the Third National Health and Nutrition Examination Study, 1988–1994. *Journal of the American Medical Association, 281,* 1006–1013.

VI

New Directions

Ambrocia and Omar Go to College: A Psychosociocultural Examination of Chicana/os in Higher Education[1]

Alberta M. Gloria
Theresa A. Segura-Herrera
University of Wisconsin–Madison

Ambrocia, a senior attending a 4-year university, was the first person in her family and neighborhood to go to college. From a lower socioeconomic family and community, she has become an educational role model in her neighborhood. She often gives academic advice to the parents of the children and adolescents in her community. Ambrocia described her role simply, yet eloquently: "The parents can see in me opportunities and possibilities for their own children to go to school as well."

She also indicated that being a role model for her three younger brothers and her community is "a lot of pressure," but that she "loves school and wants to succeed. The pressure [to succeed] is a positive motivator" for her to continue with her studies despite her feelings of isolation on campus and her daily experience of "culture clash" between her academic and cultural contexts.

Ambrocia is one of several Chicana/o college students whose educational experiences in higher education are described in this chapter. The narratives are poignant and illustrate the successes and struggles that many Chicana/o students encounter in their educational journeys.

In reviewing the current literature and the state of education for Chicana/os in higher education, a holistic and psychosociocultural approach (Gloria & Rodriguez, 2000) serves as the basis for accurately understanding the interrelationships of Chicana/o students within the environmental context and culture of higher education. An interdisciplinary approach heightens clarity and increases sophistication of the issue, and thus the intent of this chapter to merge educationally and psychologically based literatures to more holistically examine how the psychological functioning and environmental context of higher education affects Chicana/o students' educational status and tenure.

This chapter first reviews the educational status of Latina/os in the United States. Second, a review of prominent issues that serve as a model for understanding

---

[1] This chapter is dedicated to those Chicana/o college students who have persevered through numerous psychosociocultural challenges to succeed academically. *No te achicopales.*

Chicana/o student experiences in higher education is presented. Major constructs to be discussed include acculturation and ethnic identity, distress and adjustment, social supports, university and campus climate, and balance of cultures and contexts. Next, a review of proposed approaches for providing psychoeducational support services and counseling to Chicana/o college students follows. The last section of the chapter provides a directory of resources for faculty, staff, counselors, and parents of Chicana/o college students.

To illustrate the concepts and research presented, the narratives of 11 Chicana/o students (eight undergraduates and three graduates) are interwoven throughout the text. The students ranged in class standing (freshman to second-year graduate student), higher education setting (2-year community college vs. 4-year institution), entry into higher education (transitioned directly from high school vs. transferred from a community college), and location of university (e.g., Southwest, Midwest). Students requested that they be identified by their real names as they described their educational experiences to let readers know that their experiences were real. The students who are highlighted throughout the chapter are Ambrocia, Anabel, Bobby, Jorge, Jose, Magally, Monica, Nancy, Noel, Omar, and Veronica.

One student narrative was provided via e-mail; all other interviews were conducted by phone. Each of the students were asked the same questions about their education (e.g., What is your most salient educational experience?, How have you survived or managed your educational experiences?). Because their educational histories are varied, the information selected from the narratives is not intended to reflect all perspectives or to stereotype the issues and experiences of Chicana/o students, but rather to illuminate the constructs presented.

TERMINOLOGY

Before beginning our discussion, an overview of the terminology used throughout the chapter is warranted. Although the use of a single term (e.g., *Latina/o* or *Hispanic*) to describe over 38 million racially, ethnically, and culturally diverse individuals is inadequate (Gloria, Ruiz, & Castillo, 2004), governmental and educational agencies must use unifying labels or identifiers (either self-selected or other-imposed). Discourse over inclusive and nonoffensive term(s) to describe "Latina/os" continues (Oboler, 1995). As a result of personal preference, generational status, geography, nationality, acculturation, ethnic identity, and traditionality (Barón, 1991), use of terms (e.g., *Hispanic*) may elicit disdain (due to their negative colonial implications) or comfort (due to regional acceptance) from individuals or groups of individuals (García & Marotta, 1997). Padilla (1995) insisted that social and cultural politics should be secondary to the psychological implications of self-referents. As such, the term *Chicana/o* is used to refer to persons of Mexican descent living in the U.S. and the term *Latina/o* is used to refer to individuals from Mexico, Cuba, Puerto Rico, the Dominican Republic, and South and Central America who currently reside in the U.S. Despite the limitations to this terminology, the labels used are not intended to negate or minimize the varied histories and realities, but to provide clarity of reference.

Although each student is of Mexican descent (either born in Mexico, born in the U.S. but with parents born in Mexico, or both students and parents born in the U.S.), the 11 college students self-identified differently as "Mexican," "Mexican American," "Chicano," or "Chicana." Veronica and Ambrocia's responses illustrated the socio-cultural and sociocontextual complexity of self-referents. Ambrocia stated, "I self-identify as both Mexican American and Chicana . . . it varies on who I am talking to or what context I'm in." Similarly, Veronica indicated, "If I'm asked on paper to designate an ethnicity, I'll choose Mexican American, but I prefer Mexican."

THE STATUS OF LATINA/OS IN HIGHER EDUCATION

With Latina/os comprising 32.8 million or 12% of the total U.S. population and representing one of the fastest growing U.S. racial and ethnic groups (Therrien & Ramirez, 2000), it is reasonable to assume that they would also have a strong presence and large attendance in the educational system. If the proposition that all cultural groups (e.g., ethnic, socioeconomic) should participate in higher education at rates equal to their presence in the general population, then Latina/os are dismally underrepresented in higher education (Chahin, 1993).

In general, the undereducation of Latina/os is high; over one quarter have less than a ninth-grade education and approximately two in five have not graduated from high school (Therrien & Ramirez, 2000). Students leave the educational pipeline early; Latina/o children comprise the largest percentage of elementary- and secondary-level children, yet their presence in high school and college is not proportionally reflected (U.S. Department of Education, National Center for Education Statistics [NCES], 2000b). Debate has ensued as to whether Latina/o students drop out or are in effect pushed out or forced out of school. The question of whether students are pushed out stems from the fact that Latina/o elementary and secondary students are frequently tracked into non-college-bound classes, erroneously misplaced into special education classrooms due to language or interactive styles, supported by a limited number of teachers who are bilingual or who are trained to incorporate culture into the curriculum, and often held to low academic expectations by teachers (Gay, 2001). Furthermore, Latina/o elementary students are more likely to be held back or experience delayed schooling, a predictor of student dropout (President's Advisory Commission of Educational Excellence for Hispanic Americans, 1996).

Given that a greater number of Latina/os (ages 16 to 24) were born outside of the U.S. and that first and later generation Latina/os are two to three times more likely to drop out of high school than their non-Latina/o counterparts, the need to address environmental contexts (incorporating culturally relevant curriculum) is warranted (U.S. Department of Education, NCES, 2000b). In addition to low teacher expectations, Latina/o students are subject to stereotypes, societal biases, and personal prejudices and racism from within educational systems. As a result, Secada et al. (1998) cogently argued, "dropping out [of school for Hispanics] is not a random act" (p. 7).

According to recent Census information on Latina/o adult education, more than half (56%) had a high school education or more, over one quarter (29%) had some college, and about one in ten (11%) had completed a bachelor's degree or more (Newburger & Curry, 2000). Despite educational attainment gains regarding high school and college attendance (5% and 6% increase since 1989, respectively), no substantial change in the percentage of earned bachelor's degrees has occurred. For young Hispanics (ages 25 to 29), the percentage of individuals earning a bachelor's degree has not increased over the past decade (10% in 1989 versus 9% in 1999; Newburger & Curry, 2000).

Regarding college enrollment, more Latina/os enroll part time (45%) than their African American (40%) and White (39%) counterparts. As a result, Latina/os (35%) are more likely than African Americans (32%) and Whites (25%) to take 6 or more years to earn a bachelor's degree (U.S. Department of Education, NCES, 1997). Latina/os often enter higher education via community colleges or junior colleges and transfer to 4-year institutions, yet research has indicated that students who begin their higher education at a 2-year college are far less likely to earn a bachelor's degree than those students who begin at a 4-year college (U.S. Department of Education, NCES). Because of location (e.g., in the community), cost, and flexibility of course offerings, more than half of undergraduate Latina/os are enrolled in community colleges (President's Advisory Commission of Educational Excellence for Hispanic Americans, 2000). Two primary reasons for community college attendance and retention are financial aid and academic support (Avalos & Pavel, 1993; Nora, 1990).

For the last two decades, approximately 45 to 55% of Latina/os transitioned immediately from high school to college (U.S. Department of Education, NCES, 1997) and had the lowest enrollments at research universities versus other educational institutions (U.S. Department of Education, NCES, 2000b). Of the total 1,168,023 bachelor's degrees conferred in the 1996 to 1997 school year, Latina/os earned 5.5%, with Latinas earning slightly more (5.7%, 35,934) than their male counterparts (5.2%, 26,007). For more than two decades (1976 to 1997) the percentage of degrees conferred has increased 3.1% for Latinos and 3.7% for Latinas (U.S. Department of Education, NCES, 2000a). Moreover, slightly more than 50% of all Latina/os enrolled in higher education attended in California and Texas and close to three fourths of Latina/os enrolled in higher education were in California, Texas, New York, Florida, and Illinois. Finally, most Latina/o students were first-generation college students or the first in their families to attend college (President's Advisory Commission of Educational Excellence for Hispanic Americans, 2000).

When examining within-group differences, however, educational attainment varies among subgroups. Specifically, people of Cuban descent and "Other Hispanics" were most likely (73.0% and 71.6%, respectively) and those of Mexican descent were least likely (51.0%) to have had a high school education. Almost two thirds (64.3%) of individuals of Puerto Rican and Central and South American descent had a high school education (Therrien & Ramirez, 2000). In a 10-year review (1980 to 1990) of educational attainment of Chicana/os, Cubans, and Puerto Ricans in the U.S., Aguirre and Martinez (1993) indicated that Chicana/os consistently had the lowest percentage of (a) high school completion or (b) 4 or more years of college completion (for 1980, 1985, and 1990) and did not make relative aggregate educational gains compared to Cubans and Puerto Ricans.

Individuals of Mexican descent had the lowest rate of college completion (5%) and those of Cuban descent had the highest (20%). The college completion of individuals of Puerto Rican and Central and South American descent was 10% and 16%, respectively (Aguirre & Martinez, 1993). Three of the eleven (27%) students described in this chapter had parents who had completed a 4-year college degree. It is evident from these data that Latina/os are not adequately represented in higher education. With the Latina/o population more than doubling from 1990 to 2000 (22.4 million to 35.3 million; Guzmán, 2001) and a census projection that, in less than 50 years, at least one in four persons will be Latina/o (U.S. Bureau of the Census, 1995), research, programming, and educational support are clearly needed to ensure their entry into, persistence in, and graduation from higher education.

RESEARCH ON CHICANA/OS IN HIGHER EDUCATION

Because education constitutes the primary vehicle for social and financial mobility, Seda and Bixler-Marquez (1994) argued that a comprehensive examination of Latina/o education must occur at the micro and macro levels, examining culture and family, socioeconomics, and community contexts. Without such examinations, continued "undereducation of the Chicano [and Chicana] population serves to reinforce the subordinate position of the population with the country's opportunity structure" (Aguirre & Martinez, 1993, p. 9). As such, both qualitative and quantitative investigations of educational nonsuccess and success are needed to guide educational programming and policy, as retention and persistence issues for Latina/os are complex and multidimensional (Hernandez, 2000).

In a review of the literature regarding Latina/o dropouts, Ortiz and Guss (1995) noted that traditional dropout research blamed students as "deviant, deficient, or negligent with regard to education and schooling" (p. 5). Mehan (1997) similarly noted that few studies contextualized dropping out of school for Latina/os within the larger social, political, and economic arenas for students and educational institutions. More specifically, research on Latina/o students has largely neglected school policy and practice, social influences of race and ethnicity, students' alienation and isolation, school curriculum and climate, and quality of interactions among teachers, students, and parents. Attention to experiences and perceptions within the educational climate would more accurately provide a contextual understanding of Latina/o students' decisions regarding academic persistence (Ortiz & Guss).

In a review of research articles (1990 to 2000) regarding the educational experiences of African American and Latina/o college students, Gloria and Castellanos (2003) found that racism and identity (e.g., racial and ethnic), campus environment, alienation and social relationships (e.g., with faculty and peers), and self-beliefs (e.g., self-esteem, self-efficacy) were most frequently examined relative to educational persistence. They noted that few of the articles took a comprehensive approach to context (e.g., academic environment and social milieu of the setting), student self-beliefs and perceptions, and cultural aspects in their investigations. The majority of the studies were quantitative and, as Attinasi and Nora (1992) contended, unable to fully capture the complexities of multiple realities and interrelated issues for diverse students. As such, this chapter's review of salient educational concepts begins with a conceptual model (one that is supported by the students' narratives and the

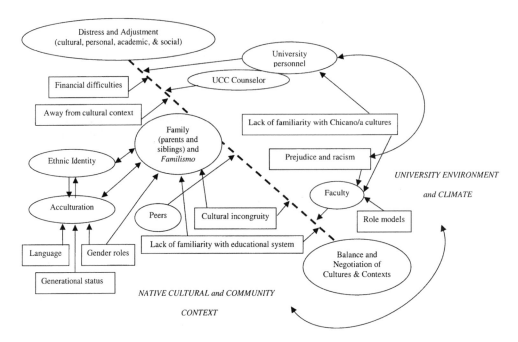

FIG. 19.1.   Conceptual model of educational issues for Chicana/o students in higher education.

academic literature) showing how student issues are interrelated. Our structural overview of issues involved in balancing and negotiating the environmental context of higher education is not comprehensive or inclusive of all Chicana/o student experiences. Instead, this framework is intended to generate further investigation and subsequent understanding of student educational issues and needs, as shown in Fig. 19.1.

Educational Issues for Chicana/os

Ethnic identity and acculturation, along with related variables of generational status, language, and gender roles within the family, provide insight into defining, measuring, and explaining the experience of Chicana/os in higher education. Several authors (Barón, 1991; Constantine, Gloria, & Barón, in press; Gloria & Rodriguez, 2000) addressed the importance of assessing ethnic identity and acculturation in understanding the issues that inform Latina/o students' interactions (e.g., with faculty and peers) and perceptions (e.g., feelings of isolation and alienation) within the university environment.

Although mistakenly used interchangeably, ethnic identity and acculturation are distinct but interrelated constructs (Gloria & Rodriguez, 2000; Keefe & Padilla, 1987). Specifically, ethnic identity is a multidimensional and dynamic process that informs an individual's feelings (e.g., self-esteem, sense of pride, and belonging), behaviors (e.g., social affiliations, marital, language, and food preferences), knowledge, and values placed on identifying with one's ethnic group (Bernal & Martinelli, 1993). Ethnic identity represents how individuals view and identify themselves as members of their ethnic group as well as how they perceive their ethnic group within society. In contrast, acculturation is a multifaceted and bidirectional process of interactions between one's native and host cultures, in which behavioral and attitudinal changes result from contact with the dominant culture and influence adherence to one's native culture, values, and beliefs (Sodowsky, Lai, & Plake, 1991).

A number of factors affect ethnic identity and acculturation for Chicana/o students, including generational status, language, adherence to familismo (value and centrality of family), and prescribed gender roles. Generational status, the length of time residing in the U.S., is central to educational issues, as two thirds of Latina/o youth are first or second generation with exposure to another language (i.e., Spanish) prior to entering the U.S. school system (Constantine et al., in press). Because Latina/os are mostly first-generation Americans, the majority of students are subsequently first-generation college students (first in their families to enter higher education; President's Advisory Commission of Educational Excellence for Hispanic Americans, 2000). Furthermore, those students whose first language is Spanish are more likely to drop out of school than their native English-speaking counterparts. As a result of generational status, the degree to which individuals adhere to values such as familismo or fulfill culturally-related gender roles has direct relevance for Chicana/o college students.

The value of family is central to adherence to cultural traits, and values correspond with different levels in acculturation. Familismo "is typified by strong feelings of loyalty, unity, solidarity, commitment and reciprocity . . . interdependence, cooperation and affiliation [in which] the family needs precede individual needs" (Gloria et al., 2004). Chicana/o families consist of related nuclear and extended family members as well as nonrelated members such as *compadres* (godparents, translated as coparents). Simply stated by Bobby, "It all starts and ends with the family." It is this natural support system from whom Chicana/o students often seek help with struggles experienced on and off campus (Gloria & Rodriguez, 2000). Many Latina/o parents, however, are frequently unaware of educational practices and expectations of their children (Aguirre & Martinez, 1993; Solberg & Villareal, 1997) and subsequently are uncertain about how to help (Hyslop, 2000).

Nancy is a first-generation college student and the first of 10 siblings to go to college. She stated, "Getting a feel for what college was like was overwhelming. I didn't know what the expectations were as a college student, how classes were like. It was overwhelming with home and school stuff. It was overwhelming to not see others like myself in the classroom. I felt bad that when I would see . . . meet others like me, I would see them doing poorly. . . . I felt like maybe I'd do poorly too." Describing her daily return home from school, she stated, "I didn't have my own space to do homework. This was a new experience and I'd come home and there was no one to relate to me. My friends were not at the same school—no one was there." Like other students, Nancy indicated, "My parents didn't know what to tell me to guide me through the college experience."

Veronica, a first-year graduate student, relayed how language adds to the complexity of understanding expectations regarding school for students and their parents: "I think it's hard for all students to figure this [referring to school expectations] out because parents can't always tell you what to expect, but it's harder for Mexican students especially when [their] parents are just learning to get a better handle on Spanish and then some English." Veronica spoke of the Mexican immigrants who come from rural areas and poor backgrounds who often do not know how to read or write in Spanish, much less English.

As indicated by Nancy and Veronica, first-generation college students often find it difficult to inform their parents of educational expectations, as they frequently are unaware of the expectations themselves. Students often feel misunderstood, not only in their new college environment, but also by their family support system.

> For example, Ambrocia stated, "My immediate family was supportive, however, the rest of the family questioned my intentions and what I was doing. They wondered if I was going out and messing around." Because of limited finances she was unable to call home every day to tell her parents about what she was doing academically: "It was difficult to help my parents understand what it was that I was going through."

Similarly, having a cultural emphasis on family, within a context (i.e., higher education) in which it is typically not included (Hernandez, 2000), Chicana/o students must often manage or juggle the needs of their families (including their own value of familismo) and those of the educational system (Fiske, 1988; Gloria & Rodriguez, 2000). For example, choosing to participate in family events can increase distress for Chicana/o students who may be struggling with academics as they feel torn between giving more time to their studies or "being loyal" to their family's desires. In contrast, decreased participation in family events may be perceived by some families as an insult, rejection, or betrayal, or as "selling out" for not spending time with their less educated family. Known as cultural incongruity (Gloria & Robinson Kurpius, 1996), Chicana/o students must balance and negotiate cultures and contexts (e.g., values and expectations) in finding their cultural fit within the educational environment. Furthermore, cultural, personal, and academic distress is intensified for students who leave home to go to school, as the ability (e.g., transportation, time, funds) to travel is often limited.

> Jose indicated that he survived his educational experiences by "adapting [to the context] and developing two different lives." As the first in his family to obtain a college degree, he indicated that "one part of my life involved my family and communicating with them, the other involved my education and adapting to a new environment. It was easy to see that whenever I would go back home, I would switch the way I spoke and how I acted. On the other hand, when I returned to school I would switch again. I felt like a chameleon, always having to blend into my environment. Once I became good at doing it, managing my educational experiences became easy."

Within many Chicano families, males and females are socialized into well-defined gender roles (e.g., machismo, *marianismo*, *hembrismo*) that are expected to be fulfilled and upheld (Arredondo, 1991). These gender roles, however, have been stereotypically depicted and negatively misinterpreted (Gloria et al., 2003) within multiple contexts (e.g., mass media, psychology). An accurate understanding of gender roles and how they are manifested is needed to assess the internal and external pressures and distress faced by Mexican American college students (Barón, 1991; Constantine & Barón, 1997). For example, the desirable aspects of protecting and being a responsible provider, a central value of respect and bravery, form the basis of machismo. These cultural attributes have been overpathologized and commonly equated with negative qualities of egotism, control, sexual aggressiveness, or promiscuity (Gloria et al.). Because paid work is highly valued among Mexican American families (Arredondo), Chicano college students often encounter gender role conflicts regarding school and work. That is, by choosing to pursue higher education, they may feel guilty or be criticized for not fulfilling the role of responsible family provider (i.e., earning money to contribute and to sustain their family).

The female gender role includes marianismo and hembrismo. Marianismo is rooted in the devotion to La Virgen de Guadalupe and perpetuates an ideal woman who, like La Virgen, exemplifies divinity, *aguantando* (endurance to suffering), and moral and spiritual superiority to her male counterpart (Arredondo, 1991). The female role of hembrismo (taken from the word *hembra*, meaning "female") connotes a Chicana version of Superwoman, who is expected to proficiently fulfill multiple roles both in and out of the home (Constantine et al., in press). The positive cultural aspects of marianismo and hembrismo have been minimized and negative stereotypes maximized. The negative portrayals of women as passive, weak, submissive, and selfless unfortunately overshadow the positive aspects of being strong, dependable, trustworthy, and dedicated caretakers of their families (Arredondo; Niemann, 2001). In particular, a great deal of family responsibility, specifically, fulfilling the role of surrogate mother, often falls on the eldest daughter in many Chicano families.

> Nancy, the oldest of 10 children, was expected to help her family financially while in school: "I had to pay bills, take a more active role with the kids [her brothers and sisters]. I was and still am the disciplinarian. If someone [was] sick I'd take them to the doctor. I didn't think about it too much at the time, all I knew was that it had to get done. Now I do think more about what I'm doing and I'm tired—mentally—about all the stuff I have to do."

Similarly, Chicanas may not receive the same encouragement to be educated from their families when they postpone creating and maintaining families of their own, as do Chicanos.

> Veronica, a first-generation college student who was married and had dropped out of school (but planned to return), described her challenge in confronting expected family roles. She stated, "I got little to no encouragement from my father due to his more traditional ideas about women." "My father has old-school Mexican mentality," which she ascribed to "why he didn't see the purpose of me going to school [referring to staying at home and raising a family]. Had my older brothers and sister gone, it would have been totally different. No one paved the way for me. . . . It was like a mountain. I had to pave my way through it myself to study."
>
> Veronica also reported that, for 1 year, she had lived on campus due to the long commute between school and home. "This [living away from home] helped my Dad to see that nothing was going to stop me [from going to school]. Even though he never came out and said 'go forward' [with college education], he didn't say anything about not continuing with school either."

In addition to the distress of balancing and negotiating the cultures and contexts of home and school, additional factors such as finances, finding on-campus support systems (e.g., peers) or role models, and negotiating the campus climate (e.g., prejudice or racism) affect Chicana/o student distress and adjustment (i.e., cultural, personal, academic, and social) in higher education (e.g., Cervantes, 1988; Hernandez, 2000; Hurtado & Carter, 1997; Hurtado, Carter, & Spuler, 1996; Solberg & Villareal, 1997). First, difficulties in financing a college education directly affect retention and completion of college for Chicana/o students. Hernandez reported that Mexican American college students consistently ranked financing their college education as one of their greatest educational concerns. Latina/o students borrow less than other racial or ethnic groups to pay for their education; almost half of first-year college students receive grants (e.g., federal and state) and almost a third receive loans (White House Initiative on Educational Excellence for Hispanic Americans, 2000). Despite the availability of monies to finance their education, academic financial support typically does not consider the economic needs of the student's family (Gloria & Castellanos, 2003). Rather than incur debt, many Latina/o students hold full-time jobs (75% of which are off campus) to pay for school and help support their families (Haro, Rodriguez, & Gonzales, 1994). As a result of working, Chicana/o students delay or discontinue their educational pursuits.

> Monica, a senior and second-generation college student, attended college part time because of the high cost of tuition. She worked three jobs to pay the tuition. She indicated, "I realize that it's taken longer to finish [school], but it works financially [to have three jobs] and it allows me to have a life outside of school and to gain work experience in my primary interests."

Along with the direct stress of college finances, Mexican American students may feel pressure or obligation (depending on level of adherence to familismo) to contribute to the family income as these students often symbolize hope for increased earning potential (i.e., family member with a college degree; Muñoz, 1986). More recent employment statistics for Latina/o college students indicated that 62% were employed while attending college, with males having a higher rate of employment than females (Jamieson, Curry, & Martinez, 2001). Experiences and comments by Omar and Bobby related the difficulties of financing higher education.

> Omar, a junior and first-generation college student, described the difficulty of paying for school. He stated, "So far I've gone through 16 years of school with no [financial] problems. My parents have been well-off enough to put us through school. We had no struggles financially. . . . I just had to go to school. In college I've helped out to complete my end of the bargain . . . but it's getting harder now. My parents have guided me through this experience and now they can't afford it. School is more expensive now. Tuition is getting more expensive . . . paying for books, transportation. Tuition is four times higher now and I have to work to pay these off and I need extra money. Next semester I have to pay for it all off myself. I would say that my biggest struggle has been money to pay for college."
>
> In describing how he managed work and school, Omar indicated, "I have to work more now and how will I do two things at once? I need to cut down on work to focus on school. I cut down a couple of hours per week at work, but it's still not enough time to focus on studying . . . and then the bills come faster and faster."

Bobby, a second-generation college student, talked about how he thought Mexican American students had limited opportunities. He stated, "A lot of Mexican Americans cannot afford the cost of an education and they just settle for second best and in their heads they know that they can do better. . . . A lot of the time family and financial restraints hold them back from pursuing their dream."

Students from lower socioeconomic status are typically less prepared for college (U.S. Department of Education, NCES, 2000a) and subsequently at higher risk for dropping out (Vasquez, 1982). That is, Chicana/o students are frequently not socialized or expected to go to college (Gay, 2001; Retish & Kavanaugh, 1992).

Describing her experiences with her lack of study skills, Veronica simply stated, "I was not as prepared as my peers. . . . Like, on the first day of class [referring to first day of college], if I had pen and paper I was lucky." She relayed that she watched students around her to figure out what she should be doing: "Say someone else took out paper and a pen, or took notes, so did I. I knew that we would get more pressure [work], but I didn't know what to expect on a daily basis. I just lived day to day as it came in order to survive. I didn't know how to study but my friends dragged me to the library." Veronica suggested that "there should be a manual for the first day of college . . . like *Chicken Soup for the College-Bound on the First Day* for Mexican students."

In learning to survive her educational environment, Veronica looked to other students to help and support her through school. Social support, such as faculty members who are role models or mentors and a supportive peer network, are central to Chicana/o students' college adjustment and academic persistence (Aguirre & Martinez, 1993; Gándara, 1995; Gloria, 1999; Nora & Cabrera, 1996). Much like Ambrocia's narrative earlier in the chapter, seeing someone who has educationally succeeded provides validation, motivation, and inspiration for students' own educational pursuits (Gloria & Rodriguez, 2000).

In addressing the need for university role models, Magally believed that "there needs to be more positive influences that are Hispanic, that they [students] can connect to. This makes it more real for us . . . that it's possible to reach higher education."

Now a senior, Nancy indicated that her sophomore year had been better than her freshman year in that it was less overwhelming: "The year was better because of the Mexican American professor in my Latin American studies class. It was cool to have a positive role model. It gave me an extra push that I need. It was nice to see that a Mexican American was doing well in his field. It filled a void, 'cause I didn't know any Latinos doing well."

When mentored, Latina/o students are more likely to succeed academically than those who are not (Gándara, 1995). Although university personnel frequently serve as mentors for Chicana/o students, the dearth of Latina/o faculty (Aguirre & Martinez, 1993) and administrators (de los Santos & Rigual, 1994) often limits these necessary interactions. Specifically, Latina/o faculty comprised 3% of the full-time faculty in 1995 (U.S. Department of Education, NCES, 2000b), representing a 1:76 Hispanic faculty to Hispanic student ratio (Hispanic Association of Colleges and Universities, 1995). Faculty-student interactions are of particular importance as

Latina/o students who reported a higher number of faculty interactions perceived less discrimination in the classroom and on campus (Nora & Cabrera, 1996).

> Addressing the importance of having a Mexican American mentor, Nancy indicated that "having that person that knows my accent, knows where I come from, my mannerisms, understands me when I talk in Spanish—like having a bond with somebody."

> Anabel, a first-year Mexican American graduate student, indicated that she found that she "had to work hard to make sure that professors took [her] seriously." She credited her relationship with faculty members as bolstering her belief in herself. For example, in her last semester of undergraduate work, she was on a research team with other Mexican American women students. She stated, "The relationship with him [the professor] made me feel like what I had to say was important. We [the research team] gave a presentation and the way we felt after the presentation. . . . It had such an impact on the audience, like it all made sense and what we had to say was significant."

In navigating the educational environment that is often unwelcoming for Chicana/os (Cervantes, 1988; Gloria & Rodriguez, 2000), students also look to peers and siblings for support.

> Describing his peer supports, Noel, a freshman attending a community college, "saw who were [his] true friends and not [his] true friends. [He] noticed their achievements and who [he] felt more connected to." He stated, "Through connections with my friends I saw people who were trying hard [in school]. I found out who I was and this helped me with my transition [from high school to college] and setting my goals of how I want to live the rest of my life."

> Nancy indicated that, as a senior in college, "I can help my younger brothers and sisters as they go through the college experience."

In managing feelings of isolation and alienation on campus and dealing with the prejudice and racism inherent in academia (Feagin, Vera, & Imani, 1996), older Latina/o students often mentor their younger siblings and younger Latina/o students outside their family of origin (Fiske, 1988). Answering questions and showing them the ropes, identifying and relying on peer support networks can decrease stress and isolation for Chicana/os and Chicanas (Gloria, 1999; Gloria & Rodriguez, 2000; Hernandez, 2000).

> Magally, a first-generation college student currently in her second year of graduate school, described her need for support in the educational environment in which she perceived there to be few Mexican American students. She stated, "Within the realm of what education offers, this opportunity allowed me to befriend people of other backgrounds and to learn about our similarities and differences. . . . It taught me that people are more alike than different. An education provides that, especially in higher levels of education because you don't see too many of us [Mexican Americans] there in the first place."

Social supports are also needed as Chicana/o students contend with negative perceptions and stereotypes regarding their cultures (e.g., gender roles) and abilities from other students, university personnel, and society in general (Fiske, 1988; Retish & Kavanaugh, 1992).

> Addressing the perceptions held by others about Mexican American college students, Bobby stated, "When you graduate in our society it opens up the possibilities for more opportunities, especially for us as Mexican Americans because our culture is known for labor. We are not . . . recognized as leaders. It's [the recognition is] based on what we can do with our hands, not what we can do with our minds."

> Anabel described how Mexican American women are often perceived educationally by faculty: "It's like we have a complex that we have to prove something because we're women and Latinas . . . that somehow we're made to feel as students like we're less adequate."

Ultimately, Chicana/o students need to find adequate cultural, personal, academic, and social support to navigate educational obstacles and balance the contexts of home and school.

FRAMEWORKS OF COUNSELING AND PSYCHOEDUCATIONAL SUPPORT FOR CHICANA/OS IN HIGHER EDUCATION

> Jorge was a freshman who began his higher education at a large university but transferred to a community college because he "didn't like the environment . . . it was too big." As a first-generation college student, he described the impersonal nature of the campus and his subsequent lack of connections. Similarly, he experienced feeling overwhelmed; he believed that he was unprepared to go to college. Feeling like he had to work twice as hard to be perceived as equal, Jorge, like many Chicana/o students, might benefit from the services of a university counselor who has specific knowledge of the culture as well as an openness to learning about it.

Despite the emergent educational and psychological literature pertaining to Chicana/o college students, there are relatively few counseling or psychoeducational support frameworks for them. In a chapter on counseling Mexican American college students, Constantine et al. (in press) reviewed several theoretical counseling frameworks. The following outline expands Constantine et al.'s work by including both theoretical and atheoretical approaches with Chicana/o college students. Because of the limited Chicana/o-focused approaches, models intended for Latina/o college students are also included. Although psychoeducational services (e.g., support groups) to promote academic persistence for Latina/o high school students have been developed (e.g., Ortiz & Guss, 1995), only those models developed specifically for college students are reviewed.

Ruiz and Casas (1976) developed the first counseling framework specifically for Chicana/o students. The model urged that counselors who work with Chicana/o students have four qualities: bilingualism, biculturality, image awareness, and outreach skills. The authors asserted that counselors must have command of both English and Spanish, be familiar and comfortable with both Chicana/o and Anglo cultures, and possess skills in providing outreach services to Chicana/o communities on campus.

Furthermore, counselors need to be aware of how they are perceived by clients (i.e., image awareness), and ideally see themselves as change agents responsive to the sociocultural issues of Chicana/os. Ruiz and Casas also recommended that counselors: (a) actively and behaviorally direct clients toward resolution, (b) focus on a limited number of issues, (c) rank client concerns based on the amount of stress associated with each concern, and (d) behaviorally contract with clients for specific therapeutic objectives. Although this model encouraged counselors to take a community-psychology approach and teach Chicana/o students how to resist and eliminate prejudicial practices, the underlying motives of students' presenting issues were not addressed. The model was developed, delivered, and intended for Chicana/os, however, the availability of Chicana/o counselors for students who prefer a counselor of the same race or ethnicity may be a limiting factor.

Ruiz, Casas, and Padilla (1977) used a behaviorally focused, contractual- and intervention-based framework that considers the underutilization of mental health services by Chicana/os. Among the stated environmental and societal causes of underutilization were institutional policies that discourage self-referral, limited Spanish fluency among those who work with Spanish-speaking people, and differences in cultural or class values that limit communication between the counselor and client. The model proposed techniques to help counselors communicate more effectively with Chicana/o college students. Recommendations were organized around the following themes: (a) characteristics of ethnic identification, (b) prerequisites for a behavioristic counseling model, (c) high-frequency problems reported by Chicana/o students, and (d) counselor responses to specific problems.

More than a decade later, a broader and more psychologically inclusive framework for counseling male Hispanic college students was introduced by Barón (1991). Emphasizing the interrelated constructs of acculturation, ethnic identity development, and machismo, the model can be used in either individual or group counseling. Barón presented the interaction of these concepts for an individual counseling case and a 12-session group intervention for male Hispanics (the majority of whom were of Mexican ancestry). The process-oriented group discussed ethnic identity, feelings regarding personal incidents of racism and internalized racism, personal power and responsibility, and seeking support. The concept of machismo entered the group conversation early to help group members confront the implications of support seeking (e.g., admitting a need for help) and being comfortable displaying and sharing emotions. As a result, the group integrated Chicano identity formation and served as a vehicle for intellectual and emotional insights and educational persistence and success.

An 8-week psychoeducational support group for Latinas was described by Capello (1994) that addressed personal, cultural, and social issues experienced by Latina students. Organized by students, the group met to better cope with the lack of cultural diversity expressed in the academic environment (e.g., college curriculum). They discussed feelings of marginalization, cultural values, and issues related to students' interactions with faculty and staff (e.g., respect and authority), quasi-parenting obligations, and education-related survival strategies. By learning about Latina/o culture and history, reading literature by Latina writers, and exploring cultural stereotypes, group members developed agency in their educational pursuits and a community of modeling, sharing, and support.

The foundations for Barón and Constantine (1997) and Constantine and Barón (1997) were extended from Barón's (1991) counseling model. In these models, the authors presented an integrated framework of counseling for Latina/o students in which core psychosocial and cultural constructs were assessed through a standard clinical interview. Specific constructs that were assessed included ethnic identity development, level of acculturation, and gender role socialization. In particular, the construct of machismo was addressed relative to male-female differences and sexual orientation. Providing dimensionality to the model, Barón and Constantine proposed that the psychosocial and cultural constructs be examined cognitively, affectively, and behaviorally. The authors addressed "interactive culture strain," which they described as the emotional distress or conflict experienced when individuals attempt to integrate various developmental challenges related to acculturation, ethnic identity development, and gender role socialization.

In developing a theoretically based psychoeducational support group for Chicana college students, Gloria (1999) integrated Yalom's (1995) therapeutic change factors and Chicana cultural values with academic persistence issues of Chicanas in higher education. Familismo, *personalismo* (personalism), *respeto* (respect), *simpatía* (a pleasant demeanor), *dignidad* (dignity), and *confianza* (trust) were discussed to better understand how these cultural values might affect the groups' dynamics. To decrease feelings of campus alienation and isolation for Chicana college students, Gloria recommended that group leaders actively participate in Chicana/o communities, establish cohesive alliances among group members to validate educational and emotional experiences, develop strategies for balancing home and school demands, promote awareness and understanding of value systems, develop interpersonal skills to address strategies regarding campus racism and discrimination, and create a "university family." Furthermore, each of Yalom's therapeutic factors (e.g., instillation of hope, imparting of information) was addressed within the psychoeducational group to advance Chicana students' educational experiences.

In Gloria and Rodriguez (2000), a psychosociocultural model for university counseling center staff who provide services to Latina/o university students was emphasized in the dynamic and interdependent relationships of psychological concerns, social support systems, cultural factors, and university environmental contexts. Gloria and Rodriguez contended that addressing the dynamic and interdependent relationships of these constructs is necessary to provide more comprehensive and context-specific counseling. A set of minimal competencies was delivered for each dimension to create a structure for university counseling center service providers. This model was the first to specifically target counseling center staff as primary agents for increasing the academic persistence of Latina/o students. In particular, the authors argued that counseling center staff have the psychological skills and training and the ethical requirements to seek out culturally relevant training and information about their clientele, knowledge of the campus and academic climate in which the students reside, and potential for personal and immediate access to students.

In extending the previous models of counseling for Chicana/o students to include a psychosociocultural perspective, Constantine et al. (in press) applied Atkinson, Thompson, and Grant's (1993) three-dimensional model of counseling racial and ethnic minority individuals to Mexican American college students. The model considered the locus of the problem's etiology, the client's level of acculturation, and the goals of helping. Using vignettes of Mexican American college students and practical examples, the authors described how counselors would function with different roles, (i.e., adviser, advocate, facilitator of indigenous support systems, facilitator of indigenous healing systems, consultant, change agent, counselor, and psychotherapist) they may assume with Mexican American college students to provide personal, academic, and educational support. Importantly, Constantine et al. recommended that counselors examine their biases or reservations in performing multiple roles, using "alternative counseling services," and possibly contending with the organizational culture and norms of their counseling center.

VOICES OF CHICANA/O STUDENTS

Each of the Chicana/o students who told their educational stories for this chapter identified individual experiences and perspectives. The themes that emerged from the students' narratives are presented here.

The most salient theme of the integration of Chicana/o culture and values within educational pursuits was not directly identified, but clearly implied. The consistent identification of solidarity and loyalty of students to their families evidenced the centrality of family in students' pursuits. Similarly, values such as personalismo (i.e., a communication style that emphasizes personal interactions of self-worth, respect, and dignity, and manifests reciprocity with perceived equals and deference with perceived authority figures; Paniagua, 1994) were salient as Anabel, Bobby, and Magally relayed the importance of interacting with faculty and other university personnel in a manner congruent with their cultures and contexts. The common thread of culture was also evidenced through nuances and actions described by the students, as well as in interaction with the chapter authors.

Regardless of setting (e.g., 4-year university or community college), class standing (i.e., undergraduate or graduate), or university composition (e.g., predominantly White institution with small minority student representation in Midwest, predominantly White institution with large minority student representation in Southwest), each of the students experienced educational struggles related to university climate. In particular, Anabel, Jorge, and Veronica reported that they had to work harder than other students to prove themselves, as they confronted prejudices and stereotypes regarding Chicana/o students. It was also the consensus among the students that university personnel, including faculty members, often do not understand the culture or world view of Chicana/os. Several of the students (i.e., Ambrocia, Magally, Monica, and Bobby) recommended that university personnel move out of their respective settings (e.g., offices and departments) to learn more about the needs of Chicana/o students. At a minimum, the students (i.e., Bobby, Jose, and Magally) suggested that faculty and staff open themselves up to learning about Chicana/o culture as a way to help students in the classroom, in faculty-student interactions, and on campus in general.

Managing social and educational obstacles and challenges, each of the students were self-determined and motivated to succeed. Although they identified obstacles, the focus was on finding ways to succeed by being creative and taking initiative. For example, Veronica stressed the need for students to seek out information and others who could help answer questions. Other students reported that they learned from their parents and families the importance of hard work and sacrifice to earn their college degrees. Similarly, students (e.g., Jose, Nancy, and Veronica) identified needing to balance their home and school contexts, reflecting the negotiation of contexts as a major construct in their educational experiences.

Next, parents were identified as primary supports of the students' educations, with mothers being the most supportive (especially for the women). Parental support ranged from small gestures (e.g., bus money to get to school for Anabel) to considerable support (e.g., paying for costly tuition expenses for Omar or purchasing cars for Magally and Veronica). For several of the students (e.g., Anabel and Omar), parents were willing to do anything within their means to help their children succeed academically. At the same time, many of the parents and families did not know what was expected of their sons and daughters in college and could not advise or recommend actions or strategies to deal with academic issues and concerns. As a result, students (in particular, Ambrocia, Anabel, and Monica) recommended that university personnel inform Chicana/o parents and elementary, secondary, and high school students about the possibilities and options of higher education. The students believed that, if they had known about college earlier in their educational tenure, they would not have been as overwhelmed or uncertain about what to expect there. Accordingly, a directory of resources and information was complied for potential use by university personnel and Chicana/o students and their parents.

DIRECTORY OF RESOURCES FOR CHICANA/OS IN HIGHER EDUCATION

The following directory of resources is not intended to be comprehensive or exclusive. An enormous number of possible resources and links were found, but due to space constraints, only the resources that are directly relevant are included. Moreover, those sites that have resource pages (i.e., directories of other links specifically for Chicana/os and Latina/os) were selected in order to provide the broadest access to information. Following are synopses of websites or citations of resources that university personnel (e.g., academic advisors, counselors, faculty, university administrators), parents, and students can access for free or minimal charge:

1. Internet Sites Related to Latina/o Educational Issues:
   • White House Initiative on Educational Excellence for Hispanic Americans: The White House Initiative was developed to advance human potential, strengthen the capacity to provide high-quality education, and increase opportunities for Hispanic Americans to participate in and benefit from Federal education programs (http://www.yesican.gov).
   • Hispanic Association of Colleges and Universities (HACU): HACU promotes access to and quality of postsecondary opportunities for Hispanic students (http://www.hacu.net/).
   • Julian Samora Research Institute (JSRI): The JSRI disseminates research and evaluation related to the social, economic, educational, and political

conditions of Latina/o communities. Research findings are provided to academic staff and faculty, government officials, community leaders, and executives in the private sector through publications, public policy seminars, workshops, and private consultations. The JSRI also focuses on Latina/o leadership development, empowerment, and education (http://www.jsri.msu.edu).

• Latino Education Directory: The Latino Education Directory is funded by the U.S. Department of Education. This site provides information about federal programming, colleges and universities that have Latino programs and departments, scholarly resources (e.g., ERIC documents, Latino journals, and educational materials), and national, international, and nongovernmental organizations for Latina/os. (http://www.ael.org/eric/maed).

• Pew Hispanic Center (PEW): This center's mission is to improve understanding of the diverse Hispanic population in the U.S. by chronicling Latina/os' growing impact on the nation. The site disseminates research to policymakers, business leaders, academic institutions, and the media. Information areas include demography, economics, education, identity, immigration, health, and military. The site also provides press briefings on important social, educational, and political issues for Hispanics (http://www.pewhispanic.org).

2. Internet Sites for Chicana/o Literature, Art, and Culture

• Chicano Latino Network (CLNet): The CLNet is a search directory of Chicana/o and Latina/o sites and links. The site features directories to "bronze pages" (one-page biographies of Chicanos and Latinos), job announcements and advertisements, on-line publications, and access to Chicano resources in university libraries, museums (i.e., art, dance, pictorial essays, film, and theater), and communities (i.e., education, housing, environment, insurance, legal labor, social services, and cultural customs and traditions; http://clnet.sscnet.ucla.edu/).

• Chicano and Chicana Space: This site, developed and sponsored by the Hispanic Research Center at Arizona State University, provides resources for teachers and students regarding Chicana/o art and culture. Historic artwork and current artwork by middle and high school students are displayed (http://mati.eas.asu.edu/ChicanArte/).

• *Hispanic Culture Review* (HCR): The *Hispanic Culture Review* is published once or twice a year by George Mason University students. It contains essays, fiction, and poetry written in English or Spanish that focus on topics related to Hispanics. Past issues of *HCR* are also available online (http://www.gmu.edu/org/hcr/).

• Making Face, Making Soul . . . A Chicana Feminist Homepage: This homepage provides information and links specifically for Chicanas regarding art, literature, academics, history, current events, religions, mass media, and many other topics (http://chicanas.com/).

3. Journals and Magazines

• *Hispanic Journal of Behavioral Sciences* (HJBS): Edited by Amado Padilla, the *HJSB* is a multidisciplinary and comprehensive journal that is published quarterly on topics for Hispanic populations, including cultural assimilation, communication barriers, intergroup relations, employment discrimination, substance abuse, AIDS prevention, family dynamics, and minority poverty (http://www.sagepub.com/journal.aspx?pid=66).

• *Hispanic Outlook in Higher Education (HOHE)*: Published 26 times a year, *HOHE* reaches educators, administrators, students, student service and community-based organizations, and corporations. The magazine focuses on communication in academic circles, the importance of positive learning experiences, the contributions of both Hispanic and non-Hispanic role models, constructive observations on policies and procedures in academia, and issues confronting Hispanics on college campuses (http://www.HispanicOutlook .com).

• *The Voice:* The national monthly newsletter of the Hispanic Association of Colleges and Universities, *The Voice* posts job announcements and also provides up-to-date information about current issues affecting Hispanic education students (http://www.hacu.net/).

4. Government and Educational Documents and Reports
• *Chicanos in Higher Education: Issues and Dilemmas for the 21st Century* (Aguirre, & Martinez, 1993).
• *Status and Trends in the Education of Hispanics* (2003). National Center for Education Statistics, NCES 2003-008. Available on-line at http://nces.ed.gov/ pubs2003/2003008.pdf.
• *Latinos in Higher Education: Many Enroll, Too Few Graduate* (2002). Report by Richard Fry for Pew Hispanic Center. Available on-line at http://www .pewhispanic.org.
• *No More Excuses: The Final Report of the Hispanic Dropout Project* (Secada et al., 1998), available on-line: http://www.ncela.gwu.edu/miscpubs/hdp/.
• *Our Nation on the Fault Line: Hispanic American Education* (President's Advisory Commission of Educational Excellence for Hispanic Americans, 1996), available on-line: http://www.ed.gov/pubs/FaultLine.
• *We, the American Hispanics* (U.S. Department of Commerce, Bureau of the Census, 1993), available on-line: http://www.census.gov/apsd/wepeople/ we-2r.pdf.

5. Student Organizations
• Latino Sororities and Fraternities: Each of the following organizations are nationally based and have chapters at various universities throughout the U.S. Although the mission of each is slightly different, their primary goals are achieving personal growth through leadership and academic excellence, making significant contributions to Latina/o communities and celebrating Latina/o culture.
  • Sigma Lambda Gamma National Sorority, Inc.
  • Sigma Lambda Upsilon/Señoritas Latinas Unidas Sorority, Inc.
  • Alpha Rho Lambda Sorority, Inc.
  • Lambda Theta Alpha Latin Sorority, Inc.
  • Mu Sigma Upsilon Sorority, Inc.

- Omega Delta Phi Fraternity, Inc.
- Lambda Alpha Upsilon Fraternity, Inc.
- Lambda Sigma Upsilon Latino Fraternity, Inc.
- Sigma Lambda Beta International Fraternity, Inc.
- Phi Iota Alpha Fraternity, Inc.
- Sigma Lambda Beta International Fraternity, Inc.
- Gamma Zeta Alpha Fraternity, Inc.
- Lambda Upsilon Lambda Fraternity, Inc.

• Movimiento Estudiantil Chicano and Chicana de Aztlán (MEChA): MEChA is a national student organization based on fundamental principles of self-determination in gaining socioeconomic justice, strong nationalist identity in building a program of self-determination, and a focus on education in ways that preserve Chicana/o culture. MEChA strives to ensure feelings of community and security for Chicana/o students on campus.

6. Student Fellowships and Scholarships

• HispanicScholarship.com: This site, sponsored by DaimlerChrylser Corporation, provides a resource of over 500 different scholarships available to undergraduate and graduate Hispanic students. Scholarships can be selected by academic level (i.e., freshman, undergraduate, graduate, all levels), 12 different academic fields, or state. The site provides scholarship contact names and phone numbers, e-mail and postal addresses, application deadline dates, website addresses, and brief descriptions of scholarships (http://www.HispanicScholarship.com).

• Hispanic College Fund, Inc. (HCF): The HCF is a scholarship created by a group of highly committed Hispanic business leaders to facilitate the next generation of Hispanic business leaders in America. Scholarships are awarded to full-time students pursuing bachelor's degrees in business or business-related majors (http://www.hispanicfund.org/).

• National Hispanic Scholarship (NHS): The NHS, sponsored by over 200 major U.S. companies, has given over 45,000 scholarships totaling nearly 60 million dollars. This site features information including tips for raising a college-bound student, strategies for selecting and applying to college, recommendations of the top 25 colleges and universities for Hispanics, strategies for choosing a major or career, applying for financial aid, finding scholarships, and accessing Hispanic student organizations. The site also features access to a Latino-CollegeChat room for college students to connect with each other (http://www.hsf.net/).

DIRECTIONS FOR THE FUTURE EDUCATION OF CHICANA/O COLLEGE STUDENTS

In ensuring the education of Chicana/o students, academic institutions and students and their families must become active educational partners. Chicana/o students need to take the initiative in finding the social, personal, psychological, cultural, and academic supports necessary to support their retention and persistence to graduation. With family and community context central to most Chicana/o students, they need to involve their parents, families, and communities in their individual educational pursuits.

In partnership with students, educational institutions need to educate about education, taking a proactive approach with Chicana/o students. Beginning with elementary and secondary school children and their parents, institutions of higher education can increase parents' and children's familiarity and comfort level with the process of higher education preparation. This process of early student preparation for higher education could include workshops on classes for college-bound students, enhancing study skills (e.g., how to take notes), strategies for studying for exams and taking tests, and exploring different academic majors.

> For example, Monica emphasized the importance of early preparation for Chicana/o students. She indicated, "So many [Chicana/o] high school students don't know what they want. There are so many jobs out there that they don't even know they exist, and if [the jobs were] advertised, people would know about them as options." She wishes she had had help in determining her major and what profession she wants: "It's a way to have students begin thinking about what they want to study once in college."

Providing this educational information (in both English and Spanish) can instill hope and positive self-beliefs regarding the possibility of higher education. For high school students, universities could also provide continuous programming regarding how to search, apply, and pay for college.

> Nancy suggested that "programs at the high school level that would help college-bound students understand what college is like, how to handle challenges, even if it's broad. It would help to better deal with college. This would help because Mexican American parents a lot of times don't have college educations and are unable to help guide their kids. My parent didn't know what to tell me to guide me [through the college experience]."

Once on campus, first-year or new students (e.g., community college transfer students) could be offered workshops or single-credit adjustment courses that address faculty and classroom expectations, availability of campus support services and resources, and general college adjustment issues. As indicated by Ortiz and Guss (1995), Chicana/o students and their families need to be "taught" the rules and mastery skills of higher education. Although university systems typically leave family out of the educational process, their inclusion (in particular parents) can increase meaningful and culturally relevant interactions for student adjustment and persistence (Hernandez, 2000).

Although universities unknowingly or inadvertently create obstacles for Chicana/o students, they continue to succeed educationally. Through self-determination, motivation, positive self-belief, and hard work, students have navigated and continue to survive their educational environments.

> Nancy spoke of these issues as she stated, "Overall, I have a lot of self-motivation. My mother helped develop that motivation, but it had to come from me. A lot comes from within."

It is these positive aspects of students' adjustment and navigation that warrant more specific investigation. In addition to exploring the rationale and decisions for student dropout, the means and mechanisms by which students stay in school also need to be examined (e.g., personal strength, positive self-beliefs). Taking a more positive approach will decrease the emphasis on student failure (Hernandez, 2000), focusing on students' experiences and educational perceptions (Gloria, 1997) and their academic successes (Arellano & Padilla, 1996).

In addressing the issues for Chicana/o college students and their environmental contexts, research should be interdisciplinary and holistic in order to understand accurately the select subgroup of Chicana/os on college campuses (Gloria & Rodriguez, 2000). Similarly, the methods by which issues are investigated need to be sophisticated and comprehensive to tap into the complexities or multiple realities experienced by many Chicana/o students (Attinasi & Nora, 1992; Hernandez, 2000). For example, an extended case study investigation (Burawoy, 1998) based on the literature of occupational therapy and counseling psychology could serve as the foundation for a study of the interrelationship of ethnic identity, acculturation level, perception of the university environment, and student's choice of leisure activities (e.g., gaining of personal and social support), relative to decisions regarding persistence.

Ultimately, university personnel (e.g., faculty, staff, administrators) need to be accountable and address their biases and stereotypes regarding Chicana/o students, recognizing that each student has unique needs and different cultural affiliations.

> Magally indicated that "professors should get to know [Hispanic] students—what they know, how they live, what they celebrate—overall more knowledge about their students' cultural backgrounds."

In particular, university counseling center staff can serve as liaisons between students and the larger campus environment, between students and faculty, and between faculty and administration regarding Chicana/o educational issues (e.g., scholarships, curriculum changes, direction in student programming). Similarly, counseling center staff can provide support services that are psychosocioculturally based to facilitate Chicana/o adjustment, personal and social well-being, and academic persistence to graduation.

Providing words of encouragement for continued education, Jorge recounted his father's sage advice: "*Siempre 'pa delante, nunca 'pa tras*—so keep going forward with your chin and head up."

REFERENCES

Aguirre, A., Jr., & Martinez, R. O. (1993). *Chicanos in higher education: Issues and dilemmas for the 21st century* (ASHE-ERIC Higher Education Report No. 3, pp. 17–51). Washington, DC: George Washington University, School of Education and Human Development.

Arellano, A. R., & Padilla, A. M. (1996). Academic invulnerability among a select group of Latino university students. *Hispanic Journal of Behavioral Sciences, 18,* 485–507.

Arredondo, P. (1991). Counseling Latinas. In C. C. Lee & B. L. Richardson (Eds.), *Multicultural issues in counseling: New approaches to diversity* (pp. 143–156). Alexandria, VA: American Association for Counseling and Development.

Atkinson, D. R., Thompson, C. E., & Grant, S. K. (1993). A three-dimensional model for counseling racial/ethnic minorities. *The Counseling Psychologist, 21,* 257–277.

Attinasi, L. C., Jr., & Nora, A. (1992). Diverse students and complex issues: A case of multiple methods in college student research. In F. K. Stage & Associates (Eds.), *Diverse methods for research and assessment of college students* (pp. 13–27). Alexandria, VA: American Counseling Association.

Avalos, J., & Pavel, M. D. (1993). *Improving the performance of the Hispanic community college student.* Los Angeles, CA: Educational Resources Information Center. (ERIC Document Reproduction Service No. EDO-JC-93-03)

Barón, A., & Constantine, M. G. (1997). A conceptual framework for conducting psychotherapy with Mexican-American college students. In J. G. Garcia & M. C. Zea (Eds.), *Psychological interventions and research with Latino populations* (pp. 108–124). New York: Allyn and Bacon.

Barón, A., Jr. (1991). Counseling Chicano college students. In C. C. Lee & B. L. Richardson (Eds.), *Multicultural issues in counseling: New approaches to diversity* (pp. 171–184). Alexandria, VA: American Association for Counseling and Development.

Bernal, M. E., & Martinelli, P. C. (1993). *Mexican American identity.* Encino, CA: Floricanto Press.

Burawoy, M. (1998). The extended case method. *Sociological Theory, 16*, 4–33.

Capello, D. C. (1994). Beyond financial aid: Counseling Latina students. *Journal of Multicultural Counseling and Development, 22*, 28–36.

Castillo, A. (1994). *Massacre of the dreamers: Essays on Xicanisma.* New York: Plume/Penguin Books.

Cervantes, O. F. (1988). The realities that Latinos, Chicanos, and other ethnic minority students encounter in graduate school. *Journal of La Raza Studies, 2*, 34–41.

Chahin, J. (1993, EDO-RC-93-5). *Hispanics in higher education: Trends in participation.* (ERIC Document Reproduction Service NO. ED 357 911) U.S. Department of Education, Office of Educational Research and Improvement.

Closing the Hispanic faculty gap. (1995, Jan.–Feb.). *Hispanic Association of Colleges and Universities, 1*, 7.

Comas-Díaz, L. (2001). Hispanics, Latinos, or Americanos: The evolution of identity. *Cultural Diversity and Ethnic Minority Psychology, 7*(2), 115–120.

Constantine, M. G., & Barón, A. (1997). Assessing and counseling Chicano(a) college students: A conceptual and practical framework. In C. Lee (Ed.), *Multicultural issues in counseling: New approaches to diversity* (2nd ed., pp. 295–314). Alexandria, VA: American Counseling Association.

Constantine, M. G., Gloria, A. M., & Barón. A. (in press). Counseling Mexican American college students. In C. Lee (Ed.), *Multicultural issues in counseling: New approaches to diversity* (3rd ed.). Alexandria, VA: American Counseling Association.

de los Santos, A., Jr., & Rigual, A. (1994). Progress of Hispanics in American higher education. In J. J. Justiz, R. Wilson, & L. G. Björk (Eds.), *Minorities in higher education* (pp. 173–194). Phoenix, AZ: Oryx Press.

Dernersesian, A. C. (1993). And, yes . . . the earth did part: On the splitting of Chicana/o subjectivity. In A. de la Torre & B. M. Pesquera (Eds.), *Building with our hands: New directions in Chicana studies* (pp. 34–56). Los Angeles: University of California Press.

Falicov, C. J. (1998). *Latino families in therapy: A guide to multicultural practice.* New York: Guilford Press.

Feagin, J. R., Vera, H., & Imani, N. (1996). *The agony of education: Black students at White colleges and universities.* New York: Routledge.

Fiske, E. B. (1988). The undergraduate Hispanic experience: A case of juggling two cultures. *Change, 20*, 29–33.

Gándara, P. (1995). *Over the ivy walls: The educational mobility of low income Chicanos.* Albany: State University of New York Press.

García, J. G., & Marotta, S. (1997). Characterization of the Latino population. In J. G. García & M. C. Zea (Eds.), *Psychological interventions and research with Latino populations* (pp. 1–14). Boston: Allyn and Bacon.

Gay, G. (2001). Educational equality for students of color. In J. A. Banks & C. A. McGee Banks (Eds.), *Multicultural education: Issues and perspectives* (4th ed., pp. 197–224). New York: Wiley and Sons.

Gloria, A. M. (1997). Chicana academic persistence: Creating a university-based community. *Education and Urban Society, 30*, 107–121.

Gloria, A. M. (1999). Apoyando estudiantes Chicanas: Therapeutic factors in Chicana college student support groups. *Journal for Specialists in Group Work, 24*, 246–259.

Gloria, A. M. (2001). The cultural construction of Latinas: Practice implications of multiple realities and identities. In D. B. Pope-Davis & H. L. K. Coleman (Eds.), *The intersection between race, gender, and class: Implications for multicultural counseling* (pp. 3–24). Thousand Oaks, CA: Sage.

Gloria, A. M., & Castellanos, J. (2003). Latino and African American students at predominantly White institutions: A psychosociocultural perspective of educational interactions and academic persistence. In J. Castellanos & L. Jones (Eds.), *The majority in the minority: Retaining Latina/o faculty, administrators, and students* (pp. 71–92). Sterling, VA: Stylus.

Gloria, A. M., & Robinson Kurpius, S. E. (1996). The validation of the Cultural Congruity Scale and the University Environment Scale with Chicano/a students. *Hispanic Journal of Behavioral Sciences, 18,* 533–549.

Gloria, A. M., & Rodriguez, E. R. (2000). Counseling Latino university students: Psychosociocultural issues for consideration. *Journal of Counseling and Development, 78,* 145–154.

Gloria, A. M., Ruiz, E. L., & Castillo, E. M. (2004). Counseling Latinos and Latinas: A psychosociocultural approach. In P. S. Richards & T. Smith (Eds.), *Practicing multiculturalism: Internalizing and affirming diversity in counseling and psychology* (pp. 167–184). Boston: Allyn and Bacon.

Gonzales, P. B. (1997). The categorical meaning of Spanish American identity among blue-collar New Mexicans, circa 1983. *Hispanic Journal of Behavioral Sciences, 19,* 123–136.

Guzmán, B. (2001). *The Hispanic population: Census Brief 2000* (Census Brief No. C2KBR/01-3). Washington, DC: U.S. Census Bureau.

Haro, R. P., Rodriguez, G., Jr., & Gonzales, J. L., Jr. (1994, HE028138). *Latino persistence in higher education: A 1994 survey of University of California and California State University Chicano/Latino students.* San Francisco: Latino Issues Forum (ERIC Document Reproduction Service No. ED 380 023)

Hernandez, J. C. (2000). Understanding the retention of Latino college students. *Journal of College Student Development, 41,* 575–588.

Hurtado, S., & Carter, D. F. (1997). Effects of college transition and perceptions of the campus racial climate on Latino college students' sense of belonging. *Sociology of Education, 70,* 324–345.

Hurtado, S., Carter, D. F., & Spuler, A. (1996). Latino student transition to college: Assessing difficulties and factors in successful college adjustment. *Research in Higher Education, 37,* 135–157.

Hyslop, N. (2000). *Hispanic parental involvement in home literacy.* Bloomington, IN: CS217298 Clearinghouse on Reading, English, and Communication (ERIC Document Reproduction Service No. EDO CS 00 09)

Jamieson, A., Curry, A., & Martinez, G. (2001). *School enrollment in the United States: Social and economic characteristics of students. October 1999* (Current Population Report No. P20-533). Washington, DC: U.S. Census Bureau.

Keefe S. E., & Padilla, A. M. (1987). *Chicano ethnicity.* Albuquerque: University of New Mexico Press.

Mehan, H. (1997). *Contextual factors surrounding Hispanic dropouts.* Washington, DC: U.S. Department of Education.

Muñoz, D. G. (1986). Identifying areas of stress for Chicano undergraduates. In M. A. Olivas (Ed.), *Latino college students* (pp. 131–156). New York: Teachers College Press.

Newburger, E. C., & Curry, A. (2000). *Educational attainment in the United States: March 1999* (Current Population Report No. P20-528). Washington, DC: U.S. Census Bureau.

Niemann, Y. F. (2001). Stereotypes about Chicanas and Chicanos: Implications for counseling. *The Counseling Psychologist, 29,* 55–90.

Nora, A. (1990). Campus-based aid programs as determinates of retention among Hispanic community college students. *Journal of Higher Education, 61,* 312–327.

Nora, A., & Cabrera, A. F. (1996). The role of perceptions of prejudice and discrimination on the adjustment of minority students to college. *Journal of Higher Education, 67,* 119–147.

Oboler, S. (1995). *Ethnic labels, Latino lives: Identity and the politics of (re)presentation in the United States.* Minneapolis: University of Minnesota Press.

Ortiz, D. L., & Guss, T. O. (1995). *Counseling implications for male Hispanic dropouts: Forging a prevention program.* #CG026503 U.S. Department of Education. (ERIC Document Reproduction No. ED 386 671)

Padilla, A. M. (1995). *Hispanic psychology: Critical issues in theory and research.* Thousand Oaks, CA: Sage.

Paniagua, F. A. (1994). *Assessing and treating culturally diverse clients: A practical guide.* Thousand Oaks, CA: Sage.

President's Advisory Commission of Educational Excellence for Hispanic Americans. (1996). *Our nation on the fault line: Hispanic American education, September 1996. A report to the President of the U.S., the Nation, and the Secretary of Education.* Washington, DC: U.S. Department of Education.

President's Advisory Commission of Educational Excellence for Hispanic Americans. (2000). *Creating the will: Hispanics achieving academic excellence (2000). A report to the President of the U.S., the Nation, and the Secretary of Education.* Washington, DC: U.S. Department of Education.

Retish, P. M., & Kavanaugh, P. C. (1992). Myth: America's public schools are educating Mexican American students. *Journal of Multicultural Counseling and Development, 20,* 89–96.

Ruiz, R. A., & Casas, J. M. (1976). Culturally relevant and behavioristic counseling for Chicano college students. In P. B. Pedersen, J. G. Draguns, W. J. Lonner, & J. E. Trimble (Eds.), *Counseling across cultures* (pp. 181–202). Honolulu: University of Hawai'i Press.

Ruiz, R. A., Casas, J. M., & Padilla, A. M. (1977). *Culturally relevant behavioristic counseling* (2nd ed.). Los Angeles: University of California.

Secada, W. G., Chavez-Chavez, R., Garcia, E., Muñoz, C., Oakes, J., Santiago-Santiago, I., & Slavin, R. (1998). *No more excuses: The final report of the Hispanic dropout project.* Washington, DC: U.S. Department of Education.

Seda, M., & Bixler-Marquez, B. (1994). The ecology of a Chicano student at risk. *Journal of Educational Issues of Language Minority Students, 13,* 195–208.

Sodowsky, G. R., Lai, E. W. M., & Plake, B. S. (1991). Moderating effects of sociocultural variables on acculturation attitudes of Hispanics and Asian Americans. *Journal of Counseling and Development, 70,* 194–204.

Solberg, V. S., & Villareal, P. (1997). Examination of self-efficacy, social support, and stress as predictors of psychological and physical distress among Hispanic college students. *Hispanic Journal of Behavioral Sciences, 19,* 182–201.

Therrien, M., & Ramirez, R. R. (2000). *The Hispanic population in the United States: March 2000* (Current Population Report No. P20-535). Washington, DC: U.S. Census Bureau.

U.S. Bureau of the Census. (1995). *The nation's Hispanic population: 1994* (Statistical Brief No. SB/95-25). Washington, DC: U.S. Government Printing Office.

U.S. Department of Commerce. (1993). *We the American . . . Hispanics.* Economics and Statistics Administration. U.S. Bureau of the Census. WE-2R.

U.S. Department of Education, National Center for Education Statistics. (1997). *Minorities in higher education* (NCES No. 97-372). Washington, DC: U.S. Government Printing Office.

U.S. Department of Education, National Center for Education Statistics. (2000a). *The condition of education 1999* (NCES No. 2000-009). Washington, DC: U.S. Government Printing Office.

U.S. Department of Education, National Center for Education Statistics. (2000b). *The condition of education 2000* (NCES No. 2000-062). Washington, DC: U.S. Government Printing Office.

Vasquez, M. J. (1982). Confronting barriers to the participation of Mexican American women in higher education. *Hispanic Journal of Behavioral Sciences, 4,* 147–163.

White House Initiative on Educational Excellence for Hispanic Americans. (2000). *Latinos in education: Early childhood, elementary, secondary, undergraduate, graduate.* Washington, DC: U.S. Department of Education.

Yalom, I. D. (1995). *The theory and practice of group psychotherapy* (4th ed.). New York: Basic Books.

Cultural Competency: Teaching, Training, and the Delivery of Services for Chicana/os

Brian W. McNeill
Washington State University

Loreto R. Prieto
The University of Akron

Fernando Ortiz
Washington State University

Cynthia A. Yamokoski
The University of Akron

As noted in the recent report of the Surgeon General (Department of Health and Human Services, 2001), "culture counts" in the conceptualization and implementation of services to minority populations. That is, cultural factors affect all aspects of psychological health and illness, as well as how and whether people seek help, types of help they seek, types of social supports and coping skills they use, the stigma attached to seeking psychological services, and, most importantly, the meanings people associate with their psychological problems. The Surgeon General's report provides overwhelming documentation that the best available research indicates racial and ethnic minority groups have less access to care and overall receive poorer quality mental health services. Chicana/o people are no exception.

According to Sue (1998), cultural competence, along with multiculturalism, in general refers to the belief that people should not only appreciate and recognize other cultural groups but also be able to deliver effective psychological interventions to members of a particular culture. In other words, cultural competence is equal to effectiveness in counseling and psychotherapy with culturally diverse clients. Consequently, the development of cultural competence starts with the training that practitioners receive through coursework, supervision, and other activities. Thus, this chapter examines crucial variables in providing culturally relevant services to Chicana/os, reviews the development and need for cultural competencies in the training of mental health practitioners relevant to working with Chicana/o populations, and provides recommendations for specific training activities and coursework for preparation in working with Chicana/os.

CULTURALLY COMPETENT SERVICES FOR CHICANA/OS

As noted by Sue (1998), the impetus for cultural competence has been the inadequacy of services for members of ethnic minority groups including Chicana/os, particularly in the area of cultural and linguistic mismatches that occur between clients and providers. Sue also stressed that these cultural differences affect the validity of assessment procedures, development of therapist-client rapport, the therapeutic relationship, and treatment effectiveness. In reviewing the literature on Chicana/os' use of mental health services, Prieto, McNeill, Walls, and Gomez (2001) concluded that Chicana/os are likely to underutilize conventional mental health services, instead preferring family or nontraditional helpers, and that both level of identification with indigenous culture and level of acculturation to the majority culture appear to affect use of services and preferences for an ethnically similar counselor. However, these authors noted the methodological problems associated with research, including the overreliance on analogue designs with college student populations, as well as a lack of ecological or external validity in assessing such preferences.

The few studies that focus on real-world clients and design and implementation of culturally relevant services for Chicana/o populations indicate that such variables as ethnic or language match and ethnic-specific programs make a difference. Theoretically speaking, proponents of ethnic matching hypothesize that these variables play an important role in the psychotherapeutic process because of the well-documented literature in social psychology that indicates the importance of attitude similarity in the social influence process (Hurtado, 1994; VandeCreek & Merrill, 1990). Sue, Fujino, Hu, Takeuchi, and Zane (1991) proposed that, from the cultural responsiveness hypothesis, the efficacy of psychotherapy is, among many factors, a function of the extent to which therapists can communicate in the language of clients and understand their cultural background. Under these conditions, therapists are presumably better able to assess the situation of clients, modify treatment strategies to suit clients, avoid group stereotypes, and form rapport.

In their review of the research on psychotherapy outcomes with ethnic and racial minorities, Sue, Zane, and Young (1994) noted that, with respect to Latina/o Americans, the available evidence suggests that ethnic and language match are important variables in explaining positive outcomes for Chicana/os; specifically, ethnic match has been found to be a significant predictor of both dropout rates and total number of sessions attended for Mexican American adolescents (Yeh, Eastman, & Cheung, 1994). Moreover, Sue et al. (1991) found that ethnic match was correlated with a greater number of treatment sessions across all ethnic groups including Chicana/os, and language match was a predictor of both length and outcome of treatment. Ethnic match has also been found to affect rapport between client and therapist as frequency of self-disclosure was found to be greater when Latina/os were ethnically matched with another Latina/o (LeVine & Franco, 1981). Geiger (1994) examined the utilization rates of Los Angeles County Mental Health Service outpatients over a 5-year period, as well as demographic characteristics of clients. Ethnic matching of therapists and clients did not result in a greater number of treatment sessions, lower dropout rates, or outcomes for anxiety disorders for Chicana/o adult populations.

In her analysis of service data from one fiscal year (1992 to 1993) that were reported to management by all mental health agencies funded by a county public mental health authority in California, Jerrell (1998) looked at ethnic match between client and outpatient therapist as a variable that affects the delivery of mental health services for children and adolescents; 48% were Latina/o, Asian, and African American cases seen during the fiscal year. She concluded that those who were served by staff of the same ethnic background (match) stayed in treatment longer. Not only did these clients stay longer in outpatient care, but they also tended "to use less of some types of intensive care (i.e., subacute day treatment) when they [had] an ethnically matched outpatient therapist" (p. 300).

Other studies focused specifically on language as an important variable in predicting successful outcomes in the therapeutic process with Mexican Americans. Researchers working with Mexican American populations whose primary language was Spanish found that, when these patients were evaluated with the aid of an interpreter, clinically relevant interpreter-related distortions led to misevaluation of the patients' mental status (Marcos, 1988; Marcos, Urcayo, Kesselman, & Albert, 1973). It was shown that the process of matching bilingual and ethnically similar therapists and interviewers resulted in different levels of rapport (Hurtado, 1994) and therapeutic outcomes (Kline, Acosta, Austin, & Johnson, 1980). Spanish-speaking Mexican American clients who used an interpreter believed they received more help and were understood better than bilingual Mexican American clients who spoke to the therapist in English (Acosta & Cristo, 1981).

Although these studies are not without limitations (e.g., accounting for level of acculturation, identifying Latina/o subgroups; see Prieto et al., 2001), they provide enough evidence of the importance of linguistic and ethnic match in the psychotherapeutic process among Chicana/os to warrant their inclusion and coverage in graduate education and training addressing the needs of Chicana/o populations.

Broad Competency Issues in Education, Clinical Training, and Research

Early models for training in issues of diversity (e.g., Pedersen, 1981; Sue et al., 1982) emphasized the importance of cultural awareness, skills, and knowledge. In the case of Chicana/os, Sandoval and De La Roza (1986) promoted the knowledge of cultural characteristics, values, and their clinical implications. In the interim time period, accrediting bodies, such as the American Psychological Association (APA), have implemented requirements for programs in clinical, counseling, and school psychology at the predoctoral, internship, and postdoctoral levels. For example, current APA criteria for accreditation state that programs "engage in actions that indicate respect for and understanding of cultural and individual diversity" (p. 4) including but not limited to ethnicity, gender, language, national origin and race. *Domain D: Cultural and Individual Differences and Diversity* (APA, 2000) explicitly requires programs to recognize the importance of cultural and individual differences and diversity in the training of psychologists, including systematic efforts to attract and retain students and faculty from differing ethnic, racial, and personal backgrounds in the program, and to provide students with relevant knowledge and experiences regarding cultural diversity as related to the science and practice of professional psychology (APA, 2000). However, as noted by the APA (2000), the "avenues by which these goals are achieved are to be developed by the program" (p. 6). Thus, the interpretation, implementation, and emphasis of these standards is left up to individual programs.

Consequently, multicultural scholars have proposed various models to guide programs in the promotion of multicultural competencies (MCC) and implementation of accreditation standards. For example, Ridly, Mendoza, and Kanitz (1994) expanded Copeland's (1982) recommendations for multicultural training (MCT) and provided a comprehensive model of MCT. Included within this model were descriptions of the typical methods by which programs address multicultural training. In the workshop design, workshops outside of program coursework or content are implemented to cover MCT. In the separate course design, the program's curriculum includes one to three unrelated course offerings to address issues of diversity. The interdisciplinary design proposes that trainees select and take courses outside their specialty area (e.g., ethnic studies, anthropology, sociology) in order to obtain knowledge in cultural diversity. The area of concentration design consists of a core of interrelated courses covering multicultural issues in assessment and testing, individual counseling, family systems, and so on. The integration design involves the infusion of MCT into all areas of the training program, including coursework and practicum experiences. As most recently noted by Abreu, Chung, and Atkinson (2000), these various program designs as ordered previously represent increasing adherence to training standards promoted by the APA. These authors also noted that the integration design is the most holistic model, and thus viewed as ideal for training program implementation. Indeed, the current model for training programs in counseling psychology takes these standards a step further by including the area of individual and cultural diversity as an "essential" curricular area that should be evident in course content, practica, and research experiences, and by asserting that professional core courses should address diversity issues (Murdock, Alcorn, Heesacker, & Stoltenberg, 1998). However, according to Abreu et al., there is little evidence that programs are responding accordingly, despite indications that exposure to training in working with culturally diverse groups is predictive of self-perceived cultural competence by clinical and counseling psychologists (Allison, Echemendia, Crawford, & Robinson, 1996), as well as of treatment outcome (Yutrzenka, 1995).

Although we certainly realize that any number of programs fall short of attaining the goals and ideals of the integration model in preparing students for work with diverse populations, it is for this very reason that there is a need to provide recommendations and guidelines for infusion of knowledge, skills, and values related to work with Chicana/o and Latina/o populations. We also realize that programs may find it difficult to implement extensive cultural content for all cultural groups. However, it is possible that certain programs with high concentrations of Chicana/o faculty and students or located in areas with high Chicana/o populations might develop specialized coursework and infuse course and training content relevant to working with Chicana/os into programs. Consequently, we review and provide recommendations for programs that may wish to implement such recommendations.

Understandably, most multicultural didactic coursework and training in applied psychology has focused on trainees' acquisition of basic, molar competencies, such as gaining an awareness of cultural biases, establishing a foundational knowledge base concerning the characteristics of other cultures, and learning fundamental skills regarding culturally sensitive behaviors when working with diverse people (cf. Sue & Sue, 1999). Such didactic coursework has been at best inconsistently utilized in applied psychology doctoral programs (Allison, Crawford, Echemendia, Robinson, & Knepp, 1994; Bernal & Castro, 1994) and, when utilized, has met with variable success with respect to bringing about cultural sensitivity in trainees. Furthermore, rarely has an infused approach been taken to curricula (cf. Ridly et al., 1994); rather, courses in multiculturalism or cross-cultural psychology, if offered at all, tend to be either elective or restricted to a "tag-on" single survey course that is not integrated with other coursework. Coursework specific to Chicana/os is all but non-existent— an example of such a course is offered later in the chapter.

With respect to clinical didactics (e.g., practicum training and supervision), virtually no research-supported approaches have been established regarding effective training techniques for supervisors to aid in trainees' acquisition of cultural competencies. Therefore, there are few empirically supported specifics in the literature to help guide instructors or supervisors in helping students to develop competencies particular to Chicana/o populations, or any racially or ethnically diverse populations for that matter. In one of the few publications on this topic, McNeill, Hom, and Perez (1995) indicated that supervisors need to be knowledgeable about multicultural issues and recognize the majority culture influence on counseling theories and interventions. Faculty and supervisors need to be open to multicultural issues and be responsible for setting an atmosphere of tolerance and respect when working with diverse trainees.

As mentioned earlier, several agents, including the APA, APA Division 17 (Counseling Psychology), and various psychology scholars have drafted or endorsed position papers for psychology (and related professions) concerning general cultural considerations for training programs, researchers, and clinical practitioners to attend to, such as Sue et al. (1982), Sue, Arredondo, and McDavis (1992), APA (1993), Arredondo et al. (1996), and most recently Sue (2001). As noted, these general papers tended to focus exclusively on the broad domain of multicultural psychology and emphasized the typical triad of culturally sensitive awareness, knowledge, and skills or the need to stop exploiting underrepresented groups in research efforts. Although these efforts are significant, their conceptualizations of cultural competence largely remain a set of guiding principles that lack empirical validation (Department of Health and Human Services, 2001) and mechanisms for implementation or enforcement. In addition, these guidelines have been criticized for not adequately addressing considerations of social justice (Vera & Speight, 2003).

In addition to these publications, task forces and committees have been implemented by the APA in order to address racial and ethnic issues. Historically, these have included the 1963 Ad Hoc Committee on Equality of Opportunity in Psychology and the 1974 APA Minority Fellowship program. In 1978, the birth of the APA Ad Hoc Committee on Minority Affairs took place, articulating curriculum issues as one area for reform, foreshadowing later accreditation requirements regarding diversity training. In 1979, the APA Office of Ethnic Minority Affairs came into being and the APA began to include diversity-related criteria for accreditation of graduate programs. In 1980, the APA Board of Ethnic Minority Affairs (BEMA) was established; the next year, BEMA itself established a task force on ethnic minority education and training. BEMA remained active over the next decade, until it was retired following APA restructuring in 1990, when the APA Committee on Ethnic Minority Affairs (CEMA) was founded. In 1994, the Commission on Ethnic Minority Recruitment, Retention, and Training in Psychology (CEMRRAT) was established and charged with encouraging multicultural education and training as well as exploring issues and barriers to recruitment, retention, and training of ethnic minorities in psychology (CEMRRAT, 1997). However, despite this organization-based activity at higher levels of APA administration, little programmatic or comprehensive attention has been paid to the specific competencies needed for working with Chicana/o populations.

To meet this void, several scholars have issued landmark papers more directly related to Chicana/o issues, including Padilla et al.'s (1991) *amicus curiae,* representing the APA Board of Directors' and Council of Representatives' opposition to the legal adoption of English-only laws in the United States, legislation that, in our view, represented a direct assault on the culture of U.S. Spanish-speaking peoples. In addition, Rogler and associates at the Fordham University Hispanic Research Center published a series of articles in the *American Psychologist* concerning culturally sensitive services for Latina/os (Rogler, Malgady, Costantino, & Blumenthal, 1987), biases in assessment and psychological evaluation with Latina/os (Malgady, Rogler, Costantino, 1987), and the interface between acculturation and Latina/o mental health (Rogler, Cortes, & Malgady, 1991). These articles also spoke to the specific situation and needs of Latina/os, including Chicana/os, particularly the critical role of the Spanish language (and bilinguality), acculturation, and assessment issues in working Chicana/o clientele. Affirming this focus, Velásquez (1997) edited a special issue of the *Journal of Counseling and Development* devoted to counseling Chicana/os and, most recently, in *The Counseling Psychologist* (see McNeill et al., 2001), a series of articles focused on these three domains as well as the domains of ethnic identity and the stereotyping of Chicanao/s. The works authored and cited by Arredondo (chap. 12, this volume), including Arredondo (1991), Padilla (1995), and Santiago-Rivera et al. (2002) were all foundational works concerning specific competencies helping professionals need when working with Chicana/os.

Further addressing the specific needs of Chicana/os, Martinez (1977), Martinez and Mendoza (1984), Marín and Marín (1991), Geisinger (1992), Sánchez (1993), Marcos (1994), Padilla (1995), Garcia and Zea (1997), Velásquez, Ayala, and Mendoza (1998), and Koss-Chioino and Vargas (1999) have also helped to underscore the role of language, acculturation, and assessment issues in working with Chicana/o clientele. These frequently identified domains of language, acculturation, and assessment issues, although different from the earlier mentioned traditional triad of knowledge, skills, and awareness (cf. Sue & Sue, 1999) cited by most multicultural scholars and position-paper authors, have been repeatedly discussed in the literature concerning Chicana/os as cornerstones to understanding and effectively working with this population. We now briefly explore the primary issues within each of these domains.

Training Considerations Regarding Acculturation, Language, and Assessment With Chicana/os

With the Chicana/o population of the United States increasing at a rate unmatched by any other minority, mental health professionals must enhance their efficacy in the treatment of this population. In order to focus on improving students' training to work with Chicana/os, rather than simply increasing their awareness of differences among and between racial and ethnic groups, we recommend that clinicians who work with Chicana/os possess the following general competencies: the ability to accurately assess cultural and ethnic world views of clients (e.g., Barón & Constantine, 1997; Delgado-Romero, 2001), to conduct complete, valid psychological assessments of their clinical difficulties (e.g., Cuéllar & Gonzalez, 2000), and to understand the role of indigenous language in the treatment of Chicana/o clientele.

Acculturation and Worldview. Underlying the effects associated with ethnic matching may be the knowledge and understanding of diverse world views (Sue, 1998). In working with Chicana/o and Latina/o clients, Delgado-Romero (2001) suggests evaluating their racial and ethnic identity development both to gather information and to form a therapeutic alliance (see Pizaro & Vera, 2001; Vera & Quintana, chap. 3, this volume) for a comprehensive summary of ethnic identity models and conceptualizations for Chicana/os). In beginning this assessment, counselors should address how clients collectively and individually identify themselves. It is also important to pay attention to how the clients pronounce their names and ask them what they would like to be called (in traditional Spanish cultures, individuals use both paternal surname and mother's maiden name). Thus, in prepracticum courses or in clinical practica, trainees can be taught to focus on utilizing basic counseling and history-taking skills that convey sensitivity to Chicana/o clientele.

Following questions regarding ethnic identity, counselors should assess the client's level of acculturation (Cuéllar, Siles, & Bracamontes, chap. 2, this volume; Paniagua, 1998). This type of assessment is important due to the fact that the relationship between acculturation and mental illness varies with age; an inverse relationship exists for Chicana/o adults and older adults, whereas a direct relationship exists for young adults and older women (Bean, Perry, & Bedell, 2001). When Chicana/os identify with both their original culture and the majority culture, the healthiest level of functioning is possible (cf. Falicov, 1996; LaFromboise, Coleman, & Gerton, 1993). Trainees should be cognizant of the fact that the genesis of the construct of acculturation has shifted from more of an initial unidimensional assimilation construct (either indigenous or majority culture identification) to a bidimensional construct (an orthogonal level of indigenous and majority culture identification; cf. LaFromboise et al.). Significantly, recent research has shown that, for Chicana/os, retention of indigenous cultural values (i.e., enculturation or ethnic identity) affects counseling variables at least as much as subscription to majority culture values does (cf. Ramos-Sanchez, Atkinson, & Fraga, 1999; Ruelas, Atkinson, & Ramos-Sanchez, 1998).

Related to clients' level of acculturation or ethnic identity is their immigration history and affiliated attitudes. Clinically, it is important for counselors to inquire about the Chicano client's "migration narrative" (i.e., circumstances of immigration, how long he or she has been in the United States, who was left behind, stresses involved). Migration history plays an important role in Chicana/o mental health. Considerable stress appears to be associated with immigrating to the United States; specific national origin has been associated with level of immigration-related stress and foreign-born immigrants may have lower rates of mental illness (Bean et al., 2001). First-generation immigrants are also vulnerable to mental health problems due to psychological and economic hardship, complicated by the fact that concepts of several mental health problems (i.e. depression, anxiety, psychosis) are not readily understood by their home culture (Gonzalez, 1997). Additionally, an illegal immigrant's fear of detection results in negative consequences for the use of mental health services. Immigrating to a new country and culture often results in psychosomatic illnesses in Chicana/os, but these illnesses appear to decrease as they gain language and cultural competence (Falicov, 1996).

A variety of other factors are important in Chicana/o clients' assessment due to their influence on the expectations and results of treatment, including: gender role identity (Paniagua, 1998; Romero, 2001), value orientations (Altarriba & Bauer, 1998), world views (Altarriba & Bauer), family structure (Delgado-Romero, 2001), socio-economic status (Altarriba & Bauer), social support (Gloria & Rodriguez, 2000), and, most importantly, personal and situational factors (Constantine & Ladany, 2000). An assessment of these domains can be achieved by having trainees informally ask clients relevant open-ended questions.

Language. Use of the Spanish language is a cornerstone of Chicana/o culture, although many Chicana/os in the U.S. are either bilingual or have lost their indigenous language altogether, often by the second or third generation. Competent trainees and clinicians do not have to be Spanish speakers themselves, but should have a network of referral services for Spanish-speaking clientele should the need arise for a Spanish-speaking or bilingual clinician or translator. Developing a referral network may be more difficult in some geographic areas than others and, overall, securing a Spanish-speaking or bilingual mental health professional can be a difficult task. Linguistic barriers for Spanish-speaking Chicana/os seeking mental health services have been outlined in the literature (e.g., Altarriba & Santiago-Rivera, 1994; Preciado & Henry, 1997; Santiago-Rivera, 1995) and clearly there is a need for bilingual service providers. Training more Chicana/o or Spanish-speaking mental health professionals is a must, especially given research findings indicating that mental health services delivered in Spanish can increase service utilization by Chicana/o clientele (Snowden & Hu, 1997; Sue et al., 1991).

Not surprisingly, use of the Spanish language has remained a critical issue with regard to difficulties in serving Chicana/os' mental health needs (cf. Altarriba & Santiago-Rivera, 1994; Malgady et al., 1987). Obviously, language use can influence the treatment process. For example, the cognitive processes involved in the use of English as a second language (especially adult acquired) can inhibit Spanish-speaking clients' affective experiences in the interview (Altarriba & Santiago-Rivera; Bamford, 1991; Marcos, 1994). That is, using a nonnative language may distance clients from their emotions as they translate their experiences from one language to another.

Chicana/os' language preferences have a substantial impact on both client and clinician perceptions and experiences during counseling. Coupled with cultural characteristics noted as often being typical of Chicana/os (e.g., a tendency to be silent, to avert eye contact, to defer to the clinician as a demonstration of respect; Malgady et al., 1987), the potential for both verbal and nonverbal communication factors to have a negative impact on clinician diagnostic judgments appears to be high. Competent trainees and clinicians are aware of typical behavioral characteristics and culturally based communication styles utilized by Chicana/os during therapy and avoid pathologizing these behaviors. Malgady et al. identified several elements in need of assessment when dealing with Spanish-speaking Chicana/o clientele, including language preference while under psychological distress, the interaction of all their acquired languages, previous experience with mental health interviews, and age when English was acquired. Furthermore, Malgady et al. asserted that these variables may have an interactive effect on each other. Moreover, the use of Spanish or English by Chicana/o clients may have differential effects on expression and experience of affect (Altarriba & Santiago-Rivera, 1994; Santiago-Rivera & Altarriba, 2002).

Assessment. Although often thought of as only consisting of paper-and-pencil tests, assessment procedures with Chicana/os call for a much more broadly defined process and content. We encourage trainees and clinicians to understand certain context variables before undertaking assessment procedures with Chicana/os, as this understanding will help to develop well-rounded competency in this area.

Cultural formulations are vital to the assessment of Chicana/o clients because culture is a ubiquitous factor whose influence is central to identity, self-concept, and adaptation (Cuéllar & Gonzalez, 2000). Therefore, the ability to conduct an extensive and comprehensive assessment is a key competency for counselors working with Chicana/o clients. The traditional clinical interview must be modified when working with Chicana/os to gather further information about their cultural and ethnic identities, including acculturation, and their effects on additional interpersonal and intrapersonal domains. Assessing these constructs assists in determining appropriate themes to address with Chicana/os and in implementing the most effective interventions possible (Barón & Constantine, 1997). Due to Chicana/os' value of personalismo, this assessment should be conducted through informal questioning rather than more formal interview techniques or questionnaires (Gloria & Rodriguez, 2000).

In addition, given Chicana/os' beliefs about health and illness, religion and spirituality are the key belief systems to assess in determining a diagnosis or focus of treatment (Falicov, 1998). After establishing a therapeutic alliance with Chicana/o clients, it is important to explore these beliefs in religion and health and how clients view them as possible resources and avenues of support (Falicov). Cuéllar, Arnold, and Gonzalez (as cited in Cuéllar & Gonzalez, 2000) developed the Folk Belief Subscale to assess the extent to which Mexican Americans rely on traditional folk beliefs and healing practices. Useful information may be obtained through the clinical interview by inquiring about what patients believe is wrong with themselves, what is causing them to feel that way, and what they believe should be done about it (Cuéllar & Gonzalez). Although assessment for beliefs in folk medicine is important with Chicana/o clients, counselors should be aware that studies of various subgroups of Mexican Americans indicate that from 7% to 44% of them consult *curanderos* and other traditional folk healers (Keegan, 1996; Macias & Morales, 2000; Risser

& Mazur, 1995; Skaer, Robison, Sclar, & Harding, 1996), suggesting many within-group differences based on acculturation, enculturation, and socioeconomic factors. Furthermore, Prieto, McNeill, Walls, and Gómez (2001) cautioned clinicians to not overgeneralize or overdiagnose the existence of culture-bound syndromes in Chicana/os, and to attend to known (and often small and ethnic group-specific) prevalence and incidence rates for Chicana/os with respect to these disorders. In summary, the competent assessment of mental health difficulties for Chicana/os involves a complex interaction between physical, psychological, and spiritual factors.

Assessment of mental health difficulties in Chicana/os also calls for an understanding of the fact that *la familia* plays an all-important part in the genesis, maintenance, and context of most psychological distress. Family is also an important force in the seeking of mental health services. Chicana/o clients from a traditional cultural environment are likely to consult with their family in times of trouble and may find it difficult to rely on professional counselors for help. When Chicana/os do seek mental health assistance, they are often reluctant to reveal all of their thoughts and feelings, perhaps due to the guilt associated with seeking help outside of the family (Altarriba & Bauer, 1998). Family members are used as referents for attitudes and behavior, individual needs are secondary to family, and Chicana/os do not value individuation from their parents and families to the degree that the dominant culture does. Failure to acknowledge family in counseling may lead to resistance or premature termination of services (Gloria & Rodgriguez, 2000). In fact, family therapy is often a recommended treatment modality for Chicana/o clients (e.g., Bean et al., 2001; Paniagua, 1998).

In addition to diagnostic issues, consideration of an appropriate treatment modality can also be helpful during competent assessment procedures when working with Chicana/os. For example, cognitive-behavioral therapy (CBT) seems to be supportive of many Chicana/o values (e.g., present focused, de-emphasis on affective expression); therefore, CBT is widely accepted as a treatment modality for this group (Bean et al., 2001; Organista, 2000; Paniagua, 1998; Perez, 1999). The problem-focused nature of CBT and its directive behavior-change techniques are consistent with the needs and desires of Chicana/o clients (Perez). Current research indicates that Chicana/os may be at higher risk for problems such as depression, anxiety, and somatization disorders compared to the general public, yet they tend to underutilize mental health services (Prieto et al., 2001). However, it is well known that Chicana/os overutilize physicians for emotional and psychological problems (Organista). By implementing more consistent and congruent therapies, such as CBT, perhaps Chicana/o clients will increase their utilization of mental health services. It is important to note that, although the CBT approach would seem to be a very comprehensive and culturally sensitive treatment program, little outcome research has actually been conducted on its use with Chicana/os.

Falicov (1996) suggested several general tips for competently working with Chicana/o clients. Chicana/os are more likely to self-disclose when the therapist uses "culturally syntonic conversational modes" (e.g., proverbs, metaphors, humor). An emotive tone is more beneficial than an efficient, structured, behavioral, or contractual approach; Chicana/os do not tend to respond as well if they are asked to directly describe or explain their feelings and reactions. Experiential approaches ("telling it like it is") and interpretations of nonverbals can inhibit Chicana/o clients. Another suggestion is for therapists to take a real interest in clients and be person oriented rather than task oriented; Chicana/os usually are not comfortable with the strict scheduling of times to be intimate or express affection. In addition, Chicana/os may feel that it is impolite to disagree with their therapist.

With respect to formal psychological testing, Prieto et al. (2001) lamented that scholars have for some time discussed the difficulties associated with using traditional psychological tests for evaluating persons from racially and ethnically diverse groups, including Chicana/os (e.g., Dana, 1993, 2000; Sandoval, Frisby, Geisinger, Scheuneman, & Grenier, 1998; Suzuki & Kugler, 1995). Several factors can play into the performance (or lack thereof) for Chicana/os undergoing traditional psychological testing. Certain context variables are important for the competent trainee and clinician to consider. Psychometric concerns rank high, including potential item bias, the use of inappropriate norm or reference groups by test publishers, the differential validity of tests for clients of color, the effects of culture-bound epistemological or social constructive sets, and how this set of factors might bias test results and clinicians' interpretations of them.

Orientation to time and familiarity with test taking and test-taking strategies have also been discussed as factors affecting Chicana/os' general performance on standardized tests (Pennack-Roman, 1992). These factors are relevant with respect to the immediacy of examinees' responses and to the development of problem-solving heuristics and response sets in the testing situation.

Acculturation has been shown to affect test scores for Chicana/os; for example, less acculturated Chicana/os sometimes generated more pathological scores on diagnostic instruments such as the MMPI-2 (cf. Velásquez et al., 1998). As discussed in previous reviews concerning Chicana/o mental health issues (e.g., Rogler et al., 1991), acculturative stress may actually be more salient to the development of mental health difficulties for Chicana/os than acculturation per se, and may also be more salient with regard to the pathology or distress-oriented elevations typically seen on certain tests. Progress in the theory and measurement of Chicana/o racial and ethnic identity and acculturation has allowed researchers and clinicians to better understand the relation of indigenous cultural perspectives, biculturality, and acculturative stress to the development of mental health difficulties in Chicana/os (Padilla, 1995). This advance has enabled competent professionals to better understand and more accurately select, administer, interpret, and therapeutically use results from psychological assessments with Chicana/os.

Translations of common psychological tests have been evolving for a long time. However, efforts at validating such translated versions have had serious shortcomings in their methodology. Because translated versions of tests may tend to overpathologize Chicana/o clients, any translations of English-normed instruments into Spanish should be used with a high degree of caution by clinicians until research demonstrates clearly that these instruments are valid and comparable to their English counterparts. We recommend that any English-normed test, if translated, utilize samples of actual Chicana/o bilinguals as opposed to nonnative European American Spanish speakers as normative subject pools or as consultants. Native Spanish speakers whose ethnicity and life experiences are grounded within the Chicana/o culture are more likely to understand semantic nuances and culture-based constructions than non-Chicana/o translators who learned and use Spanish as a second language and have little or no direct experience with the Chicana/o culture. Moreover, in developing Spanish translations of instruments, we recommend the use of back-translation trials to ensure semantic equivalence of the English and Spanish versions of the instrument (cf. suggestions made by Geisinger, 1994).

Finally, the competent trainee and clinician seek out information regarding behaviors associated with specific test scores for Chicana/os. Without consideration of Chicana/o specific behavioral correlates, many test scores may not be accurately interpreted in a clinical setting, especially when using normative data standards derived from European American samples. In addition, when employing formal tests, the competent trainee and clinician should also administer relevant emic or culture-specific tests to obtain information on various aspects of Chicana/os' life experiences that influence their mental health status (e.g., acculturation or acculturative stress).

In order to be culturally competent in the aforementioned three domains of acculturation and world view, understanding language usage, and assessment, as well as other relevant areas when working with Chicana/os, counselors must extend their knowledge beyond cultural differences and address how to best deliver effective services to specific populations (Johnson, 1987). Competence does not result from solely having the necessary ingredients; rather, trainees and clinicians need to provide services that are perceived as culturally competent by Chicana/o consumers (Dana, Behn, & Gonwa, 1992). When working with Chicana/os, counselors who seek collaboration with more traditional healers (e.g. physicians, priests, curanderos) and who display competencies in understanding Chicana/os' acculturation and world views, language usage, and assessment procedures should be able to integrate the proper ingredients and provide effective and culturally sensitive treatment for their clients.

We now consider the content and structure of a course in Chicana/o psychology, both as a way to convey the aforementioned areas of competency as well as to provide an example of how to construct and implement an ethnic group-specific course into training curricula.

COURSEWORK IN CHICANA/O PSYCHOLOGY

The Course

McNeill (1999) conducted an informal assessment of samples of course offerings in the western region of the U.S., obtained through college catalogs and departmental descriptions that indicated that, although courses such as "Minority Mental Health Issues," "Counseling Diverse Populations," "Cross-Cultural Psychology," and "Multicultural Counseling" are increasingly more common in graduate-level counseling and clinical psychology and social work programs, courses addressing the needs of specific cultural groups are offered less often. In fact, it appears that, in the western region, only a handful of courses in Asian American or African American psychology exist and only five in the psychology or health issues of Chicana/o or Latina/o populations.

As illustrated in the Appendix, the course recently developed by Brian McNeill at Washington State University has a number of objectives, including examination of the current psychosocial literature related to Chicana/o and Latina/o populations, issues of acculturation and ethnic identity, and the relationship of these variables to underutilization of psychological services. This course essentially builds on the previous work of others (e.g., Vasquez & Barón, 1988) in addressing the traditional MCC areas of skills, knowledge, and awareness and is periodically updated based on an evolving literature. Culturally appropriate counseling models and strategies for intervention are also covered. In addition, perhaps most importantly (and usually most controversially), the current sociopolitical environment, including issues of racism, ethnocentrism, and political power, is identified and discussed. Course requirements are varied accordingly for undergraduate versus graduate course credit because this is the only course on campus with this content. The intent is to offer advanced undergraduates the experience of a graduate seminar format, while attracting graduate students from various departments and programs. It is also important for the instructor to identify and describe his own biases and perceptions, or the lenses through which the issues involved in the course are viewed. Following is an overview of the course from McNeill's point of view.

At the beginning of the course, I spend a few minutes talking about myself, my ethnic background, and the effects of my sense of identity on my perceptions of the world and the way these viewpoints affect the issues covered in the course. As a child of an Anglo father of Scottish descent and a Chicana mother, I have viewed the issues of racism, discrimination, and prejudice from both sides, so to speak. Because I have an Anglo surname, often others around me are unaware of my Chicano ethnic background and I have often been exposed to the negative aspects of Anglo culture where ethnic slurs, jokes, and comments, are disclosed on an everyday basis without considering their offensiveness. At the same time, when I enter a Mexican market to buy supplies, I am often addressed in Spanish and, not fully understanding, encountered with looks and reactions that seem to say, "What is wrong with you?" My grandmother, an immigrant from Baja California Sur in Mexico, was clearly more comfortable in Spanish than in English, despite living in the United States for most of her life. My grandfather, though born in Mexico, was a Chicano from Arizona who spoke both Spanish and English with a Mexican accent. My mother was punished for speaking Spanish when she first went to school. She met and married my father in the great mix of cultures in Los Angeles, California in the 1940s and 1950s. We had large extended families on both my maternal and paternal sides and the emphasis on *familia* was common to both as we led our very middle-class existence. My Mexican familia faced many of the issues confronting Latina/os during this period of time in Los Angeles, including discrimination, loss of Spanish-language skills, self-consciousness over skin color, and identification as "Spanish" versus "Mexican." Thus, my sense of identity and perspective was formed around these experiences growing up in the Los Angeles area, and may be very different from that of a first-generation Chicano from the barrio in Chicago or southwestern Washington.

My lenses, or perceptions, also extend to the sociopolitical context of the course in that, in my view, racism directed toward Latina/os is still alive and well. The variety of anti-immigration, anti-bilingual education, and English-only legislation originating in California, as well as other states, serves as my evidence that I introduce to the class. Unfortunately, there is never a lack of examples of racism directed toward Chicana/os and Latina/os on both the individual and institutional levels. I also emphasize that these are my perceptions, and that, although others may disagree, what is most often dealt with in psychology are peoples' perceptions, beliefs, and viewpoints, along with their effects on behavior, as opposed to concrete realities. This conception of reality is often difficult for students to initially grasp as they are seeking a single truth to explain complex phenomena. Many times, the initial reaction of the students is to argue that introducing a sociopolitical context is inappropriate and that psychologists should strive to be objective and neutral. Thus, I introduce a number of genetic and environmental deficit theories and models from the history of psychology and the negative views of minorities that represent anything but objectivity and neutrality (e.g., Glaser & Moynihan, 1963; Jensen, 1973). At this point, the concept of cultural relativism is also introduced, along with the ecological paradigm as espoused through the community psychology of Rappaport (1997), whose values included respect for human diversity, the right to be different, and the belief that human problems are those of person-environment fit, rather than of incompetent people or inferior psychological and cultural environments. The history section of the recent "Chicano!" series (Galán, 1996) shown by the Public Broadcasting System also sets the stage for the sociopolitical context.

The history of Chicana/o psychology is then covered, including both Hispanic and indigenous origins and practices. The elders associated with Chicana/o psychology are also introduced and, of course, my lectures draw primarily from the classic text *Chicano Psychology* by Martinez and Mendoza (1984). At this point, it is usually necessary to talk a bit about terminology and self-identification. Consequently, I introduce concepts of race, ethnicity, and power as precursors to the usage of such terms as *Hispanic, Latina/o, Chicana/o, La Raza,* and *Mestiza/o*. Because this is a course in Chicana/o and Latina/o psychology, I spend some time discussing the historical background demographics of the four main Latina/o groups in the United States, Chicana/os or Mexican Americans, Cuban Americans, Central Americans, and Puerto Ricans. However, given the current demographics in the state of Washington and neighboring western states, the emphasis in this course is on Chicana/o or Mexican American populations. A similar course located in the Northeast or Southeast might emphasize Puerto Rican or Cuban American populations, respectively. My coverage of demographic information includes population distribution, geography, educational attainment, employment, earnings, poverty, generational immigration, family type, size, and income, language status, and socioeconomic status.

Course coverage then moves to cultural characteristics and descriptors including gender roles (e.g., machismo, *marianismo*), Chicana feminist theory, interpersonal communication styles (e.g., *personalismo, confianza, simpatía*), family dynamics (e.g., *la familia, compadrazco, respeto, fatalismo*), and religion and folk beliefs (e.g., Catholicism, *curanderismo*). The popular movie "Mi Familia" illustrated many cultural and ethnic aspects within a sociohistorical framework and also demonstrated various levels of acculturation and ethnic identity in the variety of characters, thus setting the stage for a discussion of these concepts. Chicana/o students enrolled in the class and I find it necessary and a little fun to translate some of the dialogue and Chicana/o slang used throughout the film for other students in the class (e.g., *cabron, carnal, pachuco, gabacho*, etc.). We then turn to coverage of models of Chicana/o and Latina/o ethnic identity development while introducing and operationalizing concepts of ethnic identity, enculturation, and acculturation. Specific models of Chicana/o and

Latina/o identity development by Cuéllar, Arnold, and Maldonado (1995), Bernal and Knight (1993), Ruiz, (1990), and Marín, (1992), as well as more generic identity development models by Atkinson, Morten, and Sue (1982) and Phinney (1993) are covered in some depth. As the anthropologist Michael M. J. Fischer (cited in Sánchez, 1993) stated in regard to ethnicity:

> Ethnicity is not something that is simply passed on from generation to generation, taught and learned; it is something dynamic, often unsuccessfully repressed or avoided. It can be potent even when not consciously taught; it is something that institutionalized teaching easily makes chauvinist, sterile, and superficial, something that emerges in full—often liberating—flower only through struggle. (p. 12)

The writings of Roberto Rodriguez (1997) and Richard Rodriguez (1982) illustrated Fischer's point of view perhaps better than the usual academic theorizing on ethnicity and are thus required reading for the course. *The X in La Raza* (Rodriguez, 1997) represents a call for the reaffirmation of Chicana/o or Xicana/o identity, which includes resistance, defiance, and reclaiming indigenous roots. In *Hunger of Memory*, Richard Rodriguez (1982) struggles with his Mexican identity and alienation from his family while striving for middle-class assimilation, which results in strong opinions against affirmative action and bilingual education. The videos "Mi Familia," "Challenging Hispanic Stereotypes" (Moyers, 1994) and "Biculturalism and Acculturation Among Latinos" (Cuéllar, 1991) are also used to illustrate the complexity of ethnicity and ethnic identity and to provide real first-person accounts of issues facing Chicana/o and Latina/o people, and affect students on an emotional level sometimes missing from academic readings.

The next section of the course deals with issues of education and higher education. In my view, Padilla et al. (1991) serves as an excellent single reference summary of the issues of bilingual education as related to the political motivations of the English-only movement. In my lecture for these discussions, I draw upon the dialogue between Baker (1987) and Willig (1985, 1987) and the work of Hakuta (1986) in reference to bilingual education, and Darder, Torres, and Gutiérrez (1997) for issues relevant to higher education (e.g., recruitment, retention, academic climate, etc.). The educational portion of the "Chicano!" film series, along with the film "English Only in America" (Diack, 1997) supplements readings and lectures in this area.

Because I am a counseling psychologist, the next section of the course focuses on more applied and practical issues associated with the field of Chicana/o psychology, including general health care issues such as psychological well-being, and underutilization of services, including cultural, geographical, and language barriers. We also cover various clinical issues specific to Chicana/o and Latina/o populations (e.g., *ataques de nervious, susto, mal ojo*, interventions for gang members, etc.), along with culturally appropriate models of intervention and assessment for a variety of culture-specific general clinical disorders. In addition to the required readings for the course, my lecture is supplemented by the writings of Comas-Díaz (1989), Casas and Vasquez (1996), and Velásquez and Callahan (1992). Drawing from the work of Torrey (1983) and, more recently Fisher, Jome, and Atkinson (1998), on universal healing conditions, I also cover many of the factors common to psychotherapy approaches (e.g., the therapeutic relationship, a shared world view, a ritual or procedure, client expectations, etc.) and make the case that perhaps curanderos and counselors are not so different in their intervention strategies. In addition, the moderating effects of acculturation and ethnic identity and their assessment in relation to clinical intervention are continually stressed, especially with regard to intelligence and personality assessment. Lecture and readings are supplemented by videos by Arredondo (1994) and Comas-Díaz (APA, 1996). The text *Pychological Interventions and Research with Latino Populations* by Garcia and Zea (1997) includes excellent chapters covering the previous issues.

The final part of the course covers research issues with Chicana/o and Latina/o populations in general (e.g., sample definitions, moderating variables), especially with respect to treatment outcome or preference for ethnically similar counselors as reflected in the readings by Lopez, Lopez, and Fong (1991), Lopez and Lopez (1993), and Atkinson and Wampold (1993). Because the methodological issue in these writings deals with the question of how preferences are assessed, I ask class members to place themselves in the role of a client in the setting of a first intake interview in order to assess the external validity of the methods that are advocated by the respective authors. Interestingly, the class variations often mirror the researchers' viewpoints, especially in terms of ethnicity or ethnic identification.

This single course may serve as a guide for issues that may be addressed through an integration design in professional psychology programs.

PRACTICUM AND INTERNSHIP TRAINING AND SUPERVISION

Practicum and internship placements with Chicana/o clientele in Chicana/o communities need to be developed and provided by training agencies to prepare students for culturally relevant treatment. It is only through the provision of such training experiences that students gain a hands-on appreciation of external, systemic constraints, factors affecting underutilization of psychological services, and culturally determined health-seeking practices (Prieto et al., 2001). In preparing students for work with Chicana/o clientele, supervisors who are knowledgeable of Chicana/o culture, treatment modalities, and so on must be utilized. In addition, supervisors must be trained in providing supervision and training, especially with regard to dealing with culturally diverse clients and students. The processes that trainees undergo in developing clinical skills relevant to issues of diversity have been outlined by López et al. (1989) and Stoltenberg, McNeill, and Delworth (1998), especially regarding a focus on self-awareness. As noted by González (1997), Spanish may become the "language of affect" for both Chicana/o clients and therapists. Other supervisory issues include differing levels of ethnic and cultural identity of both the supervisor and supervisee and their effect on the supervisory relationship (D'Andrea & Daniels, 1997; Stone, 1997). Chicana/o students' struggles with their own ethnic identity development (Vasquez & McKinley, 1982) and racist and discriminatory experiences in graduate programs (McNeill et al., 1995; Zuniga, 1997) should also be addressed within supervisory relationships, as supervisors must take the primary responsibility to create an environment in which these issues are viewed as relevant to supervisees' personal and professional development and are openly dealt with (Stoltenberg et al., 1998).

SPECIALIZED TRAINING PROGRAMS

An innovative program offered by Our Lady of the Lake University in San Antonio, Texas, provides an excellent example of a bilingual training program serving a large Chicana/o community in which, of 300 bilingual licensed psychologists in San Antonio, only 11 provided services in Spanish (Biever et al., 2002; Clay, 2001). This certificate program offers 21 semester hours of courses, including Latina/o Psychology, Theories of Multicultural Counseling, and Sociocultural Foundations of Counseling Mexicans and Mexican Americans, as well as rigorous training in professional and technical Spanish-language skills (Biever, Gonzalez, Servin-Lopez, & Castano, 2002). Courses are taught progressively in English, bilingually, and in Spanish. In addition, students spend at least 8 hours a week at bilingual practicum sites and a semester supervising others at a bilingual site. Optional practicum opportunities also exist in conjunction with universities in Mexico. A 4-week condensed version of the certificate program is also offered through a summer institute for bilingual psychologists. As students develop Spanish-language skills, they also become immersed in Chicana/o and Latina/o culture.

The advantages of this program are evident as Latina/os and Anglos engage in a wide range of diagnostic and therapeutic professional duties in Spanish and learn how to address situations such as family therapy sessions in which some family members speak Spanish while others choose English (Clay, 2001). Initial evaluation of this program was positive (Biever et al., 2002).

FUTURE TRAINING POSSIBILITIES AND RECOMMENDATIONS

Latina/os in Psychology

Bernal (Epilogue) documented the historical and ongoing scarcity of Chicana/o and Latina/o psychologists. Universities such as the University of Montana, Utah State University, and University of North Dakota provide innovative strategies through recruitment of American Indians into psychology (AIIP) programs; the AIIP program at Oklahoma State University serves as a useful model to potentially apply to Chicana/o and Latina/o students as well. The stated goals for this federally funded program (Chaney, 1999) are to:

- Provide outreach and recruitment for mental health careers to American Indian communities nation wide.
- Develop liaisons with tribal communities, university-affiliated programs, and other entities to promote the education of American Indian students.
- Provide stipends to undergraduate and graduate students to pursue a career in psychology.
- Provide psychological services to underserved American Indian communities by establishing training opportunities for psychology graduate students in those communities.

In addition, AIIP offers summer enrichment programs for research with faculty and graduate students in counseling, clinical, school, and experimental psychology, clinical placements with tribal health care or social service agencies, and professional development seminars with guest speakers on topics relevant to American Indian psychology (Chaney). One can easily envision a similar program with related goals and activities extended to Chicana/o students for bilingual work in Chicana/o and Latina/o communities.

Western Interstate Commission of Higher Education's Doctoral Scholars Program

The Western Interstate Commission of Higher Education's (WICHE) Doctoral Scholars Program was established in 1994 with the primary goal of increasing the representation of ethnic minorities in faculty careers in higher education. This effort has become nation wide as WICHE merged with the New England Board of Higher Education and the Southern Regional Educational Board to create a Compact for Faculty Diversity, whose mission is to address the national problem of minority underrepresentation in higher education. As described by Hill, Castillo, Ngu, and Pepion (1999), and implemented in conjunction with the counseling psychology program at the University of Utah, the program identifies doctoral students with an interest in pursuing academic careers, provides financial support, creates provisions to train and support a faculty mentor, and sponsors an annual institute to build both formal and informal support networks and promote academic mentoring and training. Thus, ethnic minority graduate students are matched with a faculty mentor and supported financially during their graduate tenure through cooperative agreements between the home department, the university, and WICHE. Increased participation in the WICHE Doctoral Scholars Program by Chicana/o and Latina/o students and faculty members could go a long way in addressing the crucial shortage of Chicana/o and Latina/o faculty members in professional psychology programs.

We have discussed a number of cultural competencies for consideration by educators and supervisors in training students or professionals to work with Chicana/o clientele. These have ranged from traditional MCC-based competencies such as knowledge, skills, and awareness (Sue & Sue, 1999) to more specific domains concerning Chicana/os' acculturation and world view, their use of the Spanish language, and the appropriate use of clinical assessment procedures and instruments. Finally, we presented a comprehensive course on Chicana/o psychology developed and offered by McNeill.

Continued efforts to meet the needs of Chicana/o clientele is critical and the points raised in this chapter offer an initial base on which researchers and clinicians can concentrate. The mental health professions can no longer afford to ignore the needs of the growing and increasingly politically and economically powerful Chicana/o population in the United States. Those professional training programs and service agencies that currently are forward thinking and culturally sensitive will be the pace setters for the future of Chicana/o mental health services, and can establish the benchmark for others to follow. We offer encouragement to all those persons and institutions who have delivered effective and culturally appropriate services to all Chicana/os and will continue to do so.

REFERENCES

Abreu, J. M., Chung, R. H. G., & Atkinson, D. R. (2000). Multicultural counseling training: Past, present, and future directions. *The Counseling Psychologist, 28,* 641–656.

Acosta, F. X., & Cristo, M. H. (1981). Development of a bilingual interpreter program: An alternative model for Spanish-speaking services. *Professional Psychology, 12,* 474–482.

Allison, K., Crawford, I., Echemendia, R., Robinson, L., & Knepp, D. (1994). Human diversity and professional competence: Training in clinical and counseling psychology revisited. *American Psychologist, 49,* 792–796.

Allison, K. W., Echemendia, R. J., Crawford, I., & Robinson, W. L. (1996). Predicting cultural competence: Implications for practice and training. *Professional Psychology: Research and Practice, 27,* 386–393.

Altarriba, J., & Bauer, L. M. (1998). Counseling Cuban Americans. In D. R. Atkinson, G. Morten, & D. W. Sue (Eds.), *Counseling American minorities* (5th ed., pp. 280–296). New York: McGraw-Hill.

Altarriba, J., & Santiago-Rivera, A. L. (1994). Current perspectives on using linguistic and cultural factors in counseling the Hispanic client. *Professional Psychology: Research and Practice, 25,* 388–397.

American Psychological Association. (1993). Guidelines for providers of psychological services to ethnic, linguistic, and culturally diverse populations. *American Psychologist, 48,* 45–48.

American Psychological Association. (Producer). (1996). *Ethnocultural psychotherapy* [Film]. (Available from American Psychological Association Psychotherapy Videotape Series)

American Psychological Association. (2000). *Guidelines and principles for accreditation of programs in professional psychology.* Washington, DC: Author.

Arredondo, P. (1991). Counseling Latinas. In C. C. Lee & B. L. Richardson (Eds.), *Multicultural issues in counseling: New approaches to diversity* (pp. 143–156). Alexandria, VA: American Association for Counseling and Development.

Arredondo, P. (Producer). (1994). *Specifics of practice for counseling with Latins* [Film]. (Available from Microtraining Associates, Inc., Box 9641, North Amherst, MA 01059–9641)

Arredondo, P., Toporek, R., Brown, S. P., & Jones, J. (1996). Operationalization of the multicultural counseling competencies. *Journal of Multicultural Counseling and Development, 24,* 42–78.

Atkinson, D. R., Morten, G., & Sue, D. W. (1983). *Counseling American minorities.* Dubuque, IA: Brown.

Baker, K. (1987). Comments on Willig's "A meta-analysis of selected studies in the effectiveness of bilingual education." *Review of Educational Research, 57,* 351–362.

Bamford, K. W. (1991). Bilingual issues in mental health assessment and treatment. *Hispanic Journal of Behavioral Sciences, 13,* 377–390.

Barón, A., & Constantine, M. G. (1997). A conceptual framework for conducting psychotherapy with Mexican-American college students. In J. G. Garcia & M. C. Zea (Eds.), *Psychological interventions and research with Latino populations* (pp. 108–124). Boston: Allyn and Bacon.

Bean, R. A., Perry, B. J., & Bedell, T. M. (2001). Developing culturally competent marriage and family therapists: Guidelines for working with Hispanic families. *Journal of Marital and Family Therapy, 27,* 43–54.

Bernal, M., & Castro, F. (1994). Are clinical psychologists prepared for service and research with ethnic minorities? Report of a decade of progress. *American Psychologist, 49,* 797–805.

Bernal, M. E., & Knight, G. P. (1993). *Ethnic identity: Formation and transmission among Hispanics and other minorities.* Albany: State University of New York Press.

Biever, J. L., Castaño, T., de los Fuentes, C. G., Servín-López, S., Sprouts, C., & Tripp, C. (2002). The role of language in training psychologists to work with Hispanic clients. *Professional Psychology: Research and Practice, 33,* 330–336.

Casas, J. M., & Vasquez, M. J. T. (1996). Counseling the Hispanic: A guiding framework for a diverse population. In P. B. Pedersen, J. G. Draguns, W. J. Lonner, & J. E. Trimble (Eds.), *Counseling across cultures* (pp. 146–176). Thousand Oaks, CA: Sage.

Clay, R. A. (2001, February). Training that's more than bilingual. *APA Monitor, 32,* 70–72.

Comas-Díaz, L. (1989). Culturally relevant issues and treatment implications for Hispanics. In D. R. Koslow & E. P. Salett (Eds.), *Crossing cultures in mental health* (pp. 31–48). Washington, DC: SIETAR International.

Constantine, M. G., & Ladany, N. (2000). Self-report multicultural competence scales: Their relation to social desirability attitudes and multicultural case conceptualization ability. *Journal of Counseling Psychology, 47,* 155–164.

Copeland, E. J. (1987). Cross-cultural awareness: A conceptual model. *Counselor Education and Supervision, 78,* 270–289.

Cuéllar, I., Arnold, B., & Maldonado, R. (1995). Acculturation rating scale for Mexican Americans-II: A revision of the original ARMSA Scale. *Hispanic Journal of Behavioral Sciences, 17,* 1–12.

Cuéllar, I., & Gonzalez, G. (2000). Cultural identity description and cultural formulation for Hispanics. In R. H. Dana (Ed.), *Handbook of cross-cultural and multicultural personality assessment* (pp. 605–621). Mahwah, NJ: Lawrence Erlbaum Associates.

Cuéllar, L. (Producer). (1991). *Biculturalism and acculturation among Latinos* [Film]. (Available from Films for the Humanities and Sciences, Box 2053, Princeton, NJ, 0543–2053)

Dana, R. H. (1993). *Multicultural assessment perspectives for professional psychology.* Boston: Allyn and Bacon.

Dana, R. H. (2000). Psychological assessment in the diagnosis and treatment of ethnic group members. In J. Aponte & J. Whol (Eds.), *Psychological interventions and cultural diversity* (2nd ed., pp. 59–74). Needham Heights, MA: Allyn and Bacon.

Dana, R. H., Behn, J. D., & Gonwa, T. (1992). A checklist for the examination of cultural competence in social service agencies. *Research on Social Work Practice, 2,* 220–233.

Darder, A., Torres, R. D., & Gutiérrez, H. (Eds.). (1997). *Latinos and education: A critical reader.* New York: Routledge.

Delgado-Romero, E. A. (2001). Counseling a Hispanic/Latino client—Mr. X. *Journal of Mental Health Counseling, 23,* 207–221.

Department of Health and Human Services, U.S. Public Health Service. (2001). *Mental health: Culture, race, and ethnicity. A Supplement to mental health: A report of the Surgeon General.*

Diack, A. (Producer). (1997). *English only in America?* [Film]. (Available from Films for the Humanities and Sciences, Box 2053, Princeton, NJ 0543–2053)

Falicov, C. J. (1996). Mexican families. In M. McGoldrick, J. Giordano, & J. K. Pearce (Eds.), *Ethnicity and family therapy* (2nd ed., pp. 169–182). New York: Guilford Press.

Falicov, C. J. (1998). *Latino families in therapy: A guide to multicultural practice.* New York: Guilford Press.

Fischer, A. R., Jome, L. M., & Atkinson, D. R. (1998). Reconceptualizing multicultural counseling: Universal healing conditions in a culturally specific context. *The Counseling Psychologist, 26,* 525–588.

Galán, H. (Producer). (1996). *Chicano!* [Film] (Available from the Public Broadcasting System)

Garcia, J. G., & Zea, M. C. (Eds.). (1997). *Psychological interventions and research with Latino populations.* Boston: Allyn and Bacon.

Geiger, L. (1994). Ethnic match and client characteristics as predictors of treatment outcome for anxiety disorders. *Dissertation Abstracts International, 54,* 4387.

Geisinger, K. F. (Ed.). (1992). *Psychological testing of Hispanics.* Washington, DC: American Psychological Association.

Geisinger, K. F. (1994). Cross-cultural normative assessment: Translation and adaptation issues influencing the normative interpretation of assessment instruments. *Psychological Assessment, 6,* 304–312.

Glaser, N., & Moynihan, D. P. (1963). *Beyond the melting pot.* Cambridge, MA: MIT Press.

Gloria, A. M., & Rodriguez, E. R. (2000). Counseling Latino university students: Psychosociocultural issues for consideration. *Journal of Counseling and Development, 78,* 145–154.

Gonzalez, G. M. (1997). The emergence of Chicanos in the twenty-first century: Implications for counseling, research, and policy. *Journal of Multicultural Counseling and Development, 25,* 94–106.

Hakuta, K. (1986). *Mirror of language: The debate on bilingualism.* New York: Basic Books.

Hill, R. D., Castillo, L. G., Ngu, L. Q., & Pepion, K. (1999). Mentoring ethnic minority students for careers in academia: The WICHE Doctoral Scholars Program. *The Counseling Psychologist, 27,* 827–845.

Hurtado, A. (1994). Does similarity breed respect? Interviewer evaluations of Mexican-descent respondents in a bilingual survey. *Public Opinion Quarterly, 58,* 77–95.

Jensen, J. R. (1973). *Educability and group differences.* New York: Harper and Row.

Jerrell, J. M. (1998). The effects of client-therapist match on service use and costs. *Administration and Policy in Mental Health, 23,* 119–126.

Johnson, S. D. (1987). Knowing that versus knowing how: Toward achieving expertise through multicultural training for counseling. *The Counseling Psychologist, 15,* 320–331.

Keegan, L. (1996). Use of alternative therapies among Mexican Americans in the Texas Rio Grande valley. *Journal of Holistic Nursing, 14,* 277–294.

Kline, F., Acosta, F. X., Austin, W., & Johnson, R. G. (1980). The misunderstood Spanish-speaking patient. *American Journal of Psychiatry, 137*, 1530–1533.

Koss-Chioino, J., & Vargas, L. (1999). *Working with Latino youth: Culture, development, and context.* San Francisco: Jossey-Bass.

LaFromboise, T., Coleman H., & Gerton, J. (1993). Psychological impact of bi-culturalism: Evidence and theory. *Psychological Bulletin, 114*, 395–412.

LeVine, E., & Franco, J. N. (1981). A reassessment of self-disclosure patterns among Anglo Americans and Hispanics. *Journal of Counseling Psychology, 28*, 522–524.

Lopez, S. R., Grover, K. P., Holland, D., Johnson, M. J., Kain, C. D., Kanel, K., Mellins, C. A., & Rhyne, M. C. (1989). Development of culturally sensitive psychotherapists. *Professional Psychology: Research and Practice, 20*, 369–376.

Macias, E. P., & Morales, L. S. (2000). Utilization of health care services among adults attending a health fair in south Los Angeles County. *Journal of Community Health, 25*, 35–46.

Malgady, R. G., Rogler, L. H., & Constantino, G. (1987). Ethnocultural and linguistic bias in mental health evaluation of Hispanics. *American Psychologist, 42*, 228–234.

Marcos, L. R. (1988). Understanding ethnicity in psychotherapy with Hispanic patients. *American Journal of Psychoanalysis, 48*, 35–42.

Marcos, L. R. (1994). The psychiatric examination of Hispanics: Across the language barrier. In R. G. Malgady & O. Rodriguez (Eds.), *Theoretical and conceptual issues in Hispanic mental health* (pp. 144–154). Melbourne, FL: Krieger.

Marcos, L. R., Urcuyo, L., Kesselman, M., & Alpert, M. (1973). The language barrier in evaluating Spanish-American patients. *Archives of General Psychiatry, 29*, 655–659.

Marín, G. (1992). Issues in the measurement of acculturation among Hispanics. In K. F. Geisinger (Ed.), *Psychological testing of Hispanics* (pp. 235–251). Washington, DC: American Psychological Association.

Marín, G., & Marín, B. (1991). *Research with Hispanic populations.* Newbury Park, CA: Sage.

Martinez, J. L. (Ed.). (1977). *Chicano psychology.* New York: Academic Press.

Martinez, J. L., & Mendoza, R. H. (Eds.). (1984). *Chicano psychology* (2nd ed.). New York: Academic Press.

McNeill, B. W. (1999). *Development of a course in Chicano/Latino psychology: An academic odyssey.* East Lansing, MI: Julian Samora Research Institute.

McNeill, B. W., Hom, K. L., & Perez, J. A. (1995). The training and supervisory needs of racial and ethnic minority students. *Journal of Multicultural Counseling and Development, 23*, 246–258.

McNeill, B. W., Prieto, L. P., Niemann, Y. F., Pizarro, M., Vera, E. M., & Gómez, S. P. (2001). Current directions in Chicana/o psychology. *The Counseling Psychologist, 29*, 5–17.

Moyers, B. (Producer). (1994). *Challenging Hispanic stereotypes: Aturo Madrid* [Film]. (Available from Films for the Humanities and Sciences, Box 2053, Princeton, NJ 0543–2053)

Murdock, N. L., Alcorn, J., Heesacker, M., & Stoltenberg, C. (1998). Model training program in counseling psychology. *The Counseling Psychologist, 26*, 658–672.

Organista, K. C. (2000). Latinos. In J. R. White & A. S. Freeman (Eds.), *Cognitive-behavioral group therapy: For specific problems and populations* (pp. 281–303). Washington, DC: American Psychological Association.

Padilla, A. M. (1995). *Hispanic psychology: Critical issues in theory and research.* Thousand Oaks, CA: Sage.

Padilla, A. M., Lindholm, K. J., Chen, A., Duran, R., Hakuta, K., Lambert, W., & Tucker, G. R. (1991). The English-only movement: Myths, reality, and implications for psychology. *American Psychologist, 46*, 120–130.

Paniagua, F. A. (1998). *Assessing and treating culturally diverse clients* (2nd ed.). Thousand Oaks, CA: Sage.

Pederson, P. B. (1981). The cultural inclusiveness of counseling. In P. B. Pederson, J. G. Draguns, W. J. Lonner, & J. E. Trimble (Eds.), *Counseling across cultures* (2nd ed., pp. 22–58). Honolulu: University of Hawaii Press.

Pennack-Roman, M. (1992). Interpreting test performance in selective admissions for Hispanic students. In K. Geisinger (Ed.), *Psychological testing of Hispanics* (pp. 99–136). Washington, DC: American Psychological Association.

Perez, J. E. (1999). Integration of cognitive-behavioral and interpersonal therapies for Latinos: An argument for technical eclecticism. *Journal of Contemporary Psychotherapy, 29*, 169–183.

Phinney, J. S. (1993). A three-stage model of ethnic identity development in adolescence. In M. E. Bernal & G. P. Knight (Eds.), *Ethnic identity: Formation and transmission among Hispanics and other minorities* (pp. 61–79). Albany: State University of New York Press.

Pizarro, M., & Vera, E. M. (2001). Chicana/o ethnic identity research: Lessons for researchers and counselors. *The Counseling Psychologist, 29*, 91–117.

Preciado, J., & Henry, M. (1997). Linguistic barriers in health education and services. In J. G. Garcia & M. C. Zea (Eds.), *Psychological interventions and research with Latino populations* (pp. 235–254). Needham Heights, MA: Allyn and Bacon.

Prieto, L. R., McNeill, B. W., Walls, R. G., & Gómez, S. P. (2001). Chicana/os and mental health services: An overview of utilization, counselor preference, and assessment issues. *The Counseling Psychologist, 29,* 18–54.

Ramos-Sanchez, L., Atkinson, D. R., & Fraga, E. D. (1999). Mexican Americans' bilingual ability, counselor bilingualism cues, counselor ethnicity, and perceived counselor credibility. *Journal of Counseling Psychology, 46,* 125–131.

Rappaport, J. (1997). *Community psychology: Values, research, and action.* New York: Holt, Reinhart, and Winston.

Ridley, C. R., Mendoza, D. W., & Kanitz, B. E. (1994). Multicultural training: Reexamination, operationalization, and integration. *The Counseling Psychologist, 22,* 227–289.

Risser, A. L., & Mazur, L. J. (1995). Use of folk remedies in a Hispanic population. *Archives of Pediatric Adolescent Medicine, 149,* 978–981.

Rogler, L. H., Cortes, D. E., & Malgady, R. G. (1991). Acculturation and mental health status among Hispanics: Convergence and new directions for research. *American Psychologist, 46,* 585–597.

Rogler, L. H., Malgady, R. G., Constantino, G., & Blumenthal, R. (1987). What do culturally sensitive mental health services mean? The case of Hispanics. *American Psychologist, 42,* 565–570.

Romero, A. J. (2001). Assessing and treating Latinos: Overview of research. In I. Cuellar & F. A. Paniagua (Eds.), *Handbook of multicultural mental health* (pp. 209–223). San Diego: Academic Press.

Ruelas, S. R., Atkinson, D. R., & Ramos-Sanchez, L. (1998). Counselor helping model, participant ethnicity and acculturation level, and perceived counselor credibility. *Journal of Counseling Psychology, 45,* 98–103.

Ruiz, A. S. (1990). Ethnic identity: Crisis and resolution. *Journal of Multicultural Counseling and Development, 18,* 29–40.

Sánchez, G. J. (1993). *Becoming Mexican American: Ethnicity, culture, and identity in Chicano Los Angeles, 1900–1945.* New York: Oxford University Press.

Sandoval, J. H., Frisby, C. L., Geisinger, K. F., Scheuneman, J. D., & Grenier, J. R. (Eds.). (1998). *Test interpretation and diversity: Achieving equity in assessment.* Washington, DC: American Psychological Association.

Sandoval, M. C., & De La Roza, H. C. (1986). A cultural perspective for serving the Hispanic client. In H. P. Lefley & P. B. Pedersen (Eds.), *Cross-cultural training for mental health professionals* (pp. 151–181). Springfield, IL: Charles C. Thomas.

Santiago-Rivera, A. L. (1995). Developing a culturally sensitive treatment modality for bilingual Spanish-speaking clients: Incorporating language and culture in counseling. *Journal of Counseling and Development, 74,* 12–17.

Santiago-Rivera, A. L., & Altarriba, J. (2002). The role of language in therapy with the Spanish-English bilingual client. *Professional Psychology: Research and Practice, 33,* 30–38.

Santiago-Rivera, A. L., Arredondo, P., & Gallardo-Cooper, M. (2002). *Counseling Latinos and la familia: A practical guide.* Thousand Oaks, CA: Sage.

Skaer, T. L., Robison, L. M., Sclar, D. A., & Harding, G. H. (1996). Utilization of curanderos among foreign-born Mexican American women attending migrant health clinics. *Journal of Cultural Diversity, 3,* 29–34.

Snowden, L. R., & Hu, T. (1997). Ethnic differences in mental health services use among the severely mentally ill. *Journal of Community Psychology, 25,* 235–247.

Stoltenberg, C. D., McNeill, B. W., & Delworth, U. (1998). *IDM supervision: An integrated development model for supervision counselors and therapists.* San Francisco: Jossey-Bass.

Sue, D. W. (1998). In search of cultural competence in psychology and counseling. *American Psychologist, 53,* 440–448.

Sue, D. W. (2001). Multidimensional facets of cultural competence. *The Counseling Psychologist, 29,* 790–821.

Sue, D. W., Arredondo, P., & McDavis, R. J. (1992). Multicultural counseling competencies and standards: A call to the profession. *Journal of Counseling and Development, 70,* 477–486.

Sue, D. W., Bernier, J. E., Durran, A., Feinberg, L., Pedersen, P., Smith, E. J., & Vasquez-Nuttall, E. (1982). Position paper: Cross-cultural counseling competencies. *The Counseling Psychologist, 10,* 45–52.

Sue, D. W., & Sue, D. (1999). *Counseling the culturally different: Theory and practice* (3rd ed.). New York: Wiley and Sons.

Sue, S., Fujino, D. C., Hu, L., Takeuchi, D. T., & Zane, N. (1991). Community mental health services for ethnic minority groups: A test of the cultural responsiveness hypothesis. *Journal of Consulting and Clinical Psychology, 59,* 533–540.

Sue, S., Zane, N., & Young, K. (1994). Research on psychotherapy with culturally diverse populations. In A. Bergin & S. Garfield (Eds.), *Handbook of psychotherapy and behavior change* (4th ed., pp. 783–817). New York: Wiley.

Suzuzki, L. A., & Kugler, J. F. (1995). Intelligence and personality assessment: Multicultural perspectives. In J. G. Ponterotto, J. M. Casas, L. A. Suzuki, & C. M. Alexander (Eds.), *Handbook of multicultural counseling* (pp. 493–515). Thousand Oaks, CA: Sage.

Torrey, E. F. (1983). *The Mind Game: Witchdoctors and Psychiatrists.* New York: Aronson.

VandeCreek, L., & Merrill, W. (1990). Mental health services for the culturally different. In G. Stricker, E. Davis-Russell, E. Bourg, E. Duran, W. R. Hammond, J. McHolland, K. Polite, & B. E. Vaughn (Eds.), *Toward ethnic diversification in psychology education and training* (pp. 195–201). Washington, DC: American Psychological Association.

Vasquez, M. J., & McKinley, D. (1982). Supervision: A conceptual model-reactions and extension. *The Counseling Psychologist, 10,* 59–63.

Vasquez, M. J. T., & Baron, A. (1988). The psychology of the Chicano experience: A sample course structure. In P. A. Bronstein & K. Quina (Eds.), *Teaching a psychology of people: Resources for gender and sociocultural awareness* (pp. 147–155). Washington, DC: American Psychological Association.

Velásquez, R. J. (Ed.). (1997). Counseling Mexican Americans/Chicanos [Special issue]. *Journal of Multicultural Counseling and Development, 25*(2).

Velásquez, R. J., Ayala, G. X., & Mendoza, S. A. (1998). *Psychodiagnostic assessment of Latina/os (MMPI, MMPI-2, and MMPI-A results): A comprehensive resource manual.* East Lansing, MI: Julian Samora Research Institute.

Velásquez, R. J., & Callahan, W. J. (1992). Psychological testing of Hispanic Americans in clinical settings: Overview issues. In K. F. Geisinger (Ed.), *Psychological testing of Hispanics* (pp. 253–265). Washington, DC: American Psychological Association.

Vera, E. M., & Speight, S. L. (2003). Multicultural competence, social justice, and counseling psychology: Expanding our roles. *The Counseling Psychologist, 31,* 253–272.

Willig, A. C. (1985). A meta-analysis of selected studies on the effectiveness of bilingual education. *Review of Educational Research, 57,* 269–317.

Willig, A. C. (1987). Examining bilingual education research through meta-analysis and narrative review: A response to Baker. *Review of Educational Research, 57,* 363–376.

Yeh, M., Eastman, K., & Cheung, M. K. (1994). Children and adolescents in community health centers: Does the ethnicity or the language of the therapist matter? *Journal of Community Psychology, 22,* 153–163.

Yutrzenka, B. A. (1995). Making a case for training in ethnic and cultural diversity in increasing treatment efficacy. *Journal of Counseling and Clinical Psychology, 63,* 197–206.

Zuniga, M. E. (1987). Mexican-American clinical training: A pilot project. *Journal of Social Work Education, 23,* 11–20.

Appendix

COPSY 457/CAC 457
CHICANA/O LATINA/O PSYCHOLOGY

Summer 2001

Instructor: Brian McNeill, Ph.D.
Office: 352 Cleveland Hall
Phone: (509) 335–6477
Classrooms: WHETS WSUTC/Pullman
E-Mail: mcneill@mail.wsu.edu
Office Hours: By appointment

Course Objectives:

1. Examine the current psychosocial research and literature relevant to the mental health and psychological well being of Chicana/o Latina/o populations, including influences of acculturation, ethnic identity, and underutilization of psychological services.
2. Examine the sociopolitical issues relevant to Chicanos/Latinos.
3. Increase awareness and understanding of culturally relevant counseling models and methods of intervention as differentiated from standard models of intervention.

Course Requirements:

1. A research paper/Literature review examining a specific issue within Chicana/o Latina/o Psychology (35%). Students will receive specific individual guidance for research papers/projects. These projects may take the form of a review of a book related to Chicana/o Latina/o populations, a term paper, research of a topical area, or other possibilities negotiated with me. Projects will be briefly presented in class.
2. Midterm or Final Examination. (35%). Students will complete a short answer/essay type exam also focused on the integration and synthesis of what you have learned over the course of the semester.
3. Course participation/involvement. (30%). All students will be required to complete weekly assigned readings prior to class and participate in class/small group discussions, etc. Please be aware that if you do not attend class, you cannot participate and your grade may be negatively effected.

Grading/Evaluation:

Grades will be assigned on a percentage basis, i.e., 93% = A, 90% = A–, 87% = B+, 83% = B, etc. Assignments are due at the beginning of the class on the day noted. I reserve the right to penalize or not accept assignments turned in after the due date. Grades of Incomplete (I) are only assigned in extreme or unusual circumstances, and in some cases may result in a penalty. Any student in this course who has a disability that prevents the fullest expression of ability should contact me personally as soon as possible so that we can discuss class requirements and accommodations.

Texts:

García, J. G., & Zéa, M. C. (1997). *Psychological interventions and research with latino populations.* Allyn & Bacon: Boston.

Rodriguez, R. (1997). *The X in La Raza II.* Roberto Rodriquez: Alburquerque.

Rodriguez, R. (1982). *Hunger of memory: The education of Richard Rodriguez.* Bantum Books: New York.

Readings:

Altarriba, J., & Santiago-Rivera, A. L. (1994). Current perspectives on using linguistic and cultural factors in counseling the Hispanic client. *Professional Psychology: Research and Practice, 25,* 388–397.

Atkinson, D. R., Casas, A., Abreu, J. (1992). Mexican-American acculturation, counselor ethnicity and cultural sensitivity, and perceived counselor competence. *Journal of Counseling Psychology, 39,* 515–520.

Atkinson, D. R., & Wampold, B. E., (1993). Mexican-Americans' initial preferences for counselors: Simple choice can be misleading comment on Lopez, Lopez, and Fong (1991). *Journal of Counseling Psychology, 40,* 245–248.

Coleman, H. L., Wampold, B. E., & Casali, S. L. (1995). Ethnic minorities' ratings of ethnically similar and European American counselors: A meta-analysis. *Journal of Counseling Psychology. 42,* 55–64.

Comas-Diaz, L., & Jacobsen, F. M. (1987). Ethnocultural identification in psychotherapy. *Psychiatry. 50,* 232–241.

Harris, M. L. (1998). Curanderismo and the DSM IV: Diagnostic and treatment implications for the Mexican-American Client. Occasional Paper No. 45. *Julian Samora Research Institute.*

Lopez, S. R., & Lopez, A. A. (1993). Mexican Americans' initial preferences for counselors: Research methodologies or researchers' values: Reply to Atkinson and Wampold (1993). *Journal of Counseling Psychology, 40,* 249–251.

Lopez, S. R., Lopez, A. A., & Fong, K. T. (1991), Mexican Americans' initial preferences for counselors: The role of ethnic factors. *Journal of Counseling Psychology, 38,* 487–496.

Malgady, R. G., Rogler, L. H., & Costantino, G. (1987). Ethnocultural and linguistic bias in mental health evaluation of hispanics. *American Psychologist, 42,* 228–234.

McNeill, B. W. (1999). Development of a course in Chicano/Latino Psychology: An Academic Odyssey.

McNeill, B. W., Prieto, L., Flores Niemann, Y., Pizarro, M., & Gómez, S. (2001). Current directions in Chicana/o psychology. *The Counseling Psychologist 29,* 5–18.

Niemann, Y. F. (2001). Stereotypes about Mexican-Americans: Implications for Counseling. *The Counseling Psychologist. 29,* 55–90.

Padilla, A. M., Lindholm, K. J., Chen, A., Duran, R., Hakuta, K., Lambert, W., Tucker, G. R. (1991). The english-only movement. *American Psychologist, 46,* 120–130.

Pizarro, M., & Vera, E. M. (2001). Reconstructing Chicana/o Identity Research: Implications for researchers and counselors. *The Counseling Psychologist. 29,* 91–117.

Prieto, L., McNeill, B. W., Walls, A., & Gómez, S. (2001). Chicana/os and mental health services: An overview of utilization, counselor preference, and assessment issues. *The Counseling Psychologist. 29,* 19–54.

Rogler, L. H., Malgady, R. G., Costantino, G., & Blumenthal, R. (1987). What do culturally sensitive mental health services mean? *American Psychologist, 42,* 565–570.

Rosado, J. W., Elias, M. J. (1993). Ecological and psychocultural mediators in the delivery of services for urban, culturally diverse Hispanic clients. *Professional Psychology: Research and Practice, 24,* 450–459.

Ruelas, S. R., Atkinson, D. R., & Ramos-Sanchez, L. (1998). Counselor helping model, participant ethnicity and acculturation level, and perceived counselor credibility. *Journal of Counseling Psychology, 45,* 98–103.

Sanchez, A. R., & Atkinson, D. R. (1983). Mexican-American cultural commitment, preference for counselor ethnicity, and willingness to use counseling. *Journal of Counseling Psychology, 30,* 215–220.

Zayas, L. H., & Solari, F. (1994). Early childhood socialization in Hispanic families: Context, cultural, and practice implications. *Professional Psychology: Research and Practice. 25,* 200–206.

Week	*Topic/Assignment*
1	Intro to course, Sociopolitical Context, Video—*Go back to Mexico!* Text-Chapter 1, McNeill (1999) Film—*Chicano History Series,* History of Chicano Psychology
	Chicano/Latino Demographics, History, (McNeill, 2001) Films—*Mexican Americans, Puerto Ricans, Central Americans*
	Family Structure, Values
	Chicano/Latino Cultural Characteristics, Gender Roles, Communication Styles, Religion, Folk Beliefs Text—Chapter 2 Film—*Mi Familia*
2	Issues of Acculturation, Ethnic Identity, Two views of Identity-Rodriguez (1997), Rodriguez (1982). Films—*Acculturation and Biculturation in Latinos, Challenging Hispanic Stereotypes.* Pizarro (2001), Niemann (2001)
	Bilingual and Higher Education, Padilla et al. (1991) Guest Speaker Films—*Chicano History Series, English Only in America?*
	Health Care Issues Text-Chapters 11–14, 5
	Psychological Well Being
3	Underutilization of Psychological Services. (Prieto, 2001)
	Sanchez & Atkinson (1983), Malgady et al. (1987), Coleman, et al. (1995).
	Culturally relevant assessment and interventions, Issues of IQ and Personality Assessment, Counselors and Curanderos: Common Factors in Treatment Atkinson, Casas, & Abreu (1992), Rogler et al. (1987) Altarriba & Santiago-Rivera (1994) Ruelas et al. (1998), Harris (1998).
4	Clinical Issues, Gang Involvement, Stereotyping, Alcohol Abuse Guest Speaker Text—Chapters 6–10, 4, Zayas & Solari (1994) Videos—Comas-Diaz, Arredondo

Models of Intervention
Comas-Diaz & Jacobsen (1987, 1991), Rosado & Ellis (1993)

Research Issues, Methodology: Lopez & Lopez (1993), Lopez, Lopez, & Fong, (1991), Atkinson & Wampold (1993)

Future Directions, Wrap up.

21

Quality de Vida: Browning Our Understanding of Quality of Life

Jason Duque Raley
J. Manuel Casas
Carla Victoria Corral
University of California, Santa Barbara

North of the U.S.-Mexico border, brown appears as the color of the future. The adjective accelerates, becomes a verb: "America is browning."

—Rodriguez (2002, p. xii)

In a recent book, essayist Richard Rodriguez (2002) offers a new way of seeing America: not as black or white but, rather, as brown. Working to understand the meaning Hispanics bring to American life, Rodriguez argues from a history of the interpenetration of European (White), African (Black), and American Indian (Red) genes, culture, and language. Latina/os are all of these and, at the same time, none of them. Increasingly, Rodriguez explains, so is America, but what does it mean to describe America in terms of *brown*? To be sure, the numbers of Brown people in America are growing. Rodriguez means for the reader to see something much less obvious. Specifically, he challenges the reader's way of thinking that lumps the world into received categories (like black and white), to look at the rich particulars of experience rather than easy generalizations about experience, and to begin seeing the complexity of not only Latina/os, but also of the world.

This idea of *brown*—as interpenetration, complexity, particularity—has helped us to better articulate our perspectives on the special subject of this chapter, the quality of life of Chicana/os and Latina/os in the United States. In fact, each of the three objectives that guide the chapter may be understood in terms of *browning*. First, as in other chapters in this volume, we focus on the increasing proportion of the U.S. population that may be described as Brown. This is the group typically labeled as Hispanic or Latina/o, sometimes further subdivided by national heritage (e.g., Cuban, Puerto Rican, Guatemalan, Chilean, etc.) and generational or political status (e.g.

455

Mexican, Mexican American, or Chicana/o).[1] Second, we develop a theoretical model of quality of life that is decidedly brown, or at least browner than the common model. In describing a browner conception of quality of life, we challenge simplistic approaches that define quality of life according to discrete, measurable variables such as socioeconomic status and education and that assume such definitions to be universally valid for persons of diverse ethnic and cultural groups. It is here that we rely most directly on Rodriguez' (2002) claims about brown as a way of understanding the world other than in terms of black and white. Finally, we argue for approaches to research and intervention that both respond to the increasing Chicana/o and Latina/o (i.e., Brown) population and reflect more careful, more complex (i.e., browner) theoretical understanding.

THE GROWING BROWN POPULATION

During the last 20 years, the racial or ethnic minority population of the United States has increased at a significant rate and is currently at 28.6% (Casas, Vasquez, & Ruiz de Esparza, 2002; U.S. Bureau of the Census, 2000b).[2] Among racial and ethnic minority groups, the Chicana/o and Latina/o rate of growth has been most significant, making them an especially notable segment of the racial and ethnic minority population. According to Census 2000, Latina/os number 35.3 million, or almost 13% of the total U.S. population (U.S. Bureau of the Census, 2001), 66% of whom are of Mexican ethnic origin. A comparison of the statistics obtained in 1990 with those obtained in 2000 clearly demonstrates that Latina/os are the fastest growing racial and ethnic group in the United States. During this 10-year period, the total U.S. population grew at a rate of 13.2%, while the Latina/o population grew at the extraordinary rate of 58% (U.S. Bureau of the Census, 2000c; U.S. Bureau of the Census, 2001). Given this rate of growth, it is likely that by the year 2050 Latina/os will number 98.2 million (U.S. Bureau of the Census, 2000a, 2000c). Based on current estimates, by the year 2050 the proportion of Latina/os in the population will impressively rise from 13% to 25%, making Latina/os the largest racial and ethnic group in the nation (National Coalition of Hispanic Health and Human Services Organizations [COSSMHO], 1999).

At the same time that their relative numbers are increasing, Chicana/os and Latina/os as a group seem to face a disproportionate number of challenges that cut across major aspects of their lives. They include, but are not limited to, socio-

---

[1] In this chapter, we use both *Hispanic* and *Latina/o* to name the group. When citing other sources, we use the authors' terminology. Where possible, our choice for describing an individual reflects that individual's expressed preference. In all other cases, we use *Latina/o*, a term that seems to best reflect contemporary preferences.

[2] The terms *racial* or *ethnic minority*, *linguistic minority*, and simply *minority* are used to designate that segment of the population that has traditionally been considered as non-White and has received differential and unequal treatment compared to the majority, White population. For a more detailed and comprehensive discussion of this term, see Ponterotto and Casas (1991). Within the context of this chapter, the individuals in the Latina/o group share a sociocultural, linguistic, and historical background and are often defined along ethnic, national, or cultural lines. Latina/os comprise a cultural, rather than racial, group.

economic status, educational achievement, health, mental health, and access to services.[3]

As of 1996, approximately 40% of all Latina/o children under the age of 17 were living in families with incomes below the poverty line and, given current education and labor market trends, poverty rates among Latino families are expected to persist (National Coalition of Hispanic Health and Human Services Organizations [COSSMHO], 1999). Latina/os continue to drop out of high school at a rate higher than that of any other major group in the United States (Kaufman, Kwon, Klein, & Chapman, 2000). Latina/o children under the age of 18 are almost twice as likely as African American children and three times as likely as non-Hispanic White children to be in poor to marginal health (National Coalition of Hispanic Health and Human Services Organizations [COSSMHO], 1999). According to 1996 Medical Expenditure Panel Survey, Latina/o-headed families were more likely to report significant barriers to health care than their African American or non-Hispanic White counterparts (National Coalition of Hispanic Health and Human Services Organizations [COSSMHO], 1999). Though the national incidence of teen pregnancy has declined, it remains highest among Latina girls (National Coalition of Hispanic Health and Human Services Organizations [COSSMHO], 1999). High-risk behaviors such as gang activity, substance use, and gun-related violence and other intentional injuries are often mentioned in statistics focusing on Latina/o youth.

We report these statistics because we believe that they are both true and important. They are true in the sense that they accurately capture some piece of reality, however circumscribed; they are important in that they reveal, in broad strokes, the relative position of Latina/os as a group in U.S. society. In short, the educational and socioeconomic achievements of Latina/os are increasing slowly, if at all, in contrast to the rapid increase in the number of Latina/os in the general population. Occupational, economic, and educational levels are symbols of status and power in the United States; whether or not a group has power or status can affect the well-being and access to opportunities for individual group members (McNeill et al., 2001; Sherif, 1982). The acknowledgement of the value of these statistics comes with a warning: They neither describe nor predict the experience or behavior of any given Brown person. Useful in the aggregate, such statistics do not tell us about what is actually going on for individuals.

Although the statistics justify our prolonged attention to the needs of Chicana/os and Latina/os (and our frustration with the reality they portray), we must also admit that they are insufficiently informative and, moreover, easy to misinterpret. The prominent and growing presence of Latina/os in the U.S., together with the number and nature of challenges they face, is forcing an increasing number of professionals (e.g., educators, researchers, social workers, and physical and mental health service providers) to think about their work with Chicana/os and Latina/os in mind. Latina/os may be different from these professionals in important ways, including ethnicity, language, and values and expectations for ways of being in the world. The

---

[3]For more comprehensive and in-depth demographic and statistical information relative to the problems (quality of life factors) that impact the Latina/o, the reader is referred to U.S. Bureau of the Census (2000a, 200b, 2000c), and especially National Coalition of Hispanic Health and Human Services Organizations (1999).

problem comes when professionals further presume that relevant dimensions of difference (or of similarity) include the same discrete categories as those just mentioned for Latina/os as a population group (e.g., socioeconomic status, education, health and mental health, etc.).

To be clear, the presumption of difference according to such measures exposes at least three problems for professionals:

1. Statistically significant group differences in socioeconomic, educational, and health categories do not necessarily reflect or claim to reflect the needs of particular individuals. Except as possible guides for inquiry, statistically significant group differences are not very useful to the professional who must recognize and respond to the local needs of a person.

2. Without careful thought, or in the absence of alternative information, professionals may find it easy to think of group conditions as sources of individual pathologies. For example, the fact that Chicana/o and Latina/o youth drop out of high school at a higher rate than their non-Chicana/o and Latina/o peers could encourage the characterization of an individual as at risk for dropping out, even without direct evidence to support such a characterization.

3. Statistically significant or not, big, discrete categories are not easy to operationalize, at least not in a way that is useful to professionals. In other words, even if they are closely associated with each other (and with Latina/os), categorical measures like socioeconomic status, education, and health resist fitting together into some explanatory model.

In the face of the problems that come from a reliance on statistical averages, professionals must turn to other ways of understanding the real, complicated lives of Chicana/os and Latina/os. Quality of life offers one way to talk and write about real, Brown lives in terms that reflect both a concern for justice and a desire to meet the needs of individuals.

SO WHAT IS QUALITY OF LIFE?

In their concern for understanding human behavior and experience, psychologists have long worried about the common-sense concept of quality of life (QOL). Historically viewed as life satisfaction or subjective well-being, QOL in psychological research is now sometimes referred to as *overall quality of life* or *global quality of life.* This is meant to distinguish the psychologist's use of the term from its widespread use among medical and other health professionals, many of whom concern themselves with *health-related quality of life,* especially the QOL for the sick or terminally ill. According to its use in medical fields, QOL offers a way for providers to think about patients' overall well-being, especially where chronic pain or infirmity may be managed but not eliminated. Even as its global, common-sense understanding makes QOL a powerful concept, researchers have struggled to face the challenge of defining, operationalizing, and measuring it in ways that both admit its complexity and make it available for analysis. While some researchers have sought to describe broad domains of QOL, others have defined more specific dimensions. Moreover, some researchers have grounded their conceptions of QOL in specific, existing psychological theory, and others have developed their conceptions from a collection of theories or, in some cases, derived them from existing data. In any case, researchers in psychology have undertaken several important efforts to define and operationalize overall QOL.

In exploring the philosophical underpinnings of QOL, McCall (1975) argued that the best approach is to measure the extent to which people's "happiness requirements" are met. Flanagan (1978, 1982) identified 15 dimensions of QOL: family relationships, religion and understanding life, passive recreation, having children, health and safety needs, friends, active recreation, creative expression, socializing, spouse relationship, learning, material comforts, work, community activities, public affairs, and an overall QOL. Flanagan's (1982) original 15-item Quality of Life Scale was derived from 6,500 critical incidents reported in interviews with 3,200 American adults of all ages and health status. Fujii (1999) discussed a theoretical model based on general needs theories (i.e., Alderfer, 1969; Maslow, 1954; Sirgy, 1986) that specifies four domains of QOL: physical, psychological, support, and existential.

A few researchers focused specifically on the QOL for Latina/os. To assess overall QOL, Mezzich et al. (2000) tried to validate a Spanish version of the health-related Quality of Life Index developed by Ferrans and Powers (1985, 1992). Designed to measure both overall QOL in general and the QOL in four specific domains (health and functioning, psychological and spiritual, social and economic, and family), the index notably measured QOL in terms of both satisfaction and importance. Lang, Muñoz, Bernal, and Sorensen (1982) examined a bicultural Latina/o community to determine the QOL and psychological well-being of its members. They described QOL as dependent on such factors as family, work, having children, physical health, education, spousal relationship, and religion.

When discussing QOL, researchers have consistently focused on the categories of socioeconomic status, education, physical health, mental health, environmental factors, delinquency and violence, and access to services. These contemporary efforts to operationalize QOL provide a beginning framework that is an essential foundation for future work, including our own. At the same time, we find these typical understandings suffering from at least three serious weaknesses.

First, most approaches to defining QOL are driven by the great value attributed to measurement. Most definitions, in fact, are developed with a particular end in mind, such as a valid survey. As a result, QOL must be defined as a set of categories— labeled by researchers as *domains* or *dimensions*—that are mutually distinct and that exert independent influence on QOL. Although some research strives to measure the relative importance of the categories (Ferrans & Powers, 1985) for QOL, the likely interrelationships among such categories are neither measured nor acknowledged. Second, typical research approaches to QOL are not obviously based on any clear theory of individuals and their environment. This weakness seems especially significant given that QOL refers not to the individual mind but to the individual's physical, emotional, social, spiritual, and embodied environments. Third, most approaches appear to ignore the role of culture. The values and expectations, shared practices, and "webs of significance" (Geertz, 1983) that enmesh any individual's experience as a member of a larger community are, simply put, left out. Consequently, the conventional definition of QOL assumes a certain homogeneity of experience, an assumption that is not borne out in the real world. At the very least, it must be acknowledged that experience is shaped by the culture or cultures in which persons find themselves; to ignore this fact leaves professionals practically and theoretically impoverished. This last weakness is especially conspicuous in work with Latina/os. If Rodriguez (2002) is correct that Hispanics (his preferred term) are a cultural rather than a racial group, bound together by a sense of shared history and experience far more than any sense of shared genes, then we must find ways to inject a consideration of culture into an understanding of QOL.

TOWARD A BROWN UNDERSTANDING OF QUALITY OF LIFE

In the end, many common approaches to QOL are driven by the demand for measurable domains, may lack some articulate theory of the person and environment, and are bereft of adequate consideration of culture. We propose that an adequate conception of QOL should address these weaknesses without sacrificing the valuable contributions of existing work, including the identification of domains for inquiry, ease of operationalization, and the analyzability of research data. Most importantly, we hope to conceptualize QOL in ways that make it both available for researchers and useful for practice. Finally, we strive for an approach to QOL that is brown: However it is defined, QOL must provide a way to address the needs of Latina/os that reflects the complexity of lived experience.

Our working, brown definition of QOL builds on a theory of the person and his or her environment, striving especially to represent the complexity of the environment and the interdependence of any person's multiple contexts. Because we begin with a concern for the ubiquitous influence of culture, we strive to represent this influence in our emerging theory of the person. In what follows, we first present our efforts in this regard, then we put our model to the test, working with an existing case study to compare the yield of our definition of QOL to that of more common understandings.

The environment should not be treated as if it were a collection of independent influences on individuals, nor the individual be considered an independent actor exerting his or her agency within or upon the environment. Instead, one should begin with the idea that any individual is embedded in a life space that includes an individual in interaction with the environment, where the individual and the environment are interdependent and mutually constitutive. This present thinking rests heavily on the foundations laid by Lewin (1936), whose field theory includes the claim that "every psychological event depends on the state of the person and at the same time on the environment, although their relative importance is different in different cases" (p. 12).

Individuals live and grow both within and across multiple contexts, and these contexts may be organized along a kind of micro-macro continuum. In describing his theory of the ecology of human development, Bronfenbrenner (1977, 1979, 1993) - described the "progressive, mutual accommodation, throughout the life span, between a growing human organism and the environments in which it lives" (1977, p. 514). Noting the self-evident fact that people interact with different environments over a life span, and even over the course of a single day, Bronfenbrenner (1977) described the various levels of systems and structures that make up these environments. These include a hierarchy of the following: the *microsystem,* consisting of the immediate physical setting and its collection of individual actors; the *mesosystem,* comprising the interrelations among settings; the *exosystem,* an extension of the mesosystem "embracing other specific social structures, both formal and informal . . . that impinge upon or encompass the [individual's] immediate settings" (1977, p. 515); and the *macrosystem,* which includes the overarching patterns of the culture or subculture. Working from the foundation laid by Bronfenbrenner, we suggest that these various systems be understood as levels of context, preliminarily defined as follows:

1. Interpersonal contexts, including both the number and quality of relationships, as well as the more immediate contexts of ongoing, emergent interactions.
2. Social contexts, where individuals must manage their lives in multiple social systems (cf. Hartup, 1979, for a discussion of the interrelated peer, family, and school "social worlds" of children) and networks (Stanton-Salazar, 1997).
3. Institutional contexts, including schools, local governments, and the maze of everyday bureaucracies.
4. Economic and political contexts, where one's place in the larger economic system and relative access to resources are deeply consequential.

The interdependent relationships among these contexts are more important than their independent influences on individual behavior and experience. Although they must be considered separately in many phases of research, when QOL is included in any theoretical model of human experience or behavior, it must be kept in mind that these contexts never exist independently of each other.

To summarize, we turn to Lewin's (1935) famous equation, depicting in rough mathematical terms the contention that individual behavior (*B*) is a function (*f*) of the individual person (*P*) in interaction with his or her psychological environment (*E*):

$$B = f(P, E)$$

With preemptive apologies to Lewin, we might adapt this equation for our own purposes, so that quality of life (*QOL*) is represented as a function (*f*) of an individual person (*P*) in interaction with his or her multiple (*n*) environments (*E*):

$$QOL = f(P, E_n)$$

Lewin also depicted the (*P, E*) part of his equation as in Fig. 21.1. For Lewin, the person and his or her psychological environment were a single entity. Again, we might

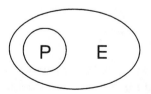

FIG. 21.1.   Lewin's model of a person in interaction with his or her psychological environment.

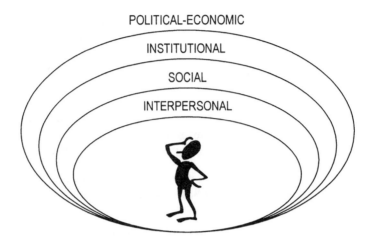

FIG. 21.2.   A person in interaction with his or her multiple, mutually constituted environments.

represent the (P, E_n) part of our own equation as in Fig. 21.2. We hope to capture the following points in our graphic-visual representation in Fig. 21.2. First, the individual person still rests at the center of the drawing and is always already embedded in a set of contexts. These contexts are nested circles, all of which share a side. By presenting these circles as sharing a side, we intend to convey our understanding that contexts are mutually constituted, as parts of each other.

What about *culture?* We presume that any individual's QOL is always already situated in culture (personal, local, global, etc.). This cultural situatedness of QOL means that a person's individual history as a member of various ethnic, linguistic, national, class, or other groups always affects the relative influence of any context and, most importantly, the way the various contexts are interdependent in any given case. Where is culture in our picture? Though the black-and-white illustration in Fig. 21.2 can never show it, culture would be much like the shifting color of the lines and figures—always present, but never separable in any way from the whole.

Earlier, we expressed our hopes for a concept of QOL that would be useful for both research and practice, reflect the needs of Chicana/os and Latina/os, and sufficiently reflect the complexity of real life. Although these hopes have guided us along the way, a better test lies in the answer to the following questions: What story does a brown QOL help us tell? How does it compare to the story told by statistics about Latina/os? What follows is an attempt to answer those questions by considering a small story of the life of a real person, Liliana, a participant in a 3-year study of youth language and learning by Raley (2003).

QUALITY OF LIFE AND LILIANA: A COMPARATIVE CASE STUDY

Wedged between a major commuter freeway and the San Francisco Bay, Bayview is a geographically bounded community of 25,000; a significant majority of its residents are African American, Latina/o, Pacific Islander, and South Asian. The city's history is difficult, marked most prominently by its social and economic isolation from the steadily increasing wealth of the Silicon Valley. Residents suffer from a basic lack of services—Bayview has no supermarket or bank—as well as potholed streets and "hot spots" where drug dealing goes on openly. Unless young people in Bayview play basketball, there are not many places to go and not much to do. Moreover, many residents find it difficult to shake the persistently negative image of their community, fossilized in the early 1990s when the national media labeled Bayview the "murder capital of the nation."

Raley met Liliana in his first few days at Pacifica Prep, in the second month of her first year there. He had spent some time with the juniors and several sophomore students, but was seeing the freshmen for the first time. Most of the freshmen students were wary with him around, though all were polite and friendly. Liliana was cool, even sullen. Her posture was contradictory, her face implacably set against any attempts to be social.

Liliana had lived in Bayview for most of the time since her family immigrated illegally from Mexico. At 18, Liliana was of average height and build. Her hair, permed into tight waves and neatly parted in the middle, always looked slightly wet and nearly black. Two strands on either side of the part, right in the front, broke off purposefully from the rest, curled over her face, reached her collarbones. Her once-solid eyebrows were plucked into narrow, sparse curves. She almost always wore long skirts, though when very hot she wore shorts.

Liliana's family was economically poor. She had met but did not have ongoing contact with her biological father, who was "somewhere in Mexico." Her mother and two older sisters were deeply committed to their Apostolic Christian church, but Liliana did not attend regularly. Liliana once rescued an older sister from a drug overdose, leveraging her own connections with local gang members to secure transportation to a nearby hospital. Liliana spoke reverently of her grandmother, currently living in a neighborhood near her own, but Liliana and her grandmother had only recently started speaking to each other again when the grandmother suffered a serious illness.

Kicked out of two middle schools for her "bad attitude," dismal attendance record, and a series of straight-F report cards, Liliana had spent the second half of her seventh grade year at home or with gang members in a nearby neighborhood. Though she had done very well in elementary school, she more or less checked out of school altogether when she got to middle school. When a school administrator encouraged Liliana's mother to send her to live with relatives in Mexico, Liliana packed her bags and planned to run away from home. In the winter of what would have been Liliana's eighth-grade year, her mother sent her to Birchwood, a small, private academy located near Bayview. Though the small classrooms and ramps (instead of stairs) helped Liliana conclude that Birchwood was a school for "mental patients," and despite Liliana's best efforts to break the behavioral contracts set out for her by the school's administration, she barely completed the last two thirds of her eighth-grade year there.

Such is the story statistics might help tell. Liliana was poor. Her mother was single and poorly educated, and Liliana herself struggled in school. She had been violent and delinquent. Her future, at least by the eighth grade, did not look good. Yet that story does not help in understanding where Liliana is today, nor does it offer a way to talk about her development over the last 4 years of high school. In 2001, Liliana was finishing up her senior year at Pacifica College Prep School. She smiled often when she spoke of her graduation and her departure for premedical study at an Ivy League university. And, through all the angst of American adolescence, she was almost undeniably happy. So what was going on for Liliana, and how can QOL help in understanding it? Specifically, what is going on in Liliana's environments and her relationship to them?

Like most Pacifica students, Liliana arrived at school just before 8:00 in the morning and often stayed later than the 5:00 dismissal time. She maintained a *B* average. As part of her long days, Liliana stayed involved in a school-based youth entrepreneur organization and was a photographer and assistant yearbook editor. Liliana also worked several hours a week in the pharmacy and cosmetics areas of a local drugstore. One summer, she decided to take a break from her drugstore job to devote her time to an internship at a local technology company. After she completed the first month's work in less than a day, her superiors gave her increasingly difficult assignments and responsibility.

In all of these places, but perhaps especially at school, Liliana developed deep, lasting relationships with peers and with adults. Pacifica is small—the size of the student body hovered around 70 during the duration of the research—and students and teachers have ample opportunity to know each other in both academic and nonacademic settings. Students and teachers alike describe the school as being "like family"; perhaps more than anyone else, Liliana was consistently fierce in her defense of the school and her activities there.

Earlier, we mentioned that Liliana and her grandmother had only recently started speaking to each other again when the grandmother suffered a serious illness. Liliana's youngest sister and brother were the product of a relationship between Liliana's mother and an African American man; because her grandmother would not touch or even speak to Liliana's mixed-race siblings, Liliana had decided not to maintain any semblance of cordial relations. Liliana initiated the more recent change in this relationship, even creating situations where the grandmother's prejudices would be indirectly challenged.

Liliana's sense of humor engaged both young people and adults, her penetrating insights guided conversations among peers as well as many classroom discussions, and she was well liked by students and the staff who know her well. She continued to defy authority when she felt that it was unjustifiably imposed, she was occasionally impatient with what she perceived to be the irrelevance of other people's emotions or reasoning, and she sometimes balked at homework and tutoring sessions. In the end, though, and by almost any measure, Liliana was, by 2001, thriving. Her ultimate goal was to be a surgeon, she said, because it is hard and interesting and because she can help people.

Liliana still has a low socioeconomic status, her mother's schooling is still limited, and she still lives in the former murder capital, but what does this statistical, black-and-white version of QOL say about the extent to which Liliana's health and "happiness requirements" (McCall, 1975) are met? Not much. A more adequate account comes from our working, brown understanding of QOL. It would highlight, for example, the interdependent relations among the contexts of her school (institutional, social); family, friends, and work (social); and working and friendship relations (interpersonal). Although space does not permit it here, a brown account of QOL would look into the real-life conversations that form the interactional contexts for Liliana's daily life. It would also explore the cultural value placed on family relationships as a possible keystone for improvement of Liliana's own QOL.

IMPLICATIONS FOR RESEARCH AND PRACTICE

A brown conception of QOL seems to call also for a new, browner approach to research and practice. Such an approach, we argue here, would include both quantitative and qualitative methodologies, a focus on the local and particular, and continued conversation between researchers and practitioners.

A great deal has already been written about quantitative approaches to psychological research. Quantitative methods are the default methodological position, requiring no defense. We therefore do not say much about quantitative approaches, discussing instead the strengths of qualitative approaches to understanding QOL and the need for researchers to "tack back and forth" (Geertz, 1983) between quantitative and qualitative methods.

In a long discussion of qualitative research methods in multicultural counseling, Morrow, Rakhsha, and Castañeda (2001, pp. 582–583) offered the following characteristics that make qualitative research a "natural" approach:

- It includes context as an essential component.
- It addresses the researcher's processes of self-awareness and self-reflection.
- It is uniquely able to capture the meanings participants give to their experiences.
- It can be used within the paradigms of participants, using the stories, folk wisdom, and common sense of ordinary people.
- Its methods provide the opportunity for voices that were previously silenced to be heard and lives that were marginalized to be brought to center.
- it provides an opportunity to explore previously unexplored or undefined constructs.
- It may address questions that cannot be answered using traditional methods.

Without belaboring the point, we are convinced that these same characteristics that make qualitative research a nice fit for multicultural counseling studies also make qualitative methods an essential part of research on a brown QOL.

We also recognize that qualitative methods sometimes range far afield from conventional assumptions about what counts as science. With that in mind, we argue that quantitative and qualitative approaches should be complementary. Although we may not want qualitative and quantitative research methods to melt into each other—epistemological differences would make such synthesis unlikely—we can surely hope that they coexist and inform one another. Whereas individual researchers might find this task daunting, we can certainly imagine psychology as a science "tacking back and forth" between qualitative and quantitative approaches.

Those concerned with understanding and improving QOL for any person or population should direct their focus to the details of the local situation, including the person and his or her environment. Qualitative approaches to research often focus on the local, but the complementary contribution of quantitative data should not be discounted. In any case, researchers and practitioners alike should strive to identify the multiple, overlapping contexts that make up a person's environment, and especially to understand the shifting, culturally situated relations among these contexts. Although concern for the relative social, economic, or educational standing of any group is essential, any group measures used do not tell very much about QOL for any real person. The focus must be on the local and the particular.

Finally, researchers and practitioners share responsibility for breaking down the boundary that is commonly viewed to separate research and practice. Just as qualitative and quantitative approaches to data collection and analysis ought to be reimagined as complementary efforts, so should the work of researchers and practitioners be mutually informing. Talking across the gap is, of course, no mean feat, though this is mostly attributable to a stubborn (and erroneous) belief that theory and practice are naturally independent of each other. To any extent that research and practice can join in conversation, the understanding of and ability to improve quality of life—not only for Chicana/os and Latina/os but also for any and all persons—will reap the benefits.

We began this chapter with a quote from Richard Rodriguez' *Brown: The Last Discovery of America* (2002), directing attention to the demographic browning of America. We end it with two short quotes from the same book that, while underscoring the browning process, reflect the beliefs that underlie professionals' emerging understanding of QOL as it concerns the Chicana/o and Latina/o:

"One should deplore any loss of uniquity in a world that has so little" (Rodriguez, 2002, p. 120). We have struggled here to preserve a sense of the individual, but have been troubled by the nagging awareness that people are, in fact, members of groups who share ideas and values. They rely on the same understandings and expectations. Together, they act out common practices. They recognize each other. Just as it is essential to discover the unique qualities of individual experience, so it cannot be assumed which pieces of experience—including QOL—are shared by members of a group. What we call the working or emerging definition of QOL is, in this way, decidedly brown. It presumes that the QOL of any individual is uniquely determined, that the substance and relationship among his or her contexts is unique, and that culture is always important, but that the way in which it is important for any individual is uniquely shaped.

"America's brilliance is a lack of subtlety. Most Americans are soft on geography. We like puzzles with great big pieces, pie-crust coasts. And we're not too fussy about the midlands" (Rodriguez, 2002, p. 117). No less than the rest of America, perhaps even more so, social science is often brilliant in its lack of subtlety. Where statisticians have already divided a population into great big pieces, social science works with them; where they do not yet exist, social science devises new ways to make them. Not only do these great big pieces inaccurately describe the increasingly brown world in which we live, but a reliance on them may actually keep professionals from seeing the rich complexity of the lives of real persons. A sufficiently complex understanding of QOL, one that is responsive to the needs of an increasingly Brown population, will have to spend some time in the midlands, where it is harder to find great big pieces and pie-crust coasts, and where there are real live people in every direction.

REFERENCES

Alderfer, C. P. (1969). An empirical test of a new theory of human needs. *Organizational Behavior and Human Performance, 4*, 142–175.

Bergner, M. (1989). Quality of life, health status, and clinical research. *Medical Care, 27*, S148–S156.

Bronfenbrenner, U. (1977). Toward an experimental ecology of human development. *American Psychologist, 32*, 513–531.

Bronfenbrenner, U. (1979). *The ecology of human development.* Cambridge, MA: Harvard University Press.

Bronfenbrenner, U. (1993). The ecology of cognitive development: Research models and fugitive findings. In R. H. Wozniak & K. W. Fischer (Eds.), *Development in context: Acting and thinking in specific environments* (pp. 3–44). Hillsdale, NJ: Lawrence Erlbaum Associates.

Cella, D. F. (1994). Quality of life: Concepts and definition. *Journal of Pain Symptom Management, 9*, 186–192.

Casas, J. M., Vasquez, M. J. T., & Ruiz de Esparza, C. A. (2002). Counseling the Latina(o): A guiding framework for a diverse population. In P. B. Pedersen, J. G. Draguns, W. J. Lonner, & J. E. Trimble (Eds.), *Counseling across cultures* (5th ed., pp. 133–159). Thousand Oaks, CA: Sage.

Ferrans, C., & Powers, M. (1985). Quality of life index: Development and psychometric properties. *Advances in Nursing Science, 8*, 15–24.

Ferrans, C., & Powers, M. (1992). Psychometric assessment of the Quality of Life Index. *Research in Nursing and Health, 15*, 29–38.

Flanagan, J. C. (1978). A research approach to improving our quality of life. *American Psychologist, 33*, 138–147.

Flanagan, J. C. (1982). Measurement of quality of life: Current state of the art. *Archives of Physical Medicine and Rehabilitation, 63*(2), 56–59.

Fujii, M. (1999). *The constructs of quality of life for cancer patients: Exploring factors that affect QOL.* Unpublished doctoral dissertation, Washington University, St. Louis, MO.

Geertz, C. (1983). *Local knowledge: Further essays in interpretive anthropology.* New York: Basic Books.

Hall, C. S., & Lindzey, G. (1978). *Theories of personality* (3rd ed.). New York: Wiley and Sons.

Hartup, W. W. (1979). The social worlds of childhood. *American Psychologist, 34*, 944–950.

Kaufman, P., Kwon, J. Y., Klein, S., & Chapman, C. D. (2000). *Dropout rates in the United States: 1998* (Statistical Analysis Report No. 2000022). Washington, DC: National Center for Education Statistics.

Lang, J. G., Muñoz, R. F., Bernal, G., & Sorenson, J. L. (1982). Quality of life and psychological well-being in a bicultural Latino community. *Hispanic Journal of Behavioral Sciences, 4*, 433–450.

Lewin, K. (1935). *A dynamic theory of personality.* New York: McGraw-Hill.

Lewin, K. (1936). *Principles of topological psychology.* New York: McGraw-Hill.

Maslow, A. (1954). *Motivation and personality.* New York: Harper and Brothers.

McCall, S. (1975). Quality of life. *Social Indicators Research, 2*, 229–248.

McNeill, B. W., Prieto, L. R., Niemann, Y. F., Pizarro, M., Vera, E. M., & Gómez, S. P. (2001). Current directions in Chicana/o psychology. *The Counseling Psychologist, 29*, 5–17.

Mezzich, J. E., Ruiperez, M. A., Perez, C., Yoon, G., Liu, J., & Mahmud, S. (2000). The Spanish version of the Quality of Life Index: Presentation and validation. *Journal of Nervous and Mental Disease, 188*, 301–305.

Morrow, S. L., Rakhsha, G., & Castañeda, C. L. (2001). Qualitative research methods for multicultural counseling. In J. G. Ponterotto, J. M. Casas, L. A. Suziki, & C. M. Alexander (Eds.), *Handbook of multicultural counseling* (2nd ed.). Thousand Oaks, CA: Sage.

National Coalition of Hispanic Health and Human Services Organizations (COSSMHO). (1999). *The state of Hispanic girls.* Washington, DC: COSSMHO Press.

Ponterotto, J. G., & Casas, J. M. (1991). *Handbook of racial/ethnic minority counseling research.* Springfield, IL: Charles Thomas.

Raley, J. D. (2003). *Safe spaces?: A study of trust, risk, and learning at the margins.* Unpublished doctoral dissertation, Stanford University, Stanford, CA.

Rodriguez, R. (2002). *Brown: The last discovery of America.* New York: Viking.

Sherif, C. W. (1982). Needed concepts in the study of gender identity. *Psychology of Women Quarterly, 6*, 375–398.

Sirgy, M. J. (1986). A quality of life theory derived from Maslow's developmental perspective: "Quality" is related to progressive satisfaction of a hierarchy of needs, lower order and higher. *American Journal of Economics and Sociology, 45,* 329–342.

Stanton-Salazar, R. D. (1997). A social capital framework for understanding the socialization of racial minority children and youths. *Harvard Educational Review, 67*(1), 1–39.

U.S. Bureau of the Census. (2000a). *Census Bureau projects doubling of nation's population by 2100* [On-line]. Available: http://www.census.gov/Press-Release/www/2000/cb00-05.html.

U.S. Bureau of the Census. (2000b). *Current population survey: March 1999.* Washington, DC: U.S. Government Printing Office.

U.S. Bureau of the Census. (2000c). *Resident population estimates of the United States by sex, race, and Hispanic origin* [On-line]. Available: http://www.census.gov/population/estimates/nation/intfile3–1.txt.

U.S. Bureau of the Census. (2001). *Census 2000 Redistricting* (Public Law 94–171) [On-line]. Available: http://www.census.gov.

Epilogue

Challenges and Opportunities for Chicana/o Psychologists: Past, Present, and Future[1]

Martha E. Bernal

Twenty-five years ago, I caught sight of my first psychologist of Mexican descent at the Conference of Chicano Psychologists, held in 1973 at the University of California, Riverside. Two psychology professors, Al Castañeda and Manuel Ramirez III, organized that conference. As I recall, approximately 40 Chicana/o psychologists and graduate students attended, reflecting the number that existed at the time. Because I had received my Ph.D. from Indiana University in 1962, 11 years had passed before I realized that other psychologists of my own ethnic background really existed.

When I walked into that meeting for the first time, however, it was not their existence that astounded me, for I had already seen the program. It was their competence that struck me so forcefully. I sat there and listened to Chicana/o psychologists who were articulate, intelligent, and knowledgeable as they presented their papers, and it was a revelation. Here I was, already *una muchachona* (a mature woman) and I had been so assimilated into the racist views of Anglo American culture that I had internalized the expectation that Chicana/o psychologists simply were not competent. That experience upset me because of what it revealed about my own internalized racism. It also made me aware of how my feelings of shame about being Mexican were bred in my native environment of West Texas and nurtured by many years of being the only Chicana among White people. My internalized racism converted into a loss of pride in my own ethnic group and a rejection

[1]This chapter is based on an invited address by Martha Bernal to the audience attending the Innovations in Chicana/o Psychology conference at Michigan State University in 1998. At the time of her death on September 28, 2001, Dr. Bernal had been working with editor Brian McNeill to update the statistics and figures included in this manuscript. Thus, in order to honor the integrity of her words and as a beginning to this chapter, only minor changes have been made and the first-person narrative retained as a strong message to Chicana/o psychologists, past, present, and future.

of my ethnic identity. Yet, the experience also exhilarated me because I had found
a group of fellow Chicana/os in my professional world. I know that my experience
was not unique, because my Chicana/o psychology peers of that era shared my
feelings.

Today, it is apparent that certain changes have occurred because a large body of
Chicana/o psychologists exists, and all of us are proud of being among peers whom
we know, and whose competence (and indeed excellence) we respect and admire.
But are these changes sufficient to powerfully affect our presence in psychology? Are
they sufficient to improve the conditions that foster *nuestro orgullo en ser* (our pride in
being) Chicana/os? These are questions explored in this epilogue. I begin by examining the theoretical relationship between representation of Chicana/os in psychology
and ethnic pride.

ETHNIC PRIDE AND CHICANA/O REPRESENTATION
IN PSYCHOLOGY

How are the representations of Chicana/os in psychology and ethnic pride related?
This question requires a review of social theory. Nonetheless, I attempt to demonstrate this relationship by extrapolating from Tajfel's (1978, 1982) social identity theory and Festinger's (1954) theory of social comparison process.

Our aggregate social identities, multiple and plural in each individual, are a major
part of the Chicana/o self-concept and provide the framework we use to define and
evaluate ourselves. Consider ethnic identity as one of many social identities that
exist for each of us. The basic premises of social identity theory are that: (a) we cate-
gorize our social world into units composed of similar objects, called *in-groups* and
units composed of dissimilar others, called *out-groups;* (b) we assign attributes to in-
groups and out-groups and can thereby infer the characteristics of individuals based
on group membership; (c) in part, these attributes result from engaging in a process
of social comparison (i.e., by comparing ourselves to out-groups, we make evaluations of our own group); and (d) we strive for a positive self-concept and self-worth,
which are derived from our membership in the in-group and from the values and
attributes that we assign to our group and to other groups.

Thus, when we think of ourselves as Chicana/os, there are values and attributes
that we assign to ourselves and to other ethnic or racial groups. When we evaluate
ourselves favorably in relation to out-groups, such as White or Black Americans, our
self-concept and self-worth are strengthened. Because ethnic pride is another way of
stating that we value our group membership, our Chicana/o pride is also strengthened when we evaluate ourselves favorably.

I refer back to our in-group, Chicana/o psychologists. There are two social conditions that must be met to compare us favorably to others, and thus strengthen our
Chicana/o *orgullo* (pride). One of these conditions is the existence of a Chicana/o psychologist in-group, meaning a critical mass. Without the existence of this in-group,
very little is possible. We cannot compare ourselves to out-groups in order to form
positive evaluations of our group, and our sense of pride suffers when others evaluate us negatively. Of course, we have the alternative of joining a group that is valued

and taking on its group identity (as I did at one time in my career), but there are also many problems with that solution. For example, when I assimilated into the White culture, I internalized negative views of my ethnic heritage.

Another condition necessary for ethnic pride is the positive evaluations made by out-groups toward Chicana/o psychologists. If there is a large in-group to influence out-groups' evaluations of us, we can subsequently promote positive evaluations that result in favorable comparisons between our group and out-groups. These comparisons correct the negative stereotypes and prejudices that we have all experienced, and thus lead to strengthening our sense of ethnic pride and status among other groups.

According to this theory, our numbers in psychology are critical to our Chicana/o pride. Hence, the need to increase the numbers of Chicana/os is crucial because our ethnic pride affects us in very personal and important ways. For example, it was my renewed ethnic identity and sense of pride in being Chicana that led to my decision, over 20 years ago, to stop conducting mainstream research and teaching mainstream courses, and begin to work in the area of minority mental health. Our ethnic identity and corresponding ethnic pride serve important functions in supporting and protecting our ethnic group, and determine the degree to which we want to serve our people. I now discuss the probable consequences of a strong ethnic identity and pride.

If you are a Chicana/o seeking admission to graduate school in psychology, you are likely to be highly identified with your ethnic group. Furthermore, the strength of your ethnic identity is related to the importance you place on the availability of multicultural training when selecting possible training programs. This phenomenon was observed in a national survey of clinical psychology graduate students that my students and I recently conducted (Bernal et al., 1998). I predict that, if you are a Chicana/o graduate student, you will seek research and clinical training addressing Chicana/os. Furthermore, if you are a Chicana/o psychologist, the degree of commitment to your people will direct you to scientific, educational, or professional work that involves them. You will also realize that you possess the a wealth of life experience that, as a Chicana/o, provides you with unique insights into the human potential of our people, as well as an understanding of many of the human problems and institutional obstacles that they face. Finally, you will also realize that you possess the cultural sensitivity to promote your Chicana/o clients' potential and help alleviate their burdens.

Of course, there are other important reasons for increasing our numbers. These reasons stem from the growth of the population of Latina/os in 1997, representing roughly 12% of the entire U.S. population, with Chicana/os comprising 66.1% of all Latina/os (Therrien & Ramirez, 2000). Because a large portion of our profession commits itself to serving the public by providing direct services, there is an increasing need for culturally competent psychologists. Similarly, the need for Chicana/os as educators, role models for youth, and behavioral scientists will also increase.

Thus, we are challenged to enlarge our numbers and proportions in psychology and, in doing so, we have the opportunity to engage in activities that lead to our increased pride. Ultimately, those activities become entwined with our need to strive for excellence in our practice and science.

CHALLENGES AND OPPORTUNITIES
OF THE PAST THREE DECADES

Chicana/o Representation in Psychology, 1970 to 1980

There was the time when our representation in psychology was *mas que un chorrito* (but a trickle). I think back to November, 1979, to the National Conference of Hispanic Psychologists, an exciting convention initiated by the Spanish Speaking Mental Health Research Center at the University of California, Los Angeles (UCLA, under the direction of Amado Padilla). The National Institute of Mental Health, held at Lake Arrowhead, CA, also supported this conference. Approximately 60 participants attended and about half were of Mexican descent.

As one of the speakers, I summarized the status of Hispanics in psychology (Bernal, 1980) and pointed to the representation of Hispanic psychologists as the major challenge facing us. Table E1 highlights the underrepresentation of Hispanics in doctoral clinical psychology programs, an area of psychology where Hispanics have always been, and still are, most numerous. The data were taken from various surveys with different instruments, response rates, and sampling methods, therefore, they must be cautiously interpreted. Moreover, the data in the 1970 and 1977–1978 columns pertain to accredited clinical programs, whereas data for the 1972 and 1976 columns pertain to both accredited and unaccredited programs. All Hispanic groups were lumped together for the sake of comparison to more recent data, because the American Psychological Association (APA) does not separate data for distinct Hispanic groups.

Most evident in Table E1 are: (a) very low numbers of Hispanic faculty, most of whom were Chicana/os, representing less than 1% of all faculty in clinical psychology between 1970 and 1977–1978; (b) very low percentages of Hispanic graduate students, increasing from .65% in 1970 to 3.4% in 1977–1978. Approximately half of these students were Chicana/os.

TABLE E1

Hispanic Faculty and Graduate Students in Doctoral Clinical Psychology Programs, 1970 to 1978

	1970[a]	1972[b]	1976[c]	1977–1978[d]
	n	n	n	n
Hispanic faculty	4 (.38%)	2 (.16%)	10 (.78%)	22 (.65%)
Total faculty	1,041	1,251	1,275	3,334
Minority Fellowship Program implemented, 1974				
Hispanic graduate students	25 (.65%)	75 (1.58%)	130 (2.18%)	207 (3.4%)
Total graduate students	3,858	4,759	5,958	6,109

[a]Boxley and Wagner (1971) mail survey of APA-accredited Ph.D. clinical programs; $N = 103$, response rate = 79%. [b]Padilla, Boxley, and Wagner (1973) mail survey of all Ph.D. clinical programs; $N = 114$, response rate = 79%. [c]Padilla (1977) mail survey of all Ph.D. clinical programs; $N = 128$, response rate = 77%. Includes part-time and graduate student instructors. [d]Vidato (1979) survey; includes only APA-accredited clinical programs.

The 1970s posed many challenges, such as the need to increase the numbers of Hispanic graduate students, new faculty, researchers, and health service providers. We were fortunate that, as a result of activities within the APA involving ethnic minority psychologists, the APA Minority Fellowship Program (MFP) was established in 1974 with Dalmas Taylor as Director. Table E1 illustrates the probable impact that the MFP had on our numbers in 1977 to 1978 and thereafter. We owe a great debt to Taylor and to James Jones, his successor.

Another challenge we faced was the need to improve the training of psychologists to enable them to conduct research and render services in a culturally sensitive manner. With only a sprinkling of Chicana/o faculty, however, there was little opportunity for introducing this training in our university programs, or for improving and supporting the admission of Chicana/o students. The one exception was an early effort in 1972 by Manuel Ramirez and Bob Singer, who obtained funding from the National Institute of Mental Health (NIMH) and initiated a program the at University of California, Riverside that focused on the training of Chicana/os.

CHRONOLOGY OF CHICANA/O ACHIEVEMENT

Despite their small numbers, our Chicana/o pioneers in psychology were resourceful. They seized opportunities for forming a small critical mass capable of reducing our isolation and powerlessness, building our professional networks, honing our scientific skills, and intensifying our search for an improved scientific understanding of Hispanics. The NIMH and the APA sponsored many of these opportunities.

In the early 1970s, Chicana/o psychologists launched a series of events. The Association of Psychologists por La Raza was founded during the 1970 APA convention by Ed Casavantes, Al Casteneda, Al Ramirez, Manuel Ramirez, and Rene Ruiz. In 1972, the first-ever Symposium on Chicano Psychology, organized by Ed Casavantes, Rene Ruiz, Ernesto Bernal, and Amado Padilla, was held during the APA convention. A number of Chicana/os participated as Hispanic representatives in the APA's National Conference on Levels and Patterns of Professional Training in 1973. At this Conference, a task group on Professional Training and Minority Groups was formed and recommended to the APA to create an Office and Board of Ethnic Minority Affairs. In that same year, the NIMH-supported Conference of Chicano Psychologists (organized by Castañeda and Ramirez) was held at the University of California, Riverside. Also in 1973, the Spanish Speaking Mental Health Research Center was established at UCLA under the direction of Padilla with funding from the NIMH. In 1974, the first symposium on Chicano psychology at the University of California, Irvine, was organized by Joe Martinez and funded by the Ford Foundation. Martinez (1977) also edited and published the conference proceedings in the first psychology book with the word *Chicano* in its title, *Chicano Psychology*. It was the first comprehensive collection of the work of active Chicano psychologists and others doing research about Chicanos. Also in 1974, a group of ethnic minority psychologists established the APA Minority Fellowship Program with funding from the NIMH.

In the later 1970s, other events and conferences continued to affect the status of Chicana/os in American psychology. In 1977, the Hispanic Research Center at

Fordham University, under the direction of Lloyd Rogler, was established with NIMH funding. Chicana/o representatives participated in the 1978 Dulles conference, entitled "Expanding the Roles of Culturally Diverse Peoples in the Profession of Psychology," under the leadership of Dalmas Taylor. The APA Board of Social and Ethical Responsibility and the NIMH convened the conference. Conference participants also recommended the establishment of an APA Office and Board of Ethnic Minority Affairs. An immediate outcome of this conference was the establishment of the APA Ad Hoc Committee on Minority Affairs in 1978, which laid the groundwork for implementation of the recommendations of both the Vail Conference on Training in Clinical Psychology and the Dulles conference.

In 1979, the NIMH-funded National Conference of Hispanic Psychologists (organized by Padilla) was held at Lake Arrowhead, CA, and united a multiethnic group of Hispanic psychologists and led to the establishment of a National Hispanic Psychological Association with Carlos Albizu-Miranda as its first president. Also in 1979, the first issue of the *Hispanic Journal of Behavioral Sciences,* under the editorship of Padilla, was printed and became a powerful influence on the scientific development of Chicana/o psychology. Finally, two highly important developments took place at the end of the decade: In 1979, the Office of Ethnic Minority Affairs was established at APA (with Esteban Olmedo as its first director) and, in 1980, the Board of Ethnic Minority Affairs was established. A small number of Chicana/o psychologists joined with other ethnic psychologists to bring about these achievements.

These activities resulted in a book, a journal, two Hispanic research centers, a National Hispanic Psychological Association, and a small, but significant, network of Latina/o psychologists scattered across the country. Within APA, the MFP provided support for ethnic minority graduate students (including Chicana/os), a board representing our concerns, and a permanent office at APA for implementation of activities, and enabled us to address our concerns.

THE REPRESENTATION OF CHICANA/OS IN PSYCHOLOGY, 1980 TO THE PRESENT

I now turn to the representation of Chicana/os in psychology and examine our impact, progress, presence in psychology since 1980. You may notice that I focus exclusively on academics, not service providers. The reason for this omission is simple: There are no comparable data on health professionals that can be used to trace the growth of Chicana/os in psychology over time. Keep in mind also that faculty members are necessary for the training of health professionals in psychology.

Hispanic Faculty

A quick look at updated data from the APA Office of Accreditation for accredited clinical programs (Wicherski & Kohout, 1994; Wicherski, Kohout, & Fritz, 1990; Wicherski, Williams, & Kohout, 1998), comparable to the older data I reviewed, illustrates the trend of Hispanic faculty representation from that date to the present. Remember that, during this period, data collected by APA on Hispanics was not dis-

TABLE E2
Full-Time Faculty in APA-Accredited Clinical Psychology Programs
by Gender and Hispanic Ethnicity, 1989 to 1998

	1989–1990[a]	1993–1994[b]	1997–1998[c]	2000–2001[d]
Total faculty	1,231	1,222	1,231	1,140
Men	915 (74%)	868 (71%)	790 (64%)	706 (62%)
Women	316 (26%)	354 (29%)	441 (36%)	434 (38%)
Total Hispanic faculty	16 (1.3%)	25 (2.0%)	41 (3.3%)	35 (3.4%)
Men	10 (62.5%)	15 (60%)	21 (51%)	20 (57%)
Women	6 (37.5%)	10 (40%)	21 (49%)	15 (43%)

[a]Wicherski, Kohout, and Fritz (1990). [b]Wicherski and Kohout (1994).
[c]Wicherski, Williams, and Kohout (1998). [d]APA, 2001.

aggregated by Hispanic subgroups. Consequently, the number of Chicana/os in accredited clinical programs is unknown.

Table E2 illustrates the numbers and percentage of full-time faculty in accredited clinical psychology programs by gender and Hispanic ethnicity from 1989 to 2000. The total faculty number increased slightly from 1997–1998 to 2000–2001. Similarly, the percentage of women steadily increased, although males continued to dominate academic programs. Note the low numbers and percentages of Hispanic faculty members, increasing at a very slow rate. Most recently, Hispanic men and women were equally represented.

One might ask, "Is the situation better if we examine data that include all graduate departments of psychology, not just accredited clinical programs?" Figure E1 displays the percentages of Hispanics in psychology through 15 acadamic years, from 1981–1982 to 2000–2001. The data were taken from the annual *APA Surveys of Graduate Departments of Psychology* (APA, 2000, 2001) and the numbers were rounded out. Hispanics constituted only 1% of graduate department faculty until 1992, when they

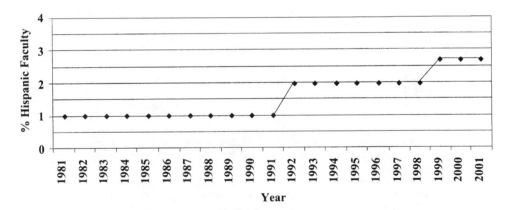

FIG. E1. Hispanic faculty representation in U.S. graduate departments of psychology, 1981 to 2000. Figures for 1981 and 1983 include both full- and part-time faculty, thereafter, only full-time faculty are reported. Information from *Surveys of Graduate Departments of Psychology, 1981–82 through 2000–01 Faculty Salary Survey*, by American Psychological Association and Council of Graduated Departments of Psychology.

rose to 2.7%. To give some idea of the representation of Hispanic faculty, in 2000–2001, there were 177 Hispanic faculty and 6,460 total faculty. However, the response rates for these annual surveys conducted by the APA varied and, in all cases, the numbers on which these percentages are based underreport the numbers of faculty because they are from a subset of the population.

Why is our representation among faculty so low? I have long hypothesized that our graduate students see the kinds of *vidas freneticas* (frenzied lives) we lead in academia and deliberately choose not to become like us. However, I would like to explore alternative reasons for Chicana/os not entering academia. The pool of Chicana/o graduate students must be an important determinant. According to a study by Russo, Olmedo, Stapp, and Fulcher (1981), approximately 10% of new ethnic minority doctorates are likely to accept university positions. This means, of course, that the pool of Chicana/o graduate students has to be quite large in order to yield a reasonable number of potential faculty members. We now turn to the status of our representation among graduate students.

Hispanic Students

The student data were taken from the *Surveys of Graduate Departments of Psychology* (APA, 1996b). Table E3 illustrates full-time graduate students in all U.S. graduate departments of psychology for the academic years between 1984–1985 and 1995–1996. The first evident trend is that, whereas the proportional representation of all female students increases, the representation of all male students decreases until there are twice as many women as men in psychology by 1995–1996. Focusing on Hispanic students, their representation in psychology reached 6.6% by 1995–1996,

TABLE E3
Full-Time Graduate Students in All U.S. Graduate Departments of Psychology
by Gender and Hispanic Ethnicity, 1984 to 1996

	1984–1985	*1987–1988*	*1991–1992*	*1995–1996*
Total graduate students	17,331	17,745	20,510	23,078
Men	43%	38%	37%	32%
Women	57%	62%	64%	68%
Total Hispanic students	610	622	939	1,526
Hispanic	3.6%	4.0%	4.6%	6.6%
Men	39%	36%	36%	30%
Women	61%	64%	64%	70%

Note. Information from *Survey of Graduate Departments of Psychology*, by American Psychological Association and Council of Graduate Departments of Psychology.

The categories for race and ethnicity on the survey instrument were: White (not Hispanic origin) and Hispanic (regardless of race). These data were based on information provided by departments of all kinds that responded to the survey and that reported demographic data on full-time doctoral students. Response rates may be different for each year. Students for whom demographic data were unavailable were excluded from these surveys. Because the numbers vary and are not representative of all students, only percentage figures are provided for comparison across years.

TABLE E4
New Doctorates in Psychology Earned by Puerto Rican, Mexican American,
and Other Hispanics in U.S. Universities, 1996 to 2000

	Total Doctorates	Mexican American	Puerto Rican	Other Hispanics	All Hispanics
1996	3,340	37 (1.1%)	48 (1.4%)	86 (2.6%)	171 (5.1%)
2000	3,623	60 (1.6%)	60 (1.6%)	74 (2.04%)	194 (5.35%)

Note. Information from *National Research Council Summary Report of Doctorate Recipients from Universities.*

but only increased by 3% over an 11-year period. The proportional representation of men and women closely follows the national trend.

How many of these Hispanic students actually completed their doctorates in psychology? Table E4 presents 1996 and 2000 data collected by the National Research Council (2000) on doctorates earned by Hispanics in psychology. All Hispanics constituted 5.1% of new doctorates in 1996 and 5.35% in 2000 and, when disaggregated, the percentage for Mexican Americans is lower than or equal to Puerto Ricans and other Hispanics. This is the case despite the fact that Mexican Americans represent about 60% of Hispanics in the country. The origin or descent of most other Hispanics tends to be Latin American countries, including Cuba. This trend of higher percentages for other Hispanics, as opposed to Chicana/os, has been the case for the past two decades.

I end my discussion of Hispanic representation in psychology by examining the constricting pipeline of Hispanics in the field of psychology. Figure E2 compares proportions of Hispanics based on enrollment in graduate school, earned doctorates, and faculty members in graduate and undergraduate departments.

Based on 1999–2000 data from two different sources, I have plotted the proportions of each group in Fig. E2. In comparison to the 2000 population estimate of 12% (Therrien & Ramirez, 2000), Hispanics are underrepresented in all three levels: 7.2% were in graduate school (APA, 1996b), 5.3% were doctoral recipients (Hoffer et al., 2001), and 2.7% were faculty (APA, 2000b). Moreover, whereas the number of doctorates earned by Hispanics was 1.9 percentage points below the number of those who enrolled in graduate school, the percentage of Hispanic faculty was even lower. However, Fig. E2 does not imply that only 2.7% of 7.2% graduate students became faculty: It only demonstrates levels of representation in the same year. These data

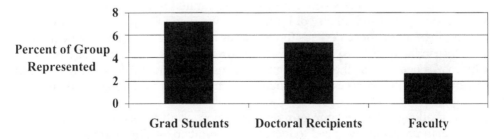

FIG. E2.   Hispanics in the field of psychology, 1999 to 2000. Information from U.S. Bureau of the Census, National Research Council, and American Psychological Association.

suggest that, in order to increase faculty representation, the proportions of graduate school enrollees need to significantly increase.

We could enlarge Fig. E2 by adding two earlier levels of the pipeline, bachelor's-level recipients and college entrants, in order to view the postsecondary trend in the constricting educational pipeline of Hispanics in psychology. Such a pipeline for 1997–1998 data has been presented elsewhere for all ethnic minorities (U.S. Department of Education, 2001). That educational pipeline also reveals underrepresentation at every level, with the greatest constriction occurring at the level of bachelor's completion, pointing to an urgent need to increase the retention rates of Hispanic undergraduates.

CHALLENGES FOR THE FUTURE

Increasing the Representation of Chicana/os in the Educational Pipeline

I believe that our efforts to increase Chicana/o representation and to promote positive evaluations of Chicana/os in psychology have been fruitful over the past two decades. Over time, the effects of every Chicana/o student we admit, encourage, train, or supervise increases the Chicana/o presence in psychology. Similarly, our presentations, publications, and discussions on this topic in committee meetings and conferences, as well as our lobbying efforts, also have an impact. We are visible in student bodies, faculties, service settings, industrial organizations, state and regional associations, and certainly national associations. We have a degree of influence at the national level through APA's Division 45 and the Committee on Ethnic Minority Concerns. We have friends and allies in other divisions, boards, and committees of the APA, in its Council of Representatives and its Board of Directions with whom we work toward common goals that affect us. Although our representation is low relative to APA's total membership, at least 1,767 (2.1%) Hispanic psychologists with doctoral degrees were members of the APA in 2000 (APA, 2000b), a much larger critical mass than 20 or 30 years ago, when our Chicana/o pioneers accomplished so much.

However, with some exceptions, our presence is too often of a token nature: a few graduate students in a program, a faculty member or two in a department, a professional in a service setting, a single person on a national committee, a few individuals in a state association, and so on. Because of this limited representation, we have not yet had the degree and quality of influence in the field of psychology that is necessary for maximum effect. Perhaps too few of us have placed ourselves in positions of influence in the field of psychology. Perhaps we need to do much more. In the future, Chicana/os need to use their training and status as psychologists to bring about the forceful action that is necessary to change the trajectory of the trends shown in this epilogue.

The challenge is to enlarge our representation at all levels of this educational pipeline. In particular, we need to increase the numbers of Chicana/o students completing their degrees in psychology at both the graduate and undergraduate levels.

The challenge, however, is characterized by circular effects: In order to have more Chicana/o undergraduate students complete their degrees and to admit more into graduate school, we need more Chicana/o faculty and larger pools of students. Breaking into that circularity means knowing where and how to intervene, which has not been easy. For the past 30 years, I have been saying that we must increase our representation in the profession, and so have others. Yet, here I am saying the same thing again, *como una sorda que no oye lo que ella mismo dice* (like a deaf woman who cannot hear her own words).

Resources for Increasing Chicana/o Representation

In 2002, more is known about what needs to be done to increase Hispanic representation in psychology than ever before and those who want to make a contribution can start by informing themselves. There are excellent resources developed by the Commission on Ethnic Minority Recruitment, Retention, and Training (CEMRRAT of the APA, which was active between 1994 and 1996). CEMRRAT was composed of 16 members who were experts from federal research, mental health agencies, and various domains and levels of postsecondary education. More importantly, each member had previously worked in various capacities to affect ethnic minority representation in psychology and all were disillusioned with our lack of progress, but not so much that they were unwilling to make another concerted effort. Members of the commission were selected by former APA President Ron Fox from among APA members who expressed interest. Their charge was "to assess the status of and barriers to the participation of persons of color in American Psychology, and to develop a five-year plan to guide the Association's efforts [(to increase ethnic minority recruitment, retention, and training]" (APA, 1997, p. 1).

CEMRRAT's report on its work, published by the APA in a volume entitled *Visions and Transformations: The Final Report* (APA, 1997) provided a wealth of information, including the following:

- A review and synthesis of the existing data regarding ethnic minority recruitment, retention, and graduation, and multicultural education and training in psychology.
- A description of the components that affect successful ethnic minority recruitment, retention, and training in psychology.
- The exploration of the nature of barriers and obstacles that prohibit significant ethnic minority recruitment, retention, and training in psychology.
- Recommendations for the development and implementation of innovative ethnic minority recruitment, retention, and training models.
- A 5-year plan of action for the APA addressing ethnic minority recruitment, retention, and training.

The following publications were also included:

- *Valuing Diversity in Faculty:* A guide for program administrators that provided a conceptual background for understanding the value of diversity in academia and described innovative ways for preparing the program and campus climate for successful recruitment and retention of ethnic minority faculty.

- *How to Recruit and Hire Ethnic Minority Faculty,* a how-to booklet that outlined strategies for use by psychology programs and search committees in recruiting ethnic minority faculty.
- *Surviving and Thriving in Academia* (in collaboration with the APA Committee on Women in Psychology) suggested strategies for use when searching for faculty positions, dealing with the recruitment visit, negotiating salary terms, and shaping one's academic career.
- *Diversity and Accreditation Questions and Actions Directors of Clinical, Counseling, and School Psychology Programs Should Consider When Assessing the Degree to which their program complies with Accreditation Domain D: Cultural and Individual Differences and Diversity,* for inclusion in the Committee on Accreditations site visitor handbook.
- *Psychology Education and Careers Guidebook for College Students of Color Applying to Graduate and Professional Programs,* a guide for ethnic minority undergraduate applicants.
- *Psychology Education and Careers: Resources for Psychology Training Programs Recruiting Students of Color,* for use by graduate and professional programs in psychology.
Psychology Education and Careers Guidebook for High School Students of Color, a set of tips for high school students.

I urge those who are concerned, who have not already done so, to become involved in the governance structure of organizations such as the APA or American Psychological Society (APS). Through service on boards and committees, one can influence their composition and agenda, and thus help effect changes that can increase Chicana/o representation in psychology. Now, and in the future, Chicana/os are especially needed in the APA governance structure to implement CEMRRAT's 5-year plan for activities and linkages that will ensure an increase in the proportion of people of color in psychology.

By the year 2050, Hispanics will constitute 22.5% of the U.S. population, approximately equal to the percentages of ethnic minorities and Anglos. As this population continues to grow, ethnic polarization will increase. The vast social problems of our people will also increase, such as low educational achievement, high rates of substance abuse, crime, incarceration, poverty, and poor physical and mental health care. In addition, national trends toward mean-spiritedness and violence in the form of hate and bias crimes, English-only advocacy, and political coalitions for denying ethnic minorities opportunities for advancement are likely to harden. Chicana/os in all fields of psychology possess skills applicable to many of these challenges. We need the strength of numbers and a strong sense of identity and *orgullo* (pride). We also need a strong commitment to serving Chicana/os, Latina/os, and, ultimately, all citizens, without fear of losing status or identity. As Chicana/os we need to fulfill the vision of our pioneers. We also need to finish building the foundation of Chicana/o psychology.

REFERENCES

American Psychological Association. (1996). *Graduate study in psychology.* Washington, DC: Author.

American Psychological Association. (1997). *APA directory survey, 1997.* Washington, DC: Author.

American Psychological Association. (2000a). *APA directory survey, 2000.* Washington, DC: Author.

American Psychological Association. (2000b). *Faculty salary survey.* Washington, DC: American Psychological Association and Council of Graduate Departments.

Bernal, M. E. (1980). Hispanic issues in psychology: Curricula and training. *Hispanic Journal of Behavioral Sciences, 2,* 129–146.

Bernal, M. E., Sirolli, A. A., Weisser, S. K., Ruiz, J. A., Chamberlain, V. J., & Knight, G. P. (1998). The relevance of multicultural training to students: Applications to clinical psychology programs. *Cultural Diversity and Ethnic Minority Psychology, 5,* 43–55.

Boxley, R., & Wagner, N. (1971). Clinical psychology training programs and minority groups: A survey. *Professional Psychology, 2,* 75–81.

Festinger, L. (1954). A theory of social comparison process. *Human Relations, 7,* 117–140.

Hoffer, T. B., Dugoni, B. L., Sanderson, A. R., Senderson, S., Ghadialy, R., & Rocque, P. (2001). *Doctorate recipients from United States universities: Summary Report 2000.* Chicago: National Opinion Research Center.

Martinez, J. L., Jr. (1977). *Chicano psychology.* New York: Academic Press.

National Research Council. (1996). *Summary report: Doctorate recipients from U.S. universities (selected years).* Washington, DC: Author.

Padilla, E. R. (1977). Hispanics in clinical psychology: 1970–76. In E. L. Olmedo & S. Lopez (Eds.), *Hispanic mental health professionals.* Los Angeles: Spanish Speaking Mental Health Research Center, University of California.

Padilla, E. R., Boxley R., & Wagner, N. (1973). The desegregation of clinical psychology training. *Professional Psychology, 4,* 259–264.

Russo, N. F., Olmedo, E. L., Stapp, J., & Fulcher, R. (1981). Women and minorities in psychology. *American Psychologist, 36,* 136–138.

Tajfel, H. (1978). *Differentiation between social groups: Studies in the social psychology of intergroup relations* (European Monographs in Social Psychology, No. 14). London: Academic Press.

Tajfel, H. (1982). *Social identity and intergroup relations.* New York: Cambridge University Press.

Therrien, M., & Ramirez, R. (2000). *The Hispanic population in the United States: March 2000* (Current Population Report No. 70-535). Washington, DC: U.S. Bureau of the Census.

U.S. Bureau of the Census. (1995). *Statistical abstract of the United States.* Washington, DC: U.S. Government Printing Office.

U.S. Department of Education. (2000). *Psychology degree recipients by sex and race ethnicity (U.S. citizens only) 1997–98.* Washington, DC: U.S. Department of Education.

Vidato, D. (1979). *A data report on the 1977–78 academic year and trends of APA accredited programs: Student and faculty distributions.* Unpublished manuscript.

Wicherski, M., & Kohout, J., (1994). [Faculty in graduate departments of psychology and ethnicity.] Unpublished raw data.

Wicherski, M., Kohout, J., & Fritz, D. (1990). [Faculty in graduate departments of psychology by ethnicity.] Unpublished raw data.

Wicherski, M., Williams, S., & Kohout, J. (1998). [Faculty in graduate departments of psychology by ethnicity.] Unpublished raw data.

About the Editors and Contributors

Roberto J. Velásquez is an associate professor of psychology at San Diego State University. He teaches courses on Chicana/o psychology and Cuba's mental health system and currently maintains a private practice in Chula Vista, California with predominantly Spanish-speaking indigent clients. He also serves as a consultant to the County of San Diego Department of Social Services, Linda Vista Health Center, Angels Foster Care Agency, and Casa Pacifica Adult Day Health Care Program.

Leticia M. Arellano is currently an assistant professor of psychology at the University of La Verne and the director of research for the Institute for Multicultural Research and Campus Diversity. Her research interests include Latina mental health, stress and Latina professionals, multicultural counseling competences, and multiracial feminism.

Brian W. McNeill is a professor and codirector of training in the counseling psychology program at Washington State University. His current professional and research interests include Chicana/o psychology, clinical supervision, multicultural counseling, and training issues. He developed the first course in Chicana/o and Latina/o psychology at Washington State University.

Patricia Arredondo is an associate professor of counseling psychology at Arizona State University and president of Empowerment Workshops, Inc. of Boston. She was president of the Association for Multicultural Counseling and Development and the Society for the Psychological Study of Ethnic Minority Issues. Her extensive publications focused on organizational diversity initiatives, immigrant and Latina/o issues in counseling, the development and application of multicultural competencies, and counselor education and professional development. She was the author of *Successful Diversity Management Initiatives* (1996), coauthor of *Counseling Latinos* and *La familia: A Practical Guide* (2002), and coeditor of *Key Words in Multicultural Interventions*.

Christina Ayala-Alcantar is an assistant professor of Chicana/o Studies at California State University, Northridge. Her research focuses on Latinas' sexuality and multiracial feminism.

Louise Baca is an associate professor of clinical psychology at the Arizona School of Professional Psychology/Argosy University. She was previously the assistant director of the Multicultural Advancement Program at Arizona State University

483

where she provided counseling and conducted research on culturally responsive treatment modalities.

Manuel Barrera, Jr. is a professor of psychology at Arizona State University and Senior Research Scientist at the Oregon Research Institute. Dr. Barrera was recently the acting director of clinical training in the Department of Psychology. His research interests include adolescent problem behavior, social support, and the management of chronic illness. Dr. Barrera has published over 70 empirically based articles and book chapters and has chaired 43 master's theses and doctoral dissertations. He has been honored for his numerous contributions as a teacher, scholar, and mentor by Arizona State University. He has also been honored as a fellow by divisions 27 (Community Psychology) and 45 (Psychological Study of Ethnic Minority Issues) of the American Psychological Association. He has served on the editorial boards for the *American Journal of Community Psychology, Hispanic Journal of Behavioral Sciences, Journal of Personality Assessment, Psychological Assessment, Journal of Social and Personal Relationships, Journal of Consulting and Clinical Psychology,* and *Psychological Bulletin.* Over the years, Dr. Barrera has received research funding from the National Institute for Drug Abuse and the National Institute of Mental Health.

Martha E. Bernal, who died on September 28, 2002, at age 70, was a Professor Emeritus of psychology at Arizona State University. After earning her doctorate from Indiana University in 1962, Dr. Bernal received a U.S. Public Health Service Postdoctoral Fellowship and completed research training in human psychophysiology at University of California–Los Angeles Health Services Center. While at the University of Denver, Dr. Bernal received a National Research Service Award from NIMH in 1979 to examine multicultural curricula for psychologists. As the director, she implemented a number of strategies to increase the presence of ethnic minority students and faculty.

Dr. Bernal was also active in various state and national organizations, including the American Psychological Association. Her leadership was demonstrated in the Board of Ethnic Minority Affairs, Commission on Ethnic Minority, Recruitment, and Training (CEMRRAT), CEMRRAT 2 Task Force, and the Board for the Advancement of Psychology in the Public Interest. She also assisted in the development of the Hispanic Psychological Association and served as its president and treasurer. Dr. Bernal was the recipient of several professional awards and distinctions, such as the APA's Distinguished Contribution to Psychology in the Public Interest Award, the Distinguished Life Achievement Award from APA's Division 45, the Carolyn Attneave Award, and the Hispanic Research Center Lifetime Award from ASU, and was honored as one of four "Pioneer Senior Women of Color" at the first National Multicultural Conference and Summit in 1991.

Erika Bracamontes is currently a second-year medical student at the College of Human Medicine at Michigan State University. She was a graduate assistant at the Julian Samora Institute where she worked closely with its director, Israel Cuéllar.

Maria Patricia Burton is an undergraduate psychology major at San Diego State University and works for the San Diego Unified School District, where she provides assessment services for second language learners, primarily Latina/o children.

J. Manuel Casas is currently a professor in the Counseling, Clinical, and School Psychology Program at the University of California, Santa Barbara. He has published widely in professional journals (more than 60 articles) in the area of cross-cultural counseling and education. His most recent research and publications have focused on Hispanic families and children who are at risk for experiencing educational and psychosocial problems, including drug and alcohol abuse. Dr. Casas has served on the editorial boards of a number of journals, including *The Counseling Psychologist, Hispanic Journal of Behavioral Sciences, Journal of Multicultural Counseling and Development,* and *Cultural Diversity and Ethnic Minority Psychology.* He is the coauthor of the *Handbook of Racial/Ethnic Minority Counseling Research* (1991) and coeditor of the *Handbook of Multicultural Counseling* (2001).

Dr. Casas has been honored as a fellow of APA Division 17 (counseling psychology) and of the Rockefeller Foundation, received the California Association of School Psychologists research award, and served as chairperson of Division 17's Committee on Ethnic Minority Affairs. He is also the recipient of numerous grants related to research on drug and alcohol use, high-risk students, and public policy related to Latina/os. For all of these accomplishments, Dr. Casas was honored as a distinguished scholar in the field of Chicana/o psychology by the Julian Samora Research Institute at the 1998 Innovations in Chicana/o Psychology conference at Michigan State University.

Jeanett Castellanos is a lecturer at the University of California, Irvine in both social science and Chicana/o studies. Her research interests include skills in cultural competency, the underutilization of psychotherapy among minorities, and coping strategies leading to resilience among ethnic minority clients.

Joseph M. Cervantes is a diplomate in clinical psychology and an associate professor in the Department of Counseling at California State University, Fullerton. His research interests include the role of spirituality and indigenous healing in the counseling process. He maintains a private practice focused on children, adolescents, and families in Orange, CA.

Richard C. Cervantes is currently a senior research fellow at the Center for Behavioral Research and Services at California State University, Long Beach. He served as research psychologist at the University of California–Los Angeles Spanish Speaking Mental Health Research Center (1984 to 1989), and more recently held a full-time faculty appointment in the University of Southern California School of Medicine Department of Psychiatry and the Behavioral Sciences (1990 to 1995). He has evaluated a number of community-based prevention programs, including two Community Partnership programs funded by the U.S. Center for Substance Abuse Prevention, the Centers for Disease Control and Prevention, the California Endowment, and the California Community Foundation.

Carla Victoria Corral is an assistant researcher at the University of California, Santa Barbara. Her clinical and research interests focus on the provision of culturally sensitive and appropriate psychological, health, and educational services to racial and ethnic minority populations, especially Latina/o and multiracial families and children

Israel Cuéllar is a professor in the Michigan State University Department of Psychology and became the Julian Samora Research Institute's director in August, 2001. Before joining Michigan State University, he worked as a clinical psychologist for state and community mental health agencies in Texas and was a professor in the Department of Psychology and Anthropology at the University of Texas–

Pan American in Edinburg, Texas. His areas of expertise include mental health, multicultural psychology, acculturation, and community health.

Dr. Cuéllar developed the Acculturation Rating Scale for Mexican Americans–II (ARSMA–II), a paradigmatic measure for assigning degree of multicultural integration in persons living in multicultural contexts. Prior to his current position at the Julian Samora Research Institute, Dr. Cuéllar provided continuous rural mental health services for 16 years to residents of Starr County, arguably the poorest county, with the highest percentage of Hispanics (97.5%) in the United States. He has been a member of the American Psychological Association for 16 years and received the Distinguished Contribution to Science award from the Texas Psychological Association in 2000. He served as the director of the Bilingual/Bicultural Adult Psychiatric Inpatient Unit of the San Antonio State Hospital from 1977 to 1984. He edited, along with Freddy A. Paniagua, the *Handbook of Multicultural Mental Health: Assessment and Treatment of Diverse Populations* (2000).

María Félix-Ortiz has held faculty positions at the University of Southern California and the University of California, Los Angeles, and was a research associate for the Hispanic Research Center at the University of Texas, San Antonio. Her research interests include the etiology and prevention of drug use and abuse, especially among Latina/o youth, cultural factors in drug use, and in the use of assisted mutual support groups to extend mental health services and staff support.

A. Cristina Fernandez is a doctoral student in clinical psychology at Arizona State University. Her research interests include child and adolescent development, mental health, prevention, public policy, and the interface of these issues with minority populations.

Yolanda Flores Niemann is an associate professor of comparative American cultures and director of Latina/o Outreach at Washington State University, Tri-Cities. She is also an affiliate faculty in women's studies and graduate faculty in American studies. Her research interests include effects of stereotypes across various domains, including identity and risky behavior, the psychological effects of tokenism, overcoming obstacles to Latina/o higher education, identity issues in the change from from Mexican to Mexican American, and the use of stereotypes as justification for discrimination.

Yvette G. Flores-Ortiz is currently an associate professor of psychology in Chicana/o studies at the University of California, Davis and codirector of the Chicana/Latina Research Center. Her areas of research include family violence, Latina mental health, and HIV prevention. Dr. Flores-Ortiz has published extensively in the areas of Latina/o mental health, family therapy, the treatment of domestic violence, and feminist psychology.

Maria Garrido is a clinical psychologist in private practice and is an adjunct associate professor of psychology at the University of Rhode Island. Her research interests include culturally appropriate psychological assessment.

Alberta M. Gloria is an associate professor in the Department of Counseling Psychology at the University of Wisconsin, Madison. Her primary research interest is in examining psychosociocultural factors for Chicana/o students in higher education. Her work has addressed issues of cultural congruity, campus environment, and psychoeducational services for these students. Other research interests include professional development issues for counselors in training.

Nancy A. Gonzales is an associate professor in the Department of Psychology and the Program for Prevention Research at Arizona State University. Her research interests include contextual influences on adolescent development and mental health, acculturation and enculturation of Mexican American families, and prevention.

Felipe González Castro is a professor of clinical psychology in the Department of Psychology at Arizona State University. Dr. Castro has conducted research in the areas of health promotion and health education with Latina/os and with other ethnic and racial minorities in the U.S. He has studied the use of community-based peer health interventions to reduce the risk of cancer among Hispanic women and to promote tobacco avoidance among Latina/o and other minority youth. His current work includes the study of the intergenerational (parent-youth) transmission of multiple risk behaviors, including drug abuse and HIV risks among Mexican American injection-drug-using fathers and their adolescent children.

Martin Harris is currently the director of the graduate program in clinical psychology at Vanguard University of Southern California in Costa Mesa. Dr. Harris' research and clinical interests include psychopharmacology, cross-cultural psychology, and cultural psychiatry.

Nilda Teresa Hernandez is self-employed and focusing on developing culturally relevant care. She reviews for Substance Abuse and Mental Health Services Administration on the Performance Measures Cross-Cultural Standing Review Committee.

Patricia Hernandez received her master's degree from the Arizona School of Professional Psychology and is currently pursuing a doctorate in psychology from Argosy University, Phoenix.

Steven R. López is a professor of psychology and psychiatry at University of California, Los Angeles. His main area of research addresses how sociocultural factors relate to the psychopathology, assessment, and intervention of Latina/os and other ethnic minority groups. He is currently ivestigating the behaviors that underlie Mexican American family warmth in an effort to identify what families do to prevent relapse. In addition to his research, Dr. López maintained a clinical practice for several years in both public and private mental health facilities.

Vera Lopez is an assistant professor in the School of Justice Studies at Arizona State University. Her research interests include juvenile delinquency, fathering, and the development of prevention programming for children.

Kurt C. Organista is an associate professor of social welfare and the director of the Center for Latino Policy Research at the University of California, Berkeley. He teaches courses on psychopathology, stress and coping, and human diversity competent practice, including social work with Latina/o populations. He is interested in Latina/o health and mental health and conducts research in the areas of HIV and AIDS prevention with Mexican migrant laborers and the treatment of depression in Latina/os.

Fernando Ortiz is currently a graduate student in the doctoral program in counseling psychology at Washington State University (WSU). He is also a graduate research assistant for the Personality and Culture Project at WSU, a cross-cultural research project measuring self-construal and individualism-collectivism across cultures. Other research interests include multicultural issues in counseling and mental health.

Loreto R. Prieto is an assistant professor in the Collaborative Program in Counseling Psychology at the University of Akron. He has research interests in multicultural issues, psychological testing and assessment, and clinical training and supervision.

Stephen M. Quintana is Chair of the Department of Counseling Psychology at the University of Wisconsin, Madison. His research focuses on ethnic perspective-taking abilities of Mexican American and other children of color.

Jason Duque Raley is an assistant professor at the University of California, Santa Barbara. His current work explores the relationships among culture, learning, and social interaction, as well as the epistemology and practice of qualitative research. As codirector of the Center for the Study of Teacher Learning in Practice, he focuses on the contribution of contemporary learning theories to the understanding of teaching and learning in schools.

Manuel Ramirez III is a professor of psychology at the University of Texas, Austin. He is a fellow of Division 45 of the APA and was named Distinguished Minority Researcher by the American Educational Research Association. He taught the first organized course in Chicana/o Psychology ever offered at a university in 1967. Together with Al Castañeda, he organized and chaired the first conference on Chicana/o psychology held at University of California–Riverside in May, 1973. He coauthored with Al Castañeda *Cultural Democracy, Bicognitive Development and Education* (1974). Dr. Ramirez is also author of *Multicultural/Multiracial Psychology* (1998) and *Multicultural Psychotherapy: An Approach to Individual and Cultural Differences* (1999). His current research is on acculturation and mental health of families residing on the U.S.-Mexico border of South Texas. Dr. Ramirez is the recipient of numerous federal grants, such as the Hogg Foundation for Mental Health and the U.S. Office of Education, and directed several federal programs in California and Texas.

Dr. Ramirez has over 100 professional publications, including articles, book chapters, books, reports, and monographs. As an educator he has mentored a multitude of graduate and undergraduate students, including Dr. Alex Gonzalez, President of California State University, San Marcos, and Dr. Ray Buriel, Professor of Psychology and Chicano Studies, Pomona College. Dr. Ramirez is a fellow of the American Psychological Association, and has a fellowship established in his honor, the Minority Student Fellowship from the Texas Psychological Association.

Teresa Renteria is a recent graduate of the Graduate Program in Clinical Psychology at Vanguard University. Teresa serves as an adjunct faculty to the Department of Clinical Psychology. Teresa's research and clinical practice are in cross cultural psychology.

Richard A. Rodriguez is currently the director of counseling and psychological services at a multicultural center at the University of Colorado, Boulder, after holding the same position at Sonoma State University for 3 years. Before that, Dr. Rodriguez was the director of Multicultural Affairs and an assistant professor at the California School of Professional Psychology, Alameda, where he taught intercultural awareness development and clinical issues with lesbians and gay men of color. His areas of clinical expertise and research include Chicana/o and Latina/o mental health, ethnic, racial, and cultural identity development, HIV and AIDS, and adult survivors of childhood sexual abuse.

Theresa A. Segura-Herrera is currently a first-year doctoral student in the Department of Counseling Psychology at the University of Wisconsin, Madison. She has worked as a case manager, counselor, and research interviewer in various inner-city community settings with Latina/os and other racial and ethnic minorities. Some of her current professional and academic areas of interest include diverse aspects of the Mexican immigrant experience, the study of mental health service delivery to Latina/os in diverse settings, the implementation of culturally sensitive and appropriate mental health services for Latina/os, examination of ethnic and racial minorities' experiences in higher education, and the development of preventive intervention programs for at-risk youth and their families.

Roxana I. Siles is currently a second-year medical student at Michigan State University College of Human Medicine where she is the cochair of the Latino Midwest Medical Student Association. Her research interest is in the study of health disparities pertaining to the Latina/o population. Prior to entering medical school, Ms. Siles worked as a medical assistant at the Cristo Rey Community Health Clinic and joined a team of volunteer physicians to provide free health care services at Mid-Michigan migrant camps.

Lisa I. Sweatt is an assistant professor in the Department of Psychology and Child Development at California Polytechnic State University, San Luis Obispo. Her research and scholarly interests include childhood trauma, violence prevention and intervention, and multicultural counseling and training.

Melba J. T. Vasquez is a psychologist in independent practice in Austin, TX. She served as a counseling center psychologist for the first 13 years of her career, including as training director at two different universities (Colorado State University and University of Texas, Austin). She was president of the American Psychological Association's Division 17 (counseling psychology) from 2001 to 2002 and is a member of the Committee for the Advancement of Professional Practice. While president of APA's Division 35 (Society for the Psychology of Women), she helped to cohost the National Multicultural Conference and Summit (NMCS) in January, 1999, as well as the second NMCS in January, 2001. She has served on the APA's Policy and Planning Board and Ethics Committee, as well as on the Ethics Committee Task Forces (ECTF) for revision of the APA's 1981 and 1992 ethics codes. She has served as chair of the Board of Professional Affairs and of the Board for the Advancement of Psychology in the Public Interest. Dr. Vasquez is currently in independent practice and the executive director of Vasquez & Associates Mental Health Services in Austin.

Dr. Vasquez has published over 100 articles, chapters, and professional papers on a variety of psychological issues such as clinical therapy, service provision, feminism, and cultural diversity. She co-authored *Ethics in Psychotherapy and Counseling: A Practical Guide* (1991, 1998). In addition to actively publishing, Dr. Vasquez serves on numerous editorial boards and is currently the associate editor of *Cultural Diversity and Ethnic Minority Psychology*. She has participated in the governance of the APA and various other professional organizations. She has received numerous professional awards, such as the Distinguished Career Contributions to Service Award from APA's Division 45, the Janet E. Helms Award for Mentoring and Scholarship, the Distinguished Leader of Women in Psychology Award, and the APA's Senior Career Award for Distinguished Contribution to

Psychology in the Public Interest. In addition, Dr. Vasquez holds fellow status within seven divisions of the APA.

Elizabeth M. Vera is an associate professor of counseling psychology at Loyola University, Chicago. Her research interests include resiliency in urban adolescents, ethnic identity development of Chicana/o children, and the impact of similarity and difference in the counseling relationship. She teaches graduate courses in prevention and outreach, the psychology of adolescence, family therapy, and human development.

Amy Weisman is an assistant professor of psychology at the University of Miami. Her research focuses on cultural and family factors that influence the course of chronic mental illness, attributions of control, religious beliefs and values, and other sociocultural factors (e.g., self-construal, acculturation) that may be associated with relatives' emotional reactions to family members suffering from schizophrenia or bipolar disorder. Dr. Weisman is also interested in family-focused psychotherapy outcome research.

Jerre White currently serves as the director of clinical training within the Department of Clinical Psychology at Vanguard University of Southern California. Dr. White has expertise in psychological testing and measurement, legal and ethical issues, and child psychopathology, maintains a private practice, and serves as a professional consultant to various agencies Orange County.

Cynthia A. Yamokoski is a doctoral student in the Collaborative Program in Counseling Psychology at the University of Akron. Her current research interests include diversity, client-therapist interactions, developmental psychopathology, and history and philosophy of psychology.

About Other Pioneers
in Chicana/o Psychology

Raymond Buriel currently serves as a professor of psychology and Chicano studies at Pomona College in Claremont, CA, where he has taught a variety of courses, including Psychology of the Chicano, Field Research in Chicano Studies, Comparative Ethnic Psychology, and Psychology of Multicultural Education. Dr. Buriel served on the editorial boards of the *Hispanic Journal of Behavioral Sciences, Harvard Journal of Hispanic Policy,* and *Revista Inter Americana de Psicologia,* and as a reviewer to the *American Psychologist, Developmental Psychology,* and *The Journal of Educational Psychology.* As a scholar, Dr. Buriel has contributed extensively to the literature of Chicana/o psychology in the areas of ethnic identity, academic achievement in Chicana/o students, and Chicano families. His current research focuses on language brokering among Chicana/os and child care in Latina/o communities. Dr. Buriel is also the recipient of various federal grants, such as the Pew National Institute of Child Health and Human Development Science Program Grant, the Ford Foundation Internship and General Education Grant, and the NICHD Families First Project Grant. For his teaching excellence, he received the Haynes Foundation Faculty Fellowship and the Wig Distinguished Teaching Award, and was made a Tomas Rivera Center for Policy Studies' Center scholar.

Amado Padilla is currently a full professor in the School of Education at Stanford University. Prior to working at Stanford University, he was a professor in the Department of Psychology at the University of California, Los Angeles from 1978 to 1988 and was the founder and director of the Spanish Speaking Mental Health Research Center there from 1976 to 1989. Dr. Padilla is currently chair of the Committee on Language, Literacy, and Culture at Stanford University. Dr. Padilla has published over 160 articles and book chapters and several books, including *Hispanic Mental Health Research: A Reference Guide* (1981), *Crossing Cultures in Therapy: Pluralistic Counseling for the Hispanic* (1980), *Acculturation: Theory, Models, and Some New Findings, Chicano Ethnicity* (1987), and *Hispanic Psychology: Critical Issues in Theory and Research* (1995). Dr. Padilla was the founder and editor of the *Hispanic Journal of Behavioral Sciences.* He has been a consultant to numerous local, state, national, and international organizations. He has been honored for his contributions as a teacher, scholar, and mentor by professional organizations, including the APA, who awarded him the Lifetime Achievement Award in 1996. He has also

491

been honored as a fellow by divisions 26 (History of Psychology), 27 (Community Psychology), and 45 (Psychological Study of Ethnic Minority Issues) of the APA.

Rene A. Ruiz, also known as Art, passed away on December 13, 1982. He began his teaching career as a lecturer and then assistant professor in the Department of Psychiatry at the University of Kansas. He then joined the faculty in the Department of Psychology at the University of Arizona as an associate professor. He later taught at the University of Missouri. His last academic position was as a full professor in the Department of Counseling and Educational Psychology at New Mexico State University, where he eventually served as Chair. From 1977 to 1979, Dr. Ruiz was a visiting scholar at the Spanish Speaking Mental Health Research Center at the University of California, Los Angeles.

Dr. Ruiz was a member of numerous state and national organizations, including the APA. He was also instrumental in the creation of the National Hispanic Psychological Association. During his career, he published more than 60 book chapters and research articles. He co-authored two books, *Latino Mental Health* (1973) and *Chicano Aging and Mental Health* (1981). The former reviewed all research conducted with Latina/os up until that period in history, and inspired many young Chicana/o psychologists to fill the gaps that he identified.

Nelly Salgado de Snyder is currently the director of the Community Health and Social Welfare Unit at the Mexican National Institute of Public Health Center for Health Systems Research in Morelos, Mexico. Dr. Salgado de Snyder is a Fulbright New Century Scholar and is currently examining the interplay between age, poverty, and health among persons of Mexican origin. Her research also focuses on addressing health needs and services among individuals from rural Mexican communities on the impact of Mexico-U.S. migration. Dr. Salgado de Snyder is a member of the Mexican Academy of Scientific Research and holds fellow status in the APA.

Dr. Salgado de Snyder is an educator who provides training and instruction on various areas of mental health throughout California and Mexico. Similarly, she has conducted numerous national and international workshops and presented professional papers and presentations. She has published well over 80 articles, chapters, and professional papers. She also serves on various national and international editorial boards. She recently served as the guest editor for a special issue on Latina women in the *Hispanic Journal of Behavioral Sciences* (1999). Dr. Salgado de Snyder has also trainied and mentored many young scholars in psychology.

Maria Nieto Senour is currently a full professor in the Department of Counseling and School of Psychology at San Diego State University. She has made hundreds of presentations to colleagues and members of the community focusing on social justice, educational attainment, and community organization.

Dr. Nieto Senour is currently the director of the Community-Based Block Program within the Department of Counseling and School of Psychology, which offers a master's degree in counseling. The program has been in existence for over two decades and offers all of its training, including courses, in the community. Dr. Nieto Senour has been involved in countless committees and is a member of the academic senate. Dr. Nieto Senour currently holds public office as a trustee for the San Diego Community College District and has been elected to four terms. She has mentored hundreds of students into the counseling profession.

Author Index

Subject Index